LEARNING TO CODE
WITH ICD-9-CM

LEARNING TO CODE WITH ICD-9-CM

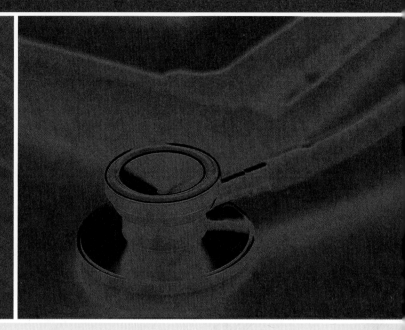

Thomas J. Falen, M.A., R.H.I.A., L.H.R.M., CPUR/CPUM, EMT-B

University of Central Florida
Department of Health Professions
Orlando, Florida

Contributing Authors:

Aaron Liberman, Ph.D.

University of Central Florida
Department of Health Professions
Orlando, Florida

Cynthia S. Falen, R.H.I.T., C.C.S.

Coding Compliance Consultant
Medical Audit Resource Services, Inc.
Tavares, Florida

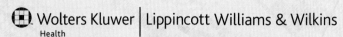
Wolters Kluwer | Lippincott Williams & Wilkins
Health

Philadelphia · Baltimore · New York · London
Buenos Aires · Hong Kong · Sydney · Tokyo

Publisher: Julie K. Stegman
Development Manager: Nancy Peterson
Development Editor: Lonnie Christiansen
Development Assistant: Elizabeth Connolly
Editorial Manager: Eric Branger
Associate Managing Editor: Erin M. Cosyn
Designer: Candice Carta-Myers
Compositor: Aptara, Inc.
Printer: RR Donnelly–Willard

Copyright © 2009 Wolters Kluwer Health | Lippincott Williams & Wilkins

351 West Camden Street
Baltimore, MD 21201

530 Walnut Street
Philadelphia, PA 19106

ISSN 1945-2357

Printed in the United States of America

To purchase additional copies of this book, call our customer service department at **(800) 638-3030** or fax orders to **(301) 824-7390**. International customers should call **(301) 714-2324**.

Visit Lippincott Williams & Wilkins on the Internet: http://www.LWW.com.
Lippincott Williams & Wilkins customer service representatives are available from 8:30 am to 6:00 pm, EST.

09
1 2 3 4 5 6 7 8 9 10

Dedication

Thomas Falen recognizes his father, the late Walter Falen, and his mother, Evelyn Falen for their love and devotion as parents. Tom dedicates this book to his lovely children Kristin and Molly Falen, who are the light of his life, and to his devoted wife Cynthia Falen, R.H.I.T., C.C.S., who is both his inspiration and his greatest source of moral support. These are the people who encouraged Tom in his determination to make a significant difference in his profession through the completion of this book.

Preface

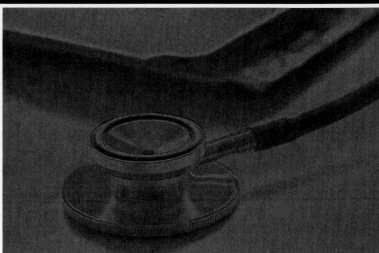

Following the advent of the Medicare Program there was a general acknowledgement of the critical role that would be fulfilled by medical coding specialists. As Medicare's expectations of providers and the organizations they represented heightened, the importance of accuracy in submissions for reimbursement continued to increase and intensify. Once DRGs were enacted, the focus of the Medicare Program experienced a sea-change shift of emphasis from access to care to accountability for each clinical service provided; this served to re-emphasize the crucial role to be played by medical coders.

During the 1990s concerns over alleged Medicare fraud and abuse once again highlighted the necessity of having medical coding specialists who could accurately represent the services being provided and submit billing statements that respected the expectau. ~f a demanding Medicare reimbursement program. Today, the ever-increasing ꞊ ꞊ssociated with the Medicare Program continue to presage renewed efforts to sι꞊ ꞊d control improper and dishonest billing practices. Thus, the importance of honesι ꞊ ' accurate billings continues to represent a first priority of virtually every healthcare provider organization.

Our purpose in preparing this text is to respond to a national demand for the training of technically competent medical coding professionals as decision makers. It is our goal to facilitate the training of medical coding professionals by teaching them to code using 'real-world' medical record examples. In the process, these specialists will develop a high level of administrative sensitivity and an understanding of the uses of coding information to increase an organization's potential for financial success, corporate compliance, and quality performance in an increasingly regulated and litigious healthcare marketplace.

The courses for which this textbook is intended are broadly based and include students studying at both the undergraduate and graduate levels of health information management, health care informatics, and health services administration. In addition, the book is applicable for students in vocational and technical schools who are being trained in ICD-9-CM medical coding of patient diagnoses, systems, and procedures. The book also can be used as a supplemental text in health services administration courses. Because of its real-world emphasis, the book also will be useful to individuals serving as coding specialists in hospitals and outpatient medical practices.

The text is comprehensive, but easy to read. The focus throughout the text is on providing examples that will facilitate the training of the reader to code effectively and correctly. Many coding texts in use today provide only short exercises without actual examples that highlight medical record documentation. The authors have sought to fill this void and to develop in each student skills that will translate into marketable talents for the array and multiplicity of jobs that are available in healthcare organizations of all sizes and types.

Health Services Administration programs are increasingly sensitive to the need for medical coding as a means of better understanding the impact of on performance improvement and meeting the requirements of corporate compliance. The content of this text provides the information and means necessary to better facilitate the sequence of translating that understanding into better administrative practices.

The book is organized to first provide essential background information about coding conventions and guidelines. This is followed by chapters that specifically address the various signs, symptoms and procedures/treatment for diseases, disorders, and injuries. The final chapter of the text equates Health Information Management to Managed Care. Throughout the text the authors have employed Red Flags to denote particularly important problems and challenges for coders that will require special attention.

This workbook is to be used in conjunction with the most current copy of the International Classification of Diseases and Procedures, 9th Revision, Clinical Modification (ICD-9-CM, volumes 1, 2, and 3). ICD-9-CM is officially published by the U.S. Government Printing Office as a three-voume set and many commercial publishers reproduce all three volumes within one book.

We are delighted to have had this opportunity to work closely with our publisher, Lippincott Williams & Wilkins, and the very competent professional staff representing the organization, in developing a textbook that is both relevant to the needs of the health services professions and crucial in meeting the ever increasing expectations of a vigilant and wary public.

Thomas Falen, M.A., R.H.I.A., L.H.R.M.
Aaron Liberman, Ph.D.
Cynthia Falen, R.H.I.T., C.C.S.

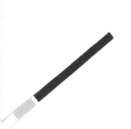

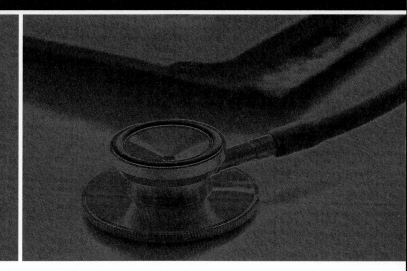

User's Guide

This User's Guide shows you how to put the features of *Learning to Code with ICD-9-CM* to work for you.

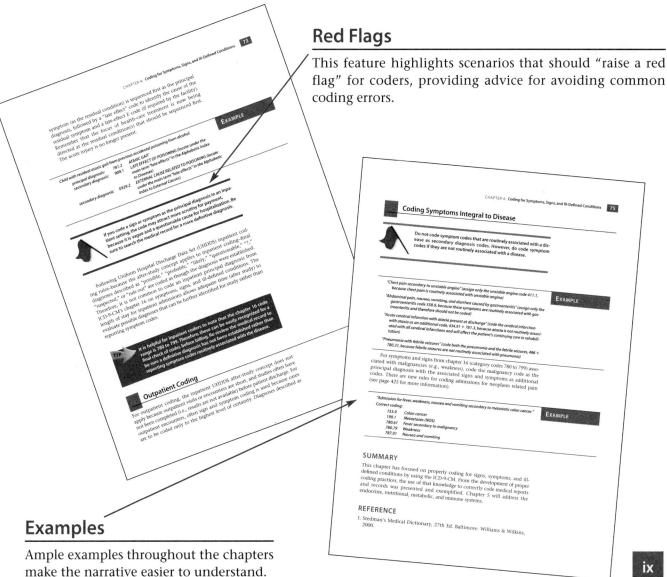

Red Flags

This feature highlights scenarios that should "raise a red flag" for coders, providing advice for avoiding common coding errors.

Examples

Ample examples throughout the chapters make the narrative easier to understand.

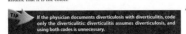

Page excerpt (152)

152   PART II: Coding for Specific Diseases and Disorders

When you are locating the code for diverticulosis, carefully review the subterms (essential modifiers) for:

- the site of the inflamed sacs
- whether the diverticulosis is with or without diverticulitis
- whether it is associated with hemorrhage (bleeding)

When a physician documents diverticulosis without specifying the site, assume that it is the colon.

> **TIP**   If the physician documents diverticulosis with diverticulitis, code only the diverticulitis: diverticulitis assumes diverticulosis, and using both codes is unnecessary.

EXAMPLE
Diverticulosis of colon: 562.10
Diverticulosis with diverticulitis: 562.11
Diverticulosis with bleeding: 562.12
Diverticulosis with diverticulitis with bleeding: 562.13
Diverticulosis of esophagus, acquired: 530.6
Diverticulosis of esophagus, acquired, with hemorrhage: 530.6 + 530.82

Diverticulosis of the colon is commonly diagnosed through colonoscopy or barium enema. Conservative treatment for diverticulosis, with or without diverticulitis, routinely includes intravenous fluids, intravenous antibiotics (to prevent infection), and soft diet. Severe acute diverticulitis may include bleeding or perforation that could indicate the need for a colon resection and temporary colostomy to let the bowel rest and heal. After treatment, the physician would schedule an admission for a take-down (removal) colostomy (principal diagnosis code V55.3). You can locate the diagnosis code for take-down colostomy under "attention to" in the Disease Index (volume 2). The procedure code is located in the procedure index under "take-down, colostomy" (code 46.52).

Gastrointestinal Ulcers

An ulcer is an open sore on the skin or epithelial tissue that lines the internal organs (Figure 7.3). Gastric (stomach) and duodenal (first part of the small intestine) ulcers are common examples of GI ulcers and are often associated with GI bleeding. For gastric and duodenal ulcers (category codes 531 and 532, respectively), the fourth digit indicates whether the ulcer is acute or chronic and whether it has an associated bleed or perforation. The fifth digit indicates whether the ulcer is with or without obstruction.

EXAMPLE
Acute bleeding gastric ulcer with perforation and obstruction: 531.21
Acute bleeding duodenal ulcer with perforation and obstruction: 532.21

Tips

Coding tips throughout the text provide practical "pearls" to assist beginning coders.

ICD-9-CM Excerpts

Excerpts provide a "snapshot" from the ICD-9-CM codebook.

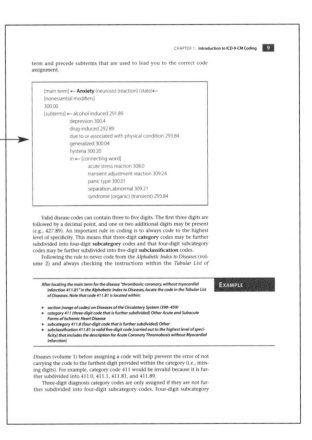

Page excerpt (9)

CHAPTER 1: Introduction to ICD-9-CM Coding   **9**

term and precede subterms that are used to lead you to the correct code assignment.

```
[main term] ← Anxiety (neurosis) (reaction) (state)←
[nonessential modifiers]
300.00
[subterms] ← alcohol-induced 291.89
        depression 300.4
        drug-induced 292.89
        due to or associated with physical condition 293.84
        generalized 300.04
        hysteria 300.20
        in ← [connecting word]
            acute stress reaction 308.0
            transient adjustment reaction 309.24
            panic type 300.01
            separation, abnormal 309.21
            syndrome (organic) (transient) 293.84
```

Valid disease codes can contain three to five digits. The first three digits are followed by a decimal point, and one or two additional digits may be present (e.g., 427.89). An important rule in coding is to always code to the highest level of specificity. This means that three-digit **category** codes may be further subdivided into four-digit **subcategory** codes and that four-digit subcategory codes may be further subdivided into five-digit **subclassification** codes.

Following the rule to never code from the *Alphabetic Index to Diseases* (volume 2) and always checking the instructions within the *Tabular List of*

> **EXAMPLE**
> After locating the main term for the disease "thrombosis; coronary, without myocardial infarction 411.81" in the Alphabetic Index to Diseases, locate the code in the Tabular List of Diseases. Note that code 411.81 is located within:
>
> - *section (range of codes) on Diseases of the Circulatory System (390–459)*
> - *category 411 (three-digit code that is further subdivided) Other Acute and Subacute Forms of Ischemic Heart Disease*
> - *subcategory 411.8 (four-digit code that is further subdivided) Other*
> - *subclassification 411.81 (a valid five-digit code [carried out to the highest level of specificity] that includes the description for Acute Coronary Thrombosis without Myocardial Infarction)*

Diseases (volume 1) before assigning a code will help prevent the error of not carrying the code to the furthest digit provided within the category (i.e., missing digits). For example, category code 411 would be invalid because it is further subdivided into 411.0, 411.1, 411.81, and 411.89.

Three-digit diagnosis category codes are only assigned if they are not further subdivided into four-digit subcategory codes. Four-digit subcategory

---

Page excerpt (193)

CHAPTER 8: Coding for Respiratory System Diseases   **193**

Word Parts and Meanings of Respiratory System Medical Terms

Word Part	Meaning	Example	Definition of Example
bronch/o, bronch/i	Bronchus	bronchogenic	Originating in the bronchus
-centesis	puncture, tap	thoracentesis	Puncture of the chest
-ostomy	an opening into the body, usually created for elimination of body waste	tracheostomy	Incision of the trachea through the neck, usually to establish an airway in cases of tracheal obstruction
-pnea	Breathing	orthopnea	Difficulty in breathing except in an upright (ortho-) position
Pleur/o	Pleura	pleural effusion	Increased amounts of fluid within the pleural cavity, usually due to inflammation
Pneumon/o	Lung	pneumonectomy	Surgical removal of a lung or lung tissue
-sis	an abnormal condition	atelectasis	Incomplete expansion of a lung or part of a lung; lung collapse

Respiratory infections are usually noted through physicians' documentation, laboratory work (such as a culture and sensitivity report), and chest radiographs. In addition, physicians' orders and medication administration records reveal treatments for respiratory diseases, such as the administration of intravenous antibiotics. Be sure to review the patient's medical record to determine or substantiate a diagnosis of respiratory disease.

Pneumonia

Pneumonia, also called **pneumonitis**, is an inflammation of the lungs in which the lung sacs (alveoli) may fill with pus or other inflammatory debris. It is frequently caused by a bacterial infection. There are many different types of pneumonias, and some universal coding conventions (mentioned in Chapter 2)—such as (1) **mandatory dual coding**, in which two codes are required to describe the condition (e.g., pneumonia attributable to aspergillosis, 117.3 + [484.5]), or (2) **combination codes**, in which one code describes both the type of pneumonia and the organism (e.g., *Staphylococcus aureus* pneumonia, 482.41)—are often applied in this section.

 Be particularly attentive when the physician documentation shows unspecified or community-acquired pneumonia without further documentation (e.g., pneumonia, not otherwise specified [NOS], 486). A reporting of pneumonia, unspecified, may not reveal the actual organism causing the infection or give an accurate clinical presentation of the patient. You should thoroughly review all laboratory work (especially culture and sensitivity reports) and query the physician if you need more information and additional supporting documentation to identify the specific type of pneumonia, if possible.

Always query the physician for the responsible organism (if known) in order to use the most precise pneumonia code. If the offending organism is unknown, use code 486 for unspecified pneumonia.

Table of Word Parts and Meanings

Understanding medical terminology is critical to accurate coding. Tables that review word parts and meanings of medical terms are included in each disease specific chapter to assist in your understanding

Illustrations

Illustrations showing human anatomy as well as related clinical procedures help bring complex information to life.

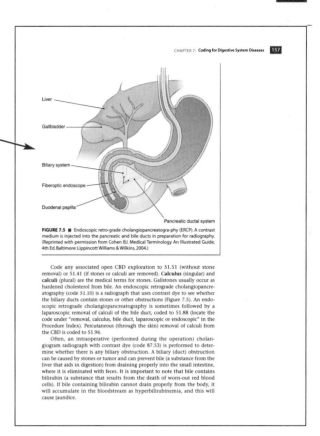

FIGURE 7.5 ■ Endoscopic retro-grade cholangiopancreatogra-phy (ERCP). A contrast medium is injected into the pancreatic and bile ducts in preparation for radiography. (Reprinted with permission from Cohen BJ. Medical Terminology An Illustrated Guide, 4th Ed. Baltimore: Lippincott Williams & Wilkins, 2004.)

Code any associated open CBD exploration to 51.51 (without stone removal) or 51.41 (if stones or calculi are removed). **Calculus** (singular) and **calculi** (plural) are the medical terms for stones. Gallstones usually occur as hardened cholesterol from bile. An endoscopic retrograde cholangiopancreatography (code 51.10) is a radiograph that uses contrast dye to see whether the biliary ducts contain stones or other obstructions (Figure 7.5). An endoscopic retrograde cholangiopancreatography is sometimes followed by a laparoscopic removal of calculi of the bile duct, coded to 51.88 (locate the code under "removal, calculus, bile duct, laparoscopic or endoscopic" in the Procedure Index). Percutaneous (through the skin) removal of calculi from the CBD is coded to 51.96.

Often, an intraoperative (performed during the operation) cholangiogram radiograph with contrast dye (code 87.53) is performed to determine whether there is any biliary obstruction. A biliary (duct) obstruction can be caused by stones or tumor and can prevent bile (a substance from the liver that aids in digestion) from draining properly into the small intestine, where it is eliminated with feces. It is important to note that bile contains bilirubin (a substance that results from the death of worn-out red blood cells). If bile containing bilirubin cannot drain properly from the body, it will accumulate in the bloodstream as hyperbilirubinemia, and this will cause jaundice.

Testing Your Comprehension

End-of-chapter review questions test your comprehension of the chapter content. Answers are provided in Appendix 6.

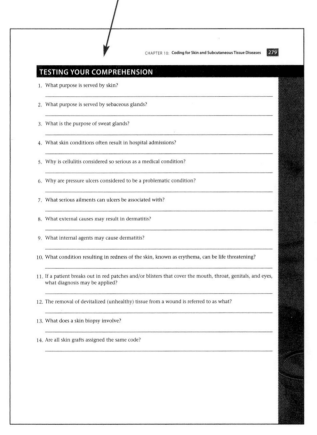

TESTING YOUR COMPREHENSION

1. What purpose is served by skin?

2. What purpose is served by sebaceous glands?

3. What is the purpose of sweat glands?

4. What skin conditions often result in hospital admissions?

5. Why is cellulitis considered so serious as a medical condition?

6. Why are pressure ulcers considered to be a problematic condition?

7. What serious ailments can ulcers be associated with?

8. What external causes may result in dermatitis?

9. What internal agents may cause dermatitis?

10. What condition resulting in redness of the skin, known as erythema, can be life threatening?

11. If a patient breaks out in red patches and/or blisters that cover the mouth, throat, genitals, and eyes, what diagnosis may be applied?

12. The removal of devitalized (unhealthy) tissue from a wound is referred to as what?

13. What does a skin biopsy involve?

14. Are all skin grafts assigned the same code?

Coding Practice I: Chapter Review Exercises

Practice exercises test your comprehension of the coding content and examples given in the chapter. These exercises give a diagnosis or procedure and ask you to provide the proper code, using the ICD-9 CM. Answer space is provided in the text. Answers are provided in Appendix 7.

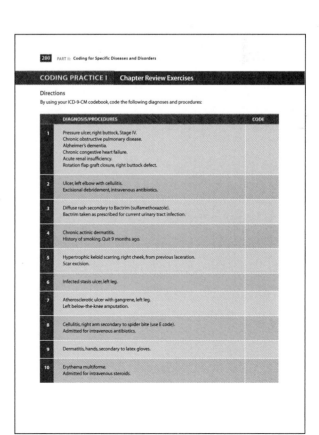

CODING PRACTICE I Chapter Review Exercises

Directions

By using your ICD-9-CM codebook, code the following diagnoses and procedures:

	DIAGNOSIS/PROCEDURES	CODE
1	Pressure ulcer, right buttock, Stage IV. Chronic obstructive pulmonary disease. Alzheimer's dementia. Chronic congestive heart failure. Acute renal insufficiency. Rotation flap graft closure, right buttock defect.	
2	Ulcer, left elbow with cellulitis. Excisional debridement, intravenous antibiotics.	
3	Diffuse rash secondary to Bactrim (sulfamethoxazole). Bactrim taken as prescribed for current urinary tract infection.	
4	Chronic actinic dermatitis. History of smoking. Quit 9 months ago.	
5	Hypertrophic keloid scarring, right cheek, from previous laceration. Scar excision.	
6	Infected stasis ulcer, left leg.	
7	Atherosclerotic ulcer with gangrene, left leg. Left below-the-knee amputation.	
8	Cellulitis, right arm secondary to spider bite (use E code). Admitted for intravenous antibiotics.	
9	Dermatitis, hands, secondary to latex gloves.	
10	Erythema multiforme. Admitted for intravenous steroids.	

Coding Practice II: Medical Record Case Studies

Case studies have you put your knowledge into practice by coding diagnoses and procedures from real-world medical records. Each case study has an answer template followed by corresponding medical reports.

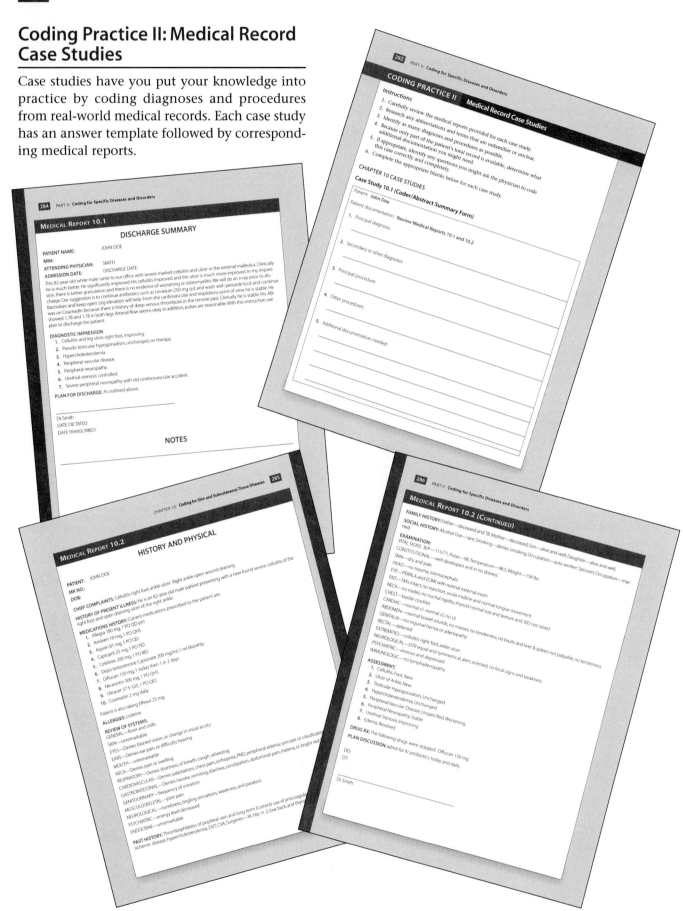

Companion Website

The companion website designed specifically for this text includes sections for instructors and students. The student section includes answers to Testing Your Comprehension and Coding Practice I: Chapter Review Exercises, as well as general coding information and updates, and links to other valuable coding resources. The companion site can be accessed at http://thepoint.lww.com/falen2009

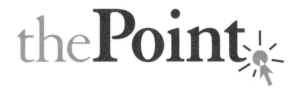

Acknowledgments

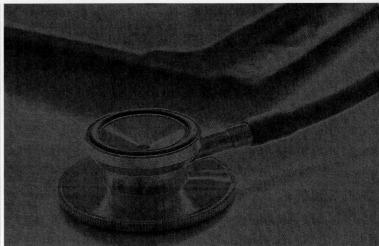

As with any creative effort there are persons who play a silent but integral role in keeping a project on course and directed toward its timely completion. I wish to express my gratitude to three faculty colleagues for their technical and inspirational contributions.

Associate Professor Tim Worrell reviewed those chapters of the book addressing the cardiovascular system and offered invaluable suggestions and insights about how to deal with a number of technical considerations. Tim is one of the most unselfish and collegial faculty members I have had the privilege of working with and my gratitude to him for his timely recommendations is deeply felt.

The late Louis Acierno, M.D., Professor Emeritus, was himself an experienced book author, in addition to having completed a distinguished career both as a practicing cardiologist and as a university professor. Lou's encouragement about the benefits this text would serve in the HIM community was most appreciated; and for this, I am forever grateful.

Aaron Liberman, Ph.D., was a contributing author to the original publication and his expertise was especially helpful in the areas of health service administration and managed care. His ongoing support for this project is invaluable. He is a respected colleague, a personal mentor, and a true friend.

Special thanks to June Woodcock, Alice Noblin, Phuong-Trang Le, and Julie Shay for their positive input in improving the quality of this book.

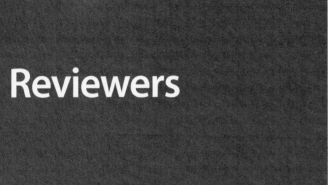

Reviewers

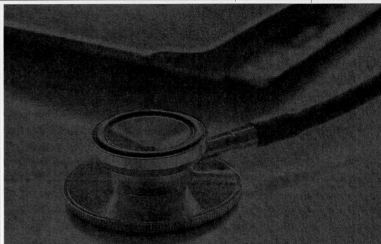

The publisher and authors gratefully acknowledge the many professionals who shared their expertise and assisted in developing this textbook, appropriately targeting our marketing efforts, creating useful ancillary products, and setting the stage for subsequent editions. These individuals include:

JODI ALBER, AAS, LVT
Clinical Coordinator Veterinary
  Technology
Baker College
Jackson, MI

MYRA M. BROWN, MBA, RHIA
Associate Professor, Health Services
  and Information Management
East Carolina University
Greenville, NC

MICHELLE BUCHMAN, BSN, RNC
Springfield College
Springfield, MO

LYDIA CAVIEUX, RHIT, MPA
Director of Distance Learning and
  Continuing Education, Assistant
  Professor, Health Policy and
  Management
New York Medical College
Valhalla, NY

LISA CERRATO, MS, RHIA
HIMT Program Coordinator and
  Associate Professor
Columbus State Community College
Columbus, OH

CHRISTINE CUSANO, CMA, CPhT,
BSM
Clark University Computer Career
  Institute
Framingham, MA

JOYCE GAROZZO, MS, RHIA, CCS
Associate Professor and Director
Health Information Technology
  Program
Community College of Philadelphia
Philadelphia, PA

FRAN GELTCH, CPC, CCP
Professional Medical Coding
  Curriculum Instructor
Lippy Group for ENT
Warren, OH

ELIZABETH A. HOFFMAN, MA ED,
CMA
Medical Program Director
Baker College of Clinton Township
Clinton Township, MI

CATHY KELLEY-ARNEY, CMA, MLTC,
BSHS
National College of Business and
  Technology
Bluefield, VA

MARY W. KING, MS, RHIA
Department Head, Health
  Information Technology
Division Chair, Allied Health
Wharton County Junior College
Wharton, TX

MARY E. LARSEN, AHI, RMA, CMT
Caldwell, ID

GERALD LEVY, BA, MS, RHE
Academic Dean/Program Director-
  MBOT
Computer Career Center
Brooklyn, NY

WILSETTA McCLAIN, BBA
National Association of Health
  Professionals (NAHP), National
  Association for Certified Medical
  Billers (NACMB), American
  Association of Medical Assistants
  (AAMA), Michigan Medical
  Assistant Post Secondary Educators
  (M-MAPSE)
Roseville, MI

PAT G. MOECK, MBA, CMA
Director, Medical Assisting
  Programs
El Centro College
Dallas, TX

IRENE L. E. MUELLER, EdD, RHIA
HIA Program Director
Assistant Professor, Health Sciences
Western Carolina University
Cullowhee, NC

BARBARA FORTUNA MURRAY, EdD, RHIA
Professor, Miami-Dade Community
  College, Retired
Member, AHIMA Council on
  Certification & Certified Coding
  Specialist (CCS) Exam Committee
  (2002–2004)
Miami, FL

CINDY C. PARMAN, CPC, CPC-H, RCC
President-Elect, AAPC National
  Advisory Board
Coding Strategies, Inc.
Powder Springs, GA

BRENDA PEREZ
Member of American Academy of
  Professional Coders
Renton, WA

JANET ROCCABELLO CPC, CPA
Allied Health Supervisor
Lincoln Technical Institute
Lincoln, Rhode Island

DORY P. RINCON, MA, RHIT, CMA, CPC
City College of San Francisco
San Francisco, CA

DARCY ROY, CPC, RHE, CMA, BHO
Medical Coder/Biller Program
  Director
Brevard Community College
Cocoa, FL

SHANNON SHARPE, B.S., CCS-P, CMRS
Instructor, Medical Administrative
  Programs
Renton Technical College
Renton, WA

JANET SKWIER, BS
Instructor
Dorsey Business School
Madison Heights, MI

SHIRLEY N. SMITH, MPA, RT
Department Chair/Program
  Director
Radiation Therapy
Baker College of Jackson
Jackson, MI

JANETTE THOMAS, MPS, RHIA
Director of Learning Assistance
Alfred State College, Alfred,
  NY

JEAN TYNER, RDH, BS
Instructor, Dental Department
Florence Darlington Technical
    College
Florence, SC

CAROLE ZEGLIN MS, BS, RMA
Director Medical Assistant
    Program/Asst. Professor
Westmoreland County Community
    College
Youngwood, Pennsylvania

BERHANE M. ZEROM, CEO/PRESIDENT
Aster Technology Institute
Tacoma, WA

BRANDY G. ZIESEMER, MA, RHIA, CCS
HIM Program Manager/Instructor
Lake-Sumter Community College
Leesburg, FL

Contents in Brief

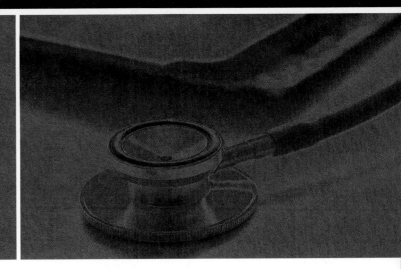

Expanded Contents

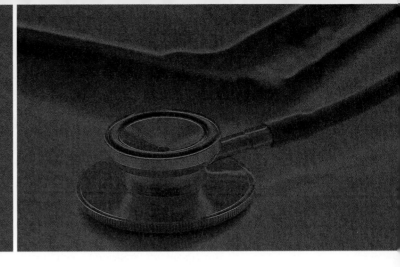

PART I

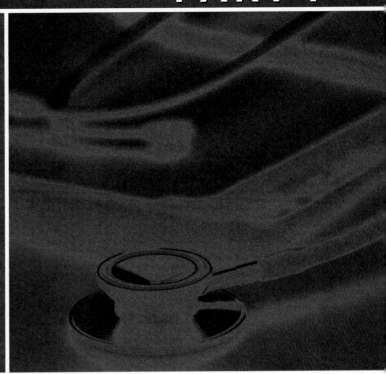

INTRODUCTION TO ICD-9-CM

CHAPTER 1

Introduction to ICD-9-CM Coding

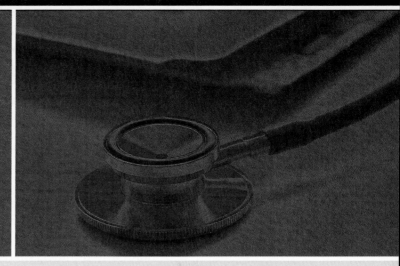

Chapter Outline

History of the ICD-9-CM
Medical Coding Simplifies Reimbursement
Other Uses of Medical Coding
Format and Content of ICD-9-CM
Coding Compliance
ICD-10-CM and ICD-10-PCS
Testing Your Comprehension

Chapter Objectives

▶ Define the International Classification of Diseases, 9th Revision, Clinical Modification (ICD-9-CM) and briefly describe the history of the ICD-9-CM classification system.

▶ Define the clinical coding system and classification system.

▶ Identify the main purposes of the ICD-9-CM classification system.

▶ Define the World Health Organization (WHO).

▶ Define prospective payment systems (PPS).

▶ Explain the format and content of the three volumes of the ICD-9-CM.

▶ Identify the American Hospital Association's *Coding Clinic* as the "official" resource for ICD-9-CM information.

▶ Define ICD-10-CM and explain considerations for its adoption.

Data on the types and number of diseases in the United States provide important information to help us understand the overall condition of our nation's health. Information contained in patients' medical records, whether paper based or electronic, holds great value in letting us know what is happening in health care. It is through the study of patient diseases and treatments that we can begin to understand, improve, and standardize quality health care; improve patients' medical outcomes; and improve patient services at reduced cost. Each individual success at the patient, provider, and institutional level (microlevel) adds to our collective health success at a national level (macrolevel).

Codes tell us the important story of each patient's health-care encounter. The quality of coded data provides us with health-care information to support our best decisions to improve the quality of patient care.

The International Classification of Diseases, 9th Revision, Clinical Modification (ICD-9-CM) is a widely used classification system for coding, classifying, and identifying patient diseases and procedures in the United States. It is a standardized medical communication tool that serves all health-care stakeholders, including physicians, health-care networks, hospitals, long-term care and outpatient facilities, insurers or other payers of care, employers, government officials, managed care organizations, patients, and countless other interested parties.

To quickly process and communicate important health-care data within this complex and dynamic health-care environment, medical coding systems transform verbal medical descriptions of patient diseases and procedures into numbers that, for the most part, are communicated electronically (e.g., diagnosis code 428.0 indicates congestive heart failure). Codes, rather than long narrative descriptions of diseases and procedures, can be quickly entered into computerized systems and processed to create health-care information. This health-care information is used for medical research to study and improve the quality of patient care, and can also be transmitted to third-party payers to facilitate payments to health-care providers. Codes also communicate to payers what medical services they are paying for. They can substantiate that the care rendered was medically necessary, health-care resources were properly utilized, and that the health-care provider's charges were reasonable.

History of the ICD-9-CM

Historically, the ICD-9-CM's *Tabular List of Diseases* (volume 1) and the *Alphabetic Index to Diseases* (volume 2) represent a clinical modification (CM) of the World Health Organization's (WHO) publication *International Classification of Diseases, 9th Revision (ICD-9)*, which was first published in 1977. The WHO collaborates with the United Nations and assists governments in strengthening their health services wherever possible.[1] Through ICD, the WHO collects international information on the diseases of member populations. However, this international version does not completely meet the needs of the United States because of its emphasis on the more acute infectious diseases seen in developing countries rather than on the chronic diseases seen in the United States (such as arteriosclerosis and hypertension).[2] For that reason, WHO's ICD-9 has been clinically modified (CM) for use in the United States as the ICD-9-CM. In 1992, WHO published ICD-10; however, the 9th version remains currently in use in the United States as ICD-9-CM for reporting and billing requirements mandated under the 1996 Health Insurance Portability and Accountability Act (HIPAA). As one exception, in 1999, the United States did implement ICD-10 for the coding of causes of death as a required content for death certificates.

The ICD-9-CM's *Alphabetic Index to Procedures* and *Tabular List of Procedures* (volume 3) was specifically developed for use in the United States and was not developed by the WHO. ICD-9-CM code revisions and new codes have been developed annually by the United States Centers for Medicare and Medicaid Services (CMS) and the National Center for Health Statistics (NCHS). In prior years, starting with patient discharges on October 1, new codes and code revisions have been implemented throughout the United States. Last year (October 1 , 2007), CMS released 142 new diagnosis codes and 39 new procedure codes with 20 revised diagnosis and procedure codes. This year (October 1, 2008), CMS released 367 new diagnosis codes and 60 new procedure codes with 94 revised diagnosis and procedure codes.

Compared to previous years, this represents a significant number of code changes. In addition, providers will be struggling with major changes to the Medicare payment structure, which will be explained in the next section.

Medical Coding Simplifies Reimbursement

Over the past several years, to control and reduce skyrocketing health-care costs, the U.S. government's Medicare and Medicaid programs and most other private third-party payers of health-care services have used medical coding systems to structure prospective payment rates to health-care providers for services to their patients. Prospective payment systems (PPS) are reimbursement formulas determined in advance of the health-care services rendered that are not based on the health-care provider's costs to treat the patient. The provider knows prospectively what the payment will be for services rendered. These payments are predetermined based on the average cost of health-care resources necessary to treat the patient's condition as revealed through diagnosis and procedure codes.

In the 1980s, the federal government, as a large payer of health-care bills, started the first major initiative to develop and implement a PPS for its Medicare population. In 1982, Congress passed the Tax Equity and Fiscal Responsibility Act (TEFRA), which required the development of a prospective patient system for reimbursement of Medicare inpatient services to hospitals. In 1983, the federal government implemented diagnosis-related groups (DRGs) as a PPS in which the amount of payment to the hospital is determined in advance of the services rendered. Originally, researchers at Yale University developed DRGs as an inpatient classification scheme to group patients who were medically similar with respect to diagnoses, treatments, and lengths of hospital stay. For the 2008 federal fiscal year (FY), the DRG system was refined to Medicare Severity-DRGs (MS-DRG). Federal fiscal years begin on October 1 and end on September 30.

In the MS-DRG system, many factors influence the hospital payment amount:

▸ principal diagnosis—sequenced first, the "condition, after study, chiefly responsible for occasioning the admission of the patient to the hospital for care"

▸ secondary diagnos(es)- MS-DRGs established a new three-tiered payment system for DRGs that includes distinguishing between a MAJOR complication or comorbidity (MCC); a REGULAR complication or comorbidity (C/C); or, NO complication or comorbidity. A **complica-**

tion is a condition that occurs after admission that affects the patient's care or length of stay (e.g., after admission, the patient develops a catheter-associated urinary tract infection); and a **comorbidity** is a pre-existing condition that affects the patient's care or length of stay (e.g., patient admitted for pneumonia with preexisting chronic systolic left heart failure).

▶ operating room procedures

▶ the patient's gender

▶ discharge status (e.g., discharged to home or transferred to a skilled nursing facility). For the federal fiscal year 2009, 273 MS-DRGs payment rates to hospitals are affected if the patient is transferred from the hospital to a PPS-exempt or skilled nursing facility, or the hospital discharge is followed by a home health agency visit. Only 190 DRGs were affected by this post-acute care transfer policy in 2007.

MS-DRGs represent classifications (groups) of diagnoses in which patients with similar conditions within the same MS-DRG group will consume similar types and amounts of hospital resources (see Appendix 1, p. 672). The federal government implemented severity of illness DRGs (MS-DRGs) to more accurately identify and stipulate the requirements of patients for health services resources. In turn, it is expected this change will establish payment rates that are more accurate.[3]

For FY2008, under the severity-adjusted DRGs, the number of diagnosis-related groups expanded from 538 DRGs to 745 MS-DRGs. For FY2009, hospitals will see few changes to MS-DRG system; however, they will see a significant expansion of quality measures and the reporting of hospital-acquired conditions (HAC). The few changes for 2009 include revisions to the descriptions for MS-DRG 245, 870, 871, 872, and a new MS-DRG 265 (see Appendix 1, MS-DRGs for 2009). Once a full rollout of the MS-DRG system is accomplished, there could be over 900 MS-DRGs. The DRG logic within the severity of illness system of reporting will better reflect the complexity and interaction of multiple diseases that cause some patients within a certain DRG category to be sicker (and need more resources) than other patients within the same category. Also, based on a patient's severity of illness level (e.g., minor, moderate, major), payments to health care providers will be more closely linked to performance that results in positive patient outcomes. The advancement of a severity adjusted reporting system even further increases the need for precise coding and complete and accurate provider documentation in order to receive fair and optimum payments under the MS-DRG system and to have the data necessary to study and improve patient care practices and outcomes.

A software application called a **grouper** assigns the MS-DRG. In the MS-DRG inpatient PPS, the rate of payment to the hospital is established in advance of the health-care services rather than being determined retrospectively after the services are provided on the basis of the provider's cost or usual and customary charge.

At patient discharge, coded diagnostic and procedural information on each Medicare patient is used to identify and assign MS-DRG payments to providers at rates that have been predetermined on the basis of the average cost of health-care resources necessary to treat the patient's condition as it falls within a MS-DRG. Each MS-DRG is assigned a relative weight to reflect the resource consumption associated with the treatment of the condition that is multiplied against a base rate, also called a blended rate (i.e., an individual hospital monetary adjustment factor for geographic status, such as urban versus rural, and local wage index). Beginning in 2007, the Centers for Medicare and Medicaid Services (CMS) began a three-year transition from a charge-based relative weight system (under DRGs) to a cost-based system (under MS-DRGs). FY 2008 began with a 50/50 (DRG/MS-DRG) payment blend, however, MS-DRGs with cost-based relative weights will be fully implemented in 2009.

It is important to note that MS-DRGs do not tell providers how to practice medicine. However, the limits in provider reimbursement within the DRG formula provide an effective and politically correct way of controlling health-care costs by controlling providers' behaviors regarding the internal utilization of hospital resources. Within each hospital, providers must practice effective, efficient, quality care at reduced cost to return a profit within the cost controls imposed under the MS-DRG PPS.

MS-DRG 195 for the treatment of simple pneumonia, with a national relative weight of 0.7301, multiplied against a given hospital's base rate of $4,922.73, would have a reimbursement of $3594.09.

EXAMPLE

Other Uses of Medical Coding

In addition to reimbursement, coded information is used by health-care facilities to determine and plan for the types of services that are needed within communities. For example, coded data revealing a high incidence of coronary artery disease within a hospital may indicate the need to recruit more cardiologists and open a diagnostic heart catheter laboratory. Coded data revealing a young community and high birth rate may indicate the need to expand the hospital's obstetrics unit and to recruit more obstetricians. Also, coded data can be analyzed to help develop and implement local, state, and national health-care policy (e.g., smoking cessation, obesity education, anti-drug policies, and early-pregnancy education) and to determine mechanisms to contain health-care costs.

Coded information helps to identify patient cases to develop **best-care practices** (also known as **critical paths** and **patient care maps**) as clinical guidelines to assist physicians in providing consistent quality care for particular diseases and to identify patient cases to further clinical research. With the growth of managed care organizations, coding also serves as the basis for disease management through various health-care settings and provider networks. For example, as a patient travels from the doctor's office to a hospital to a home health agency or skilled nursing facility, coding provides a flow of patient information to promote the continuity of patient care and preventive care services. Foremost, quality coded data provide information to help health-care administrators make good decisions to improve medical care for the patients they serve. Providing quality care to patients within their communities is the unifying mission of all health-care providers.

Format and Content of ICD-9-CM

According to Huffman, an effective (coding) classification system such as ICD-9-CM must follow three basic rules:

1. the set of categories should be derived from a "single classification principle," meaning that the classification should be organized by anatomic body sites (e.g., appendix and heart), causes of disease (e.g., infection and tumors), or names of diseases
2. the set of categories should be "exhaustive," meaning that there is a code provided for every disease and procedure (i.e., a place to code everything)
3. the categories within the classification should be "mutually exclusive" (i.e., each disease and procedure must have a unique code to retain the integrity of the data)

ICD-9-CM is "officially" published by the U.S. federal government as a three-volume set that includes the *Tabular List of Diseases* (volume 1), the *Alphabetic Index to Diseases* (volume 2), and the *Alphabetic Index to Procedures* and *Tabular List of Procedures* (volume 3). ICD-9-CM codes can be downloaded as PDF files from the CMS and NCHS websites and are also available for purchase from the U.S. Government Printing Office as a CD-ROM, which can be accessed at http://bookstore.gpo.gov. In addition, each year's new and revised codes (both proposed and final) are published in the *Federal Register*, a daily (Mon-Fri) publication of the federal government that contains proposed rules, public notices, and federal agency regulations. The Federal Register can be accessed at http://www.gpoaccess.gov//.

To ensure accurate coding, coders must first look up the name of the disease or procedure alphabetically in the indexes and then access the code numerically within the tabular sections, where there is additional information on each code. A universal coding rule states that *"a coder must never code from the index,"* because the indexes serve to point to the tabular sections, where more information is always found.

Since you must first access the index sections before using the tabular sections, many commercial publishers make the three-volume set more "user friendly" by publishing all three volumes within one book, with the *Alphabetic Index to Diseases* (volume 2) first, followed by the *Tabular List of Diseases* (volume 1); and then the *Alphabetic Index to Procedures* followed by the *Tabular List of Procedures* (both in volume 3). For this reason, this text discusses the volumes in the order in which they are presented in most commercial publications (i.e., volumes 2-1-3).

Alphabetic Index to Diseases (Volume 2)

The *Alphabetic Index to Diseases* is organized so that you can look up the main term by the name of the disease. However, ICD-9-CM is a multiaxial system, meaning that you can locate the condition under different names. For example, diseases may also be accessed by more general terms (e.g., **anomaly, disorder**, or **disease**), abbreviations, or synonyms. **Main terms** for the names of diseases in the *Alphabetic Index to Diseases* are in **bold** print.

Indented under the main term for the disease, **subterms**, also known as **essential modifiers**, can change the code assignment and must always be thoroughly reviewed, because they are essential. Located directly after the main term in parentheses, **nonessential modifiers** add information that will clarify the code selection but do not change the code assignment. Often, connecting words—such as **in**, **with**, and **due to**—are listed under the main term and precede subterms that are used to lead you to the correct code assignment.

[main term] ← **Anxiety** (neurosis) (reaction) (state)←
[nonessential modifiers]
300.00
[*subterms*] ← alcohol-induced 291.89
      depression 300.4
      drug-induced 292.89
      due to or associated with physical condition 293.84
      generalized 300.04
      hysteria 300.20
      in ← [connecting word]
            acute stress reaction 308.0
            transient adjustment reaction 309.24
            panic type 300.01
            separation, abnormal 309.21
            syndrome (organic) (transient) 293.84

Valid disease codes can contain three to five digits. The first three digits are followed by a decimal point, and one or two additional digits may be present (e.g., 427.89). An important rule in coding is to always code to the highest level of specificity. This means that three-digit **category** codes may be further subdivided into four-digit **subcategory** codes and that four-digit subcategory codes may be further subdivided into five-digit **subclassification** codes.

Following the rule to never code from the *Alphabetic Index to Diseases* (volume 2) and always checking the instructions within the *Tabular List of*

EXAMPLE

After locating the main term for the disease "thrombosis; coronary, without myocardial infarction 411.81" in the Alphabetic Index to Diseases, locate the code in the Tabular List of Diseases. Note that code 411.81 is located within:

▶ *section (range of codes) on Diseases of the Circulatory System (390–459)*
▶ *category 411 (three-digit code that is further subdivided) Other Acute and Subacute Forms of Ischemic Heart Disease*
▶ *subcategory 411.8 (four-digit code that is further subdivided) Other*
▶ *subclassification 411.81 (a valid five-digit code [carried out to the highest level of specificity] that includes the description for Acute Coronary Thromobosis without Myocardial Infarction)*

Diseases (volume 1) before assigning a code will help prevent the error of not carrying the code to the furthest digit provided within the category (i.e., missing digits). For example, category code 411 would be invalid because it is further subdivided into 411.0, 411.1, 411.81, and 411.89.

Three-digit diagnosis category codes are only assigned if they are not further subdivided into four-digit subcategory codes. Four-digit subcategory

TIP For an inexperienced coder, a good rule to follow is to assume that all the disease codes have five digits unless you can prove otherwise.

codes are only assigned if they are not further subdivided into five-digit sub-classification codes. Three-digit category codes are usually subdivided by adding another digit after a decimal point to a four-digit subcategory or five-digit subclassification code. In disease coding, five-digit codes are the most specific classification and are mandatory, if provided.

A coder should perform a final check of all disease codes before reporting them. If any disease codes have fewer than five digits, the coder should make sure to double-check the instructions in the Tabular List of Diseases (volume 1) section to ensure that they are carried out to their highest level of specificity.

A special feature of the *Alphabetic Index to Diseases* is that it includes three tables:

1. Hypertension Table
2. Neoplasm Table
3. Table of Drugs and Chemicals

These tables, or grids, provide quick and easy access to a list of related conditions often associated with these main diseases.

Additionally, the *Alphabetic Index to Diseases* (volume 2) includes an Alphabetic Index to External Cause of Injury that provides quick and easy access to a list of E-codes that describe the external circumstance for an injury (e.g., <u>fall</u> from a ladder, <u>cut</u> by broken glass). By locating the responsible drug or chemical that is listed in the Table of Drugs and Chemicals, you can use E-codes to describe the causes of poisonings (e.g., accident, suicide attempt, assault, or undetermined), and the causes of adverse effects (e.g., rash or confusion) that result from drugs taken as prescribed (e.g., for therapeutic use). E-codes coming from Alphabetic Index to External Cause of Injury or Table of Drugs and Chemicals contained within the *Alphabetic Index to Diseases* (volume 2) must be validated by a review of the E-code supplemental section provided in the *Tabular List of Diseases* (volume 1).

Tabular List of Diseases (Volume 1)

The *Tabular List of Diseases* contains 17 chapters that relate to various body systems, such as the digestive system or respiratory system. Some chapters do not relate to any specific body system but to causes of disease that can affect any or all systems, such as neoplasms (tumors) and infectious diseases. The *Tabular List of Diseases* also contains two supplementary classifications that contain alphanumeric codes. These are the V and E codes. Table 1.1 shows the organization of volume 1.

Codes within the *Tabular List of Diseases* (volume 1) are arranged numerically. To code precisely, the coder must look up the name of the disease alphabetically within the *Alphabetic Index to Diseases* (volume 2) and then locate the code numerically within the *Tabular List of Diseases* (volume 1), where there is additional information on each code.

Chapter	Description	Code Range/Section
TABLE 1.1	**Organization of Volume 1:** *Tabular List of Diseases*	
1	Infectious and parasitic diseases	001–139
2	Neoplasms	140–239
3	Endocrine, nutritional, and metabolic disease and immunity disorders	240–279
4	Diseases of the blood and blood-forming organs	280–289
5	Mental disorders	290–319
6	Diseases of the nervous system and sense organs	320–389
7	Diseases of the circulatory system	390–459
8	Diseases of the respiratory system	460–519
9	Diseases of the digestive system	520–579
10	Diseases of the genitourinary system	580–629
11	Complications of pregnancy, childbirth, and the puerperium	630–677
12	Diseases of the skin and subcutaneous tissue	680–709
13	Diseases of the musculoskeletal system and connective tissue	710–739
14	Congenital anomalies	740–759
15	Certain conditions originating in the perinatal period	760–779
16	Symptoms, signs, and ill-defined conditions	780–799
17	Injury and poisoning	800–999
18	Classification of factors influencing health status and contact with health service	V01–V89
19	Classification of external causes of injury and poisoning	E 800–E999

427.81 SINOATRIAL NODE DYSFUNCTION

Sinus bradycardia:

 Persistent

 Severe

Syndrome:

 Sick sinus

 Tachycardia-bradycardia

Excludes: sinus bradycardia, not otherwise specified (427.89)

V Codes (V01-V89)

The supplementary classifications of "Contact with Health Services" and "Factors Influencing Health Status" are preceded by a "V."

V codes can be used as a **principal diagnosis** (sequenced first) to describe the reason for contact with health services. For example, code V58.11 indicates that a patient's health-care encounter is to receive chemotherapy, code V58.0 indicates that a patient's health-care encounter is to receive radiation therapy, code V56.0 indicates that a patient's health-care encounter is to receive hemodialysis, and code V30.00 describes an admission of a live newborn infant.

V codes can be used as **secondary diagnoses** to describe other factors influencing health care. These codes do not describe disease states, yet their presence affects patient care. For example, code V45.01 describes a patient's cardiac pacemaker status, code V43.64 describes that a patient has had previous hip replacement surgery, V10.3 describes a past personal history of breast cancer, and code V27.0 describes a single live-born infant as the outcome of delivery on the mother's record.

E CODES (E800-E999)

The supplementary classification of "External Causes of Injury and Poisoning" is preceded by an "E."

E codes are never sequenced first as the principal diagnosis. They are used solely as secondary diagnoses to explain:

- ► the external cause of an injury: for example, code E884.4 sequenced as a secondary diagnosis would explain that a patient's injury (e.g., a fractured hip) was caused by a fall from a bed
- ► the external cause of a poisoning: for example, code E850.3 sequenced as a secondary diagnosis would explain that a poisoning with aspirin was accidental
- ► the adverse effect of a medication taken as prescribed: for example, code E930.0 sequenced as secondary diagnosis would explain that an adverse effect (e.g., rash) was attributed to penicillin taken as prescribed

The *Tabular List of Diseases* (volume 1) also provides four appendices that provide the following information:

1. Appendix A—Morphology of Neoplasms provides codes that describe the **histology** (tissue type) and **behavior** (e.g., benign or malignant) of neoplasms (tumors). Appendix A is most often used by hospital cancer registries.
2. Appendix B—Glossary of Mental Disorders provides definitions for various types of mental illnesses.
3. Appendix C—Classification of Drugs by the American Hospital Formulary Service (AHFS) List Number and Their ICD-9-CM Equivalents can be used to help assign the correct poisoning diagnosis codes to identify the responsible drug or chemical.
4. Appendix D—Classification of Industrial Accidents According to Agency is used by external agencies to gather statistics relating to the machinery, materials, substances, and environment involved in employment-related injuries.

Alphabetic Index to Procedures and *Tabular List of Procedures* (Volume 3)

The *Alphabetic Index to Procedures* and *Tabular List of Procedures* are both contained within volume 3. The structure for the *Alphabetic Index to Procedures* and *Tabular List of Procedures* is similar to that of the *Alphabetic Index to Diseases* (volume 2) and the *Tabular List of Diseases* (volume 1).

The *Alphabetic Index to Procedures* is organized so that you can look up the main term by the name of the procedure. However, procedures may also be accessed by more general terms (e.g., **repair, excision, removal**, and **resection**), abbreviations, eponyms (named after people; e.g., McBride), or synonyms. **Main terms** for the names of procedures in the *Alphabetic Index to Procedures* are in **bold** print. Indented under the main term, **subterms** (also known as **essential modifiers**) can change the procedure code and must always be thoroughly reviewed, because they are essential. Located directly after the main term in parentheses, **nonessential modifiers** clarify the code selection but do not change the code assignment. Often, connecting words such as **with**, **without**, **as**, or **by** are listed under the main term and are used to lead you to the correct code assignment.

[main term] ← **Colostomy** (ileo-ascending) (ileotransverse) (perineal) (transverse) ← [nonessential modifiers] 46.10

with ← [Connecting word] anterior rectal resection 48.62

    [subterms] ← delayed opening 46.14

    loop 46.03

    permanent (magnetic) 46.13

    temporary 46.11

Valid procedure codes can contain three to four digits. The first two digits are followed by a decimal point, and one or two additional digits may be present (e.g., 45.25). An important rule in coding is to always code to the highest level of specificity. This means that three-digit **subcategory** codes may be further subdivided into four-digit **subclassification** codes.

Following the rule to never code from the *Alphabetic Index to Procedures* and always checking the instructions within the *Tabular List of Procedures* before assigning a code will help prevent the error of not carrying the code to the furthest digit provided beyond the two-digit procedure category.

EXAMPLE

After locating the main term for the procedure "lysis; adhesions, peritoneum, laparoscopic 54.51" in the Alphabetic Index to Procedures, locate the code in the Tabular List of Procedures. Note that code 54.51 is located within:

▶ *section (range of codes) on Operations on the Digestive System (42–54)*
▶ *category 54 (two-digit code that is further subdivided) Other Operations on Abdominal Region*
▶ *subcategory 54.5 (three-digit code that is further subdivided) Lysis of Peritoneal Adhesions*
▶ *subclassification 54.51 (a valid four-digit code [carried out to the highest level of specificity] that includes the description Laparoscopic Lysis of Peritoneal Adhesions)*

Two-digit procedure category codes are not assigned. Three-digit subcategory codes are only assigned if they are not further subdivided into four-digit subclassification codes. Two-digit category codes are always subdivided by adding another digit after a decimal point to three-digit subcategory or four-digit subclassification code. In procedure coding, four-digit codes are the most specific classification and are mandatory, if provided.

TIP For an inexperienced coder, a good rule to follow is to assume all the procedure codes have four-digits unless you can prove otherwise.

A coder should perform a final check of all procedure codes before reporting them. If any procedure codes have fewer than four digits, the coder should double-check the instructions in the Tabular List of Procedures section to ensure that they are carried out to their highest level of specificity.

The *Tabular List of Procedures* contains 17 (00–16) chapters relating to operations or procedures on various body systems, such as the digestive system or respiratory system, and miscellaneous diagnostic and therapeutic procedures (see Table 1.2).

Codes within the *Tabular List of Procedures* are arranged numerically. To code precisely, the coder must look up the name of the procedure alphabetically in the *Alphabetic Index to Procedures* and then locate the code numerically within the *Tabular List of Procedures,* where there is additional information on each code.

39.29 OTHER (PERIPHERAL) VASCULAR SHUNT OR BYPASS

Bypass (graft):

 Axillary-brachial

 Axillary-femoral [axillofemoral] (superficial)

 Brachial

 Femoral-femoral

 Femoroperoneal

 Femoropopliteal (arteries)

 Femorotibial (anterior) (posterior)

 Popliteal

 Vascular, not otherwise specified

Excludes: peritoneovenous shunt (54.94)

TABLE 1.2	Organization of Volume 3: *Tabular List of Procedures*	
Chapter	**Description**	**Code Range/Section**
0	Procedures and interventions, not elsewhere classified	00
1	Operations on the nervous system	01–05
2	Operations on the endocrine system	06–07
3	Operations on the eye	08–16
4	Operations on the ear	18–20
5	Operations on the nose, mouth, and pharynx	21–29
6	Operations on the respiratory system	30–34
7	Operations on the cardiovascular system	35–39
8	Operations on the hemic and lymphatic system	40–41
9	Operations on the digestive system	42–54
10	Operations on the urinary system	55–59
11	Operations on the male genital organs	60–64
12	Operations on the female genital organs	65–71
13	Obstetrical procedures	72–75
14	Operations on the musculoskeletal system	76–84
15	Operations on the integumentary system	85–86
16	Miscellaneous diagnostic and therapeutic procedures	87–99

Coding Compliance

Compliance means "in good faith" to follow the laws and rules that govern you. Coding compliance derives from accurate assignment and sequencing of diagnoses and procedure codes within established rules that ensure appropriate reimbursement. This process is highly dependent on the competent training of all individuals involved in the coding process and especially those at highest risk (e.g., coders and billers). Medical coders and billers are at higher risk because they can knowingly (fraud) or unknowingly (abuse) report codes to payers that are not representative of the diagnoses and services given to patients that can result in a higher reimbursement to the provider. This is an unethical and fraudulent practice called "upcoding." As you will learn in the following chapters, medical coders must fully understand the conventions of the ICD-9-CM classification system, follow federal coding guidelines and definitions as presented through the Uniform Hospital Discharge Data Set (UHDDS), learn coding steps and rules, apply official coding rules published through the *Coding Clinic* for ICD-9-CM, and, ultimately, learn how to interpret a medical record for the process of coding. All this must be accomplished within a compliant and ethical context and an institutional culture that supports this as a matter of practice.

The *Coding Clinic* is a quarterly publication of the American Hospital Association (AHA) and is recognized by the CMS as an official source for ICD-9-CM coding advice. The *Coding Clinic* is developed through an editorial board, and coding advice is approved by representatives of the American Hospital Association, the CMS, the NCHS, and the American Health Information Management Association (AHIMA). The *Coding Clinic* is considered an invaluable resource for ICD-9-CM coding advice. In addition, the CMS and NCHS have created guidelines to assist in coding and reporting in situations for which the ICD-9-CM does not provide specific direction.

ICD-10-CM and ICD-10-PCS

The WHO published ICD-10 in 1992, and there has been considerable progress by the CMS on its clinical modification (CM) for adaptation for use in the United States as ICD-10-CM. It will eventually replace volumes 1 and 2 of ICD-9-CM. In addition, each year and continuing with 2009 ICD-9-CM changes released by CMS, the ever-increasing specificity and detail of codes indicates we are moving closer to adopting ICD-10-CM.

ICD-10-PCS is being developed as a procedural coding system to replace volume 3 of ICD-9-CM, which will be implemented with ICD-10-CM. This new alphanumeric coding system provides an expansion of new codes and increased detail that will provide a significant improvement over the three volumes of ICD-9-CM in current use. However, it will require substantial reengineering of PPS decision trees and logic, including MS-DRGs and ambulatory payment classifications (APCs). Therefore, ICD-10-CM will have a profound effect on hospital reporting under MS-DRGs that are an inpatient PPS (IPPS) and on APCs that are an outpatient PPS (OPPS) used in the hospital setting.

The implementation of ICD-10-CM will require the mapping of the new ICD-10-CM codes to the older ICD-9-CM legacy systems. This coded information is critical to health-care finance, case management, utilization review, quality improvement, and patient case-mix studies, which describe the type and volume of patients treated by the facility. Medical coding is a vehicle of communication that provides for the continuity of patient care through various health-care settings, providers, and networks, and it is also the mechanism for provider reimbursement. Therefore, ICD-10-CM's adaptation will require precise planning, at great cost, and implementation may be several years in the future. Also, we must remain aware that problems that have occurred with ICD-9-CM in regard to the quality of physicians' documentation for coding will extend to ICD-10-CM and limit the ability to benefit from the full utility of the new classification. Although it is widely accepted among health information professionals that ICD-10-CM is a better classification that allows us to capture more clinical detail, ICD-10-CM's success depends on a corresponding increase in the level of detail within physicians' documentation. Moreover, the WHO has already begun working on ICD-11, and there is a possibility that the United States will skip ICD-10 and convert directly to ICD-11. However, there is also a possibility that it may be cost-effective to develop software that more accurately maps the refined United States' ICD-9-CM system to ICD-10 or 11. As the CMS adds more detail to the ICD-9-CM codes each year, it may eventually mirror the detail of the ICD-10 system, at which point precise conversion (i.e., electronic crosswalk) may be possible, as well as more economically feasible.

EXAMPLE	*Comparison of ICD-9-CM to increased detail of ICD-10-CM*

ICD-9-CM: 440.24 *Atherosclerosis of the extremities with gangrene*

ICD-10CM: I70.26 *Atherosclerosis of native arteries of extremities with gangrene*

I70.261 *Atherosclerosis of native arteries of extremities with gangrene, right leg*

I70.262 *Atherosclerosis of native arteries of extremities with gangrene, left leg*

I70.263 *Atherosclerosis of native arteries of extremities with gangrene, bilateral legs*

I70.268 *Atherosclerosis of native arteries of extremities with gangrene, other extremity*

I70.269 *Atherosclerosis of native arteries of extremities with gangrene, unspec. extremity*

"There is not yet an anticipated implementation date for the ICD-10-CM. Implementation will be based on an as yet to be defined process for adoption of standards under the federal **Health Insurance Portability and Accountability Act** [HIPAA] of 1996 (Public Law 104-191). There will be a two-year implementation window once the final notice to implement ICD-10-CM has been published in the Federal Register."[4]

Therefore, an amendment to HIPAA law will be required to make ICD-10-CM the official coding standard. Under the Title II "Administrative Simplification" provisions of HIPAA, federal standards mandate the simplification of the electronic transfer of medical data for health-care providers, health plans, and health-care clearinghouses. The "Administrative Simplification" provision includes four parts that include requirements for:

1. Electronic Health Transaction Standards including standard code sets
2. Unique Identifiers for patients, providers, employers, and health plans
3. Security and Electronic Signature Standards for health information maintained or transmitted electronically
4. Privacy and Confidentiality Standards for protected health information (PHI)

Within the provision for electronic health transaction standards, health-care organizations must use standard code sets for all health transactions. Currently, ICD-9-CM and Current Procedural Terminology (CPT) published by the American Medical Association (AMA)/HCPCS are the uniform code sets that have been selected under HIPAA. The Healthcare Common Procedure Coding System (HCPCS) was developed by the CMS to meet the needs of the federal Medicare and Medicaid reimbursement programs. HCPCS has two levels, including Level I HCPCS (published by the AMA as CPT) and Level II (developed by the CMS for providers to report and bill for Medicare and Medicaid services not found in CPT, such as nonphysician services and medical supplies).

CPT codes consist of five digits (e.g., 45378: colonoscopy with biopsy), and HCPCS Levels II and III consists of alphanumeric codes (e.g., A0429: ambulance service, emergency service with basic life support). Two-digit and alphanumeric code modifiers are available that can be appended to CPT/HCPCS codes that do not change the basic definition of the code but explain a special circumstance that affected the service in some way (e.g., 50: bilateral procedure).

It will be years before ICD-10-CM will actually be used in hospitals. However, by learning the concepts of ICD-9-CM now, students will be better prepared to learn ICD-10-CM when it is approved.

Currently, all three volumes (1-2-3) of the ICD-9-CM are used to report and bill for hospital inpatient services being reimbursed under MS-DRGs. Hospital outpatient encounters are reported and billed using ICD-9-CM diagnosis codes (volumes 1-2) and the Current Procedural Terminology (CPT)/HCPCS for coding procedures and services that are reimbursed under APCs. Physicians use ICD-9-CM diagnosis codes and CPT/HCPCS procedure codes to report and bill for their services in health-care settings in which they provide patient care (e.g., office, hospital). Based on the reported CPT/HCPCS service codes, predetermined payment rates to physicians are based on a resource based relative value scale (RBRVS) that establishes the physician's fees for Medicare patients.

Although CPT/HCPCS is used to report procedures and services in hospital outpatient settings and for reporting physician services, ICD-9-CM is fundamentally required to report the diagnoses that establish the "medical necessity" for both inpatient and outpatient services. ICD-9-CM is used by providers in all health-care settings (hospitals, physician's offices, long-term care facilities, clinics, etc.), which explains why it is of primary importance to begin your training in medical coding systems with learning to code using the ICD-9-CM.

Additionally, hospitals use the Uniform Bill 04 (UB-04 or CMS 1450; formerly UB-92) and physicians use the CMS 1500 as standardized billing forms to report required patient information to Medicare, Medicaid, and other third party payers (Figures 1.1, 1.2 and 1.3). The patient data contained within the claim forms include ICD-9-CM diagnosis codes and procedure codes (ICD-9-CM and/or CPT/HCPCS) that are electronically abstracted by providers and transmitted as a bit stream of data to a fiscal intermediaries, carriers, insurance companies, or health plans for payment (i.e., application to application electronic claims submission/processing). Essentially, the forms outline and identify the core data and fields required for reporting patient information to Medicare, Medicaid and other third party payers. These forms are often produced in hardcopy (i.e., printed out) for both internal and external auditing functions. In addition, paper forms are sometimes produced for a particular private payer; however, the CMS only accepts paper claims from institutional providers excluded from the mandatory electronic claims submission requirements.

The electronic exchange of data between a provider and insurance company is called electronic data interchange (EDI). Sometimes a provider contracts with a clearinghouse to assist in the processing of electronic claims due to the varied data formats required by different insurance companies and health-care plans. However, the Title II, Administrative Simplification provisions of HIPAA are intended to implement national transaction standards to simplify, improve, and reduce the cost of health-care administration and redirect the money saved to more patient-care focused activities. The national transaction standards implemented by HIPAA will reduce the many different electronic formats providers and plans (insurance companies) use today. For example, Accredited Standards Committee (HIPAA ASC) 837 Institutional electronic claim format is the electronic version of the UB-04 form that is used by providers who submit claims electronically.

Hospitals use the UB-04 to report both inpatient and outpatient services and bill Medicare Part A for claims paid under MS-DRGs and APCs and to report services to other insurance companies for payment. The UB-04 provides fields to report ICD-9-CM diagnosis and procedure codes, and CPT/HCPCS that includes:

- ▶ an admitting diagnosis in field 69
- ▶ eighteen diagnoses including the patient's principal and secondary diagnoses in fields 67, 67A-H, and 67 I-Q
- ▶ six ICD-9-CM procedure codes including the principal procedure and secondary procedures in fields 74, 74 a-e
- ▶ CPT/HCPCS codes for outpatient services in field 44

It is important to note that in February 2005, the National Uniform Billing Committee (NUBC) approved a conversion of the UB-92 form to a new UB-04 format (Figure 1.1). As of May 23, 2007, Medicare no longer accepted the UB-92. The UB-04 marked an important milestone for transition to new data elements that are required for electronic claims submission to Medicare (see http://www.nubc.org).

In contrast to the UB-92 billing form, the newer UB-04 accepts more diagnosis codes and expands the diagnosis and procedure fields to accept ICD-10-CM and ICD-10-PCS. In addition, the UB-04 incorporates the National Provider Identifier (NPI) to better align the paper claim format with the electronic claim requirements mandated by the Health Insurance Portability and Accountability Act of 1996. It also provides a new field to indicate whether or not diagnoses submitted on inpatient claims were present on admission (POA). The POA indicators include Y = Yes; N = No; U = No information in the record; W = Clinically undetermined; and, (-) = Exempt from POA reporting. POA indicators help identify comorbidities (conditions present on admission) from complications (conditions that develop after admission) that can help to red flag quality of care issues. Mandated by CMS, Medicare adopted the POA indicators for inclusion in its pay-for-performance system, and all hospitals were required to report POA indicators for inpatient discharges starting October 1, 2007.

Physicians use the CMS-1500 to report their services and bill Medicare Part B for claims that are paid under RBRVS and other insurance companies for payment. The CMS-1500 provides fields to report ICD-9-CM diagnosis and CPT/HCPCS procedure codes that includes:

- ▶ four ICD-9-CM diagnoses including a primary diagnosis and other diagnoses in field 21
- ▶ six CPT/HCPCS codes in column D of field 24

This is an image of the new UB-04 Form

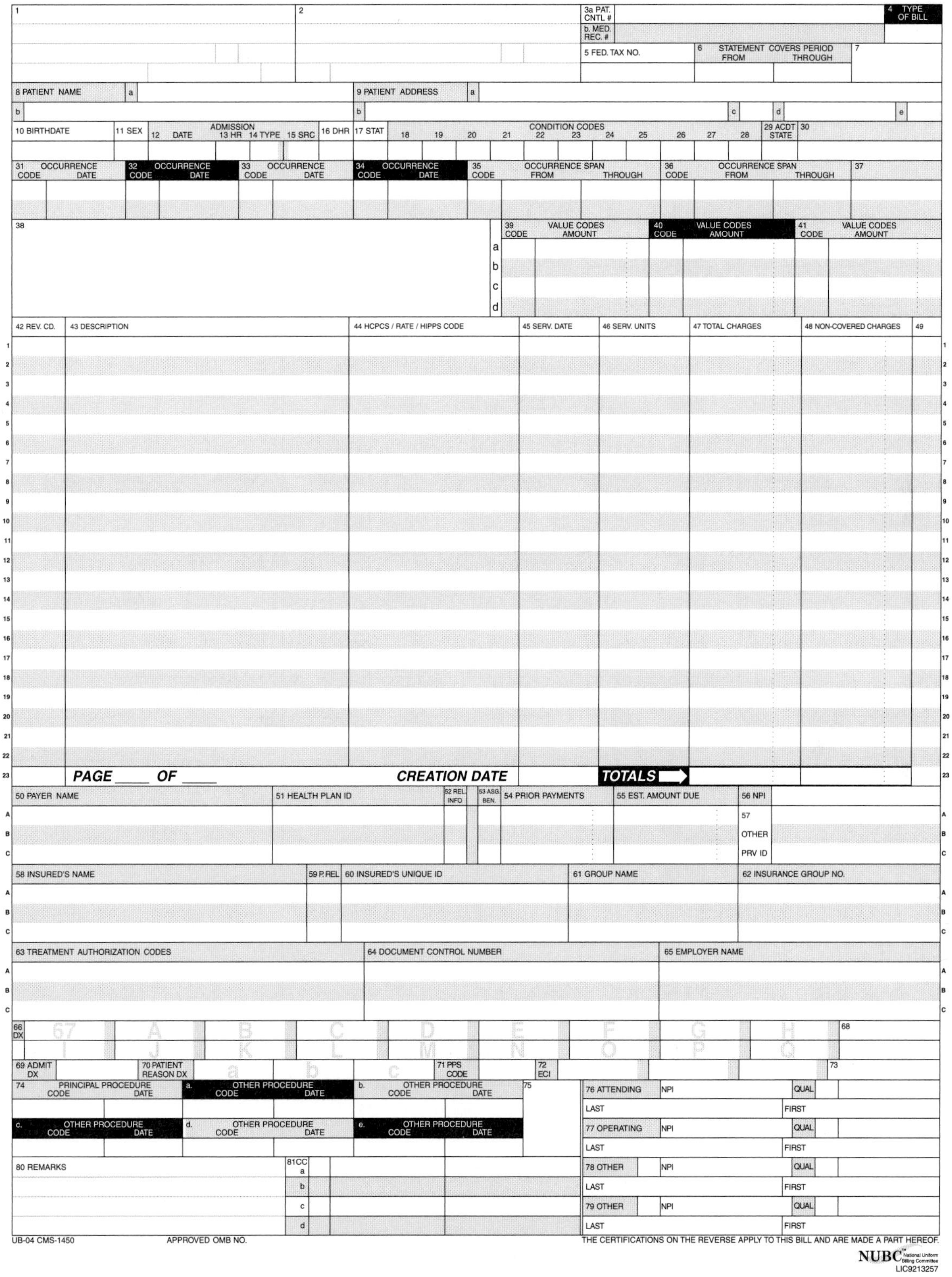
1
2
3a PAT. CNTL #
b. MED. REC. #
4 TYPE OF BILL
5 FED. TAX NO.
6 STATEMENT COVERS PERIOD FROM THROUGH
7
8 PATIENT NAME a
b
9 PATIENT ADDRESS a
b c d e
10 BIRTHDATE
11 SEX
ADMISSION 12 DATE 13 HR 14 TYPE 15 SRC
16 DHR
17 STAT
CONDITION CODES 18 19 20 21 22 23 24 25 26 27 28
29 ACDT STATE
30
31 OCCURRENCE CODE DATE
32 OCCURRENCE CODE DATE
33 OCCURRENCE CODE DATE
34 OCCURRENCE CODE DATE
35 OCCURRENCE SPAN CODE FROM THROUGH
36 OCCURRENCE SPAN CODE FROM THROUGH
37
38
39 VALUE CODES CODE AMOUNT
40 VALUE CODES CODE AMOUNT
41 VALUE CODES CODE AMOUNT
a b c d
42 REV. CD.
43 DESCRIPTION
44 HCPCS / RATE / HIPPS CODE
45 SERV. DATE
46 SERV. UNITS
47 TOTAL CHARGES
48 NON-COVERED CHARGES
49
1 2 3 4 5 6 7 8 9 10 11 12 13 14 15 16 17 18 19 20 21 22 23
PAGE ____ OF ____
CREATION DATE
TOTALS
50 PAYER NAME
51 HEALTH PLAN ID
52 REL. INFO
53 ASG. BEN.
54 PRIOR PAYMENTS
55 EST. AMOUNT DUE
56 NPI
57 OTHER PRV ID
A B C
58 INSURED'S NAME
59 P. REL
60 INSURED'S UNIQUE ID
61 GROUP NAME
62 INSURANCE GROUP NO.
A B C
63 TREATMENT AUTHORIZATION CODES
64 DOCUMENT CONTROL NUMBER
65 EMPLOYER NAME
A B C
66 DX
67 A B C D E F G H
I J K L M N O P Q
68
69 ADMIT DX
70 PATIENT REASON DX a b c
71 PPS CODE
72 ECI
73
74 PRINCIPAL PROCEDURE CODE DATE
a. OTHER PROCEDURE CODE DATE
b. OTHER PROCEDURE CODE DATE
75
c. OTHER PROCEDURE CODE DATE
d. OTHER PROCEDURE CODE DATE
e. OTHER PROCEDURE CODE DATE
76 ATTENDING NPI QUAL
LAST FIRST
77 OPERATING NPI QUAL
LAST FIRST
80 REMARKS
81CC a b c d
78 OTHER NPI QUAL
LAST FIRST
79 OTHER NPI QUAL
LAST FIRST
UB-04 CMS-1450
APPROVED OMB NO.
THE CERTIFICATIONS ON THE REVERSE APPLY TO THIS BILL AND ARE MADE A PART HEREOF.
NUBC National Uniform Billing Committee
LIC9213257

FIGURE 1.1 ■ Uniform Bill 04 (UB-04, or CMS 1450; formerly UB-92) is the newer version of the standard billing form used by hospitals. (Reprinted courtesy of the U.S. Department of Health and Human Services, Centers for Medicare and Medicaid Services.) A sample form as well as additional information regarding the UB-04 is available for download from the CMS website Medicare Learning Network: http://www.cms.hhs.gov/MLNProducts/downloads/ub04 fact_sheet_050207.pdf; and more information on the UB-04 and the UB-92 is available through the NUBC website at http://www.nubc.org.

1500

HEALTH INSURANCE CLAIM FORM

APPROVED BY NATIONAL UNIFORM CLAIM COMMITTEE 08/05

[ ] PICA | | | | | | PICA [ ]

1. MEDICARE (Medicare #)   MEDICAID (Medicaid #)   TRICARE CHAMPUS (Sponsor's SSN)   CHAMPVA (Member ID#)   GROUP HEALTH PLAN (SSN or ID)   FECA BLK LUNG (SSN)   OTHER (ID) | 1a. INSURED'S I.D. NUMBER (For Program in Item 1)

2. PATIENT'S NAME (Last Name, First Name, Middle Initial) | 3. PATIENT'S BIRTH DATE MM DD YY   SEX M [ ] F [ ] | 4. INSURED'S NAME (Last Name, First Name, Middle Initial)

5. PATIENT'S ADDRESS (No., Street) | 6. PATIENT RELATIONSHIP TO INSURED Self [ ] Spouse [ ] Child [ ] Other [ ] | 7. INSURED'S ADDRESS (No., Street)

CITY | STATE | 8. PATIENT STATUS Single [ ] Married [ ] Other [ ] | CITY | STATE

ZIP CODE | TELEPHONE (Include Area Code) ( ) | Employed [ ] Full-Time Student [ ] Part-Time Student [ ] | ZIP CODE | TELEPHONE (Include Area Code) ( )

9. OTHER INSURED'S NAME (Last Name, First Name, Middle Initial) | 10. IS PATIENT'S CONDITION RELATED TO: | 11. INSURED'S POLICY GROUP OR FECA NUMBER

a. OTHER INSURED'S POLICY OR GROUP NUMBER | a. EMPLOYMENT? (Current or Previous) YES [ ] NO [ ] | a. INSURED'S DATE OF BIRTH MM DD YY   SEX M [ ] F [ ]

b. OTHER INSURED'S DATE OF BIRTH MM DD YY   SEX M [ ] F [ ] | b. AUTO ACCIDENT? YES [ ] NO [ ]   PLACE (State) | b. EMPLOYER'S NAME OR SCHOOL NAME

c. EMPLOYER'S NAME OR SCHOOL NAME | c. OTHER ACCIDENT? YES [ ] NO [ ] | c. INSURANCE PLAN NAME OR PROGRAM NAME

d. INSURANCE PLAN NAME OR PROGRAM NAME | 10d. RESERVED FOR LOCAL USE | d. IS THERE ANOTHER HEALTH BENEFIT PLAN? YES [ ] NO [ ] If yes, return to and complete item 9 a-d.

READ BACK OF FORM BEFORE COMPLETING & SIGNING THIS FORM.
12. PATIENT'S OR AUTHORIZED PERSON'S SIGNATURE I authorize the release of any medical or other information necessary to process this claim. I also request payment of government benefits either to myself or to the party who accepts assignment below.

SIGNED _____ DATE _____ | 13. INSURED'S OR AUTHORIZED PERSON'S SIGNATURE I authorize payment of medical benefits to the undersigned physician or supplier for services described below.

SIGNED _____

14. DATE OF CURRENT: MM DD YY   ILLNESS (First symptom) OR INJURY (Accident) OR PREGNANCY(LMP) | 15. IF PATIENT HAS HAD SAME OR SIMILAR ILLNESS. GIVE FIRST DATE MM DD YY | 16. DATES PATIENT UNABLE TO WORK IN CURRENT OCCUPATION MM DD YY   MM DD YY FROM   TO

17. NAME OF REFERRING PROVIDER OR OTHER SOURCE | 17a. | 17b. NPI | 18. HOSPITALIZATION DATES RELATED TO CURRENT SERVICES MM DD YY   MM DD YY FROM   TO

19. RESERVED FOR LOCAL USE | 20. OUTSIDE LAB? YES [ ] NO [ ] $ CHARGES

21. DIAGNOSIS OR NATURE OF ILLNESS OR INJURY (Relate Items 1, 2, 3 or 4 to Item 24E by Line)
1. ____.____   3. ____.____
2. ____.____   4. ____.____
| 22. MEDICAID RESUBMISSION CODE   ORIGINAL REF. NO.
23. PRIOR AUTHORIZATION NUMBER

24. A. DATE(S) OF SERVICE From MM DD YY To MM DD YY	B. PLACE OF SERVICE	C. EMG	D. PROCEDURES, SERVICES, OR SUPPLIES (Explain Unusual Circumstances) CPT/HCPCS MODIFIER	E. DIAGNOSIS POINTER	F. $ CHARGES	G. DAYS OR UNITS	H. EPSDT Family Plan	I. ID. QUAL.	J. RENDERING PROVIDER ID. #
1								NPI	
2								NPI	
3								NPI	
4								NPI	
5								NPI	
6								NPI	

25. FEDERAL TAX I.D. NUMBER   SSN [ ] EIN [ ] | 26. PATIENT'S ACCOUNT NO. | 27. ACCEPT ASSIGNMENT? (For govt. claims, see back) YES [ ] NO [ ] | 28. TOTAL CHARGE $ | 29. AMOUNT PAID $ | 30. BALANCE DUE $

31. SIGNATURE OF PHYSICIAN OR SUPPLIER INCLUDING DEGREES OR CREDENTIALS (I certify that the statements on the reverse apply to this bill and are made a part thereof.)

SIGNED _____ DATE _____ | 32. SERVICE FACILITY LOCATION INFORMATION
a. NPI   b. | 33. BILLING PROVIDER INFO & PH # ( )
a. NPI   b.

NUCC Instruction Manual available at: www.nucc.org | APPROVED OMB-0938-0999 FORM CMS-1500 (08-05)

(Right margin labels:) CARRIER → | PATIENT AND INSURED INFORMATION → | PHYSICIAN OR SUPPLIER INFORMATION →

FIGURE 1.2 ■ Health Insurance Claim Form CMS-1500 is the standard billing form used by physicians. (Reprinted courtesy of U.S. Department of Health and Human Services, Centers for Medicare and Medicaid Services.)

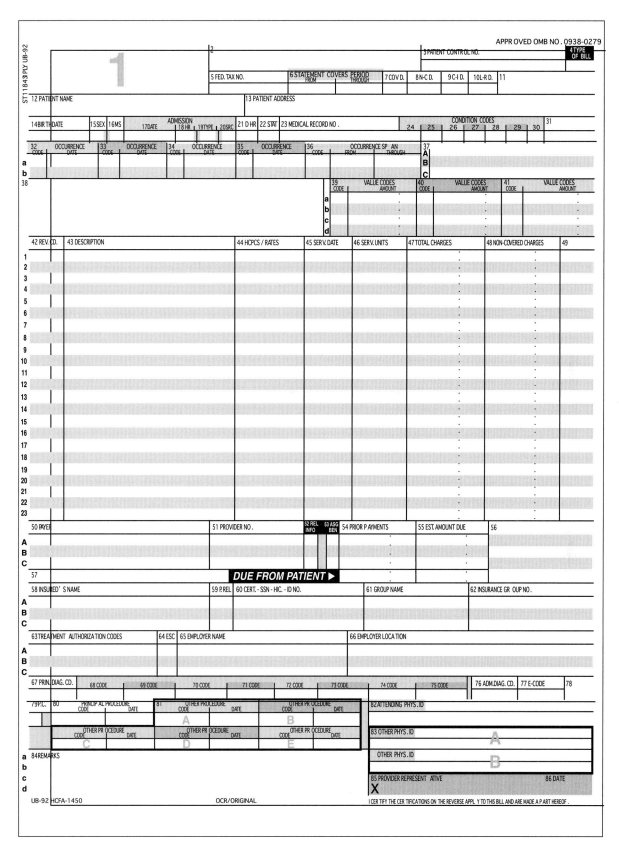

FIGURE 1.3 ■ Uniform Bill 92 (UB-92, or HCFA-1450) was formerly the standard billing form used by hospitals. This form was replaced by the newer UB-04 (Reprinted courtesy of U.S. Department of Health and Human Services, Centers for Medicare and Medicaid Services.)

SUMMARY

Medical records contain valuable information about a patient's medical history. Classification systems such as the ICD-9-CM, translate verbal descriptions from these medical records into numbers—codes that tell an important story. Codes are a standard form of medical communication that allow us to identify diseases and procedures, as well as study health-care trends, facilitate payment, substantiate the medical necessity of care rendered, and help validate that the provider's charges are reasonable.

The ICD-9-CM classification system is used throughout the United States in inpatient and outpatient facilities for medical coding. The three volumes—*Tabular List of Diseases* (volume 1), the *Alphabetic Index to Diseases* (volume 2), and the *Alphabetic Index to Procedures* and *Tabular List of Procedures* (volume 3)—provide the information you need to properly code from medical records. The various conventions and guidelines that apply to the ICD-9-CM classification system are discussed in the following chapter.

REFERENCES

1. Huffman EK. Health Information Management. Cofer J, ed. Berwyn, IL: Physicians' Record Co., 1994:27–28, 322.
2. Bowman E. Coding, classification, and reimbursement systems. In: Abdelhak M, Grostick S, Hanken MA, et al., eds. Health Information Management: Management of a Strategic Resource. Philadelphia: WB Saunders, 1996:231.
3. Ingenix 2007 Prospective Payment System Alert. July 2006 Update.
4. National Center for Health Statistics. About the International Classification of Diseases, Tenth Revision, Clinical Modification (ICD-10-CM). Available at: http://www.cdc.gov/ nchs/about/otheract/icd9/abticd10. htm. Accessed May 9, 2002.

TESTING YOUR COMPREHENSION

1. What standard coding sets are used to provide data in order to understand, standardize, and improve health care, improve medical outcomes, and improve patient services at a reduced cost to the consumer?

_____

2. What does ICD-9-CM mean?

_____

3. Why was ICD-9-CM developed specifically for use in the United States?

_____

4. What was the first prospective payment system developed under the Medicare program?

_____

5. Under the MS-DRG system, several factors influence the amount paid. Name them.

_____

6. What is the established formula for calculating a MS-DRG?

_____

7. Identify Huffman's three basic rules of an effective coding classification system.

_____

8. What is an example of a universal rule of coding that is presented in Chapter 1?

_____

9. What could be indented under the main term referred to in a code?

_____

10. What is the purpose of a nonessential modifier?

_____

11. What is the list that contains 17 chapters relating to various body systems?

_____

12. V codes in the *Tabular List of Diseases* indicate what two things?

_____

13. E codes are used to indicate what three things?

_____

14. What three tables are available in the *Alphabetic Index to Diseases* (volume 2) that provide coders with easy access to related conditions associated with three main diseases?

_____

15. What classification system did the World Health Organization originally publish in 1992?

_____

16. What is the standard billing form used by hospitals?

_____

17. What is the standard billing form used by physicians?

_____

18. What code set(s) is/are used for reporting hospital inpatient services?

_____

19. What code set(s) is/are used for reporting hospital outpatient services?

_____

20. What code set(s) is/are used by physicians for reporting their services?

_____

21. Is ICD-10 used in the United States at all?

_____

CHAPTER 2

Coding Conventions, Rules, and Guidelines

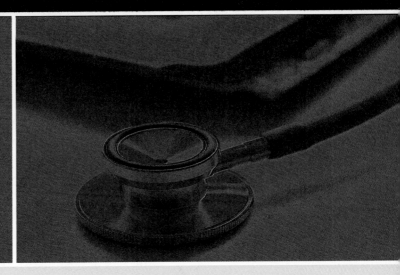

Chapter Outline

Coding Conventions
Uniform Hospital Discharge Data Set
General Coding Guidelines
V and E Codes (Supplementary Classifications)
Testing Your Comprehension
Coding Practice I: Chapter Review Exercises

Chapter Objectives

▶ Identify common conventions used in the three volumes of the ICD-9-CM.
▶ Explain the Uniform Hospital Discharge Data Set (UHDDS) rules and definitions that are most important to the coding process.
▶ Describe the basic steps to locating a diagnosis code through the *Alphabetic Index to Diseases* and the *Tabular List of Diseases*.
▶ List general diagnosis-coding guidelines.
▶ Identify three diagnosis-coding concepts that help a coder correctly convey the story of a patient's care.
▶ Describe the basic steps to locating a procedure code through the *Alphabetic Index to Procedures* and the *Tabular List of Procedures*.
▶ Apply general procedure-coding guidelines.
▶ Describe the purposes of V and E codes (supplementary classifications).

The accuracy of diagnosis and procedure codes reported for each patient is critically important. Inaccurate coding misrepresents the care of the patient, can impede studies to improve patient care, and can result in lost revenue for the health-care provider or in fraudulent overbilling. Health information management professionals must code diagnoses and procedures as documented by physicians within the patient's health record from medical reports, such as the patient's history and physical examination, operative report, progress notes, and discharge summary.

However, in real-world settings, physicians are often unfamiliar with coding conventions, guidelines, and definitions, including the coding rules presented in the Uniform Hospital Discharge Data Set (UHDDS). Therefore, it is important for coders to be up-to-date on all the information needed for accurate coding to ensure correct and ethical reporting of patients' medical information.

Accurate coding requires the correct sequencing of the patient's principal diagnosis and all secondary diagnoses that affect patient care, the correct sequencing of the principal procedure and any other significant procedures, and the correct use of ICD-9-CM coding rules and conventions. To this end, coders validate the sequencing and reporting of patient diagnoses and procedures documented by the physician by knowing and applying established coding rules.

Before advancing to the process of coding from patients' medical records (the source document), this chapter describes how to locate codes by using the ICD-9-CM codebook.

Coding Conventions

To use the ICD-9-CM classification system correctly, coders must learn ICD-9-CM conventions, including the abbreviations, symbols, notes, phrases, and punctuation used in the ICD-9-CM codebook. Understanding the conventions in the three volumes of the ICD-9-CM is important in facilitating precise coding. Conventions occur both in the alphabetic indexes to diseases and procedures and in the tabular lists for diseases and procedures.

ICD-9-CM Disease and Procedure Index Conventions

Following are conventions used in the ICD-9-CM *Alphabetic Index to Diseases* and *Alphabetic Index to Procedures*:

1. **Main terms** are in **bold print.** Listed in alphabetic order, main terms for locating diseases or procedures appear in bold print.
   *Locate the main term **Pneumonia** in the Alphabetic Index to Diseases*
   *Locate the main term **Bypass** in the Alphabetic Index to Procedures*
2. **Subterms** are also called **essential modifiers** and are indented under the main terms in the alphabetic indexes. They do affect code assignment.
   Locate the following in the Alphabetic Index to Diseases:
   Anemia
      blood loss (chronic) 280.0
        acute 285.1
   Locate the following in the Alphabetic Index to Procedures:
   Repair
      abdominal wall 54.72
3. **Nonessential modifiers** are contained within parentheses; they immediately follow main terms and sometimes follow subterms in the indexes to enclose supplementary words. Nonessential modifiers may be either present or absent in the statement of the diagnosis or procedure without affecting the code assignment.

Locate the following in the Alphabetic Index to Diseases:
Hernia, hernial *(acquired) (recurrent) 553.9*
   with gangrene (obstructed) NEC 551.9
Locate the following in the Alphabetic Index to Procedures:
Incision *(and drainage)*
   groin region (abdominal wall) (inguinal) 54.0

4. **General instructional notes** appear in all three ICD-9-CM volumes to provide instructions for correct code assignment. General notes within the indexes appear as italic print within boxes.

   Locate the following in the Alphabetic Index to Diseases:
   Fracture
   Note—For fracture of any of the following sites with fracture of other bones—see Fracture multiple.
   "Closed" includes the following descriptions of fractures, with or without delayed healing, unless they are specified as open or compound: comminuted, depressed, elevated, fissured, greenstick, impacted, linear, march, simple, slipped epiphysis, spiral, unspecified.
   "Open" includes the following descriptions of fractures, with or without delayed healing: compound, infected, missile, puncture, with foreign body.
   For late effect of fracture, see Late, effect, fracture, by site.
   Locate the following in the Alphabetic Index to Procedures:
   Examination *(for)*
   Note—Use the following fourth-digit subclassification with categories 90–91 to identify type of examination:
      1 bacterial smear
      2 culture
      3 culture and sensitivity
      4 parasitology
      5 toxicology
      6 cell block and Papanicolaou smear
      9 other microscopic examination

5. **NEC** means "not elsewhere classified." NEC indicates that the physician's documentation was specific; however, a more precise classification code was not available. NEC codes usually have a fourth or fifth digit of 8. NEC codes should be used only if a more specific code is not available.

   Locate the following in the Alphabetic Index to Diseases:
   Dysrhythmia
      specified type NEC 427.89

6. **Cross-references: see** and **see also. See** is a command that directs the coder to look elsewhere. The coder must refer to an alternative main term. **See also** directs the coder to look under another main term if all the information sought cannot be located under the first main term accessed.

   Locate the following in the Alphabetic Index to Diseases:
   Nerve—*see condition*
   Depressive reaction—*see also Reaction, depression*
   Locate the following in the Alphabetic Index to Procedures:
   Herniorrhaphy—*see Repair, hernia*
   Resection—*see also Excision, by site*

7. **Relational terms** (connecting words)—such as **with, due to, as,** and **by**—are connecting words listed under the main term in the indexes. They are used to lead you to the correct code assignment. **Due to**

expresses a causal relationship between conditions (i.e., a particular condition is caused by another underlying condition).

Locate the following in the Alphabetic Index to Diseases:

Bronchitis *(diffuse) (hypostatic) (infectious) (inflammatory) (simple) 490*
  with
    emphysema—see Emphysema
    influenza, flu, or grippe 487.1
    obstruction airway, chronic 491.20
      with acute exacerbation 491.21
Complications
  Infection and inflammation
    due to (presence of) any device, implant, or graft classified to 996.0–996.5 NEC
    996.60

Locate the following in the Alphabetic Index to Procedures:

Repair
  aneurysm (false) (true) 39.52
    by or with
      clipping 39.51

8. Slanted brackets (*[ ]*) are used to display the manifestation code when mandatory dual coding is required (i.e., two codes are required: the first code identifies the underlying condition, and the second code identifies the manifestation). Slanted brackets indicate that the codes must be sequenced exactly in that order. Italicized manifestation codes in slanted brackets in the index and tabular materials can never be sequenced as principal diagnoses. The underlying condition must be sequenced first unless directed otherwise by notes. Slanted brackets are also used in the procedure index to denote that mandatory dual coding is required to express the complete procedure.

    Locate the following in the Alphabetic Index to Diseases:

    Retinopathy *(background) 362.10*
      diabetic 250.5 [362.01]

    Locate the following in the Alphabetic Index to Procedures:

    Lithotripsy
      bladder
        with ultrasonic fragmentation 57.0 [59.95]

ICD-9-CM Disease and Procedure Tabular Conventions

Following are conventions used in the ICD-9-CM *Tabular List of Diseases* and *Tabular List of Procedures*:

1. **Category**, **subcategory**, and **subclassification** codes are listed in numerical order and **bold print**.

    Locate the following in the Tabular List of Diseases:

    426   Conduction disorders
      426.0   Atrioventricular block, complete
      426.1   Atrioventricular block, other and unspecified
        426.10   Atrioventricular block, unspecified

    Locate the following in the Tabular List of Procedures:

    79   Reduction of Fracture and Dislocation
      79.7   Closed Reduction of Dislocation
        79.75   Closed Reduction of Dislocation of Hip

2. **General instructional notes** appear in all three volumes to provide instructions in correct code assignment (i.e., general notes give more information about the code selected). Look at the beginning of a section or under category notes.

   Locate the following in the Tabular List of Diseases:

   715   Osteoarthrosis and allied disorders
   NOTE: Localized, in the subcategories below, includes
   bilateral involvement of the same site.

3. "Includes" notes explain the content of a particular classification code.

   Locate the following in the Tabular List of Diseases:

   401   Essential hypertension

Includes	*High blood pressure*

   Hyperpiesia
   Hyperpiesis
   Hypertension (arterial) (essential) (primary) (systemic)
   Hypertensive vascular:
    Degeneration
    Disease

4. "Excludes" notes are the opposite of "includes" notes. "Excludes" notes literally mean to look elsewhere for the code. The "excludes" term is italicized and enclosed in a box.

   Locate the following in the Tabular List of Diseases:

   401 Essential hypertension

Excludes	*Elevated blood pressure without*

    diagnosis of hypertension (796.2)
    pulmonary hypertension (416.0–416.9)
    that involving vessels of:
     brain (430–438)
     eye (362.11)

5. "Code first underlying condition" signifies that the code for the underlying condition must be sequenced first before the italicized manifestation of the disease code.

   Locate the following in the Tabular List of Diseases:

   443.81   Peripheral angiopathy in diseases classified elsewhere
    Code first underlying disease as:
     Diabetes mellitus (250.7)

6. "Use additional code" is required to convey the patient's condition completely.

   Locate the following in the Tabular List of Diseases:

   599.0   Urinary tract infection, site not specified
   Use additional code to identify organism, such as
   Escherichia coli [E. coli] (041.4)

7. **NOS** means "not otherwise specified" and is the equivalent of unspecified. Because the physician's documentation was nonspecific, a nonspecific code is assigned. NOS codes usually have a fourth or fifth digit of 9. NOS codes should be used only if a more specific code is not available.

   Locate the following in the Tabular List of Diseases:

   414.9   Chronic ischemic heart disease, unspecified
    Ischemic heart disease, not otherwise specified

8. Brackets enclose synonyms, abbreviations, alternative wording, or explanatory phrases.

Locate the following in the Tabular List of Diseases:

496 Chronic airway obstruction, not elsewhere classified
> *NOTE: This code is not to be used with any code from categories 491–493*
> *Chronic:*
>> *Nonspecific lung disease*
>> *Obstructive lung disease*
>> *Obstructive pulmonary disease [COPD], not otherwise specified*

9. Braces are used by some ICD-9-CM publishers. This use is similar to the colon in that braces connect a series of terms to a common stem or root term. This is a space-saving mechanism that makes the ICD-9-CM look less busy and easier to read.

   Locate the following in the Tabular List of Diseases:

   429.4 Functional disturbances following cardiac surgery

   Cardiac insufficiency } Following cardiac
   Heart failure   surgery or due to prosthesis

10. Colons signify an incomplete term or root term or stem that must have at least one modifier after the stem present to use the code.

    Locate the following in the Tabular List of Diseases:

    518.5 Pulmonary insufficiency following trauma and surgery
    > *Pulmonary insufficiency following:*
    >> *Shock*
    >> *Surgery*
    >> *Trauma*

11. The section mark (§) indicates an earlier instructional note or footnote at the bottom of the page informing the coder of the need to assign a fifth digit to complete the code assignment.

    Locate the following in the Tabular List of Diseases:

    §642 Hypertension complicating pregnancy, childbirth, and the puerperium

12. **And** means "and/or" when given within the title to a disease or procedure description.

    Locate the following in the Tabular List of Diseases:

    415.1 Pulmonary embolism and infarction

13. **Code also** is used to indicate that a second code is needed to complete the procedure.

    Locate the following in the Tabular List of Procedures:

    36.1 Bypass anastomosis for heart revascularization
    > *Code also cardiopulmonary bypass [extracorporeal circulation] [heart-lung machine] (39.61)*

14. **Omit code** is used to indicate that a procedure is a component part of another integral procedure code and should not be coded.

    Locate the following in the Tabular List of Procedures:

    54.11 Exploratory laparotomy

    | Excludes | *Exploration incidental to intra-abdominal surgery—omit code* |

15. The lozenge symbol (♦) indicates that the code is unique to ICD-9-CM and that it does not have a counterpart in the World Health Organization's ICD-9 classification.

    Locate the following in the Tabular List of Diseases:

    ♦ 369.4 Legal blindness, as defined in U.S.A.

Uniform Hospital Discharge Data Set

The UHDDS was developed by the Secretary of the U.S. Department of Health, Education, and Welfare in 1974 (now the Department of Health and Human Services) as a minimum common core of data on individual hospital discharges in the Medicare and Medicaid programs.[1] The UHDDS has gone through several revisions since then. The UHDDS represents a federally mandated minimum data set for health-care providers to report data on each Medicare and Medicaid inpatient discharge from an acute care hospital.

The overall purpose of UHDDS is to define a set of rules and definitions for data collection from hospitals to promote uniformity and comparability of data. This allows for evaluation and planning of health-care initiatives for the United States to improve the effectiveness of patient care and the cost of that care within the nation's health-care system. Most other health-care payers also require UHDDS inpatient reporting rules.

UHDDS Rules and Definitions

The following summarizes key UHDDS rules and definitions:

1. **Principal diagnosis:** "the condition, after study, chiefly responsible for occasioning the admission of a patient to the hospital for care." For example, a patient is admitted to the hospital with severe chest pain. "After study," the chest pain was found to be attributable to an acute myocardial infarction (i.e., heart attack). Code the acute myocardial infarction as the principal diagnosis.

TIP   Remember the general rule that people are admitted to acute care hospitals for acute(severe) conditions, and this should guide your selection of a principal diagnosis.

2. **Other reportable diagnoses:** all conditions that coexist at the time of admission, that develop subsequently, or that affect the treatment received or the length of stay. Diagnoses that relate to an earlier episode of care that have no bearing on the current hospital stay are excluded. UHDDS secondary diagnoses, or "other diagnoses associated with the current hospital stay," refer to **comorbidities** (e.g., preexisting conditions that affect patient care, such as chronic systolic heart failure) and **complications** (e.g., conditions that occur after admission, such as postoperative hemorrhage, and that affect patient care) or **other conditions** that affect the patient's treatment or extend the length of stay (e.g., preexisting hypertension that must be monitored; blindness; or status post hip replacement requiring assistance with ambulation).

3. **Significant procedures** that must be reported under UHDDS are:

   ▶ surgical in nature
   ▶ carry a procedural or anesthetic risk
   ▶ require specialized training (personnel)

Examples of significant procedures include coronary artery bypass grafts, insertion of cardiac pacemakers, organ resections, heart catheterizations, upper gastrointestinal endoscopies, colonoscopies, and percutaneous endoscopic gastrostomies.

4. **Principal procedure:** a procedure performed for definitive treatment rather than one performed for diagnostic or exploratory purposes, or one that was necessary to resolve a complication. Definitive treatments (e.g., operations) should be sequenced before diagnostic studies or procedures. If there seem to be two principal procedures, the one most related to the principal diagnosis should be selected as the principal procedure. For example, during an operation, a patient had a breast biopsy (diagnostic) followed by a modified radical mastectomy (definitive treatment) for breast cancer. Sequence the modified radical mastectomy procedure first, followed by the breast biopsy, because the mastectomy represents definitive treatment for the breast cancer.

5. The UHDDS minimum data set contained in the Uniform Bill-04 (UB-04) is submitted by hospitals to bill for patient services to the Medicare fiscal intermediary or other third-party payer. The UB-04 can hold up to eighteen diagnoses and six procedure codes. Today, most submissions of the UHDDS minimum data set are performed electronically via electronic data interchange, which is a requirement under the Title II: Administrative Simplification provision of the 1996 federal Health Insurance Portability and Accountability Act (HIPAA) legislation. HIPAA was intended to reduce health-care administrative costs by standardizing electronic data interchange for medical claims submission. Final HIPAA regulations include standards for electronic transactions and coding sets. The original deadline for compliance of covered entities with the electronic standards provisions was October 16, 2002; this was extended to October 16, 2003. Covered entities include providers, health plans, and clearinghouses. The UB-04 is also known as the CMS-1450 form.

General Coding Guidelines

To accurately represent the "story" of the patient in code, a coder should carefully, systematically, and thoroughly review a patient's medical record for significant diagnoses and procedures that may have affected the patient's care. In addition to coding conventions and the definitions and rules presented in the UHDDS, coding guidelines describe the steps necessary to ensure accurate coding of patients' diagnoses and procedures from the medical record and clarify how to apply coding to problematic situations.

Diagnosis Coding

Basic steps to follow in locating the proper diagnosis code within the ICD-9-CM codebook include the following:

1. From the source document (i.e., medical record), look up the main term for the name of the disease or condition in the *Alphabetic Index to Diseases* (volume 2). Review all index notes. Search for alternate terms, if necessary.
2. Review all subterms (essential modifiers) under the main term.
3. Review all nonessential modifiers (within parentheses) after the main term.
4. Follow all cross-references (*see* or *see also*).

5. After you have located the diagnosis term and corresponding code in the index, locate the code numerically in the Disease Tabular and review the code for more information. Never code from the index. Review all instructional notes, "includes" notes, and "excludes" notes in the Disease Tabular. Assign the code to its highest level of specificity (remembering that three-digit category codes can be carried further to four-digit subcategory or five-digit subclassification codes).

TIP Beginning coders should assume that all diagnosis codes have five digits unless proven otherwise (i.e., valid diagnosis codes consist of three to five digits).

6. Select the diagnosis code.

Knowledge of three diagnosis-coding concepts can help a coder correctly convey the story of a patient's episode of care. The three concepts can be thought of as the "mechanics of coding," which includes knowing when to apply each of the three concepts as follows:

1. **Mandatory dual coding** or classification requires two codes to express the disease or condition. Sequencing is determined by ICD-9-CM convention (refer to the slanted brackets convention, described previously).

Diagnosis: Diabetic nephropathy

> *250.40* *Diabetes with renal manifestations (code first the underlying disease)*
> *[583.81]* *Nephropathy (code second the manifestation of the underlying disease)*

Diagnosis: Aspergillosis pneumonia

> *117.3* *Aspergillosis infection (code first the underlying disease)*
> *[484.6]* *Pneumonia in aspergillosis (code second the manifestation of the underlying disease)*

EXAMPLE

---

2. **Combination codes** are used in ICD-9-CM when a single code can express more than one interrelated disease process.

Klebsiella pneumonia *482.0*
Staphylococcal enteritis *008.41*

EXAMPLE

---

3. **"Use additional codes"** (as needed) is situations in which the conventions of mandatory dual coding or combination codes are not provided, yet more than one code is needed to express the patient's complete condition. Sequencing is determined by ICD-9-CM convention (refer to the "use additional code" convention, described previously) or based on the coder's best discretion.

Diagnosis: E. coli urinary tract infection

> *599.0* *Urinary tract infection (use additional code to identify organism)*
> *041.4* *with E. coli bacterial organism*

Diagnosis: Postoperative atelectasis

> *997.39* *Post-operative respiratory complication (use additional code to identify complication)*
> *518.0* *with pulmonary atelectasis (as specific complication)*

EXAMPLE

Do not code additional symptoms routinely associated with a disease. For example, gastroenteritis with abdominal pain would be coded only to gastroenteritis (code 558.9), because abdominal pain is routinely associated with gastroenteritis. However, code symptoms if they are not routinely associated with the disease. For example, in urinary tract infection (UTI) with hematuria, sequence the UTI first (code 599.0) followed by the hematuria code (code 599.70), because hematuria is not routinely associated with UTIs.

Other general ICD-9-CM diagnosis code guidelines include the following:

1. For inpatients, when final diagnoses are documented as "possible," "probable," "likely," "questionable," "?," "rule out," or "suspected" the condition should be coded as though the diagnosis were established. This rule does not apply for diagnosis coding for outpatient services, which are coded to the "highest level of certainty." Outpatient diagnosis coding often requires symptom coding because the stays are short and definitive test results are sometimes not available by patient discharge. Therefore, UHDDS rules, which are specific to inpatients only, do not apply to outpatients (i.e., the inpatient "after study" concept does not apply to outpatient services).

2. If the same condition is described as both acute (subacute) and chronic and separate subterms exist in the alphabetic diagnosis index at the same indentation level, code both and sequence the acute (subacute) code first.

EXAMPLE	*Diagnosis: Acute and chronic cystitis*
	595.0 *Acute cystitis*
	595.2 *Chronic cystitis*

3. When two or more interrelated conditions meet the definition of principal diagnosis, either condition may be sequenced first. However, if the focus of treatment is directed at one condition more than the other, that condition should be sequenced as the principal diagnosis.

4. When two or more contrasting diagnoses are documented as "either/or" or "versus," either diagnosis may be sequenced as the principal diagnosis.

5. When a symptom is followed by contrasting or comparative diagnoses (e.g., "either," "or," or "versus"), the symptom code is sequenced first as the principal diagnosis (e.g., for chest pain secondary to hiatal hernia versus costochondritis, code the chest pain symptom as the principal diagnosis, followed by the diagnosis codes for hiatal hernia and costochondritis).

6. Even though treatment may not have been performed because of unforeseen circumstances, sequence the principal diagnosis as the condition that, after study, occasioned the admission of the patient to the hospital for care.

7. If the reason for admission is a residual condition from a prior injury or disease, an adverse effect of correct medication, or a poisoning, the residual condition is sequenced first, followed by a late effect code for the cause of the residual condition, except in situations in which the disease index directs otherwise.

Procedure: Admit for excision of scar
> *709.2   Scar (as residual) tissue from old burn to arm*
> *906.7   "Late effect" of burn to arm*

Procedure Coding

Steps to follow in locating the proper procedure code within the ICD-9-CM codebook include the following:

1. From the source document (i.e., medical record), look up the main term for the name of the operation or procedure in the Alphabetic Index. Review all index notes. Search for alternate terms, if necessary.
2. Review all subterms (essential modifiers) under the main term.
3. Review all nonessential modifiers (within parentheses) after the main term.
4. Follow all cross-references (*see* or *see also*).
5. After you have located the operative or procedure term and the corresponding code in the index, locate the code numerically in the Procedure Tabular and review the code for more information. Never code from the index. Review all instructional notes, "includes" notes, and "excludes" notes in the Procedure Tabular. Assign the code to its highest level of specificity (remembering that two-digit category codes will be carried further to three-digit subcategory or four-digit subclassification codes).

TIP Remember, beginning coders should assume that all procedure codes have four digits unless proven otherwise (i.e., valid procedure codes consist of three to four digits).

6. Select the operative or procedure code.

Other general ICD-9-CM operation or procedure code guidelines include the following:

1. General terms: along with specific codes for surgical procedures (e.g., nephrectomy), many surgical codes can be located through more general terms, such as *removal, excision, incision, repair, implantation, or suture.*
2. Open versus closed biopsies: open biopsies of body tissues involve an incision, and closed biopsies (without incision) can be performed endoscopically, by needle (percutaneous aspiration), or by brush. An excisional biopsy is coded to "excision, lesion" if the entire lesion is removed.
3. Coding operative approaches: an operative approach (e.g., laparotomy or thoracotomy) is normally considered a routine part of the operation or procedure itself and, therefore, is not coded. For example, for laparotomy with appendectomy, one would code only the appendectomy because the laparotomy is an integral part of the appendectomy. However, if only a biopsy (diagnostic procedure) is performed, then the operative approach would be coded and sequenced first, with the code for the biopsy second.

EXAMPLE	*Procedure: Exploratory laparotomy with percutaneous needle liver biopsy*
	54.11 Exploratory laparotomy
	50.11 Closed (percutaneous needle) liver biopsy

4. Open versus laparoscopic procedures: because of advancing technology, many previously open procedures (i.e., those requiring large incisions) are now performed laparoscopically by advancing a scope through a small incision (e.g., laparoscopic cholecystectomy and laparoscopic appendectomy). Laparoscopic procedures are less invasive; this enables a quicker healing time and shorter hospital stay than with open procedures. Be sure to locate the appropriate subterm (essential modifier) for laparoscopic procedures. If what begins as a laparoscopic procedure is changed to an open procedure during the operation (e.g., because of a poor visual field or an anomalous finding), code to the open procedure and record **Laparoscopic surgical procedure converted to open procedure (code V64.41) as a secondary diagnosis code.**

5. Bilateral procedures: major procedures such as bilateral hip and knee replacement operations must be coded twice because there is no provision for a bilateral code within the code description.

6. Eponyms: operations and procedures can sometimes be named after the person who developed the procedure. Within the procedure index, look under the eponym name or under the main term **operation**, where many eponyms will be located (e.g., Billroth I and II, Bosworth arthroplasty, Burch procedure).

V and E Codes (Supplementary Classifications)

V codes can be used as a principal diagnosis (sequenced first) to explain the main reason for the contact with health service or can be sequenced as secondary diagnoses to describe conditions that did not bring the patient to the hospital but that represent other factors influencing health care.

V codes can explain the reason for a health-care encounter. For example, used as a principal diagnosis (sequenced first), code V58.11 signifies that a patient's main reason for the health-care encounter is to receive chemotherapy, code V58.0 signifies that a patient's main reason for the health-care encounter is to receive radiation therapy, and code V56.0 signifies that a patient's main reason for the health-care encounter is to receive hemodialysis.

V codes can also explain other factors that influence health care. For example, used as a secondary diagnosis, code V45.01 describes a patient's cardiac pacemaker status, and code V43.64 describes that a patient has had previous hip replacement surgery. Status post prosthetic heart valve replacement causing the patient to be on long-term anticoagulant therapy is coded to V43.3 and V58.61.

To locate V codes in the Disease Index, coders must look under general terms such as *admission for, encounter for, follow-up, attention to, history (of), status (post), examination, aftercare, problem, screening for, long-term use,* and *examination*. Recognition of these terms comes with increasing coder experience. A V-code tabular supplementary section is located at the end of the 17 system chapters in the *Tabular List of Diseases* (volume 1).

E codes are never sequenced first as principal diagnoses. They are solely used as secondary diagnoses to explain the external causes of injuries, poisonings, and adverse effects to drugs taken as prescribed. The E code can also describe where an accident occurred (i.e., E849.0 indicates an accident occurring at home).

E codes can report the external cause of a poisoning. Code E850.4 would signify an accidental poisoning with acetaminophen.

E codes can also report the adverse effect of a medication taken as prescribed. Code E947.8 would explain that an adverse effect such as an allergic rash was attributed to the use of a contrast dye used in a diagnostic x-ray procedure.

E codes can also report the external cause of an injury. Code E881.0 would explain that a patient's injury was attributable to a fall from a ladder, and E920.0 would explain that the patient was cut from a powered lawn mower accident.

To locate E codes, coders must:

1. Locate the Table of Drugs and Chemicals at the end of the *Alphabetic Index to Diseases* (volume 2). Rows identify the responsible drug or chemical, and columns provide E codes related to the causes of poisonings (i.e., accident, suicide attempt, assault, or undetermined) or adverse effects of medications taken as prescribed (i.e., therapeutic use).
2. Locate the External Cause of Injury Index located in the *Alphabetic Index to Diseases* (volume 2) directly after the Table of Drugs and Chemicals. The External Cause of Injury Index provides E codes that explain the external circumstances for an injury (e.g., automobile accident, falls, or struck by an object).
3. An E-code tabular supplementary section is located at the end of the 17 system chapters in the *Tabular List of Diseases* after the V-code section.

SUMMARY

This chapter has focused on the common conventions used in the three volumes of the ICD-9-CM codebook. The UHDDS rules and definitions that are most relevant and important to the coding process have been presented. The basic steps used to locate a diagnosis code in the ICD-9-CM have been reviewed. General diagnosis coding guidelines and a definition of three diagnosis coding concepts that assist a coder in correctly conveying the story of an episode of care have been presented. The basic steps in locating a procedure code and defining the procedures used also have been presented, as have the definitions of general procedure guidelines. Locating V and E codes and understanding the purposes of each also were covered in this chapter. Chapter 3 focuses on the medical record and proper documentation, which serves as the basis of all coding of clinical services.

REFERENCE

1. Department of Health, Education, and Welfare. The Uniform Hospital Discharge Data Set. 1974.

TESTING YOUR COMPREHENSION

1. Before you begin to code from a patient's medical record, what must you do?

_____

2. What does the acronym NEC mean?

_____

3. What are general instruction notes used for?

_____

4. Why are cross-references used?

_____

5. What purpose is served by slanted brackets?

_____

6. What does "code first underlying condition" mean?

_____

7. What purpose do brackets serve?

_____

8. How are braces used?

_____

9. What purpose does a colon serve?

_____

10. What is the purpose of the Uniform Hospital Discharge Data Set (UHDDS)?

_____

11. What is the principal procedure under UHDDS rules?

_____

12. What are the three diagnosis coding concepts that must be known by a coder to correctly convey the story of a patient's episode of care?

_____

13. What are the six general steps to follow in locating the proper procedure code in the ICD-9-CM codebook?

_____

14. What are the purposes of V codes?

_____

15. What are the purposes of E codes?

_____

CODING PRACTICE I | Chapter Review Exercises

Directions

By using your ICD-9-CM codebook, code the following diagnoses and procedures:

	DIAGNOSIS/PROCEDURES	CODE
1	Acute cystitis with *Escherichia coli* bacterial infection.	
2	*Staphylococcus aureus* pneumonia.	
3	Peripheral angiopathy caused by type 1 insulin-dependent diabetes mellitus.	
4	Incomplete left bundle branch heart block.	
5	Arteriosclerosis; left leg with ulceration.	
6	Friction burn, right arm, infected.	
7	Spontaneous fracture of femur secondary to aseptic necrosis.	
8	Coagulation disorder secondary to vitamin K deficiency.	
9	Hemorrhagic gastroenteritis.	
10	Acute lymphocytic leukemia, in relapse.	
11	Pernicious anemia.	
12	Acute subendocardial myocardial infarction, initial episode. Patient is on long-term anticoagulant therapy because of chronic atrial fibrillation.	
13	Diagnosis: Abdominal aortic aneurysm (AAA). Procedure: Resection of AAA with graft. Patient is status post cardiac pacemaker insertion.	
14	Acute drug-induced confusion.	

	DIAGNOSIS/PROCEDURES	CODE
15	Diagnosis: Unstable angina secondary to arteriosclerotic heart disease. Procedures: Right and left heart catheterization with coronary angiography and left ventriculogram.	
16	Acute duodenal ulcer with bleeding; blood-loss anemia.	
17	Left ventricular dysfunction with congestive heart failure.	
18	Guillain–Barré syndrome.	
19	Diagnosis: Acute cholecystitis with cholelithiasis. Procedures: Laparoscopic cholecystectomy with intraoperative cholangiogram.	
20	Diagnosis: Simple fracture of the distal radius. The patient was involved in a fight at a local tavern. Procedure: Closed reduction of radial fracture with application of cast.	
21	Diagnosis: Osteoarthritis, left hip. Procedure: Total hip replacement, left hip.	
22	Syncopal episode secondary to bradycardia versus orthostatic hypotension.	
23	Postoperative ileus.	
24	Deep venous thrombosis of leg.	
25	Upper respiratory infection, influenzal with hemoptysis.	
26	Admission for chemotherapy. The patient has primary breast cancer metastatic to the axillary lymph nodes. Procedure: Chemotherapy administration.	
27	Fractured femoral neck on the left attributable to a fall from a ladder while the patient was painting his house.	
28	Severe sprain injury, right ankle, from a twisting injury while the patient was playing racquetball.	
29	Admission for external beam radiation therapy for primary lung cancer, right upper lobe. Procedure: Administration of radiation therapy.	
30	Deep laceration to left forearm. The patient slipped with a knife while carving a Halloween pumpkin. Procedure: Suture repair of laceration to left forearm.	

CHAPTER 3

Medical Records: The Basis for All Coding

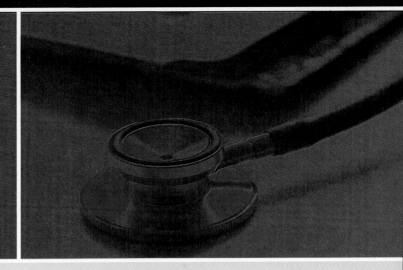

Chapter Outline

Format of Medical Records

Content of Medical Records

Incomplete Medical Records

Ten Steps for Coding From Medical Records

Testing Your Comprehension

Coding Practice I: Chapter Review Exercises

Coding Practice II: Medical Record Case Study

Chapter Objectives

▶ Identify common formats of the medical record.

▶ Describe the basic steps taken to review a medical record for coding.

▶ Identify administrative and clinical data contained in medical records that are important to the coding process.

▶ Explain problems associated with coding from incomplete medical records.

▶ Identify various medical reports important to the coding process.

▶ Demonstrate coding from medical reports by using the 10-step method.

▶ Demonstrate the use of a Coder/Abstract Summary Form and a Physician/Coder Query/Clarification Form.

The coding process begins with a careful and strategic review of the medical record (MR). Whether it describes inpatient or outpatient services, the MR tells a story of each patient's care and provides the best evidence of what physicians, hospitals, and the health-care team are doing.

This chapter explains and illustrates the typical structure and main content of a conventional MR, including various medical reports, and its importance to coders. It then presents a traditional step-by-step approach to reviewing and interpreting the MR for accurate coding. This approach serves as the basic framework on which you can build as you become more adept at coding.

Medical reports contain consistent content, much of which is dictated by laws and accrediting standards. However, from facility to facility, there is no requirement for reports to be formatted (organized or arranged) in the same manner. Over time, information requirements have been standardized through accrediting agencies such as the Joint Commission, Medicare's Conditions of Participation, and state licensure laws. Health-care providers also want to collect and share data to improve their patient services by determining how some institutions can do certain things better than others (i.e., benchmarking to improve performance). This book uses real-world examples of medical reports, so you will see different formats from various health-care facilities presented in this chapter's coding exercises and in those throughout the book.

Format of Medical Records

The formatting of an MR, whether paper based or electronic, can change from one institution to another, but the contents or data remain consistent. Similar information is usually found, although it can be found in different places within MRs from different institutions. To ensure correct coding, you should be searching for data first. Knowledge of MR formatting, although helpful, is of secondary concern.

Different MR formats that you may be exposed to include:

▶ Problem-oriented MR—contains four main parts: database, problem list, initial plans, and progress notes. This format allows a physician to focus on the whole patient in the context of addressing all problems. Writing progress notes in the problem-oriented MR is referred to as **SOAPing**, which follows all problems through a structured approach of **S**ubjective **O**bjective (data), **A**ssessment (of diagnoses), and **P**lan (for care).

▶ Source-oriented MR—forms are organized by departments or units (i.e., all laboratory, x-ray, nurses' notes, and physician's progress notes are separated), which allows for quick comparison of data over time (e.g., results of lab work, x-rays, or tests).

▶ Integrated MR—integrates various forms and caregiver notes, arranging them in strict chronological order to allow for a quick assessment of the patient at any particular moment in time.

Don't worry: you do not have to become an expert at MR formatting to become a good coder. You do need an awareness of the data you are looking for. The arrangement of data within or between pages is not as important as the information itself. Although familiarity with MR formats might help you find data more quickly, by trial and error alone, you will soon find the data and be able to code. You must become familiar with the data contained within MRs to code accurately.

Content of Medical Records

MRs contain administrative and clinical data that assist in the process of coding. Administrative data include routine patient identification such as the patient's name, age, sex, date of birth, address, religious preference, insurance data, and consent for treatment. Clinical data include diagnoses, procedures, and results of tests such as laboratory work, x-ray studies, and operations.

Although most registration data (administrative) collected at the time of patient admission contribute to accurate coding, the key information for coding is clinical (e.g., diagnosis of hepatitis or alcohol abuse and procedures such as cardiac pacemaker insertions or bowel resections).

Incomplete Medical Records

In the real world, you often must code from incomplete records to process records quickly for reimbursement. Discharge summaries (DS) and other important forms and information are often not yet available at the time of coding. Missing information can result in inaccurate coding that can cause the institution to lose money and create compliance issues (e.g., fraud and abuse), and the resulting bad data can spill over into inadequate quality-of-care reviews to evaluate patient care concerns. According to the Joint Commission, patients' histories and physicals (H&Ps) must be completed within 24 hours, and operative reports must be completed immediately. However, the overall record must be completed within 30 days, and often DS fall within this time period. Coding from incomplete records will not result in 100% coding accuracy. In the face of incomplete records, you may need to query the physician for more information or wait until an important report is available.

Just as you need to get a paycheck to pay your bills, a hospital must receive remittance (payments for services) to pay its bills. Under today's prospective payment systems, an MR must be coded before billing and remittance. It is important that health-care professionals remain aware of the effect of incomplete and untimely physician documentation and its effect on the institution's financial bottom line, performance-improvement activities (e.g., internal reviews of surgical and mortality cases), and compliance with its governing laws. Because documentation is the basis of all coding, monitoring and actions to improve the timeliness and quality of MR documentation must constantly be stressed to all who are involved in the coding and billing process.

Ten Steps for Coding from Medical Records

Before beginning the process of coding, make sure sufficient basic materials are in place, including up-to-date ICD-9-CM codebooks, a medical dictionary, and reference books for drugs, human anatomy, and the American Hospital Association's *Coding Clinic*. Have a scratch pad available to take notes as you go. Make sure you have a quiet place to code and plenty of desk space. Be aware that software products such as encoders are available to help you code and are used by many hospitals. However, before you use software, the basics are best learned starting with the ICD-9-CM codebook. The Office of Inspector General's Model Hospital Compliance Plan also prescribes not to rely

100% on computerized encoders and indicates that staff must have access to coding books.[1]

Most hospitals use hundreds of different medical report forms. This chapter does not illustrate every possible report found within a medical record, but it does introduce those most important for beginning the process of coding. The 10 steps below will give you a framework for coding from MRs.

Step 1: Review Face Sheet or Registration Record

The Face Sheet or Registration Record (Medical Report 3.1) is the front page of the MR. It contains basic patient identification data, insurance information, and sometimes clinical data such as the admitting and final diagnoses.

What to look for:

- ▶ the size of the record and the patient's length of stay, sex, age, and admitting diagnosis—all of which will give you insight into the complexity of the diagnosis
- ▶ prospective payment system payers (e.g., Medicare), which may raise compliance and reimbursement issues

Step 2: Review History and Physical, Emergency Department Report, and/or Consultant's Report

The H&P Report (see Medical Report 3.2) is usually dictated by the attending physician and then transcribed (typed) by medical transcriptionists. The history is an important form that uncovers the chief complaint (CC) of the patient, history of the present illness (HPI), review of systems (ROS), and personal, family, and social history (PFSH). This contains subjective data collected from the patient to begin the process of diagnosis by the physician. The physical examination (PE) includes a system-by-system physical examination by the provider to collect objective data on the patient's condition.

Review the H&P to determine the chief reason(s) for admission and to begin to get a feel for the possible options for the principal diagnosis (i.e., "the condition, after study, chiefly responsible for occasioning the admission of the patient to the hospital for care") and secondary diagnoses. Review the history for secondary diagnoses such as comorbidities and other diagnoses affecting patient care that need to be reported per Uniform Hospital Discharge Data Set (UHDDS) rules. Review the physical examination for abnormal findings. Altogether, the H&P enables the physician to collect both subjective and objective data on the patient to establish a provisional diagnosis and begin a plan of care for the patient.

Determine the provisional or tentative diagnoses given by the physician and plan for care. The Emergency Room or Emergency Department Report provides initial diagnosis and treatment information by the emergency room physician. If a patient is admitted through the emergency room, review the presentation of the patient and the initial treatment or orders given. Emergency room diagnoses should be considered in the context of admitting impressions and assessments.

A Consultant's Report (Medical Report 3.3) contains an expert opinion requested by the attending physician to aid in the diagnosis and treatment of the patient. Ask what the chief reason was for the consultation request by the attending physician, and note all diagnoses given by the consulting physician.

Consultation reports are usually dictated by the consultant and transcribed (typed) but can be handwritten as well.

It is helpful to think of these reports as a connected set; that is, each report that comes from a different physician serves a similar function, which is to assess the patient and begin a plan of care. Often, coders forget to review an emergency room record that may in fact have more detail than the attending physician's H&P.

Step 3: Review Operative Reports, Special Procedure Reports, and/or Pathology Reports

The Operative Report is usually dictated by the surgeon or physician and then transcribed (typed). If applicable, go to the operative report to note operations/ procedures and the preoperative and postoperative diagnoses (Medical Report 3.4). Depending on whether it is a major operation or a minor procedure, it is best to recognize that MR forms related to operations or special procedures usually exist as a set of linked forms. This operative set includes the operative report itself, the anesthesia record, special consents for surgery, the recovery room record, and pathology reports for specimen analysis.

Note the results of special procedures such as cardiac catheterizations, colonoscopies (lower endoscopies), esophagogastroduodenoscopies (upper endoscopies), and bronchoscopies, with or without biopsies.

Remember to sequence "definitive before diagnostic" procedure codes per UHDDS rules.

Note pathologic diagnoses given for any specimens removed at operation that are usually dictated by the pathologist and then transcribed (typed).

Step 4: Review Physician's Progress Notes

Physician's progress notes (Medical Report 3.5) need to be taken as often as the patient's condition warrants. Progress notes include an admit note, notes that relate to the patient's condition and progress, complications, response to treatment, and a discharge note. Review physician's progress notes for significant diagnoses, findings, and resolution of problems or complications.

Step 5: Review Laboratory, Radiology, and/or Special Test Reports

Laboratory work (Medical Report 3.6) includes several types of chemistry tests, analyses, cultures, and other examinations of body fluids or substances such as blood, urine, stool, and pus. Review laboratory, x-ray, and special tests to note any abnormal results and clarify treatments given through physician documentation. Query the physician for added documentation if this is necessary to clarify the precise code selection.

Radiology Reports (Medical Report 3.7) include x-ray studies, computed tomographic scans, nuclear medicine studies, magnetic resonance imaging, arteriograms, and so on. Review radiologic reports to note any abnormal findings and clarify through additional physician documentation within the MR (e.g., physician's progress notes or DS).

Special Test Reports (Medical Report 3.8) include electrocardiograms, echocardiograms, cardiac stress tests, and so on. Review special tests to note any abnormal findings and clarify through additional physician documentation.

Do not code from laboratory work, radiology, or special tests without additional supporting documentation from the attending physician.

Step 6: Review Physician's Orders

Physician's orders (Medical Report 3.9) are written or oral orders to nursing or ancillary personnel that direct all treatments and medications to be given to the patient. Review the doctor's orders to determine the treatments given. Sometimes doctors prescribe treatments without documenting the corresponding diagnoses or conditions (as the reasons for treatment). Therefore, you may need to query the physician to clarify a diagnosis for coding and ask the physician to add supporting documentation to the patient's MR through an addendum. Diagnosis codes establish the medical necessity for services—an important compliance issue.

Step 7: Review Medication Administration Record (MAR)

The Medication Administration Record (Medical Report 3.10) provides documentation of the drugs given to the patient, including the names of drugs, dosages, times given, and routes of administration, such as by mouth, by intramuscular injection, or intravenously. The nurse or physician administering the drug signs off on all entries. If necessary for clarity, review the MARs to determine medications given to help clarify or justify the diagnoses given by the physician.

Step 8: Review Discharge Summary or Clinical Résumé

The DS (Medical Report 3.11) is usually dictated by the attending physician and then transcribed (typed). It is a summary of the patient's course in the hospital, the patient's condition on discharge, the discharge instructions, and the plan for follow-up care. It includes all final diagnoses, as well as any significant principal procedures and/or any other procedures.

Review the DS for completeness and proper sequencing according to UHDDS reporting rules. Physicians are often unfamiliar with ICD-9-CM coding conventions and rules, so it is the coder's responsibility to ensure that the correct code assignment and sequencing are reported.

Step 9: Assign Codes

The Coder/Abstract Summary Form (Figure 3.1) is a form typically used by coders to summarize their MR review and assign and sequence the patient's codes. Assign codes by following UHDDS and coding rules and conventions in accordance with the steps in Chapter 2.

Step 10: Submit Physician/Coder Query/Clarification Form

The Physician/Coder Query/Clarification Form (Figure 3.2) is typically used as a good-faith communication tool between coders and physicians to clarify proper code assignment for a patient care episode. It is important to note that the Centers for Medicare and Medicaid Services has expressed concern that questions from coders can at times inappropriately lead physicians to add diagnoses that lead to a higher-weighted diagnosis-related group and payment. Nonetheless, Physician/Coder Query/Clarification Forms are still necessary and used, but coders must now express (within the form) the following points:

1. the coder is not seeking or expecting any particular response from the physician
2. the physician must add supporting documentation to the body of the medical record
3. the Physician/Coder Query/Clarification Form itself must be labeled as part of the permanent MR

TIP If in doubt, query the physician, remembering "if not documented, not done." Without sufficient documentation, you cannot code, because documentation is the basis of all coding. The same or similar type of query form may be used to clarify whether or not a condition was present on admission (POA) to comply with Medicare's new POA reporting requirements (Figure 3.3).

CODER/ABSTRACT SUMMARY FORM
XYZ COMMUNITY MEDICAL CENTER

Medical Record #   Acct. #:   Name:

Admission Date:	Encounter Type:
Discharge Date:	Origin:
Birthdate:	Primary Payor:
	Sex:
Admission Type:	LOS:
Admission Source:	Admission Service:
Discharge Disposition:	Discharge Service:

Admit Physician:
Discharge MD:
Consultant:

	CODE(S)	SHORT DESCRIPTION(S)
Admit Diag		
Princ Diag		
Other Diag		
Other Diag		
Other Diag		
Other Diag		
Other Diag		
Other Diag		
Other Diag		
Other Diag		

	CODE(S)	SHORT DESCRIPTION(S)
Prin Proc		
Other Proc		
Other Proc		
Other Proc		
Other Proc		
Other Proc		

I certify that the narrative description of the principal and secondary diagnoses and major procedures performed are accurate and complete to the best of my knowledge.

_____   _____
               SIGNATURE   DATE

FIGURE 3.1 ■ The Coder/Abstract Summary Form is typically used by coders to summarize their MR review and assign and sequence the patient's codes.

PHYSICIAN/CODER QUERY/CLARIFICATION FORM

Date: _____ / _____ / _____

Dear Dr.:

We need your help. Per the documentation in the medical record, the following has to be clarified in order to correctly code the patient's medical record. The fact that a question is asked does not imply that we expect or desire any particular answer. Please exercise your independent judgment when responding. We sincerely appreciate your clarification on this issue.

Coder's Name / Phone Extension #: _____

Patient Name: _____

Admit / Discharge Dates: _____ to _____

MR #: _____

The medical record reflects the following clinical findings per the following source forms:

_____

_____

_____

Please respond to the following question:

_____

_____

_____

PHYSICIAN RESPONSE:

☐ YES — If yes, please document your response in the space below and be sure to include the clarification in your documentation within the body of the medical record (i.e., progress notes, dictated report or as an addendum to a dictated report)

_____

_____

_____

_____   _____
PHYSICIAN SIGNATURE   DATE

☐ NO — If no, please check the box, and sign and date below

☐ UNABLE TO DETERMINE — If so, please check the box, and sign and date below

_____   _____
PHYSICIAN SIGNATURE   DATE

This form is a part of the Permanent Medical Record

FIGURE 3.2 ■ The Physician/Coder Query/Clarification Form is typically used as a good-faith communication tool between coders and physicians to clarify proper code assignment for a patient care episode.

PHYSICIAN DOCUMENTATION QUERY
PRESENT ON ADMISSION (POA) DIAGNOSIS CLARIFICATION

Date: _____ / _____ / _____
Med. Rec. No.: _____
Patient Name: _____
Admit Date: _____ / _____ / _____

Dear Doctor: _____

We need your help. Per documentation in the medical record, the following has to be clarified in order to correctly code your patient's record. Documentation clarification is required to meet both federal and state POA Compliance.

It is unclear whether or not the following condition or diagnosis was present on admission.

_____ (Specific diagnosis/condition)

Please select one of the following:

_____ **Y** = Yes, the condition was present on inpatient admission

_____ **N** = No, the condition was not present on admission (developed after admission)

_____ **W** = Clinically undeterminable by provider (physician)

_____ **MD Signature**

_____ / _____ / _____ **Date**

If you have any questions, please do not hesitate to contact the HIM Department (Medical Records) for assistance at # 999-9999. Thank you!

This form is a part of the Permanent Medical Record

FIGURE 3.3 ■ The Physician Documentation Query Present on Admission (POA) Diagnosis Clarification Form may be used to clarify whether or not a condition was present on admission to comply with Medicare's new POA reporting requirements.

SUMMARY

In this chapter, the common formats of the MR were identified. The basic steps in reviewing an MR for the process of coding were reviewed. The administrative and clinical data contained in MRs have been identified, and the content has been defined. Various MR forms have been identified, and the coding process has been exemplified by using the 10-step method. The uses of the Coder/Abstract Summary Form and the Physician/Coder Query/Clarification Form have also been demonstrated.

Chapter 4 focuses on how to code for signs, symptoms, and ill-defined conditions.

REFERENCE

1. Russo R, Russo JJ. Healthcare compliance plans: good business practice for the new millennium. J AHIMA 1998;69:24, 26–28, 30–31; quiz 33–34.

TESTING YOUR COMPREHENSION

1. What are the four parts of a problem-oriented medical record?

2. What is unique about the source-oriented medical record?

3. What is the unique element of the integrated medical record?

4. The Face Sheet (Registration Record) of the clinical record customarily contains what information?

5. What medical report is defined as an expert opinion requested by a physician to aid in the diagnosis and treatment of a patient?

6. Under what conditions should a coder decline to code from laboratory work, radiology, or other special tests?

7. What is used as a good-faith communication tool between the coder and the physician?

8. What are other indicators of the complexity of a diagnosis?

CODING PRACTICE I   Chapter Review Exercises

Directions

By using your ICD-9-CM codebook, code the following diagnoses and procedures:

	DIAGNOSIS/PROCEDURES	CODE
1	Cellulitis of the leg.	
2	Acute asthmatic bronchitis.	
3	Diagnosis: Open distal femur fracture. Procedure: Open reduction, internal fixation, femur fracture.	
4	Viral meningitis.	
5	Mitral valve insufficiency with aortic regurgitation.	
6	Rheumatoid arthritis.	
7	Endometriosis of the cervix.	
8	Primary thrombocytopenia.	
9	Diagnosis: Nontraumatic rotator cuff tear, right shoulder. Procedure: Rotator cuff repair.	
10	Diagnosis: Loose bodies in left knee. Procedure: Arthroscopy with removal of loose bodies, left knee.	
11	Hypoglycemic coma in patient with non-insulin-dependent diabetes mellitus.	
12	Dehydration with hyponatremia.	
13	Diagnosis: Open wound of hand. Procedure: Suture skin of hand.	
14	Alzheimer's dementia with behavioral disturbance.	
15	Decompensated congestive heart failure.	

Instructions

This is an exercise to give you practice in coding from a real-life medical record.

1. Refer to the 10 steps for coding from medical records in this chapter.

2. Follow each step and review each medical report; these are all part of this patient's medical record.

3. At step 9, begin filling in the correct codes on the Coder/Abstract Summary Form (Figure 3.1).

4. If necessary, complete a Physician/Coder Query/Clarification Form (Figure 3.2) to clarify the physician's documentation and ensure more precise coding.

MEDICAL REPORT 3.1

REGISTRATION RECORD

Thursday April 6, 2000 9:23 AM

XYZ Community Medical Center

MRUN:	0002648-650
ACCT#:	4006755706
MR#:	1234567
CAMPUS:	XYZ – COMMUNITY MEDICAL CENTER
NAME:	John Doe
ADMIT DATE/TIME:	04/06 0321
DISCHARGE DATE/TIME:	04/12 1700
PT TYPE:	INPATIENT
VISIT TYPE:	INTERNAL MEDICINE

PATIENT INFORMATION:

Patient Address:	1234 PARK AVE	DOB:	06/20/1938
Patient Address:		Age:	65Y
City:	SOMEPLACE	Sex:	M
County:		M/S:	MARRIED
State/FC:	FL	Race:	CA
Zip:	99999	Religion:	PROTESTANT
Home Phone #:	999-999-9999	Patient SSN:	
Work Phone #:		Previous Room/Bed:	8302/01 NU: 3EA
Emp. Status:	RETIRED	Privacy Code:	
Occupation:	NONE	Valuables Secured:	N
Employer:	RETIRED	LMP:	
Employer Address:		Onset of Illness:	11/30
City:		Health Program:	MEDICARE
State:			
Zip:			

NEXT OF KIN:

NOK #1:	JANE DOE	NOK #2:	
Rel to Pt:	WIFE	Rel to Pt:	
Address:	1234 PARK AVE	Address:	
City:	SOMEPLACE	City:	
State:	FL	State:	
Zip:	99999	Zip:	
Home Phone #:	999-999-9999	Home Phone #:	
Work Phone #:		Work Phone #:	

Continued

MEDICAL REPORT 3.1 (CONTINUED)

PHYSICIAN/DIAGNOSIS INFORMATION:

Admitting Physician: 000405-SMITH, MARIE Other Physician: 005500-EMRG DEPT, M

Attending Physician: 000405-SMITH, MARIE

Admitting Diagnosis: UNSTABLE ANGINA/CATH POSS ANGIOPLAST, ARRHYTHMIA

ACCIDENT INFORMATION:

Accident Date: How Occurred:

Accident Time: Where Occurred:

Accident Type:

ADVANCE DIRECTIVES:

Adv. Directive: NO

Adv. Directive Type:

Follow-Up Required: NO

NOTES

MEDICAL REPORT 3.2

PATIENT NAME: John Doe
MEDICAL RECORD NUMBER: 1234567
ACCOUNT NUMBER: 4006755706
ADMISSION DATE: 04/07
ROOM: 3507

HISTORY AND PHYSICAL

CHIEF COMPLAINT AND HISTORY OF PRESENT ILLNESS: This 65-year-old male was referred here by Dr. J. Jones.

This patient was working doing auto refurbishing and his wife states that he does a lot of sanding and preparation for painting.

I saw this patient in my office on February 29. I have since reviewed the catheterizations done by Dr. Jones on January 27, at Memorial Hospital. This shows a totally occluded RCA with a tiny distal vessel filled by collaterals and in the posterior one-half of the inferior wall line, the distribution of the RCA is akinetic and the remainder moderately hypokinetic with an overall EF of 30%. The left main has mild disease, the LAD has diffuse 50 and 75% proximal and mid narrowing, with a rather diffuse distal LAD which is not a good target for CABG. The circumflex marginal has diffuse 75% narrowing and is not a good target, the groove circumflex had 50–75% diffuse narrowing.

The patient was admitted on this occasion with rapid atrial fibrillation, with heart rates of 160. He was transferred here for consideration for possible CABG or interventional angioplasty, but after reviewing the films I did not feel that he was a good candidate.

The catheterization was done from the right arm approach since he was total occlusion of the abdominal aorta below the renal arteries.

The patient has had diabetes for 20 years and he has been a chronic heavy cigarette abuser with underlying emphysema. He also has a marked hyperlipidemia.

Since admission, he has had intermittent atrial fibrillation in spite of IV Cardizem drip, and I have started him on a low dose of beta-blocker therapy. The patient has a past history of sinus bradycardia and since admission he has been in and out of atrial fibrillation versus sinus rhythm. When he is in sinus rhythm, he has occasional marked sinus bradycardia with heart rates as low as 30 per minute. He has also had severe long pauses.

PAST MEDICAL HISTORY: PAST SURGICAL HISTORY: None.

ALLERGIES: None.

MEDICATIONS: He has been on Zocor 20 mg q.d., nitroglycerin patch, Humulin N 16 units q.d.

SOCIAL HISTORY: Noncontributory.

Continued

MEDICAL REPORT 3.2 (CONTINUED)

FAMILY HISTORY: Both parents died in their 70s with cancer. He has a 61-year-old sister that is alive and well and he has a brother who died with cancer. He has been married for 42 years and he has a 31-year-old son and a daughter who is around 30 and they are both living and well.

REVIEW OF SYSTEMS: He has a history of a marked hyperlipidemia and blood work on January 26, showed cholesterol of 317, LDL 254, triglycerides 93 and HDL 45. He has early cataracts. He denies problems with his liver, lungs, kidney, bladder, prostate, bleeding, stomach problems, neurological problems, thyroid, cancer, glaucoma, arthritis or gout. He has claudication if he walks one or two blocks, but if he rests for a few moments, he can continue without difficulty.

The patient was very combative and confused early this morning and was treated with Haldol and Valium.

PHYSICAL EXAMINATION:

GENERAL APPEARANCE: The patient is a slender individual, who is currently a little confused, but much better then earlier this morning.

VITAL SIGNS: He weighs 145 pounds.

SKIN: His skin was normal.

NECK: He has loud bilateral carotid bruits. The carotid pulses were somewhat diminished bilaterally. The thyroid was not enlarged.

HEART: Sounds were irregular due to atrial fibrillation. He has no palpable femoral pulses.

ABDOMEN: Soft, without palpable masses.

PELVIC/RECTAL: Deferred.

IMPRESSION:
1. Severe widespread atherosclerotic disease—see above. I do not feel that he is a good candidate for CABG (coronary artery bypass grafting) or interventional therapy after I reviewed the films. I feel that if we did a Rotablator on the LAD (left anterior descending) he would have a lot of difficulties, and his CX (circumflex) vessels are not candidates for bypass or interventional therapy.
2. Sick sinus syndrome with intermittent atrial fibrillation alternating with sinus bradycardia, with heart rates as low as 30.
3. COPD/Emphysema, secondary to heavy cigarette abuse in the past.
4. Diabetes for 20 years.
5. Marked hyperlipidemia.

MEDICAL REPORT 3.2 (CONTINUED)

RECOMMENDATION: I feel that the best therapy will be to control his atrial fibrillation with Cardizem, digoxin and beta-blockers, and we will need to put in a permanent AV sequential pacemaker to try to suppress his atrial fibrillation and to keep him out of marked sinus bradycardia from the medications. Medical therapy is indicated for his coronary disease and I do not feel that he is a candidate for interventional therapy.

_____

Marie Smith, M.D.

130097/tjf 04/07/2000 17:10:33 04/07 19:29:45

CC:

J. Jones, M.D.

NOTES

MEDICAL REPORT 3.3

CONSULTATION FORM

Patient's Name: John Doe

ATTENDING PHYSICIAN Smith to CONSULTANT Jones

Reason for Consultation Request: Help with diabetic management of patient

Date: 04/08   Marie Smith, MD

_____

SIGNATURE OF ATTENDING PHYSICIAN

Findings and Recommendations of Consultant:

IMP:
1. OHD CAD w/ Anterolateral 1
   Atrial Fibrillation (Paroxysmal)
   Marked sinus bradyarrhythmia +SSS
2. PVD Occlusion distal aorta & 1/10 femoral s
   w/ collateral circulation
3. CVD with BL carotid & vertebral artery ds.
4. DM2   Diabetes 20 yrs
          Rx NPH 16u Q am
          Control: Moderate
          Cxs None known
5. HLP/Marked & Chol
6. Smokes 2 $\frac{1}{2}$ ppd x 40y (60pk yrs)
7. COPD / Emphysema
8. Cataracts BL

REC:

1. Nutritional ADA Rx	4. → GLUC precautions	will F/u with you in hospital
2. Insulin Rx	5. Hbg A1C	Thanks
3. Freq Accuchecks	6. TSH	

Date: 04/08   S. Jones, MD
                        _____
                        Signature of Consultant

MEDICAL REPORT 3.4

OPERATIVE REPORT

PATIENT NAME:	John Doe
MEDICAL RECORD NUMBER:	1234567
ACCOUNT NUMBER:	4006755706
ADMISSION DATE:	04/07
ROOM:	3507
CARDIOPULMONARY	
DATE:	04/10

PRE-OP DIAGNOSIS: Tachy-brady Syndrome; Atrial Fibrillation

POST-OP DIAGNOSIS: Same

OPERATION: Dual Chamber permanent pacemaker

CLINICAL HISTORY: This is a 65-year-old gentleman with a history of tachy-brady syndrome with paroxysmal atrial fibrillation and documented bradycardia.

PROCEDURE: After informed consent was obtained, the patient was brought to the electrophysiology laboratory in a fasting state. He was prepped and draped in the usual sterile fashion with multiple layers of Betadine. Lidocaine 1% infiltration was used to achieve local anesthesia. Using sharp and blunt dissection a generator pocket was created. Over 9 French introducers, Pacesetter atrial and ventricular leads were advanced to the appropriate sites in the right atrium and right ventricle. The atrial lead was model #9999P, serial #MJ9999 with PSA values of 0.7 volts at 0.5 msec at a current of 1.4 mA. An impedance of 500 ohms and a P-wave of 2.2mV. The ventricular lead was a Pacesetter #9999P, serial #MK9999 with PSA of 0.9 volts at 0.5 msec and a current of 1.7 mA and an impedance of 520 ohms and an R-wave of 14.2mV. Both leads were secured to the fascial layer with 2-0 silk and than attached to a Pacesetter Trilogy DR Plus, model #9999 which was also secured to the fascial layer with 0-silk after the pocket had been copiously irrigated with antibiotic solution. The lower layers were closed with 2-0 Vicryl and Durabond in several layers. He tolerated the procedure exceptionally well.

CONCLUSION: Successful dual chamber permanent pacemaker implant with fluoroscopy.

A. Michaels, M.D.

131381/tjf 04/10 09:31:52 04/10 09:35:40

cc:

J. Jones, M.D.

Chart Copy

MEDICAL REPORT 3.5

PATIENT:	Doe, John
MR:	1234567
AD:	04/07
ACCT#:	4006755706
PHY:	Smith, Marie MD

PROGRESS NOTES

DATE	TIME	
4/7	8:00/A	H & P dictated. See recent office note—Very confused & combative last & night—Cath cancelled —in and out of rapid afib–High risk for PTCA or CABG—will try to settle him down and TX w/ meds—Dig, IV Cardizem strict low dose Lopressor—former brady problem. Smith
4/7	5:00/P	Less confused/agitated now—Int. afib alt w/ sinus rhythm w/ HR down to 30 at times (marked sinus brady). Needs perm A-V Seq. Pacer. I reviewed the cath films by Dr. Jones at Memorial Hospital 1-27-00–100% RCA occlus w/ collat circ from the lft, LAD—Diffuse 50–75% prox & mid w/ distal not good target, 75% diffuse cx marg & mode diffuse cx groove, akinetic post ½ of inf wall w/ EF 30% overall. Rec/CABG & med therapy. Smith
4/7		

— Endo —

Pt seen in cardiac tele DM orders written   Jones

EP/Cardiology

4/8		Asked by Dr. Smith to see pt for pacemaker. Has severe CAD & PVD. Has had Tachy-Brady Syndrome. Had rapid afib as recently as yesterday & required IV Cardizem. BP 100/50 HR 60 on IV Cardizem @10. Chest clear. W/O SS

Imp: 1. Angina
2. Severe PVD
3. Severe CAD
4. Tachy-brady Syndrome

Plan: 1. Δ to oral Cardizem
2. con't telemetry
3. Pacer Monday
4. d/c Zestril
5. add topical nitrates   Michaels

MEDICAL REPORT 3.6

J. Johnson, M.D.
Medical Director, Clinical Laboratory

PRINTED DATE: 04/07
TIME: 0012
PAGE: 2
PATIENT: Doe, John
MED REC NO: 1234567
ACCOUNT #: 4006755706
BIRTHDATE: 06/20/1938
SEX: M
PHY: Smith, Marie MD
DISCHARGE DATE:

CHEMISTRY—GENERAL

| COLLECTION | DATE | 04/06/ | | |
| | TIME | 2250 | UNITS | NORMAL RANGE |

TEST				
SODIUM		131 L	meq/L	[136–144]
POTASSIUM		5.0	meq/L	[3.6–5.1]
CHLORIDE		93 L	meq/L	[101–111]
CO2		34 H	meq/L	[22–32]
GLUCOSE RANDOM		145 H	mg/dL	[70–125]
BUN		49 H	mg/dL	[8–20]
CREATININE		1.7 H	mg/dL	[0.9–1.3]
CALCIUM		8.3 L	mg/dL	[8.9–10.3]
TOTAL PROTEIN		5.3 L	g/dL	[6.1–7.9]
ALBUMIN		2.2 L	g/dL	[3.5–4.8]
BILIRUBIN TOTAL		0.7	mg/dL	[0.4–2.0]
AST		21	IU/L	[15–41]
ALT		18	IU/L	[17–63]
ALK PHOS		81	IU/L	[38–126]
BUN/CREAT RATIO		28.8 H		[7.3–21.7]
CALCULATED OSMO		289	MOs/kg	[280–300]

L   LOW   H   HIGH

Patient: Med Rec No: CONTINUE

MEDICAL REPORT 3.7

RADIOLOGY/NUCLEAR MEDICINE REPORT

PATIENT:	Doe, John
DOB:	06/20/1938
SEX:	M
MR#:	1234567
CUR LOC:	3N 3507
REQ LOC:	5C 3513
NM#	
PT TYPE:	IP
SERVICE PROVIDED ON:	04/10 at 1003
APPROVED:	04/10 at 1637
ADM BY:	Smith, Marie MD
PROCEDURE:	Chest 1 View, Inspiration
PROC ID#:	14538822
CC TO:	

ORDERED BY:
Smith, Marie MD
600 W. Street
Somewhere, FL 99999

D: 04/10 @ 1031

XYZ COMMUNITY MEDICAL CENTER * DEPARTMENT OF RADIOLOGY
Somewhere, FL 99999 * (999) 999-9999

INTERPRETATION PROVIDED BY: Community Medical Center Radiology Group

CHEST ONE VIEW: 04/10/.

INDICATION: Status post cardiac pacemaker insertion, evaluate for pneumothorax. Cardiac pacing module is positioned at the left axilla with leads extending into the right atrium and right ventricle. No pneumothorax is visualized. There are bilateral pleural effusions of moderate size. Coarse pulmonary interstitium is seen bilaterally which may reflect chronic changes or congestive failure. Heart size is mildly enlarged.

IMPRESSION: No pneumothorax status post cardiac pacing module and left placement.

/tjf
04/10 @ 1628

_____

s/ Samuel E. Exray, M.D.

MEDICAL REPORT 3.8

PATIENT NAME:	John Doe
MEDICAL RECORD NUMBER:	1234567
ACCOUNT NUMBER:	4006755706
CARDIOPULMONARY	
DATE OF TEST:	4/10

PROCEDURE: Echocardiogram

REFERRING PHYSICIAN: Marie Smith, M.D.

INDICATION: A 65-year-old male with dyspnea, status post pacemaker.

M-MODE ECHOCARDIOGRAM: The left ventricle is dilated at 5.6 cm. End-systolic dimension is 4.3. The wall thickness is normal. Small paradoxical septal motion. The left atrium measures 3.8 cm. The aortic root is not dilated. The aortic leaflet cusp opening 1.6 cm. Right-sided chambers are normal size. There is no pericardial effusion.

TWO-DIMENSIONAL STUDY: The left ventricle is mildly dilated. Wall motion abnormalities are noted in the anteroapical segment. There is mild paradoxical septal motion. The left atrium is dilated. There is annulus calcification posteriorly. Aortic root is not dilated. The aortic leaflets show focal sclerosis. Cusp excursion appears adequate. Right-sided chambers of normal size. There is no pericardial effusion.

DOPPLER STUDY: There is trace to mild mitral insufficiency. There is also mild tricuspid insufficiency. No significant gradient across the aortic valve is noted.

IMPRESSION:

1. Abnormal echocardiogram.
2. Left ventricular chamber enlargement.
3. Depressed left ventricular function, estimated ejection fraction is about 35% with anteroapical wall motion abnormalities.
4. Aortic sclerosis.
5. Spontaneous echo contrast noted in the cavity of the left ventricle.

R. Smith, M.D.

131866/tjf 04/10 15:07:07 04/12 07:26:37

Chart copy

A1

1SPOOL – 0196   XYZ COMMUNITY MEDICAL CENTER – HOSPITAL

04/07 00:12   (QARK$N)

MEDICAL REPORT 3.9

PATIENT:	John Doe
MR:	1234567 AD 04/07
ACCT#:	4006755706
ALLERGIES:	NKA
PHYSICIAN:	Marie Smith, MD

PHYSICIAN'S ORDERS
Please use Ball Point Pen. **PRESS FIRMLY.**

Another brand of generically equivalent product may be substituted unless otherwise indicated by the physician.
◯ DO NOT USE THIS FORM UNLESS A RED NUMBER SHOWS

Date / Time Written

4/7	CARDIZEM 10 mg IV Bolus then
0135	CARDIZEM drip 10 mg/hr.

> T.O. Phillips, ARNP
> Noted by: L. Curtis, RN
> Smith 4/7

4/7	HALDOL 1 mg IVP NOW
0315	

> T.O. Phillips, ARNP
> Noted by: L. Curtis, RN
> Smith 4/7
> 0415

4/7	Cancel Heart Cath
0545	Cancel Pre-op meds
	Digoxin 0.5 mg IV NOW

> T.O. Phillips, ARNP
> Noted by: L. Curtis, RN 0640
> Smith 4/7

FORM NO 366 REV. 11/99

NOTES

MEDICAL REPORT 3.10

MEDICATION ADMINISTRATION RECORD

RUN DATE/TIME 04/07 00:00 TO 23:59   RUN FOR: 04/07

PAGE: 1

CARDIAC TELE/ 3507 C   DOE, JOHN   SEX: M   AGE: 65

ADM: 04/06

HEIGHT: 170.2 CM   WEIGHT 65.400 KG   BSA   1.76 SqM   PHYSICIAN: SMITH, MARIE MD

DX: UNSTABLE ANGINA/CATH POSS ANGIOPLAST

ALLERGIES: NKDA

     NKA

PHA ALLERGIES: UPDATE ALLERGIES BEFORE PLACING ORDERS

Rx # GENERIC NAME START/STOP DATE/TIME (TRADE NAME) SIG ROUTE	0700-1459 (7-3)	1500-2259 (3-11)	2300-0659 (11-7)

SCHEDULED MEDS

000085   INTRAVENOUS INFUSION . . . . START NACL 0.9%, 100ML, DILTIAZEM INJ (5MG/ML) 125MG, RATE – 10CC HR, CONT TIL DC'D

000086   CARDIZEM DILTIAZEM INJ (5MG/ML) 10MG, IV PUSH, NOW

000090   HALDOL HALOPERIDOL DECANOATE INJ (50MG/ML) 1MG, IVPB/SYRINGE, NOW

	INITIALS SIGNATURE		INITIALS SIGNATURE
0700-1500		1500-2300	
2300-0700		VERIFIED BY	

1. OFF THE UNIT   LU—LEFT UPPER QUAD.

2. NAUSEA   LLQ—LEFT LOWER QUAD.

3. REFUSED   RA—RIGHT ARM

* SEE NURSES NOTES   RT—RIGHT THIGH

SQ—SUBQ   RU—RIGHT UPPER QUAD.

LA—LEFT ARM   RLQ—RIGHT LOWER QUAD.

LT—LEFT THIGH

NOTES

_____

_____

MEDICAL REPORT 3.11

CLINICAL RÉSUMÉ

NAME:	John Doe
DOB:	06/20/1938
04/06:	ADMITTED XYZ COMMUNITY MEDICAL CENTER:
4/12:	DISCHARGED

DIAGNOSES:

1. Three-vessel coronary artery disease, being treated medically.

2. Tachy-brady syndrome status post permanent pacemaker implantation with Pacesetter Trilogy DR Plus model #9999. Atrial lead is a Pacesetter Tendrile DX endocardial steroid eluting screw-in lead, model #9999P, serial #MJ9999. Ventricular lead is a Pacesetter Tendrile DX model #9999P endocardial steroid eluting lead serial #MK9999. Pacemaker implanted 4/10.

3. Severe peripheral vascular disease.

4. Diabetes mellitus.

5. Recurrent atrial fibrillation

MEDICATIONS: Include Cardizem CD 120 mg daily, enteric-coated aspirin 325 mg daily, K-Dur 20mEq daily, Pepcid 20 mg b.i.d., Zocor 20 mg daily, Lasix 40 mg daily, insulin NPH as directed, nitroglycerin patch on discharge.

SUMMARY: John Doe is a 65-year-old gentleman who was referred by Dr. J. Jones for evaluation of coronary artery disease and rapid atrial fibrillation which is recurrent. He was admitted to my care. I reviewed cardiac catheterization films from 1/27 by Dr. Jones and felt with the wide spread atherosclerotic disease he was not a good candidate for coronary artery bypass grafting or interventional therapy. Medical therapy was advised. However, the patient also has a history of a sick sinus syndrome with intermittent atrial fibrillation alternating with sinus bradycardia with rates as low as 30. He was advised to proceed with permanent pacemaker implantation in an attempt to treat recurrent atrial fibrillation and to have pacemaker backup for bradycardia. He was entered into the XYZ1 study with Pacesetter and on 4/10 underwent permanent pacemaker implantation. The pacemaker implantation took place without any complications. Of note, on the morning after admission he was noted to be very confused and combative and he was in and out of rapid atrial fibrillation. At the present time, he is alert and oriented and stable from cardiac status.

FOLLOWUP: The patient will follow-up with Dr. Jones in 10-14 days and will then decide at that time if John Doe is a candidate for Coumadin. He will continue to be followed through our EP clinic and Pacesetter through the XYZ1 study to prevent atrial fibrillation study protocol.

D. Doe, A.R.N.P.

d: 04/11: 04/14 jf

_____

Marie Smith, M.D.

cc:

S. Jones, M.D.

J. Jones, M.D.

A. Michaels, M.D.

CODING FOR SPECIFIC DISEASES AND DISORDERS

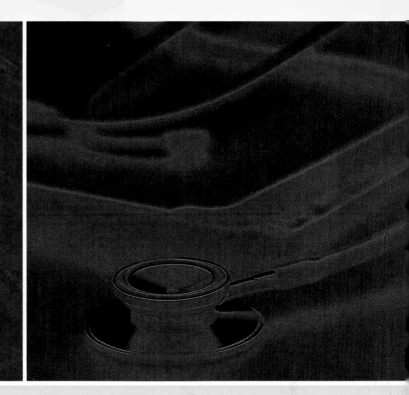

Coding for Symptoms, Signs, and Ill-Defined Conditions

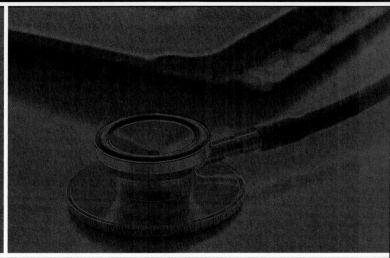

Chapter Outline

Chapter Objectives

- ▸ Differentiate between symptoms, signs, and ill-defined conditions.

- ▸ Describe two situations in which it is acceptable to use symptoms, signs, or ill-defined conditions for inpatient coding.

- ▸ Explain why it is more common to code from the ICD-9-CM's chapter on symptoms, signs, and ill-defined conditions for the provision of outpatient health-care services.

- ▸ Explain when it is appropriate to use abnormal findings codes.

- ▸ Explain when it is appropriate to use a symptom code as a secondary diagnosis.

- ▸ Correctly code for symptoms, signs, and ill-defined conditions by using the ICD-9-CM and medical records.

A **symptom** is a subjective sign of disease experienced and described by the patient. A **sign** is an objective symptom of disease discovered on examination of the patient by the physician.[1] An **ill-defined condition** is one for which a more precise diagnosis cannot be made.

Symptoms, signs, and ill-defined conditions are included in code section 780 to 799 of chapter 16 of the *Tabular List of Diseases* of ICD-9-CM. As a general rule, if the underlying condition that caused the symptom or sign is known, code the definitive diagnosis and not the symptom, sign, or ill-defined condition. This rule applies for both inpatient and outpatient coding.

Inpatient Coding

There are some acceptable instances in which symptoms, signs, and ill-defined conditions can be used for inpatient coding (as principal [PDx] or secondary diagnoses [SDx]). These rules are as follows:

1. When a symptom is followed by differential diagnoses (i.e., contrasting or comparative diagnoses), the symptom code is sequenced first as the principal diagnosis, followed by the contrasting conditions. This comparative/contrasting guideline is only for the selection of the principal diagnosis. If there is a symptom followed by contrasting or comparative diagnoses given as secondary diagnosis, code only the symptom, and do not code each contrasting condition.

TIP   *Coding Clinic* 1990, second quarter, and 1998, first quarter, provide additional information regarding symptoms followed by contrasting conditions.

EXAMPLE

As a principal diagnosis:

Chest pain secondary to angina versus GERDs

principal diagnosis:	786.50	CHEST PAIN
secondary diagnosis:	413.9	ANGINA PECTORIS
	530.81	GASTROESOPHAGEAL REFLUX DISEASE (GERD)

As a secondary diagnosis:

principal diagnosis:		Coronary artery disease, native vessels.
secondary diagnosis:		Lethargy secondary to hypothyroidism vs. iron-deficiency anemia
principal diagnosis:	414.01	CORONARY ARTERY DISEASE, NATIVE VESSELS
secondary diagnosis:	780.79	LETHARGY

2. A symptom code may be assigned as a principal diagnosis or secondary diagnosis when, after study, a definitive diagnosis is not identified and the symptom is described as "etiology unknown or undetermined," "cause unknown," or "idiopathic" (e.g., abdominal pain, etiology unknown, code 789.00).

3. A symptom code may be assigned as a principal diagnosis if a patient is transferred to another facility or signs out (discharges himself or herself) against medical advice (AMA) before a workup is completed. In these instances, an incomplete workup made it impossible to establish a definitive diagnosis before the patient's leaving AMA or transferring to another facility for care.

4. If an admission symptom is a residual condition from a prior acute injury, disease, poisoning, or adverse effect of correct medication, the

symptom (as the residual condition) is sequenced first as the principal diagnosis, followed by a "late effect" code to identify the cause of the residual symptom and a late-effect E code (if required by the facility). Remember that the focus of health-care treatment is now being directed at the residual condition(s) that should be sequenced first. The acute injury is no longer present.

			EXAMPLE
Child with residual ataxic gait from previous accidental poisoning from alcohol			
principal diagnosis:	*781.2*	*ATAXIC GAIT*	
secondary diagnosis:	*909.1*	*LATE EFFECT OF POISONING (locate under the main term "late effects" in the Alphabetic Index to Diseases)*	
secondary diagnosis:	*E929.2*	*EXTERNAL CAUSE RELATED TO POISONING (locate under the main term "late effects" in the Alphabetic Index to External Causes)*	

If you code a sign or symptom as the principal diagnosis in an inpatient setting, the code may attract more scrutiny for payment, because it is vague and a questionable cause for hospitalization. Be sure to search the medical record for a more definitive diagnosis.

Following Uniform Hospital Discharge Data Set (UHDDS) inpatient coding rules–because the after-study concept applies to inpatient coding–final diagnoses described as "possible," "probable," "likely," "questionable," "?," "suspected," or "rule out" are coded as though the diagnosis were established. Therefore, it is not common to code an inpatient principal diagnosis from ICD-9-CM's chapter 16 on symptoms, signs, and ill-defined conditions. The length of stay for inpatient admissions allows adequate time (after study) to evaluate possible diagnoses that can be further identified for study rather than reporting symptom codes.

It is helpful for inpatient coders to note that the chapter 16 code range is 780 to 799. Therefore, these can be easily recognized for a final check of codes before billing. Re-review the medical record to be sure a definitive diagnosis has not been established rather than reporting symptom codes routinely associated with the disease.

Outpatient Coding

For outpatient coding, the inpatient UHDDS after-study concept does not apply because outpatient visits or encounters are short, and studies often have not been completed (i.e., results are not available) before patient discharge. For outpatient encounters, often sign and symptom coding is used because cases are to be coded only to the highest level of certainty. Diagnoses described as "possible," "probable," "likely," "questionable," "?," "suspected," or "rule out" should not be coded for outpatient stays. Therefore, it is more common to code from chapter 16 on symptoms, signs, and ill-defined conditions to establish medical necessity for the outpatient health-care services provided.

EXAMPLE

Diagnosis coding examples for outpatient versus inpatient coding:

"Chest pain, possible angina pectoris"

Inpatient setting: code 413.9 (code only the angina pectoris)

Outpatient setting: code 786.50 (code only the chest pain)

> For both inpatient and outpatient reporting, do not code conditions as ruled out. When there is a d at the end of rule, it means that the diagnosis is no longer a possibility because the condition did not occur.

EXAMPLE

"Chest pain, etiology unknown. Acute myocardial infarction ruled out" (code only the chest pain: 786.50)

"Persistent hyponatremia, syndrome of inappropriate antidiuretic hormone ruled out" (code only the hyponatremia: 276.1)

Abnormal Findings

Abnormal laboratory, examination, and test findings without a definitive diagnosis are included in category codes 790 to 796 of chapter 16. Most of these codes can be located by looking under "Findings, abnormal, without diagnosis" in the *Alphabetic Index to Diseases* (volume 2). These codes should be used only when the physician has not documented a definitive diagnosis but does document that further workup or follow-up for the abnormal test is needed.

EXAMPLE

"Abnormal liver function tests, will follow up in office" (code 794.8)

"Abnormal electrocardiogram, will send patient home on Holter monitor for further cardiac rhythm evaluation and schedule cardiac stress test" (code 794.31)

"Elevated cancer antigen (CA-125), will refer patient to oncologist" (code 795.82)

> A coder should never code from laboratory work, radiology, or special tests without additional supporting documentation from the attending physician found within the body of the medical record (e.g., physician's progress notes or discharge summary). These codes should never be used as an inpatient principal diagnosis and are rarely used for secondary diagnosis.

Coding Symptoms Integral to Disease

Do not code symptom codes that are routinely associated with a disease as secondary diagnosis codes. However, do code symptom codes if they are not routinely associated with a disease.

EXAMPLE

"Chest pain secondary to unstable angina" (assign only the unstable angina code 411.1, because chest pain is routinely associated with unstable angina)

"Abdominal pain, nausea, vomiting, and diarrhea caused by gastroenteritis" (assign only the gastroenteritis code 558.9, because these symptoms are routinely associated with gastroenteritis and therefore should not be coded)

"Acute cerebral infarction with ataxia present at discharge" (code the cerebral infarction with ataxia as an additional code, 434.91 + 781.3, because ataxia is not routinely associated with all cerebral infarctions and will affect the patient's continuing care in rehabilitation)

"Pneumonia with febrile seizures" (code both the pneumonia and the febrile seizures, 486 + 780.31, because febrile seizures are not routinely associated with pneumonia)

For symptoms and signs from chapter 16 (category codes 780 to 799) associated with malignancies (e.g., weakness), code the malignancy code as the principal diagnosis with the associated signs and symptoms as additional codes. There are new rules for coding admissions for neoplasm related pain (see page 425 for more information).

EXAMPLE

"Admission for fever, weakness, nausea and vomiting secondary to metastatic colon cancer."
Correct coding:

153.9	*Colon cancer*
199.1	*Metastases (NOS)*
780.61	*Fever secondary to malignancy*
780.79	*Weakness*
787.01	*Nausea and vomiting*

SUMMARY

This chapter has focused on properly coding for signs, symptoms, and ill-defined conditions by using the ICD-9-CM. From the development of proper coding practices, the use of that knowledge to correctly code medical reports and records was presented and exemplified. Chapter 5 will address the endocrine, nutritional, metabolic, and immune systems.

REFERENCE

1. Stedman's Medical Dictionary, 27th Ed. Baltimore: Williams & Wilkins, 2000.

TESTING YOUR COMPREHENSION

1. Distinguish among the terms **symptoms**, **signs**, and **ill-defined conditions**.

2. Under what conditions is a symptom code normally assigned?

3. Coding a sign or symptom as a principal diagnosis may invite increased scrutiny. Why?

4. What category codes are used for abnormal laboratory, examination, and test findings without a definitive diagnosis?

5. When there is a *d* at the end of the term *rule,* one should not code the condition(s). Why?

6. What are the rules for coding symptoms as secondary diagnoses, framed as a "DO" and a "DO NOT"?

CODING PRACTICE I   Chapter Review Exercises

Directions

By using your ICD-9-CM codebook, code the following diagnoses and procedures:

	DIAGNOSIS/PROCEDURES	CODE
1	Diagnosis: Alcohol cirrhosis with massive ascites. Alcoholism, continuous. Procedure: Paracentesis.	
2	Syncopal episode of unknown etiology.	
3	Abdominal pain, cholecystitis versus colitis.	
4	Vertigo, labyrinthitis, or atypical migraine.	
5	Shortness of breath secondary to congestive heart failure and acute bronchitis.	
6	Dysuria secondary to urinary tract infection.	
7	Hemoptysis attributable to pneumonia.	
8	Hematuria secondary to cystitis.	
9	Palpitations attributable to sinus tachycardia or psychogenic arrhythmia.	
10	Nausea and vomiting secondary to adverse effect of digoxin, taken as prescribed. Compensated atrial fibrillation.	
11	Hand numbness secondary to previous injury/fracture.	
12	Ataxia secondary to late effect of near drowning.	
13	Febrile seizures.	
14	Fever, undetermined etiology, sepsis and pneumonia ruled out. Abnormal liver function tests, will follow up in office.	

	DIAGNOSIS/PROCEDURES	CODE
15	Altered mental status secondary to heat stroke.	
16	Osteoarthritis, left knee, with joint pain.	
17	Acute embolic cerebrovascular accident/infarction with aphasia at discharge.	
18	Paresthesia, right hand, of unknown etiology.	
19	Atypical chest pain of uncertain cause.	
20	Diarrhea.	
21	Epistaxis secondary to uncontrolled essential hypertension.	
22	Malaise and tremors of unknown etiology.	
23	New-adult onset diabetes mellitus with polydipsia.	
24	Failure to thrive in 6-month-old infant, etiology unknown.	
25	Syncopal episode secondary to orthostatic hypotension.	

Instructions

1. Carefully review the medical reports provided for each case study.
2. Research any abbreviations and terms that are unfamiliar or unclear.
3. Identify as many diagnoses and procedures as possible.
4. Because only part of the patient's total record is available, determine what additional documentation you might need.
5. If appropriate, identify any questions you might ask the physician to code this case correctly and completely.
6. Complete the appropriate blanks below for each case study.

CHAPTER 4 CASE STUDIES

Case Study 4.1 (Coder/Abstract Summary Form)

Patient: **John Doe**

Patient documentation: **Review Medical Report 4.1**

1. Principal diagnosis:

   _____

2. Secondary or other diagnoses:

   _____

3. Principal procedure:

   _____

4. Other procedures:

   _____

5. Additional documentation needed:

   _____

   _____

   _____

   _____

Case Study 4.1 (Continued)

6. Questions for the physician:

_____

_____

_____

_____

_____

MEDICAL REPORT 4.1

CONSULTATION REPORT

NAME: DOE, JOHN

PATIENT #: 111111

MR#: 0000123456

ROOM NUMBER: 300

CONSULTING: J. JOHNSON, M.D.

ATTENDING: P. SMITH, M.D.

ADMIT DATE: 4/1

DISCHARGE DATE:

DATE: 04/02

PRESENT ILLNESS: Mr. Doe is a 69-year-old man that I have seen in the past with history of two-vessel coronary artery bypass grafts. He had an evaluation in January where he had open grafts. He had good flow of the IMA, had total graft collaterals from the first marginal. The first marginal was noted to be open proximal to the circumflex occlusion and filled the distal right coronary artery.

It was felt at the time that he should have a bypass if he failed medical therapy. I think overall, he has done fairly well. He presents now to me with an episode of dizziness. This has been a fairly chronic problem. It is not something that is related to any history of orthostasis or problem with positioning. He says he gets dizzy and staggers when he walks. I am curious to know whether perhaps lacunar infarct noted on CT is affecting this somewhat. His cardiac rhythm has been stable as far as he is able to tell me. He has not had palpitations or pre-syncope.

He denies history of exertional angina. He has had no orthopnea, PND or edema. He has had no other significant cardiac problems.

PAST HISTORY: Non-compliance, insulin-dependent diabetes, hypothyroidism, hypertension, depression, and peripheral neuropathy.

REVIEW OF SYSTEMS: Please see the patient questionnaire reviewed by me.

SOCIAL HISTORY: Habits: He is a non-smoker. He doesn't drink significant amounts of alcohol.

PHYSICAL EXAMINATION

VITALS: Blood pressure 130/70, pulse 60.

GENERAL: He is a well-developed, well-nourished white man in no acute distress who is alert and oriented.

HEENT: Grossly normal.

NECK: Supple, there is no JVD. Carotids without bruit.

CHEST/LUNGS: Clear to auscultation and percussion.

CARDIOVASCULAR: Reveals regular rate and rhythm. No murmur, rub, or gallop is noted.

ABDOMEN: Soft, non-tender with normative bowel sounds.

EXTREMITIES: Reveals no cyanosis, clubbing, or edema.

EKG: Shows right bundle branch block, questionable old inferior MI, unchanged from prior EKG done back in January.

Continued

MEDICAL REPORT 4.1 (CONTINUED)

IMPRESSION:

1. DIZZINESS, QUESTIONABLE ETIOLOGY. HE IS CONCERNED IT WAS FROM SOME OF THE MEDICINES HE HAS GOTTEN.
2. ARTERIOSCLEROTIC CARDIOVASCULAR DISEASE, STATUS POST TWO-VESSEL CORONARY ARTERY BYPASS GRAFT WITH OCCLUSION OF THE RIGHT CORONARY GRAFT.
3. ABNORMAL CARDIAC ISOENZYMES, NONE OF SIGNIFICANT DIAGNOSTIC CHANGE TO THIS POINT. NEED REPEAT.
4. NON-COMPLIANCE.
5. INSULIN-DEPENDENT DIABETES, TYPE I.
6. HYPOTHYROIDISM.

PLAN: Get neurology to evaluate. Get supine and standing blood pressures, monitor his rhythm and will repeat his cardiac ISOs. Further recommendations will follow.
Thank you for this consultation.

_____

J. JOHNSON, M.D.

DD: 04/02

DT: 04/02

NOTES

Case Study 4.2 (Coder/Abstract Summary Form)

Patient: **Frank Smith**

Patient documentation: **Review Medical Report 4.2**

1. Principal diagnosis:

   _____

2. Secondary or other diagnoses:

   _____

3. Principal procedure:

   _____

4. Other procedures:

   _____

5. Additional documentation needed:

   _____

   _____

   _____

   _____

6. Questions for the physician:

   _____

   _____

   _____

   _____

   _____

MEDICAL REPORT 4.2

DISCHARGE SUMMARY

NAME: SMITH, FRANK

PATIENT #:   222222

ROOM NUMBER: 200

MR#:   0000123456

ATTENDING: JANE SMITH, MD

ADMIT DATE: 4/1

DISCHARGE DATE: 4/3

DISCHARGE DIAGNOSIS:

1. RESPIRATORY DISTRESS, UNCLEAR ETIOLOGY. POSSIBLE CONGESTIVE HEART FAILURE VERSUS MUCOUS PLUGGING VERSUS MILD ASPIRATION PNEUMONIA.
2. CARDIOMYOPATHY WITH LEFT VENTRICULAR HYPERTROPHY. EJECTION FRACTION OF 30%.
3. RECENT MASSIVE CEREBROVASCULAR ACCIDENT WITH RIGHT HEMIPARESIS, RIGHT UPPER EXTREMITY GREATER THAN LOWER EXTREMITY.
4. APHASIA.
5. APHAGIA.
6. CHRONIC ATRIAL FIBRILLATION.
7. MODERATE MITRAL REGURGITATION, MODERATE TRICUSPID REGURGITATION.
8. ELEVATED LIVER TRANSAMINASE WITH ALKALINE PHOSPHATASE.
9. GASTROSTOMY TUBE FEEDING.
10. PERIPHERAL VASCULAR DISEASE.
11. PROBABLE URINARY TRACT INFECTION.
12. RESOLVING PERINEAL RASH, PROBABLY YEAST.

HOSPITAL COURSE: Mr. Smith is an 84-year-old gentleman who suffered a recent CVA approximately two months ago. He was cared for at XYZ Hospital before being transferred to Rehab. The patient had been transferred into a swing bed at ABC Nursing Home approximately two days prior to developing decreased level of consciousness and respiratory distress. He was transferred to the emergency room for evaluation and admitted to ICU to rule out MI. He had EKG changes and was noted to be in chronic atrial fibrillation. The patient was admitted to ICU and had marked elevation and total CPK with peak of 1,187. However, his Troponin level remained essentially stable. He was also noted to have an elevation of alkaline phosphatase of 199, SGOT of 994 and SGPT of 680. The patient appeared dry with a BUN of 39, creatinine of 0.8. He was admitted and Dr. Heart was consulted for cardiology. He was ruled out for acute MI. The patient was found to be in euthyroid state. He remained stable hemodynamically and had no runs of V-tach or V-fib. Dr. Heart strongly recommended the patient be made **do not resuscitate (DNR).** He was found to have a previous echocardiogram at XYZ Hospital read by Dr. Heart, cardiology, which indicated moderate global hypokinesis with ejection fraction of 30%. There is moderate MR with mild to moderate TR. Atrial fibrillation was noted at that time as well.

The patient had an EEG showing no evidence of seizure. Dr. Nerve was consulted for neurology. He noted left MCA distribution, cerebrovascular accident. He has now completed rehab. He agreed not to proceed with any further testing. He recommended continuing enteric-coated aspirin, 81 mg a day. He did not recommend starting any anti-epileptics at this point.

The patient is now stabilized. He has had some improvement in labs including a BUN of 31, alkaline phosphatase of 152, SGOT 314, SGPT 417. His discharge blood count includes white blood count 8,600, hemoglobin 12.5, hematocrit 37.1, platelet count 286,000.

Patient did have evidence of hematuria which may have been traumatic. He does have 15-25 WBCs in his urine. He has been started on Levaquin 750 mg q. day for 10 days. Recommended continuing Lovenox at this time. Patient is now stable

MEDICAL REPORT 4.2 (CONTINUED)

for discharge back to ABC Nursing Home. Will review with family and would strongly recommend DNR status. Plan to repeat a UA along with labs in one week. He will continue to be followed by me at this facility and I will arrange for his transfer by ambulance. Greater than 30 minutes was spent in discharge of this patient today.

JANE SMITH, M.D.

DD: 04/03

DT: 04/04

cc: ABC NURSING HOME

NOTES

Case Study 4.3 (Coder/Abstract Summary Form)

Patient: **Ellen Parker**

Patient documentation: **Review Medical Reports 4.3 and 4.4**

1. Principal diagnosis:

   _____

2. Secondary or other diagnoses:

   _____

3. Principal procedure:

   _____

4. Other procedures:

   _____

5. Additional documentation needed:

   _____

   _____

   _____

6. Questions for the physician:

   _____

   _____

   _____

   _____

MEDICAL REPORT 4.3

DISCHARGE SUMMARY

NAME: PARKER, ELLEN

NUMBER: 999999

SEX: F

AGE: 79

ADMIT: 4/03

DISCH: 4/04

TYPE: INPT

ROOM: 100

ATTENDING PHYSICIAN: JANE SMITH, M.D.

FINAL DIAGNOSES:

(1) Tachycardia.

(2) Hypertension.

(3) Hyponatremia, chronic.

COMPLICATIONS: None.

PROCEDURE: Telemetry.

CONSULTATION: None.

HISTORY OF PATIENT: This is a 79-year-old female who was brought to the emergency room on the day of admission with the chief complaint of palpitations. She denies chest pain, paroxysmal nocturnal dyspnea, or orthopnea. She got frightened and came to the emergency room. No headache, blurred vision, or double vision.

PAST MEDICAL HISTORY: Palpitation, hypertension, hyponatremia, osteoarthritis.

PAST SURGICAL HISTORY: Denied.

ALLERGIES: None.

SOCIAL HISTORY: The patient is widowed, no tobacco or alcohol.

FAMILY HISTORY: Denied for heart disease, lung disease, diabetes mellitus, or cancer.

PHYSICAL EXAMINATION

GENERAL APPEARANCE: The physical examination reveals a well-developed elderly female.

EYES: Eyes equal and react to light. Extraocular movements intact.

EARS: Tympanic membrane intact without retraction or bulging.

NOSE: Nares patent.

OROPHARYNX: Not injected.

NECK: Supple. No jugular venous distention or bruits. No thyromegaly, no adenopathy.

LUNGS: Clear.

Continued

MEDICAL REPORT 4.3 (CONTINUED)

HEART: Regular rate and rhythm without murmur, S2 or S4.

EXTREMITIES: No clubbing, cyanosis, or edema. Pulses intact.

ABDOMEN: Soft and non-tender. Bowel sounds are present. No hepatosplenomegaly.

NEUROLOGICAL: Awake, alert and oriented to person, place and time. Cranial nerves two through twelve intact. Deep tendon reflexes are intact.

Chest x-ray is still pending.

White count 4.5, hemoglobin 10, hematocrit 30, platelet count 279,000, sodium 135 on discharge, on admission was 120. Potassium 4.1, chloride 109, glucose 89, BUN 13, creatinine 1, calcium 8.3, serum osmolarity was 263. TSH 2.3, thyroid profile normal.

Electrocardiogram on discharge was normal sinus rhythm with a heart rate of 70.

HOSPITAL COURSE: The patient was admitted to the hospital and her anti-hypertensive medication was changed to Zestoretic. She was on an IV Saline drip. She improved greatly. She was feeling 100% better by the next day and was requesting to go home. She had no further desire for work up. She had a cardiac work up recently and it was okay. She will be discharged home to close follow up.

MEDICATIONS: Her medications will include Tenormin 25 mg daily.

DIET: Diet will be as tolerated.

ACTIVITY: Her activity will be as tolerated.

Signature affixed via participation in alternative signature program

Job Number: 99999

_____

JANE SMITH, M.D.

D: 4/04

T: 4/04

NOTES

MEDICAL REPORT 4.4

HISTORY AND PHYSICAL

NAME: PARKER, ELLEN

NUMBER: 999999

SEX: F

AGE: 79

ADMIT: 4/03

DISCH: 4/04

TYPE: INPT

ROOM: 100

ATTENDING PHYSICIAN: JANE SMITH, M.D.

HISTORY OF PRESENT ILLNESS: This is a 79-year-old female brought to the emergency room on the day of admission with palpitations. She got short of breath and was afraid something was wrong. She denies chest pain, paroxysmal nocturnal dyspnea or orthopnea. No edema. No dyspnea on exertion. She has been tiring, but this is an old problem. She was brought to the emergency room where it was found that her sodium was 123 and she is admitted.

PAST MEDICAL HISTORY: Hypertension.

PAST SURGICAL HISTORY: Denied.

ALLERGIES: No known drug allergies.

MEDICATIONS: Zestoretic 20-12.5.

SOCIAL HISTORY: The patient is widowed. No tobacco or alcohol.

FAMILY HISTORY: Denies for heart disease, lung disease, diabetes, or cancer.

REVIEW OF SYSTEMS: The patient denies blurred vision, double vision, dizziness. No cough, congestion, or wheeze. She has had palpitations. No chest pain, paroxysmal nocturnal dyspnea, orthopnea, or edema. No dyspnea on exertion. No indigestion, heartburn, melena, hematochezia, hematemesis.

PHYSICAL EXAMINATION

GENERAL: A well-developed female.

HEAD, EYES, EARS, NOSE AND THROAT: Pupils equal, round and reactive to light. Extraocular muscles intact. Tympanic membranes intact without retraction or bulging. Nares patent. Oropharynx not injected.

NECK: Supple. No jugular venous distention or bruit. No thyromegaly or adenopathy.

LUNGS: Clear to auscultation without wheezes or rhonchi.

HEART: Regular rate and rhythm without murmur, S3 or S4.

EXTREMITIES: Without clubbing, cyanosis, or edema. Pulses intact.

ABDOMEN: Soft and non-tender. Bowel sounds are present. No hepatosplenomegaly.

Continued

MEDICAL REPORT 4.4 (CONTINUED)

NEUROLOGICAL: Alert and oriented to person, place, and time. Cranial nerves II-XII intact. Deep tendon reflexes intact.

ASSESSMENT: A 79-year-old female now admitted with palpitations; hyponatremia which is a chronic problem.

PLAN: Will admit, will get baseline laboratory, monitor heart rate. Will repeat cortisol levels. The patient requests that we do not perform further cardiac workup, as she has had a graded exercise test in the recent past and it was negative. Will contemplate switching her antihypertensive med to a beta blocker for rate control.

Signature affixed via participation in alternative signature program

Job Number: 99999

_____

JANE SMITH, M.D.

D: 4/04

T: 4/04

NOTES

Coding for Endocrine, Nutritional, Metabolic, and Immune Disorders

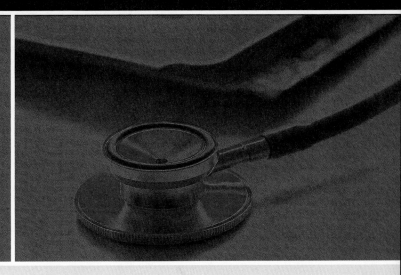

Chapter Outline

Endocrine Disorders
Nutritional Disorders
Metabolic Disorders
Immune Disorders
Testing Your Comprehension
Coding Practice I: Chapter Review Exercises
Coding Practice II: Medical Record Case Studies

Chapter Objectives

▶ Describe the pathology of common endocrine, nutritional, metabolic, and immunity disorders.

▶ Recognize the typical manifestations, complications, and treatments of common endocrine, nutritional, metabolic, and immunity disorders in terms of their implications for coding.

▶ Correctly code common endocrine, nutritional, metabolic, and immune disorders by using the ICD-9-CM and medical records.

The organs that comprise the endocrine, nutritional, metabolic, and immune systems help us to maintain a balance in the internal environment of the body—a state known as homeostasis. This balance is needed to support healthy cells.

Word Parts and Meanings of Endocrine System Medical Terms

Word Part	Meaning	Example	Definition of Example
endo-	within, into, in		
Crin/o	secrete		
endocrin/o	endocrine glands secrete substances (hormones) into the bloodstream	endocrinopathy	Disease of the endocrine glands
thyr/o, thyroid/o	thyroid gland	thyroidectomy	Surgical removal of thyroid tissue
gluc/o	glucose	hyperglycemia	Excess glucose in the bloodstream
ur/o	urine, urinary tract	glycosuria	Sugar in the urine
nephr/o	kidney	nephropathy	Disease of the kidney
-sis	an abnormal condition	ketoacidosis	Acidosis caused by an excess of ketone bodies, as in diabetes mellitus
Natri	sodium	hyponatremia	Abnormally low concentrations of sodium in the bloodstream

Cells throughout the body need to receive nutrients in the presence of oxygen and give off waste (carbon dioxide that we exhale and nitrogenous waste that we eliminate in urine). Blood is the transport system that carries nutrients to the cells and takes away waste. It also transports substances such as hormones from endocrine glands and white blood cells needed to fight infection.

This chapter explains some of the more common endocrine, metabolic, nutritional, and immune disorders you will be coding from chapter 3 of the ICD-9-CM.

Endocrine Disorders

Endocrine organs or glands secrete hormones directly into the bloodstream ("ductless glands") that help us maintain homeostasis. Although there are many endocrine glands with different functions and related diseases, this chapter highlights the most common diseases that you will be coding. These involve dysfunctions of the pancreas (islets of Langerhans), thyroid gland, and pituitary gland. To assist in your understanding, the Word Parts Box on this page reviews word parts and meanings of medical terms related to the endocrine system.

Diabetes Mellitus

Diabetes mellitus (code category 250) and its manifestations involve a reduction or complete deficiency of insulin. Insulin is a hormone produced in special cells called **beta cells** in the islets of Langerhans of the pancreas that helps us maintain a normal level of glucose (sugar) in our circulating bloodstream. The normal level of glucose in our bloodstream is between 70 and 115 mg/dL.

When we have too much glucose in our circulating blood (e.g., after a meal), insulin is secreted to help carry excess glucose from our bloodstream to the body tissues. There, it can be used in body metabolism to create cell energy; alternatively, it is stored as glycogen in the liver. Excess glucose in the bloodstream is referred to as **hyperglycemia.** Hyperglycemia can spill over into the urine as **glycosuria.** Glycosuria occurs because the excess sugar in the bloodstream is filtered through the glomerular portion of the kidneys and cannot be properly reabsorbed through the renal (kidney) tubules before the elimination of urine from the body. Abnormal laboratory findings of high blood glucose or glucose in urine may indicate diabetes mellitus.

Type 1 and Type 2 Diabetes

There are two different types of diabetes mellitus: type 1 and type 2. Type 1 diabetes mellitus is also referred to as insulin-dependent diabetes mellitus, juvenile diabetes mellitus, and ketosis-prone diabetes mellitus. This type of diabetes results from a complete lack of insulin. Individuals with type 1 diabetes require insulin injections to maintain normal glucose levels in the blood.

Note: As of October 2004, insulin-dependent diabetes mellitus (IDDM) not documented by the physician as "type 1" DM is coded to 250.00 (type 2 DM). Therefore, if the physician documents IDDM, you must clarify if this was type 1 or type 2 diabetes and have the physician document (amend the medical record) accordingly.

IDDM documentation does not mean coders can classify a patient as Type I DM; it must be documented as Type I by the physician.

Type 2 diabetes mellitus is also referred to as non-insulin-dependent diabetes mellitus, adult-onset diabetes mellitus, and mature-onset diabetes mellitus. This type of diabetes mellitus usually occurs in adults who have a deficiency of insulin or whose target tissues are no longer as responsive to the effects of insulin. Type 2 diabetes responds to diet, exercise, and oral hypoglycemic drugs such as chlorpropamide (Diabinese) and glipizide (Glucotrol).

TIP **Diabetes mellitus without further physician documentation is coded to type 2 diabetes.**

Acute (primary) complications of diabetes include chronic hyperglycemia, glycosuria, water and electrolyte loss, ketoacidosis, and coma. Long-term (secondary) complications of diabetes can include the development of neuropathy, retinopathy, nephropathy, generalized degenerative changes in large and small blood vessels, and increased susceptibility to infection.[1] Diabetics are more prone to develop atherosclerosis, which can lead to strokes, heart disease, and peripheral vascular disease.

Acute Complications of Diabetes Mellitus

Acute conditions are characterized by severe and rapid onset of symptoms associated with the disease. Diabetic ketoacidosis (code 250.1X) is an acute primary complication caused by a lack of insulin in which fat is used (i.e., catabolized) in place of sugar to produce cell energy. It usually occurs as a complication of type 1 diabetes because insulin is not available to carry sugar from the bloodstream to the cells.

A by-product of fat catabolism is an excess of substances called **ketones** in the bloodstream: this is a condition called **ketosis**. Ketones are acidic and, when they accumulate in the blood, can change the normal pH (acid/alkaline) balance of the blood and cause diabetic ketoacidosis, which can be a life-threatening condition.

Another acute primary complication of diabetes is hyperosmolarity (code 250.2X). It usually occurs as a complication of type 2 diabetes. Symptoms include confusion, weakness, seizures, excessive thirst, and coma. This condition results in high levels of blood glucose without ketones or ketoacidosis. However, high blood glucose and osmolarity draw water from body tissues (intracellular spaces) into vascular spaces, resulting in extreme dehydration. Osmolarity occurs when a lower concentration of a solute (substance dissolved in a solution) passes through a semipermeable membrane to a higher concentration of solute; this tends to balance the concentrations.

Long-Term Complications of Diabetes Mellitus

For coding long-term complications or manifestations of diabetes mellitus, the general coding rule is to code the diabetes code first, followed by the code for the complication or manifestation. The fourth digit of the diabetes category code 250 identifies the general type of complication (e.g., ophthalmic, neurological, or circulatory). The fifth digit identifies the type of diabetes (type 1 or type 2) and whether it is controlled or uncontrolled. If diabetes is controlled, blood glucose levels are maintained within the normal range through drugs, diet, exercise, or a combination of these. Uncontrolled diabetes occurs when blood glucose levels are out of the normal range (i.e., high or low). An additional (secondary) code is used to describe the specific complication associated with the diabetes (i.e., it adds more detail). As discussed in Chapter 2, this usually involves the mandatory dual coding mechanism.

EXAMPLE

Uncontrolled diabetes mellitus type 2 with moderate nonproliferative retinopathy: 250.52 + 362.05

Diabetic peripheral vascular disease: 250.70 + 443.81

Nephropathy secondary to uncontrolled insulin-dependent diabetes mellitus, Type I: 250.43 + 583.81

Diabetic ulcer, left lower leg: 250.80 + 707.10

Diabetic retinitis: 250.50 + 362.01

Acute osteomyelitis, left great toe, attributable to type 1 diabetes mellitus: 250.81 + 731.8 + 730.07

Type I diabetic gastroparesis: 250.61 + 536.3

Do not assume that a patient who is taking insulin has type 1 insulin-dependent diabetes. Often, even type 2 diabetics require insulin periodically to help regulate their diabetes. Hospital stays associated with surgery, infection, or stress can also precipitate episodes of hyperglycemia that require a brief insulin regimen. Only the physician can determine and document the type of diabetes the patient has. If you find conflicting information in the record, clarify the type of diabetes with the attending physician.

Because the type of diabetes changes the fifth digit code assignment, you should review the glucose ranges from the laboratory work to determine whether a patient might have uncontrolled diabetes that has not been sufficiently documented by the physician. If a thorough review of the record reveals a blood glucose of ≥300 mg/dL, use the Physician/Coder Query/Clarification Form to query the physician to determine whether the patient's diabetes mellitus was uncontrolled and required added monitoring and resources to treat. If so, request that the physician add supporting documentation to the record via an addendum.

Never code from the laboratory results alone without supporting physician documentation in other parts of the medical record (e.g., history and physical, progress notes, or clinical résumés).

OTHER DIABETIC-RELATED COMPLICATIONS AND MANIFESTATIONS

When a medical condition or drug causes the development of diabetes, it is called "secondary diabetes." Starting October 1, 2008, a new code category has been provided to report secondary diabetes, which is classified from 249.0X to 249.9X. Some medical conditions that may result in secondary diabetes include pancreatitis, HIV infection, Cushing syndrome, hyperthyroidism, cystic fibrosis, and depression. Drugs that have been linked to the development of secondary diabetes include diuretics, hormones, antidepressants, anticonvulsants, and certain types of chemotherapy and antihypertensive medications. However, remember Type I and Type II diabetes are still classified to category 250.XX.

Steroid-induced diabetes secondary to an adverse effect of the therapeutic use of methylprednisolone (Depo-Medrol): 249.00 + E932.0	**EXAMPLE**

Hypoglycemic reactions can occur spontaneously in nondiabetic patients as well as in diabetic patients, sometimes as a reaction to insulin administration. Spontaneous or reactive hypoglycemia in a nondiabetic patient is coded to 251.2. Spontaneous hypoglycemia in a diabetic is coded to 250.8X, and hypoglycemia with diabetic coma is coded to 250.3X. If hypoglycemia is specified as attributable to insulin, use code 251.0 with an additional E code from the Table of Drugs and Chemicals to identify the drug. Note that gestational diabetes (diabetes associated with pregnancy) is not considered "true" diabetes. This disease is covered in Chapter 15, "Complications of Pregnancy, Childbirth, and the Puerperium."

Hypothyroidism and Hyperthyroidism

The body needs thyroid hormone to maintain proper metabolism by helping body cells with their uptake of oxygen. A deficiency of thyroid hormone, known as **hypothyroidism** (category code 244), causes signs and symptoms such as low metabolic rate (i.e., slow metabolism), fatigue, mental slowness, and a loss of body heat. In contrast, an excess of thyroid hormone, known as **hyperthyroidism** (category code 242), causes signs and symptoms such as a high metabolic rate (i.e., fast metabolism), rapid heart rate, nervousness, an inability to concentrate, and excessive perspiration.

The most common form of hyperthyroidism is Graves disease (code 242.0X). Hyperthyroidism can be marked by a severe onset called a **thyrotoxic crisis** or **storm**, which changes the fifth digit assignment (e.g., Graves disease with acute crisis—assign code 242.01). Hyperthyroidism can be treated with a thyroidectomy (surgical removal of the overactive tissue) or administration of a radioactive iodine that destroys overactive thyroid tissue. Such treatment can result in a postsurgical (244.0) or postablative (244.1) hypothyroidism, which is amenable to treatment through hormone-replacement drugs such as levothyroxine (Synthroid).

Review the record and all subterms (essential modifiers) to assign the proper type of hyperthyroidism or hypothyroidism code.

Syndrome of Inappropriate Antidiuretic Hormone and Associated Hyponatremia

The pituitary gland is an endocrine gland at the base of the brain that secretes antidiuretic hormone. **Anti** means "against," and a diuretic produces urine. The condition known as **syndrome of inappropriate antidiuretic hormone** (code 253.6) occurs when the pituitary gland secretes too much antidiuretic hormone, causing the body to retain too much water. Sodium (or salt) in the body helps the body maintain a proper water volume, because salt draws water. However, an excess of antidiuretic hormone reduces salt in the circulating blood, creating a condition known as *hyponatremia*. Because hyponatremia is a common symptom of syndrome of inappropriate antidiuretic hormone, do not code it as a secondary diagnosis.

Cystic Fibrosis

Although cystic fibrosis is an exocrine disorder, it is worth mentioning here because cystic fibrosis is included in chapter 3 of the ICD-9-CM. In contrast to endocrine glands that secrete substances directly into the bloodstream, exocrine glands excrete substances through ducts to the outside of the body. Cystic fibrosis (code 277.0X) is characterized by decreased secretion of pancreatic digestive enzymes, causing improper digestion of fats and excess respiratory mucous discharge.

No cure is known for cystic fibrosis, and treatment is often directed at the presenting conditions, such as bowel obstruction (ileus), acute bronchitis, or obstructive pneumonia caused by the excessive mucus. Therapies may involve replacement of pancreatic enzymes to aid in the absorption of food or antibiotics to treat respiratory infections.

A combination code is available to express cystic fibrosis with meconium ileus (code 277.01). Because the condition of meconium ileus is included in the code description, no additional code is needed to add detail. However, general codes are available to describe pulmonary, gastrointestinal, and other manifestations associated with cystic fibrosis. These general description codes require an additional code to describe the specific manifestation associated with the underlying condition of cystic fibrosis. The acute condition that occasions the admission to the hospital should be coded as the principal diagnosis.

Cystic fibrosis with meconium ileus: 277.01 only

Cystic fibrosis with obstructive pneumonia: 486 + 277.02 (cystic fibrosis with pulmonary manifestations; patient admitted for obstructive pneumonia)

EXAMPLE

Nutritional Disorders

Commonly coded nutritional disorders include malnutrition, vitamin deficiencies, and obesity. Nutritional disorders are becoming more prevalent in our society and, as a result, are attracting more attention in the media today. One major contributing factor for the increase in nutritional disorders is the overconsumption of high-calorie, low-nutrition fast foods, which results in an increased occurrence of obesity in the population. Also, fad diets ("starvation diets"), which severely restrict the foods people consume, can lead to vitamin deficiencies and malnutrition. To respond to the increased incidence of nutritional disorders, health-care providers are increasing nutritional services.

Malnutrition

Malnutrition results from a lack of nourishment and is commonly associated with a deficient diet, an underlying organic disease such as cancer, acquired immunodeficiency syndrome, intestinal malabsorption, and feeding difficulties (e.g., poststroke dysphagia). Failure to eat or properly absorb food can result in protein-calorie malnutrition or marasmus (extreme malnutrition). These disorders are included in code categories 260 to 269. Protein-calorie malnutrition (code 263.9) is usually associated with diets high in carbohydrates (starch) and sugars but deficient in protein. For example, it may be found in teenagers who exclusively eat "junk food" diets high in sugar and carbohydrates (e.g., candy and potato chips). Kwashiorkor (code 260) is a form of severe protein deficiency noted by changes in skin and hair pigment, edema (swelling), and retarded growth. Nutritional marasmus (code 261) is an extreme form of malnutrition in which one exhibits severe tissue wasting with loss of subcutaneous fat that can be associated with wasting diseases such as disseminated (widespread) cancer.

Treatment for malnutrition can include hyperalimentation (code 99.15), which involves the intravenous (IV) administration of nutritional substances or percutaneous endoscopic gastrostomy tube placement (code 43.11) for infusion of nourishment via a tube placed through the abdominal wall directly into the stomach. Malnutrition may be the principal diagnosis or secondary diagnosis, depending on the circumstances of the admission. Eating disorders such as anorexia nervosa will be covered in Chapter 19 on mental disorders.

Vitamin and Mineral Deficiencies

Usually derived from foods, vitamins provide essential nutrients necessary to maintain good health. Vitamin-deficiency codes are rarely assigned as the principal diagnosis because they generally do not require an inpatient admission. However, you may assign a vitamin-deficiency code as a secondary diagnosis that affects the overall care of the patient. Vitamin B12 and vitamin D are commonly coded vitamin deficiencies. Vitamin B12 can be found in milk, eggs, and meat (e.g., liver), and it is necessary for the proper development of red blood cells.

Symptoms of vitamin B12 deficiency (code 266.2) include anemia, fatigue, and weight loss. An inadequate diet and alcohol abuse can cause vitamin B12 deficiency. Organic causes of B12 deficiency may include inadequate absorption of food because of malnutrition or pernicious anemia. In pernicious anemia, an individual lacks a substance called **intrinsic factor in gastric secretions** that is necessary for the absorption of B12. If a physician documents pernicious anemia with B12 deficiency, only the code for the anemia is assigned. The B12 deficiency is included in the anemia code (pernicious anemia with B12 deficiency: 281.0).

Vitamin D deficiency (category 268) has recently become more prevalent in children. This is caused by a more sedentary lifestyle (e.g., watching television or spending long hours on the computer) in which they spend less time outdoors and are not exposed to sunlight, which is a source of vitamin D. Vitamin D is necessary to promote the absorption of calcium through the small intestine into the blood, where it is used for proper bone development. Vitamin D deficiency in children can cause rickets (a metabolic bone disease) and is coded to 268.0. This can cause pain on walking and the development of deformities such as "bowlegs" or "knock knees." Vitamin D deficiency in adults may cause osteomalacia (softening of the bone) and is coded to 268.2.

Obesity, Morbid Obesity, and Overweight

Obesity is reaching epidemic proportions in the United States and is the underlying cause for numerous associated medical conditions/diseases. Obesity can lead to joint disease, heart disease, and type 2 diabetes, which can further progress to renal disease and other associated conditions. Unspecified obesity is coded to 278.00, morbid obesity is coded to 278.01, and overweight is coded to 278.02. Morbid obesity is defined as "sufficient to prevent normal activity or physiologic function, or to cause the onset of a pathologic condition."[1] Morbid obesity may be diagnosed when a person is at least twice his or her ideal body weight, 100 pounds over an ideal body weight, or has a Body Mass Index (BMI) that is greater than 39.

Starting October 1, 2005, if documented by the physician, you may use an additional V-code with subcategory 278.0X to identify Body Mass Index (V85.21-V85.4). Body Mass Index (BMI) uses a person's weight and height to calculate the total body fat in adults (over 20 years old). BMI is used to determine when added weight puts a person at a higher risk for related health disorders such as diabetes, hypertension, and heart disease. The higher the BMI, the greater the risk of developing associated health problems (e.g., BMI 26-27 = 20% overweight with a moderate health risk). In addition, because of the increasing concerns regarding weight in children (both over- and underweight), new subcategory codes (V85.5X) have been provided to indicate BMI for pediatric patients (ages 2–20 years), which is based on growth charts (percentiles for age) published by the Centers for Disease Control and Prevention (CDC).

The code for a patient's BMI may also effect the hospital's reimbursement under MS-DRGs; and as such, a coder should thoroughly review the medical record to determine if the BMI has been established and documented. The patient's BMI may be located in the nutritionist's notes or documented by a physician; however, per official coding guidelines (i.e., AHA's Coding Clinic), a coder cannot assign a BMI based solely on the patient's weight and height that were documented in the record. In order to assign a BMI code, a registered dietician or a physician must document it.

Increasing obesity counseling and treatment services will be a primary initiative of health-care providers in the future. Proper diet and exercising will be stressed; however, invasive (surgical) treatment for obesity has been increasing. Invasive treatment can include gastric bypass (44.31). Gastric bypass involves decreasing the size of the stomach and bypassing the duodenum, where most food is absorbed (i.e., reconnecting [anastomosing] the stomach to the jejunum called a gastrojejunostomy).

Metabolic Disorders

Metabolism involves all the chemical processes necessary to maintain healthy cells to support a healthy body. Commonly coded metabolic disorders include hypokalemia (low blood potassium), hyponatremia (low blood sodium), and dehydration (lack of water), which are included in code category 276.

Electrolytes: Sodium and Potassium

It is important for the body to maintain a balance of substances called *electrolytes*, such as potassium and sodium, to help us conduct electricity for the proper functioning of nerves and muscles. Muscles, including the heart, cannot contract without electricity, so there must be proper nerve-to-muscle functioning for health. Hypopotassemia (low blood potassium), more commonly called **hypokalemia** (code 276.8), can sometimes occur as a consequence of taking diuretics to control hypertension. Diuretic drugs reduce fluid in the blood through urination and waste potassium, which must be supplemented with potassium replacement drugs such as potassium chloride (K-Dur).

Volume Depletion

Starting October 1, 2005, new codes were added to provide more detail to subcategory 276.5X for Volume Depletion (abnormal loss of body fluid levels). This is because volume depletion, unspecified (276.50) can sometimes be more precisely described as dehydration (276.51), which is associated with an abnormal loss of total body water; or, hypovolemia (276.52), which is associated with an abnormal loss of blood volume.

Code 276.51, dehydration, often occurs as a complication of vomiting and diarrhea associated with gastroenteritis. Generally, if a patient is admitted with dehydration secondary to a bout of noninfectious gastroenteritis, the acute reason for inpatient hospitalization is secondary to the dehydration (e.g., the patient is given oral medication for treatment of gastroenteritis, versus IV fluids for treatment of dehydration). Oral medications could have been prescribed for outpatient use, whereas IV fluids necessitated inpatient admission. According to principal diagnosis guidelines, you should code the dehydration as the principal diagnosis and gastroenteritis as the secondary diagnosis. This rule does not apply when a patient is admitted for dehydration secondary to infectious gastroenteritis and the patient receives IV antibiotics.

EXAMPLE	*A patient is admitted with nausea, vomiting, and diarrhea consistent with noninfectious gastroenteritis and subsequent dehydration. She receives IV fluid hydration for the dehydration and diphenoxylate and atropine (Lomotil) and promethazine (Phenergan) by mouth for the diarrhea, nausea, and vomiting. In this case, the dehydration would be sequenced as the principal diagnosis because it received the focus of treatment, and the noninfectious gastroenteritis would be sequenced as an additional code. The nausea and vomiting would not be coded, because they represent symptoms routinely associated with gastroenteritis (code 276.51 + 558.9).*
	A patient is admitted with persistent nausea, vomiting, and diarrhea with dehydration. Subsequent stool cultures were positive for Clostridium difficile bacteria. If the patient was admitted for IV antibiotics (e.g., IV metronidazole [Flagyl] or IV levofloxacin [Levaquin]) and IV fluid hydration, the infectious gastroenteritis should be sequenced as the principal diagnosis, and dehydration should be sequenced as an additional code (008.45 + 276.51).

Hypercholesterolemia and Hypertriglyceridemia

Hypercholesterolemia (code 272.0) and hypertriglyceridemia (code 272.1) are disorders of lipid (fat) metabolism that are often associated with a high-fat diet. Both conditions are often seen as secondary diagnoses and comorbid conditions that, if uncontrolled, can lead to atherosclerosis (hardening of the arteries with fatty plaque). A comorbid condition is a preexisting condition that did not cause the admission to the hospital but that affects the care of the patient and requires the facility to expend more resources to treat the patient. Comorbid conditions may or may not effect your MS-DRG payment; however, they should still be reported as additional diagnosis.

Immune Disorders

On a biological cell level, the function of the immune system is to defend our body from attacks by harmful foreign invaders called **antigens**. The body produces antibodies in response to these attacks to kill antigens. Antigens can include harmful bacteria, viruses, or cancer cells. Also, in autoimmune disorders, one's own body creates antibodies against its own healthy tissues that are recognized as antigens (e.g., rheumatoid arthritis is an autoimmune disorder in which one creates abnormal antibodies that attack one's own joint tissues, which become inflamed, painful, and disfigured).

Although rarely coded, various specified and unspecified immune disorders are included in code category 279 from chapter 3 of the ICD-9-CM (e.g., selective immunoglobulin A immunodeficiency [279.01] and unspecified immunity deficiency [279.3]). These underlying immune deficiencies, whether of hereditary or acquired origin, impair the normal function of the immune system, and this can be the primary cause of other manifestations of disease. Immune disorders contained in code category 279 do not include diseases related to human immunodeficiency virus or acquired immunodeficiency syndrome, which are covered in Chapter 6 on infectious diseases.

SUMMARY

This chapter has focused on learning to code common endocrine, nutritional, metabolic, and immune disorders by using the ICD-9-CM. This has included an opportunity for you to apply this new knowledge in locating the correct codes in each of these classifications in the ICD-9-CM codebook. This is followed by an opportunity to demonstrate that you can apply your new knowledge to coding medical reports and records.

REFERENCE

1. Stedman's Medical Dictionary, 27th Ed. Baltimore: Williams & Wilkins, 2000.

TESTING YOUR COMPREHENSION

1. Should the use of insulin always be considered an indicator of type 1 insulin-dependent diabetes?

   _____

2. What is the effect of syndrome of inappropriate antidiuretic hormone?

   _____

3. What disorder is characterized by decreased secretion of pancreatic digestive enzymes?

   _____

4. What condition may occur as a consequence of taking diuretics to control hypertension?

   _____

5. Hypercholesterolemia and hypertriglyceridemia are disorders of lipid metabolism that are frequently associated with what type of diet?

   _____

6. Vomiting and diarrhea, when associated with gastroenteritis, can result in what condition?

   _____

7. What rule applies to coding long-term complications or manifestations of diabetes?

   _____

8. What is the most common type of hyperthyroidism?

   _____

9. Cystic fibrosis is characterized by decreased secretion of pancreatic digestive enzymes. What does this cause?

   _____

10. What is protein-calorie malnutrition generally associated with?

   _____

11. What is a vitamin D deficiency in adults often associated with?

   _____

12. In children, what is a vitamin D deficiency associated with?

   _____

13. "All of the chemical processes necessary to maintain healthy cells to support a healthy body" describes what process?

   _____

14. Electrolytes are essential for the proper functioning of which two body systems?

   _____

15. Comorbidity is described as a preexisting condition that does not necessarily cause admission to the hospital. However, its presence does exert a considerable influence. Describe that influence.

   _____

CODING PRACTICE I — Chapter Review Exercises

Directions

By using your ICD-9-CM codebook, code the following diagnoses and procedures:

	DIAGNOSIS/PROCEDURES	CODE
1	Diagnosis: Diabetic gastroparesis. Procedure: Insertion of a percutaneous endoscopic gastrostomy tube.	
2	Type 1 diabetic neuropathy.	
3	Adult-onset diabetes mellitus with hypoglycemia.	
4	Diagnosis: Graves disease. Procedure: Partial thyroidectomy.	
5	Postablation [destruction] hypothyroidism.	
6	Severe hyponatremia secondary to syndrome of inappropriate antidiuretic hormone.	
7	Acute congestive pneumonia; cystic fibrosis.	
8	Diagnosis: Malnutrition. Status post cerebrovascular accident with dysphagia. Procedure: Gastrostomy tube insertion.	
9	Intractable (persistent) vomiting with dehydration treated with IV fluids and oral Phenergan as needed.	
10	Diagnosis: Morbid obesity. BMI of 48. Procedure: Gastric stapling (gastroplasty).	
11	Coronary atherosclerosis. Hypercholesterolemia.	
12	Hypertensive cardiovascular disease with acute systolic heart failure. Hypokalemia.	
13	Diabetic ketoacidosis with coma. Type 1 insulin-dependent diabetes mellitus.	
14	Type 2 diabetes mellitus, uncontrolled. Atherosclerotic peripheral vascular disease (peripheral vascular disease) secondary to diabetes with gangrene, left great toe.	

	DIAGNOSIS/PROCEDURES	CODE
15	Hyperthyroidism with thyrotoxic crisis.	
16	Diabetic nephropathy. Type 1 insulin-dependent diabetes mellitus.	
17	Hypoparathyroidism with hypocalcemia.	
18	Diabetic peripheral vascular disease with ulcer of right leg.	
19	Anorexia nervosa. Severe protein-calorie malnutrition.	

20	Diagnosis: Ovarian cancer.
	        Metastases to liver, peritoneum, and colon.
	        Carcinomatosis.
	        Cachexia with severe malnutrition.
	Procedure: Exploratory laparotomy (staging).
	        Total abdominal hysterectomy with bilateral salpingo-oophorectomies.
	        Excisional biopsies of liver, peritoneum, and colon.	

Medical Record Case Studies

Instructions

1. Carefully review the medical reports provided for each case study.

2. Research any abbreviations and terms that are unfamiliar or unclear.

3. Identify as many diagnoses and procedures as possible.

4. Because only part of the patient's total record is available, determine what additional documentation you might need.

5. If appropriate, identify any questions you might ask the physician to code this case correctly and completely.

6. Complete the appropriate blanks below for each case study.

CHAPTER 5 CASE STUDIES

Case Study 5.1 (Coder/Abstract Summary Form)

Patient: **Jane Doe**

Patient documentation: **Review Medical Reports 5.1 and 5.2**

1. Principal diagnosis:

   _____

2. Secondary or other diagnoses:

   _____

3. Principal procedure:

   _____

4. Other procedures:

   _____

5. Additional documentation needed:

   _____

   _____

   _____

   _____

Case Study 5.1 (Continued)

6. Questions for the physician:

_____

_____

_____

MEDICAL REPORT 5.1

HISTORY AND PHYSICAL

PATIENT NO:	9999999
MED REC NO:	111111
NAME:	DOE, JANE
DOB:	
SS#:	999-99-9999
ADDR:	
ADDR:	
CITY:	
ROOM NO:	300
ADMISSION DATE:	
PHYSICIAN:	JOHN SMITH, M.D.

CHIEF COMPLAINT: Diarrhea and very weak.

HISTORY OF PRESENT ILLNESS: Ms. Doe is an 86-year-old lady who has lost five pounds since we saw her last. She has had diarrhea persistent for five days and is dehydrated. She is having abdominal discomfort. She is admitted for definitive therapy of this.

PAST MEDICAL HISTORY: Her past medical history is persistent for allergy to Avantin. She has had a history of glaucoma and chronic atrial fibrillation. She has had a total abdominal hysterectomy with oophorectomy, hiatal hernia repair, and pacemaker insertion and repair.

REVIEW OF SYSTEMS: She has a history of gastric reflux and chronic arthritis.

SOCIAL HISTORY: She does not smoke or drink.

FAMILY HISTORY: The family history is negative.

PHYSICAL EXAMINATION

VITAL SIGNS: Blood pressure is 120/80 and pulse 100 and regular. Weight is 95.5.

HEENT: Pupils show previous cataract surgery. Oropharynx is benign.

NECK: The neck is soft and supple. There are no carotid bruits.

LUNGS: The lungs are clear.

HEART: The heart has an irregular rate and rhythm at about 100.

ABDOMEN: The abdomen is soft with diffuse tenderness.

GENITOURINARY: Deferred.

RECTAL: Deferred.

EXTREMITIES: There are some arthritic changes of the knees. There is no clubbing, cyanosis, or edema.

NEUROLOGIC: Cranial nerves are intact. Motor and cerebellar function are normal.

MENTAL STATUS: She is anxious and says that she feels very weak.

Continued

MEDICAL REPORT 5.1 (CONTINUED)

IMPRESSION:

1. Dehydration and chronic diarrhea for five days.
2. Chronic atrial fibrillation. S/P cardiac pacer insertion.
3. History of gastric reflux.

PLAN OF CARE: Will admit and consult gastroenterology. Will rehydrate.

John Smith, M.D.
DICTATED: 07-15
TRANSCRIBED: 07-15

NOTES

MEDICAL REPORT 5.2

CONSULTATION REPORT

PATIENT NO: 9999999
MED REC NO: 111111
NAME: DOE, JANE
DOB:
SS#:   999-99-9999
ADDR:
ADDR:
CITY:
ROOM NO: 300
ADMISSION DATE:
PHYSICIAN: JOHN SMITH, M.D.

GASTROENTEROLOGY CONSULTATION

CONSULT DATE: 07-16

REASON FOR CONSULTATION: Evaluation of diarrhea.

DIAGNOSTIC IMPRESSION:
1. Diarrhea, rule out infectious causes; rule out colitis; rule out polyp.
2. Await stool studies including Clostridium difficile, ova and parasites, culture. Treat appropriately.
3. Colonoscopy. The patient requests that we hold off with colonoscopy until some of the stool studies are back so that she does not have to have the test if a diagnosis can be made some way else. Consider additional laboratories: CBC, chemistry profile, BUN, thyroid profile. IV hydration.

HISTORY: This is an 86-year-old woman who I was asked to see in consultation by Dr. Smith for evaluation of diarrhea. She has had several days now of multiple episodes of loose watery, non-bloody type of stools associated with some abdominal discomfort but no significant pain. She denies any blood in the stool. She denies any nausea or vomiting. She denies any severe cramps.

PAST HISTORY: Past history is significant for glaucoma and atrial fibrillation.

PAST SURGICAL HISTORY: Surgeries include an abdominal hysterectomy and oophorectomy, hiatal hernia repair and pacemaker insertion.

ALLERGIES: She is allergic to Avantin.

MEDICATIONS: Medications include Lanoxin, Prevacid, and Tylenol and Celexa.

SOCIAL HISTORY: Negative for tobacco or alcohol.

FAMILY HISTORY: Family history is negative for colon cancer.

REVIEW OF SYSTEMS: Review of systems is significant for dehydration, weakness, and fatigue. She denies any double vision, blurred vision, ringing in the ears. She denies any shortness of breath, coughing or chest pain. She denies any abdominal pain but has had the discomfort. No urinary tract difficulties.

Continued

MEDICAL REPORT 5.2 (CONTINUED)

PHYSICAL EXAMINATION

GENERAL: Physical examination reveals a well developed, elderly appearing, acutely ill looking, 86-year-old woman who is alert and oriented.

VITAL SIGNS: Blood pressure is 120/80, heart rate 98. She is afebrile.

HEENT: HEENT showed the head to be normocephalic and atraumatic. Sclerae were not icteric.

NECK: Supple without adenopathy.

LUNGS: Clear.

CARDIAC: The cardiac examination revealed no murmur, rub, or gallop.

ABDOMEN: The abdomen was soft. It was mildly tender diffusely. No rebound or guarding. Bowel sounds were normal.

EXTREMITIES: No cyanosis, clubbing, or edema.

LABORATORY: Laboratories show a BUN of 30 which has come down to 20. H&H is 11.0 and 32.7 with 40 neutrophils. Urinalysis shows trace leukocyte, 3+ blood, zero to two red blood cells, four to eight white cells. Fecal occult blood and other studies are still pending.

Thank you for allowing me to participate in the care of this patient. We will follow along and make additional recommendations as warranted.

_____

JOHN JONES, M.D.

DICTATED: 07-16
TRANSCRIBED: 07-16

NOTES

Case Study 5.2 (Coder/Abstract Summary Form)

Patient: **David Brown**

Patient documentation: **Review Medical Reports 5.3 and 5.4**

1. Principal diagnosis:

   _____

2. Secondary or other diagnoses:

   _____

3. Principal procedure:

   _____

4. Other procedures:

   _____

5. Additional documentation needed:

   _____

   _____

   _____

   _____

6. Questions for the physician:

   _____

   _____

   _____

   _____

   _____

MEDICAL REPORT 5.3

DISCHARGE SUMMARY

PT NAME:	BROWN, DAVID
MR#:	222222
ACCOUNT#:	9999999
AGE:	78
ROOM:	
DICTATED:	7/17
TRANSCRIBED:	7/17
DATE OF ADMISSION:	7/14
DATE OF DISCHARGE:	7/17
ATTENDING PHYSICIAN:	JOHN JONES, M.D.

DISCHARGE DIAGNOSIS: Type 2 diabetes mellitus, uncontrolled
> Hyperosmolar state
> Acute confusion
> Arterial hypertension
> Hyperlipidemia
> Senile dementia
> Hypercholesterolemia

COMPLICATIONS: None

BRIEF HISTORY: A 78-year-old male who usually goes to the VA Hospital for his health care is brought into the emergency room because of confusion. He was found to have a blood sugar higher than 600. The patient was given IV regular insulin and admitted to the hospital for further evaluation and management. Although he was confused, the neurologic examination showed no focal neurological deficits. The CT scan of the head showed no acute changes.

HOSPITAL COURSE: The patient was admitted to the hospital, given IV fluids and regular insulin as per sliding scale. He was started on IV empiric antibiotic with Claforan one-gram IV piggyback q. 8h. The chest x-ray showed no acute infiltrate. The urinalysis showed no evidence of urinary tract infection. The patient's sugar was controlled with improvement of the mental condition.

The patient has been able to ambulate and to resume regular diabetic diet. He was started on NPH insulin ten units twice a day with stabilization of his sugar around the 220 range. He is being discharged home with Home Health to continue NPH insulin twice a day that will be adjusted depending on the sugar results as well as regular insulin as per sliding scale. Glucophage will be continued as well as other prior medications. Discharge disposition/medications: Glucophage XR 500 mg two tablets q.p.m., Tenormin 50 mg b.i.d., Monopril 50 mg q.d., hydrochlorothiazide 25 mg q.d., Micro-K 8 mEq q.d., Procardia 90 mg q.d., Zocor 40 mg q.h.s., NPH insulin ten units in the morning and fifteen units in the evening, Colace 100 mg three times a day.

DIET: 1800 calorie ADA diet. Activity as tolerated. Home Health for Accu-Checks, diabetes teaching and monitor compliance with medications.

Follow-up in my office in two weeks.

JOHN JONES, M.D.

MEDICAL REPORT 5.4

HISTORY AND PHYSICAL

PT NAME:	BROWN, DAVID
MR#:	222222
ACCOUNT#:	9999999
AGE:	78
ROOM:	
DICTATED:	7/17
TRANSCRIBED:	7/17
DATE OF ADMISSION:	7/14
DATE OF DISCHARGE:	7/17
ATTENDING PHYSICIAN:	JOHN JONES, M.D.

CHIEF COMPLAINT: Confusion.

HISTORY AND PRESENT ILLNESS: This is a 78-year-old male with a history of diabetes, hypertension who was found lying on the floor by his wife and EMS was called. The patient was transported to the Emergency Room. On arrival he was confused and combative and had a blood sugar of higher than 600. The patient's initial vital signs were normal. The IV fluids and IV regular insulin were given as well as IV Haldol. The patient is being admitted in the hospital for further evaluation and management.

PAST MEDICAL HISTORY: The past medical history is unclear and from the medication list includes hypertension, hypercholesterolemia, type 2 diabetes mellitus, and osteoarthritis.

ALLERGIES: The patient has no known drug allergies.

MEDICATIONS: The patient's medications include Atenolol 50 mg b.i.d., Fosinopril 40 mg q.d., hydrochlorothiazide 25 mg q.d., KCl 10 mEq q.d., metformin 500 mg b.i.d., Procardia XL 90 mg q.d., Ranitidine 150 mg q.d., salicylate 500 mg b.i.d., Simvastatin 40 mg h.s., Terazosin 2 mg q.d.

SOCIAL HISTORY: The patient lives independently in the community with his wife. No further information is available.

FAMILY HISTORY: The family history is not able to be obtained.

REVIEW OF SYSTEMS: The review of systems is unable to be obtained. The patient was sedated after Haldol was administered.

PHYSICAL EXAMINATION: The blood pressure was 126/72, pulse 82, respiratory rate 16 and temperature 98.2. General appearance showed an elderly male drowsy but responds to questions, confused and disoriented. The neck was supple and there is no jugular venous distension. HEENT examination is unremarkable. There is no jaundice. The oral mucosa is well hydrated. The neck was supple with no jugular venous distension. The carotid pulses are two plus, no bruits, no lymphadenopathy or thyromegaly. The chest and lungs are clear to auscultation or percussion. The heart was normal S1, S2, no murmurs or friction rubs. The abdomen was obese, soft, no tenderness or distension, no hepatosplenomegaly.

LABORATORY DATA: The chest x-ray showed no acute infiltrate. The electrocardiogram has sinus arrhythmia with right bundle branch block. This lab showed an ABG with a pH of 7.36, PCO2 102, bicarbonate 21, saturation 98% on two liters nasal cannula. The complete blood count showed a white blood cell count of 7.4, hemoglobin 14.7, hematocrit 44% and MCV 78, platelets of 210,000. The neutrophils were 35, bands 5%, lymphocytes 6%. Urinalysis is negative. The glucose is four plus. The first set of cardiac enzymes is negative.

Continued

MEDICAL REPORT 5.4 (CONTINUED)

IMPRESSION:

1. Confusion.
2. Uncontrolled type 2 diabetes mellitus.
3. Arterial hypertension.
4. Hyperlipidemia.
5. Arteriosclerotic heart disease.

ASSESSMENT: This is an elderly man presenting with confusion, consider the differential diagnosis stroke verses underlying dementia due to uncontrolled hyperglycemia.

PLAN: Will admit the patient to the medical floor and give regular insulin per sliding scale, continue peripheral antibiotics, neuro checks. Will try to obtain prior history with the wife and review of old medical records.

_____

JOHN JONES, M.D.

NOTES

Case Study 5.3 (Coder/Abstract Summary Form)

Patient: **Carl Waters**

Patient documentation: **Review Medical Reports 5.5 and 5.6**

1. Principal diagnosis:

   _____

2. Secondary or other diagnoses:

   _____

3. Principal procedure:

   _____

4. Other procedures:

   _____

5. Additional documentation needed:

   _____

   _____

   _____

Case Study 5.3 (Continued)

6. Questions for the physician:

_____

_____

_____

_____

_____

_____

MEDICAL REPORT 5.5

DISCHARGE SUMMARY

PATIENT:	WATERS, CARL
MED. REC. NO.	33-33-33
DATE OF ADMISSION:	04-02
DATE OF DISCHARGE:	04-04

This is a 42-year-old white male who has been seen in my office for medical care the past six to eight months for rapidly progressive peripheral edema and almost generalized anasarca. He has developed shortness of breath and dyspnea even at rest. He has recently developed chest pain and has now become unmanageable for his fluid retention. The patient was admitted to the hospital on 04-02 for evaluation, workup, and management of this anasarca.

Consultations included nephrology for evaluation of his renal status as to the cause of this problem. Cardiology was also consulted for possible etiologic involvement of his cardiac system.

FINAL DIAGNOSES:
1. Peripheral edema and anasarca probably secondary to nephrotic syndrome which is most likely secondary to insulin-dependent diabetes mellitus, Type I.
2. Renal insufficiency with impending dialysis in the near future.
3. No significant involvement of his cardiac status even though the chest x-ray was read as bibasilar pleural effusion extending to the level of the posterior right 9th rib, questionable infiltrate could not be excluded.
4. Hypoxemia with a p02 of 80.
5. Anemia, most likely secondary to chronic disease.

DISCHARGE FOLLOW UP: To be with Dr. Smith in her office within the next seven days.

DISCHARGE DIET: 4-gram sodium diet.

DISCHARGE FOLLOW UP LABS: Was to include a CBC, chem profile, and a chest x-ray.

DISCHARGE MEDICATIONS: Include the resumption of all the medicines that he was admitted with which include the following: Zaroxolyn 10mg po b.i.d., Bumex 2mg po b.i.d., K-tab 20 meq 1 b.i.d., B-6 vitamin 50 mg q daily, Bethanechol 25 mg t.i.d., Procardia XL 60 mg q daily, Lente Insulin 30 units q a.m.

JANE SMITH, M.D.

D: 06-11

T: 06-13

MEDICAL REPORT 5.6

HISTORY AND PHYSICAL

PATIENT:	WATERS, CARL
MED. REC. NO.	33-33-33
DATE OF ADMISSION:	04-02
DATE OF DISCHARGE:	04-04

CHIEF COMPLAINT: Shortness of breath and peripheral edema and swelling.

HISTORY OF PRESENT ILLNESS: This is a 42-year-old white male who presents to my office today complaining of shortness of breath especially with exertion, mild to moderate cough for the last several days to a week. He denies any chest pain. Does smoke cigarettes one pack per day. He has no sore throat or fever, chills, or sweats. The patient does complain of slight post nasal drip but he has no history of asthma, COPD (chronic obstructive pulmonary disease), ischemic heart disease, or congestive heart failure. The patient also denies any nausea, vomiting, or stomach pain. The patient has been under the care of multiple physicians including a hematologist, nephrologist, and an endocrinologist as well as me and he has had definitive diagnosis of nephrotic syndrome for which he is being treated with diuretics to eradicate the fluid, blood transfusions to restore the anemia, and bed rest to help the nephrotic syndrome. He has progressively worsened with increasing weight gain, elevated blood pressure, and severe fatigue.

PAST MEDICAL HISTORY: Initially seen in September by Dr. Jones for peripheral edema. He obtained some blood work on him and found a sodium of 124, chloride 92, creatinine 1.4, albumin of 2.6, total protein of 5.2. Magnesium of 1.4, calcium of 8.2 and a phosphorous of 4.7. His SGPT was 295; SGOT 49; LDH 493. His cholesterol was 147. The patient was to follow-up with the office on a strict diet and better control of the insulin and he was also placed on diuretics. The patient showed no significant improvement. He had continually elevated glucoses to 368 and low hemoglobin. The patient's creatinine done at an endocrinology office in November revealed creatinine of .6, Sodium 126, with a hematocrit of 20. He had a retic count of 5.8%. The patient was seen by me on October. We had done some preliminary hemolytic evaluations including glucose 6; phosphorate D. Hydrogenase which was normal. We also did hemoglobin electrophoresis which was normal. We did Coombs' test which was negative. Haptoglobin which was less than 10.5, normal being 100 to 300. Reviewing the G6 PD, the quantitative G6 PD was 4.20, normal being 1.9 to 3.4. The patient has been on diuretics for the last several months with some improvement and then a relapse. I switched him to Bumex and 10 mg of Zaroxolyn simultaneously; therefore, his dosage was decreased. He is getting ongoing laser therapy for his retinal hemorrhages.

SURGERY: Tonsillectomy at five years old. Diabetes mellitus began approximately 1980 of which the last five to six years was insulin-dependent. Denies any history of ischemic heart disease angina, MI, etc.

MEDICATIONS: K-tab 10 mEq once a day; B6 50 mg t.k.d.; Bethanechol 25 mg t.i.d.; Zaroxolyn 5 mg per day; Bumex 1 mg t.i.d.; Procardia XL 60 mg qd.; Lente insulin 30 units per day.

ALLERGIES: None.

FAMILY HISTORY: Mother alive and well. No history of ischemic heart disease, just positive for rheumatoid arthritis. Father is alive and well. No history of ischemic heart disease. Smokes one pack per day.

PHYSICAL EXAM: Well-developed, well-nourished, pale in pallor, white male who is in mild distress secondary to fatigue.

WEIGHT: 198 pounds.

BP: 180/117.

PULSE: 90.

TEMP: 98.9.

RESPIRATIONS: 16.

HEENT: PERRLA. EOMs intact. Funduscopy revealed grade 3 retinopathy to grade 4. TMs clear. Throat clear.

MEDICAL REPORT 5.6 (CONTINUED)

NECK: There is JVD at 75 degrees. No carotid bruits. No hepatojugular reflux. Thyroid normal.

LUNGS: Significantly decreased breath sounds in the right lower lobe posteriorly. Scattered occasional rales and rhonchi present. No wheezes.

CARDIAC: Sinus tachycardia. No murmurs. Questionable S-3 gallop. No rubs. PMI not localized.

CHEST: Nontender to palpation.

ABDOMEN: Bowel sounds present. Abdomen is nontender. No hepatosplenomegaly.

EXTREMITIES: 5+ pre-tibial edema that goes up toward his scrotal area.

GENITALIA: Deferred.

RECTAL: Deferred.

NEURO: N1.

LAB: Chest x-ray in my office reveals a right effusion on his lung that goes 2/3 the way up his lung fields. Cardiac silhouette is greatly enlarged.

IMPRESSION:
1. Edema, etiology includes probably nephrotic syndrome based on the patient's presentation and his other physical findings but some of the other causes of the peripheral edema cannot be excluded whether primary or secondary and these include Budd-Chiari syndrome, pulmonary emboli, constrictive pericarditis, congestive heart failure.
2. Shortness of breath secondary to nephrotic syndrome plus new development of congestive heart failure whether secondary to nephrotic syndrome and the anemia is not clear.
3. Severe anemia, etiology is unclear. Has labeled due to anemia of chronic disease but there has been a positive G6 PD and elevated retic and decreased haptoglobin demonstrated as an outpatient.

PLAN: Fully work the patient up to evaluate the exact cause. To determine whether nephrotic syndrome is due to diabetes or whether it is due to something else that requires a renal biopsy so that definitive therapy may or may not be instituted.

JANE SMITH, M.D.
D: 04-02
T: 04-03

NOTES

Coding for Infectious and Parasitic Diseases

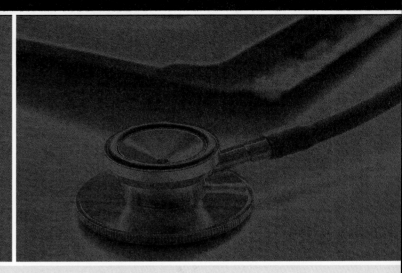

Chapter Outline

Chapter Objectives

▶ Describe the pathology of common infectious and parasitic diseases.

▶ Recognize the typical manifestations, complications, and treatments of common infectious and parasitic diseases in terms of their implications for coding.

▶ Correctly code common infectious and parasitic diseases by using the ICD-9-CM and medical records.

Infectious and parasitic diseases are included in code section 001 to 139 of chapter 1 of the Disease Tabular of the ICD-9-CM. This includes communicable (transmissible) diseases and other diseases of infectious origin. This chapter highlights some of the more common infectious diseases that cause inpatient hospital admissions. These diseases include sepsis, infectious gastroenteritis with dehydration, respiratory syncytial virus (RSV), AIDS- and HIV-related disease, viral hepatitis, meningitis, and tuberculosis. To assist in your understanding, the Word Parts Box on page 122 reviews word parts and meanings of medical terms related to infectious and parasitic diseases.

Word Parts and Meanings of Medical Terms Related to Infectious and Parasitic Diseases

Word Part	Meaning	Example	Definition of Example
-emia	condition of the blood	septicemia	Presence of pathogenic bacteria in the blood; blood poisoning
gastr/o	stomach	gastroenteritis	Inflammation of the mucous membrane of the stomach and intestine
-itis	inflammation	hepatitis	Inflammation of the liver
bacteri/o	bacterium	bacteremia	Presence of viable bacteria in the circulating blood
-penia	decrease in, deficiency of	neutropenia	Decreased number of neutrophils in the circulating blood
mening/o, meninge/o	meninges	meningitis	Inflammation of the meninges of the brain or spinal cord
immun/o	immunity, immune system	immunocompromised	Individual whose immune system is deficient

In coding infectious diseases, sometimes a single combination code designates both the organism and condition. However, at other times, two codes (i.e., dual coding) must be used to designate the condition and organism involved.

EXAMPLE

Staphylococcus aureus *pneumonia: 482.41 (single combination code)*
Clostridium difficile *enteritis: 008.45 (single combination code)*
Aspergillus *pneumonia: 117.3 + 484.6 (dual coding required)*
Urinary tract infection with **Escherichia coli** *bacteria: 599.0 + 041.4 (dual coding required)*

Septicemia

Septicemia involves an overwhelming systemic infection (i.e., an infection affecting many organs) with pathogenic (disease-causing) organisms, usually bacterial, invading the bloodstream. Septicemia is a life-threatening condition that can result in hemodynamic collapse (i.e., the cessation of systemic circulation) and multiorgan system failure if not treated immediately (e.g., by intravenous administration of broad-spectrum antibiotics). Symptoms that characterize septicemia include:

- high fever
- hypotension
- rapid heart and pulse rates
- confusion secondary to toxic encephalopathy (a brain disorder caused by the toxic effects of certain substances)
- leukocytosis (increased white blood cells) or shift to the left (**shift to the left** is a phrase commonly used by physicians that indicates that the patient has an infection [i.e., an increase in circulating immature white blood cells caused by the destruction of mature white blood cells by infection])
- renal failure
- toxic or septic shock

Septicemia is usually coded to category 038; the fourth and fifth digits identify the precise bacterial organism involved. Other specified septicemias (viral) are coded elsewhere. If sepsis or septicemia with septic shock is listed, code the sepsis or septicemia first, followed by the code for septic shock.

Remember, septic shock code 785.52 comes from chapter 16 (category codes 780 to 799), "Signs and Symptoms," and should be listed second in this situation.

Often the terms **sepsis** and **septicemia** are used interchangeably by physicians. With the October 1, 2002 coding changes, systemic inflammatory response syndrome (SIRS) codes (995.9X) were introduced that can be used as additional codes in combination with the sepsis or septicemia codes from the 038 category.

Various conditions can cause SIRS. However, the terms **sepsis** or **SIRS** must be present to assign a code from the 995.9X category. For example, *Staphylococcus* sepsis would be coded to 038.10 + 995.91, whereas *Staphylococcus* septicemia would be coded only to 038.10 unless specified, as with SIRS. Under the subclassification code 995.9X in the Disease Tabular, please refer to the inclusion note that specifies to "code first underlying condition." The addition of SIRS denotes an advanced complication of an infection, disease, or trauma that includes systemic inflammation.

Coding Clinic 2003, fourth quarter, describes SIRS more fully.

EXAMPLE

Escherichia coli *septicemia: 038.42*
Escherichia coli *sepsis: 038.42 + 995.91*
Escherichia coli *septicemia with SIRS: 038.42 + 995.91*
Escherichia coli *sepsis with septic shock: 038.42 + 995.91 + 785.52*
Acute pancreatitis with SIRS: 577.0 + 995.93

If a patient presents with septic symptoms and the physician's impression is possible clinical septicemia, the physician will order broad-spectrum intravenous antibiotics immediately because of the urgency of the clinical situation. Sometimes, because antibiotics have already been given or because of problems inherent in culturing blood, subsequent blood cultures do not grow an identifiable bacterial organism. Even if antibiotics were ordered to treat septic symptoms, you can code clinical sepsis as the principal diagnosis (code 038.9), provided that the attending physician documented the septic symptoms (revealing the severity of illness), the appropriate treatment (revealing the intensity of health-care service), and the diagnosis of "clinical sepsis or septicemia" within the medical record.

Urosepsis and Bacteremia

A "red flag" should go up when the physician documents urosepsis.

Although the ICD-9-CM classifies urosepsis as a urinary tract infection (code 599.0), physicians who document urosepsis are often referring to a urinary tract infection that invades the blood and leads to septicemia. When you see urosepsis documented by the physician, review the medical record—especially the blood and urine culture and sensitivity and physician's progress notes—to clarify the coding of septicemia. Also, query the physician if necessary. If the patient has both a urinary tract infection and septicemia, code the septicemia first and the urinary tract infection second because septicemia is a more acute cause for inpatient admission. Urinary tract infections do not often require an inpatient admission.

Bacteremia (code 790.7) is a transient septic condition covered in chapter 16, "Signs and Symptoms." Normally, bacteremia is quickly arrested by the patient's own immune response and does not require an inpatient admission. However, some physicians use the term *bacteremia* to mean sepsis or septicemia, and you should query to clarify the diagnosis for coding.

TIP   *Coding Clinic* 1998, first quarter, and 2000, second quarter, describe sepsis, urosepsis, and bacteremia more fully.

Resistant Organisms

Today's universal precautions, patient isolation, and negative air-pressure rooms all help to prevent the spread of infections in hospitals and other health-care facilities. These precautions are enforced by laws and standards of accrediting bodies, and hospitals must monitor the precautions and take action to prevent infections from occurring within the facility. Inappropriate use of antibiotics can cause pathogenic organisms to develop a resistance to those drugs. Consequently, scientists must continually research and develop new generations of antibiotics to combat the resurgence of drug-resistant organisms. Category code V09 of the ICD-9-CM helps to identify patients who present with drug-resistant infectious organisms (e.g., methicillin-resistant *Staphylococcus aureus,* code V09.0). Locate these codes under the main term "resistance" in the Disease Index. Use "resistance" codes as secondary diagnosis codes, when applicable.

Additional Codes for Bacterial and Viral Agents

When a combination code (i.e., a single code that identifies both the disease and responsible organism) is not provided, use category code 041 as an additional code to identify the precise bacterial organism responsible for the principal disease, and use category code 079 as an additional code to identify the precise virus responsible for the principal disease. List the disease first, followed by the responsible organism code.

EXAMPLE

Escherichia coli *urinary tract infection: 599.0 + 041.4*
Pneumonia attributable to Hantavirus: 480.8 + 079.81

Although rare, both 041 and 079 category codes can sometimes be used as a principal diagnosis when the physician documents a bacterial or viral infection of unspecified site, source, or nature. This can occur when the patient is immunocompromised and presents with general symptoms, such as fever and chills, that respond to antibiotic or antiviral therapy but when a specific site or source of the infection cannot be determined. An immunocompromised patient has a suppressed immune system, which results in an increased susceptibility to infections that are usually prevented through normal defenses.

TIP Often, cancer patients can become immunocompromised because a common side effect of chemotherapy is neutropenia (decreased white blood cell count). This can result in an admission for a bacterial infection in which the site of infection cannot be readily identified and would be coded to the 041 category as the principal diagnosis. The physician must identify "Bacterial Infection" as the principal diagnosis to be able to sequence a code from category 041 first, and this must be supported by additional documentation within the medical record. Similarly to category 041, category code 079 can sometimes be used as a principal diagnosis when the physician documents viral infection of unspecified nature or site.

TIP Be sure to review the Disease Tabular notes under the 041 and 079 categories in the ICD-9-CM books; they provide important coding instructions.

Infectious Gastroenteritis with Dehydration

When a patient is admitted for both infectious gastroenteritis and dehydration and is treated for both conditions (e.g., is given intravenous antibiotics for the infectious gastroenteritis and intravenous fluids for the dehydration), sequence the infectious gastroenteritis first. If only the dehydration is aggressively treated with intravenous fluids and the infectious gastroenteritis is treated with oral medication, then sequence the dehydration first. In this case, the intravenous fluids necessitate inpatient admission, whereas oral medication could be prescribed on an outpatient basis.

Respiratory Syncytial Virus

Respiratory syncytial virus (RSV) is a contagious viral infection that commonly affects the lungs. RSV often results in severe pneumonia in children and the elderly, who are more susceptible to an aggressive infection. RSV is contracted through inhaling airborne droplets or coming into contact with infected individuals. Symptoms include fever, rhinorrhea (runny nose), sore throat, dyspnea (difficult breathing), coughing, and wheezing.

Inpatient admission may be necessary to provide respiratory therapy or treatment with passive immunization (i.e., "ready-made" antibodies) to fight the disease. RSV infection of unspecified site is coded to 079.6, and combination codes are available that describe both the condition and the virus for RSV bronchiolitis (466.11) and RSV pneumonia (480.1).

AIDS- and HIV-Related Conditions

Aquired Immunodeficiency Syndrome (AIDS) is a syndrome that results in suppression of the immune system caused by Human Immunodeficiency Virus (HIV)-1. It is characterized by opportunistic infections, viruses, cancers, and neurologic disorders.

T-cell lymphocytes fight infection and disease and are important to our immune response. HIV, the virus responsible for AIDS, attaches to a CD4 protein within a T-cell lymphocyte and causes cell death.

In AIDS, the resulting destruction of T-cell lymphocytes depresses the immune system and makes the patient immunocompromised (i.e., more susceptible to opportunistic infections and cancers). The ensuing infections, such as *Pneumocystis carinii* pneumonia, often cause morbidity (disease) and mortality (death) in AIDS patients. Many drugs are available today to inhibit the growth of HIV (e.g., reverse transcriptase and protease inhibitors).

Coding Infections or Diseases Related to HIV/AIDS

For coding infections or diseases related to AIDS, AIDS-like syndrome, AIDS-related complex, or HIV, the general coding rule is to assign the AIDS code (042) first, followed by the code for the complication or manifestation. If documented because of AIDS or HIV, common related infections and diseases include:

- *Pneumocystis carinii* pneumonia—code 042 + 136.3
- *Mycobacterium avium-intracellulare*—code 042 + 031.2
- *Histoplasma* pneumonia—code 042 + 115.95
- Cytomegalovirus—code 042 + 078.5
- Pulmonary tuberculosis—code 042 + 011.90
- Kaposi's sarcoma of the skin—code 042 + 176.0
- Lymphoma—code 042 + 202.80

If a patient is admitted for a condition unrelated to AIDS or HIV (e.g., appendicitis or a fractured arm from a fall), code the condition first (as the principal diagnosis), with the AIDS code (042) and any associated conditions assigned as secondary diagnoses.

EXAMPLE

A patient is admitted for laparoscopic cholecystectomy because of acute cholecystitis with cholelithiasis. The patient has HIV-related Kaposi's sarcoma on the skin of the legs.

Principal diagnosis: 574.00
Secondary diagnosis: 042
Secondary diagnosis: 176.0
Procedure: 51.23

Unfortunately, possible social and employment stigmata can be associated with an AIDS- or HIV-related diagnosis. Because of this, there is an exception to the inpatient rule for coding possible, probable, suspected, rule-out, and questionable diagnoses as if the condition existed. This Uniform Hospital Discharge Data Set inpatient coding rule does not apply to the diagnosis of AIDS. You should ask the physician to state the diagnosis in precise terms. Physicians are not always aware of inpatient Uniform Hospital Discharge Data Set coding rules for assigning a principal diagnosis or the consequences attached.

In the case of an HIV-infected mother and possible transmission of HIV antibodies to the fetus, neonates may test positive on the enzyme-linked immunosorbent assay (ELISA), a laboratory test that looks for HIV antibodies as evidence of infection. However, because neonates carry the immune status (antibodies) of the mother only for a short while, be sure to code positive neonate testing on the enzyme-linked immunosorbent assay test to 795.71 (inconclusive HIV test) until future testing confirms or negates the neonate's true HIV status. Add code 795.71 as a secondary diagnosis code on the neonate's record. The principal diagnosis for neonates is always coded to category V30-39 and can be located in the Disease Index under "newborn" because the reason for admission on a patient born during that admission is to be born.

HIV Testing Codes

The following HIV testing or counseling codes are commonly used to explain the reason for an outpatient encounter; however, they may be used, along with HIV status codes, as secondary codes for inpatient admission, when applicable:

- ▶ HIV screening is coded to V73.59 (locate under "screening, disease, viral, specified type" in the Disease Index)
- ▶ HIV counseling is coded to V65.44 (locate under "counseling, HIV" in the Disease Index)
- ▶ an inconclusive HIV test result is coded to 795.71 (locate under "findings abnormal, serological, HIV, inconclusive" in the Disease Index)
- ▶ V08 is coded for asymptomatic HIV infection status (locate under "human immunodeficiency virus" in the Disease Index)

Viral Hepatitis

There are three main types of viral hepatitis: type A, type B, and type C. When coding viral hepatitis (category code 070), the fourth digit identifies the type of hepatitis involved, and the fifth digit identifies other manifestations of the disease.

Type A hepatitis, also called **infectious hepatitis**, is caused by contaminated food or water (commonly from stool to mouth via poor hygiene) and is usually a self-limiting (i.e., short-lived) disease that causes no significant long-term liver damage.

Type B hepatitis, also called **serum hepatitis**, is of particular concern to hospital workers who are involved in direct patient care because it can be acquired through needlesticks (i.e., parenterally) and can lead to chronic liver disease. It can also be transmitted by sharing needles, through body fluids and blood transfusions, and from mother to baby. A vaccination to prevent type B hepatitis is provided to health-care personnel who provide direct patient care, and hospitals routinely administer hepatitis B vaccinations to neonates.

For a neonate inpatient admission, use code V05.3 as a secondary diagnosis code to describe the need for a vaccination (in this case, the V code is used to describe another factor influencing health status) and 99.55 as a procedure code for the injection of the vaccine. You will find these codes under the main term "vaccination" in both the Disease Index and the Procedure Index.

Type C hepatitis, which is transmitted through blood or sexual contact, can sometimes lead to chronic hepatitis, cirrhosis, and liver failure.

A **carrier** is a person who harbors a specific infectious agent without a discernible clinical disease and who serves as a potential source of infection to others. Types B and C hepatitis can be spread by asymptomatic chronic carriers of the virus (codes V02.61 and V02.62), and you would use these codes as secondary diagnosis codes to describe other factors influencing health status. Locate these codes in the Disease Index under the main term "carrier."

Meningitis

Meningitis involves an inflammation of the meninges, the protective membranes surrounding the brain and spinal cord that comprise the central nervous system. Meningitis can be caused by bacterial, fungal, and viral organisms, and its diagnosis is often confirmed by a lumbar puncture, also called a **spinal tap**, to remove cerebrospinal fluid for culture and analysis (Figure 6.1). Symptoms of meningitis include stiff neck, fever, headache, and sensitivity to light (photophobia). More often, infants are given spinal taps if there is a suspected infection, because they cannot verbalize their symptoms and tend to run higher fevers than adults. Antibiotics are used to treat the bacterial type of meningitis; the viral type is treated symptomatically.

Various forms of bacterial, viral, and fungal meningitis can be classified with a single combination code from either chapter 1, "Infectious and Parasitic Diseases" (category 001 to 139), or chapter 6, "Diseases of the Nervous System and Sense Organs" (category 320 to 389), or can be described with dual coding from both chapters (e.g., adenoviral meningitis, 049.1; Gram-negative bacterial meningitis, 320.82; actinomycotic meningitis, 039.8 + 320.7).

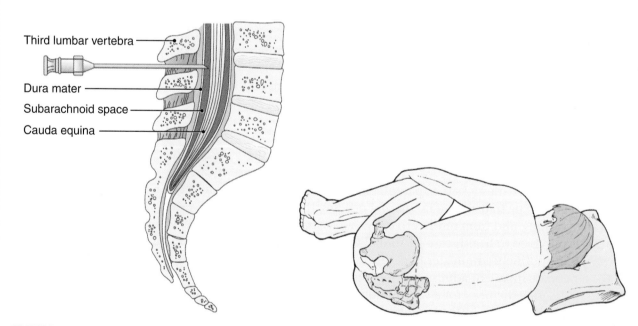

FIGURE 6.1 ■ Lumbar puncture. (Reprinted with permission from Taylor C, Lillis CA, LeMone P. Fundamentals of Nursing, 2nd Ed. Philadelphia: JB Lippincott, 1993:543.)

Tuberculosis

Tuberculosis is an infectious disease caused by tubercle bacilli (i.e., rod-shaped bacteria). Although this bacterial infection most often affects the lungs, causing swelling (tubercles) of tissue, it can affect other organs as well. Possible tuberculosis infection can be determined through a positive purified protein derivative test (PPD) (an intradermal injection that causes a localized red swollen reaction on the skin) followed by a chest radiograph. Because tuberculosis is highly contagious, all health-care workers must have an annual purified protein derivative skin test or other tuberculin testing. Immunocompromised patients, such as those with AIDS, are at greater risk for contracting tuberculosis. Symptoms that characterize tuberculosis include hemoptysis (spitting up blood), persistent cough, and weight loss.

Tuberculosis code categories 010 to 018 use a fifth-digit subclassification to identify confirmation of the disease by the type of testing performed (i.e., bacterial culture, histologic examination, tubercle bacilli found in the sputum, and so on).

Pneumonia secondary to tuberculosis confirmed by a positive tubercle bacilli culture: 011.54   **EXAMPLE**

SUMMARY

This chapter focused on learning to correctly code common infectious and parasitic diseases. The diseases included in this chapter were septicemia, infectious gastroenteritis with dehydration, RSV, AIDS- and HIV-related disease, viral hepatitis, meningitis, and tuberculosis. This chapter highlighted an ICD-9-CM convention wherein a single combination code will sometimes serve to describe a condition and its causative organism. However, in other situations, two codes must be used to describe the condition and its causative organism. Therefore, these distinct uses have been included as a part of this chapter's learning tools. Coding for services designed to facilitate the prevention of infections among hospital patients has also been discussed. Chapter 7 will focus on digestive system diseases.

TESTING YOUR COMPREHENSION

1. When coding infectious diseases, what does a combination code designate?

2. What life-threatening conditions can result from sepsis?

3. If a patient has both a urinary tract infection and septicemia, how should these be sequenced?

4. If a patient has both septicemia and septic shock, how should these be sequenced?

5. Under what condition can systemic inflammatory response syndrome (SIRS) codes (995.9X) be used as additional codes in combination with the sepsis or septicemia codes from the 038 category?

6. Under what circumstance can category 041 codes be used as a principal diagnosis?

7. How is respiratory syncytial virus contracted?

8. What occurs when HIV attaches to a CD4 protein within a T-cell lymphocyte?

9. What is the cause of type A hepatitis?

10. What is the cause of type B hepatitis, and what is the potential long-term effect?

11. What is the cause of type C hepatitis, and what are the long-term effects?

12. What are some common symptoms of meningitis?

13. What is the cause of tuberculosis?

14. What are some common symptoms of tuberculosis?

CODING PRACTICE I — Chapter Review Exercises

Directions

By using your ICD-9-CM codebook, code the following diagnoses and procedures:

	DIAGNOSIS/PROCEDURES	CODE
1	*Enterobacter aerogenes* septicemia with septic shock.	
2	Acute cystitis secondary to *Escherichia coli*.	
3	Viral infection with fever and malaise.	
4	Nausea/vomiting and hypovolemia secondary to infectious gastroenteritis (patient was given intravenous fluids/antibiotics).	
5	Dyspnea and cough secondary to respiratory syncytial virus bronchiolitis.	
6	Cytomegalovirus retinitis and thrush secondary to AIDS.	
7	Diagnosis: Acute femoral neck fracture attributable to fall from ladder. HIV-related Kaposi's sarcoma, left leg. Procedure: Open reduction, internal fixation, right femoral neck fracture.	
8	Term neonate admission (vaginal birth in hospital). HIV mother with HIV-positive status in neonate.	
9	Acute type B hepatitis with coma and type D hepatitis	
10	Meningitis secondary to Lyme disease.	
11	Candidal meningitis.	
12	Diagnosis: Acute syphilitic meningitis. Procedure: Lumbar puncture.	
13	Pulmonary tuberculosis with cavitation. Tubercle bacilli, bacterial culture positive. Methicillin-resistant *Staphylococcus aureus* patient.	
14	Fever and chills from an HIV-related histoplasmosis lung infection.	

	DIAGNOSIS/PROCEDURES	CODE
15	Diagnosis: Acute cholecystitis with cholelithiasis. Postoperative sepsis. Asymptomatic HIV infection. Procedure: Laparoscopic cholecystectomy. Intraoperative cholangiograms.	
16	Septicemia secondary to anthrax.	
17	Latent neurosyphilis with cerebellar ataxia.	
18	Gonococcal ophthalmia neonatorum.	
19	Hepatitis from cytomegalic inclusion virus.	
20	*Staphylococcus aureus* lung abscess. Hemoptysis.	
21	*Enterobacter* sepsis, septic shock, and SIRS, with acute renal failure and acute respiratory failure.	

CODING PRACTICE II — Medical Record Case Studies

Instructions

1. Carefully review the medical reports provided for each case study.
2. Research any abbreviations and terms that are unfamiliar or unclear.
3. Identify as many diagnoses and procedures as possible.
4. Because only part of the patient's total record is available, determine what additional documentation you might need.
5. If appropriate, identify any questions you might ask the physician to code this case correctly and completely.
6. Complete the appropriate blanks below for each case study.

CHAPTER 6 CASE STUDIES

Case Study 6.1

Patient: **Jane Doe**

Patient documentation: **Review Medical Report 6.1**

1. Principal diagnosis:

   _____

2. Secondary or other diagnoses:

   _____

3. Principal procedure:

   _____

4. Other procedures:

   _____

5. Additional documentation needed:

   _____

   _____

   _____

Case Study 6.1 (Continued)

6. Questions for the physician:

_____

_____

_____

_____

_____

_____

_____

_____

_____

_____

_____

_____

_____

_____

_____

_____

_____

MEDICAL REPORT 6.1

PATIENT:	Doe, Jane
PATIENT REPORT#:	001
RM#:	
ACCT#:	999999
HIST#:	99-99-99
COPIES OF REPORT SENT TO:	Dr. Smith
SEX:	F
AGE:	025
ADMIT DT:	04/03
DISCH DT:	04/09
ATTENDING MD:	Jones, John

DISCHARGE SUMMARY (PAGE 1 OF 3)

REASON FOR ADMISSION: Abnormal Liver Function Test.

BRIEF SUMMARY: Ms. Doe is a 25-year-old female who was admitted because of epigastric and right upper quadrant pain. The patient does not have a significantly abnormal liver function test at the time of admission with a bilirubin of 7.3, SGOT 591, LDH 757, and alk. phos. 188. Amylase was normal. The patient had an ultrasound of the gallbladder, which revealed a small gallbladder with thickened walls, but no stones and no dilatation of the ducts. Hepatobiliary scan was done which revealed evidence of nonvisualization of the biliary system; however, her bilirubin was significantly elevated with impairment of hepatic excretion.

The patient had no previous history of biliary tract disease. She denied she had a previous history of alcoholism and according to the patient's mother however, at this time, she does not drink excessively. The patient was not exposed to hepatitis or jaundice. She denies any previous history of any blood transfusions. History of taking some drugs in the past but these were not IV per the patient's mother. No history of recent travel abroad. No history of diarrhea or gastrointestinal upset prior to this. She had no nausea or vomiting. She had noticed yellowing of her urine color. No history of back pain or shoulder pain.

During the hospitalization, the patient was managed as per acute hepatitis of possible viral etiology. She was not on any drugs that could cause hepatitis. The patient had viral profile done which revealed evidence of positive hepatitis A IGM antibody as well as hepatitis B core antibody. Hepatitis B surface antigen was negative. Hepatitis B surface antibody was still pending, as well as hepatitis B core antibody IGM. Her liver profile during the hospitalization improved significantly. Her abdominal symptoms improved. She was placed on a liquid diet and advanced and was able to tolerate this. Her IV's were discontinued. The patient did not have any significant symptoms of pruritus, other gastrointestinal manifestations, or any other significant manifestations. The patient was ambulating.

During hospitalization, her liver profiles include bilirubin peaked at 7.3 and dropped to 6.0. Following that, her liver function including SGOT began to improve. At this time it was decided to discharge the patient and to follow her as an outpatient.

FINAL DIAGNOSES:
1. Acute Hepatitis, probably type A: however, serology for type B still pending. Possible that the patient has Type B Hepatitis but if this is acute or whether from past infection is still to be determined. Will follow obtaining the Hepatitis B surface antibody as well as Hepatitis core B antibody IGM.

DISCHARGE INSTRUCTIONS:
1. The patient is advised to avoid any sexual intercourse in view of the possibility of infecting the partner at this time. The patient is negative for Hepatitis B surface antigen. However at this time, we will await the remaining viral parameters. These will be checked as an outpatient.

Continued

MEDICAL REPORT 6.1 (CONTINUED)

2. Follow-up liver profile as an outpatient within one week.

3. The patient was advised to avoid any strenuous activity and any alcohol ingestion or taking any medications without consulting her physicians first.

4. She is to follow-up within one week or earlier if she has any undue symptoms. She will have her liver profile done before coming to the office.

5. Patient to adopt good hygienic practices and watch sharing of razor blades, or any other personal items.

6. The patient has also been advised that her husband should get viral serology done for viral hepatitis parameters.

7. Diet should consist of a very soft regular diet without any significant limitations except for alcohol.

The patient appears to understand these parameters.

JOHN JONES MD
D: 04/09
T: 04/11

NOTES

Case Study 6.2

Patient: **Frank Smith**

Patient documentation: **Review Medical Record 6.2**

1. Principal diagnosis:

   _____

2. Secondary or other diagnoses:

   _____

3. Principal procedure:

   _____

4. Other procedures:

   _____

5. Additional documentation needed:

   _____

   _____

   _____

   _____

6. Questions for the physician:

   _____

   _____

   _____

   _____

   _____

   _____

MEDICAL REPORT 6.2

HISTORY AND PHYSICAL

NAME:	Smith, Frank
ROOM:	999
ACCT#:	9999999
DATE OF ADMISSION:	7/18
ATTENDING PHYSICIAN:	Jane Smith, MD

CHIEF COMPLAINT: The patient is an 83-year-old white male with a three-day history of nausea, vomiting, and diarrhea upon eating or drinking. No blood noticed in diarrhea or vomiting. Reported possible history of fever.

ALLERGIES: Reported an allergy to penicillin. "Swells up" when exposed to penicillin. Also to wild flowers, his eyes get watery and his throat swells up.

MEDICATIONS: Poor historian of medications, reported takes pills for diabetes.

PERSONAL HISTORY: Occupations and exposure history: He was a farmer and raised chickens. Denied alcohol use. Ten-pack/year history of tobacco use, quit 40 years ago. Denied drug use.

PAST MEDICAL HISTORY: He has history of hypertension and type 2 diabetes mellitus. Reported that he was in the hospital three weeks ago with syncopal episode.

SEVERE INJURIES: Broken ribs, bruised hip, he fell two years ago and three years ago.

INFECTIONS: No reported infections.

FAMILY HISTORY: Heart attack, stroke, coronary artery disease.

SYSTEMS REVIEW

GENERAL: 40-pound weight loss over the past three years. Notices occasional fatigue, chills, night sweats, and weakness.

SKIN: Denies nail changes, itching, rashes, eruptions, eczema, hives.

HEAD: Reported a syncopal episode three weeks ago.

EYES: Wears glasses for reading and had cataract removed from right eye three months ago.

EARS: Reported decreased hearing over the past several years. Wears hearing aid.

NOSE: Reported occasional sinusitis.

THROAT: Occasional hoarseness.

RESPIRATORY: Occasional dyspnea with walking up stairs.

BREASTS: Denies masses, pain, and discharge.

CARDIOVASCULAR: Occasional palpitations and lower extremity edema.

GASTROINTESTINAL: Reported decreased appetite over the past several years. Occasional constipation. Occasional nausea and diarrhea. Recent episode of nausea, vomiting, and diarrhea for three to four days with food and water.

GENITOURINARY: Reported decreased frequency of urination, urgency, sometimes difficulty starting flow, states it takes a little longer.

ENDOCRINE: History of glycosuria.

MEDICAL REPORT 6.2 (CONTINUED)

BONES, JOINTS AND MUSCLES: Occasional stiffness bilateral lower extremities and pain in the right ribs and right hip. History of fall, fractured rib, bruised hip. Never x-rayed or followed-up.

BLOOD AND LYMPHATICS: Denies anemia, pain, bleeding tendencies, or lymph node enlargement.

NEUROLOGIC: Episode of syncope three weeks ago. He has a history of two episodes of falls, one two years ago, one three years ago, both occasions reported fractured ribs, bruised hip.

PSYCHOLOGIC: Denies anxiety, memory problems, mood disturbance or depression, emotional disturbances, drug abuse, or alcohol problems.

PHYSICAL EXAMINATION

GENERAL APPEARANCE: In no apparent distress. Mild abdominal discomfort secondary to nausea and vomiting.

SKIN: No abnormal findings.

LYMPH NODES: No cervical, post auricular, axillary, inguinal, epitrochlear, or femoral adenopathy.

HEAD: Normocephalic. Atraumatic. No tenderness or bruits.

EYES: Lids intact. No ptosis. Conjunctivae clear and sclerae white. Pupils equal, round, and reactive to light and accommodation. Extraocular muscles intact. No exophthalmos.

EARS: Reported decreased hearing over the past several years.

NOSE: Septum midline, not deviated. Mucosa pink and moist. No polyps or inflammation.

THROAT: Occasional hoarseness.

NECK: Neck is supple. No thyromegaly, jugular venous distention. Trachea midline. No carotid bruits.

CHEST: Lungs clear to auscultation. No rales, rhonchi, or wheezes.

BREASTS: No masses, discharge, or tenderness.

CARDIOVASCULAR: Regular rate and rhythm. No murmurs, thrills, heaves, rubs. Normal S1 and S2. No S3 or S4.

ABDOMEN: Right upper quadrant, right lower quadrant, left lower quadrant tenderness. Increased bowel sounds × four.

GENITALIA: No abnormal findings.

RECTUM: Already tested.

NEUROLOGIC: Cranial nerves II-XII intact. Deep tendon reflexes were equal bilaterally. Motor and sensory intact.

EXTREMITIES: No clubbing, cyanosis, edema, varicosities, amputations, phlebitis, or atrophic changes.

JOINTS: Mild arthritic deformity bilateral knees.

BACK: No paravertebral muscle spasm. Lloyd's sign was negative. No kyphosis, scoliosis or sacral base unleveling. No costovertebral angle tenderness.

IMPRESSION: Abdominal pain; nausea/vomiting/diarrhea; suspect infectious enterocolitis, diverticulitis; malnutrition and dehydration secondary to diarrhea, metabolic acidosis, renal insufficiency.

PLAN OF CARE: Admit to GMF; IV fluids, IV Levaquin/Flagyl, stool, WBC diff, enteric pathogen studies

---

JANE SMITH, MD
HISTORY AND PHYSICAL
D: 7/18
T: 7/18

Case Study 6.3

Patient: **Don Jones**

Patient documentation: **Review Medical Reports 6.3 and 6.4**

1. Principal diagnosis:

   _____

2. Secondary or other diagnoses:

   _____

3. Principal procedure:

   _____

4. Other procedures:

   _____

5. Additional documentation needed:

   _____

   _____

   _____

   _____

6. Questions for the physician:

   _____

   _____

   _____

   _____

   _____

   _____

MEDICAL REPORT 6.3

HISTORY & PHYSICAL

PATIENT:	Jones, Don
MED REC:	1111111
SEX/RACE:	M/1
PT ADM:	9999999
LOCATION:	0210
ADM DATE:	07/05

This patient is an elderly white male who was followed by Dr. Jones. The patient presents to the emergency room with poor history but apparently has had no appetite, nausea for one week, and was discharged from ABC Hospital last week for pneumonia. The patient apparently has had decreasing appetite. History is very difficult to obtain in the emergency room. The patient apparently has the smell of alcohol. He is confused, seemed to be generally weak with malaise. He also had a complaint of urinary tract infection but history is difficult to obtain. Old records revealed the patient had pneumonia, pleural effusion, bronchitis, and history of prostate CA with bone mets. Last time he was hospitalized, he was also seen by pulmonary consultation for this and has also developed congestive heart failure.

PAST MEDICAL, SURGICAL, FAMILY AND SOCIAL HISTORY: See old records.

REVIEW OF SYSTEMS: Really not a negative review of systems but difficult to really ascertain review of systems from patient. He is confused.

PHYSICAL EXAM

GENERAL: Ill appearing white male who is pleasant but not alert.

HEENT: Pupils equal, round, reactive to light and accommodation, nasopharynx is normal.

NECK: Supple, no jugular venous distention. No carotid bruits are heard.

LUNGS: Scattered rhonchi and wheezing throughout all lung fields.

HEART: Regular rate and rhythm.

ABDOMEN: Soft, nontender with normoactive bowel sounds.

EXTREMITIES: No clubbing, cyanosis, or edema.

Lab work reveals the patient had elevated white count of 12,000 hematocrit 33, abnormal urine. Chest x-ray was apparently not done. Need to rule out pneumonia. EKG which showed the patient to have anterior infarct type changes.

IMPRESSION:
1. Rule out urinary tract infection.
2. Probable exacerbated COPD.
3. Poor historian. He is confused and unable to provide adequate history.
4. History of seizures, repetitive.

PLAN: Will admit, cover with IV antibiotics, will get the chest x-ray. The patient is also anemic and will keep patient improving and will follow.

JOHN SMITH, M.D.
DD: 07/07
TD: 07/07

MEDICAL REPORT 6.4

INFECTIOUS DISEASE CONSULTATION

PATIENT:	Jones, Don
MED REC:	1111111
SEX/RACE:	M/1
PT ADM:	9999999
LOCATION:	0210
ADM DATE:	07/05

CONSULT DATE: 07/9

HISTORY: Mr. Jones is a 70-year-old male admitted on 07/5 for rule out urinary tract infection and possible COPD exacerbation. He is confused, and he is unable to provide any history. The nursing staff reports this confusion is worse over the past 3 days. He has been having fever 101°F intermittently. He has been on IV Levaquin. He cannot relay any other information.

PAST MEDICAL HISTORY: History of metastatic prostate cancer. COPD.

ALLERGIES: Methadone.

SOCIAL HISTORY: Smokes—50 years.

FAMILY HISTORY: Unobtainable.

REVIEW OF SYSTEMS: Unobtainable.

PHYSICAL EXAMINATION

VITAL SIGNS: Temperature is 96.4, blood pressure is 93/52, and pulse is 100.

HEENT: Chronically ill, awake but confused to place, time, and situation. Oriented to person.

EYES: PERRLA, conjunctiva normal.

OROPHARYNX: No teeth, erythema of soft palate.

NECK: No masses.

LUNGS: Bibasilar rales, fair air movement.

CARDIOVASCULAR: Regular, tachy, no murmur, trace edema.

ABDOMEN: Soft and nontender, no hepatosplenomegaly.

MUSCULOSKELETAL: No clubbing or cyanosis. Right upper extremity—right shoulder markedly tender, no normal ROM very severe pain on rotation. Other extremities—no joint inflammation.

SKIN: Dry skin, purpura senile, no rashes, warm and dry.

LYMPHATICS: No adenopathy of neck or axilla.

LABORATORY:
   7/6 blood culture—staphylococcus epidermidis sensitive to Vancomycin.

   7/5 cr-0.8, BUN-13, AST-23, ALT-27, WBC-12.9, H/H wnl

   7/5 Plt-661, 7/8 UA-Negative, Urine culture negative

   7/6 Uni 4, sputum culture—no growth

   7/6 Right shoulder x-ray—sclerosis on both sides of the humeral joint

   7/8 chest x-ray—consolidation of right lung, bony sclerotic lesions

MEDICAL REPORT 6.4 (CONTINUED)

IMPRESSION:

1. Staphylococcus species septicemia.
2. Acute delirium.
3. Prostate cancer history. Bone metastases.

RECOMMENDATIONS:

1. Change Levaquin to oral.
2. CT scan head.
3. D/C Restoril.
4. Vancomycin lgm IV q/12.
5. Repeat blood culture.
6. ESR.

_____

JANE SMITH, MD

D: 07/09
T: 07/09

Case Study 6.4

Patient: **Amy Parks**

Patient documentation: **Review Medical Reports 6.5 and 6.6**

1. Principal diagnosis:

   _____

2. Secondary or other diagnoses:

   _____

3. Principal procedure:

   _____

4. Other procedures:

   _____

5. Additional documentation needed:

   _____

   _____

   _____

   _____

   _____

Case Study 6.4 (Continued)

6. Questions for the physician:

_____

_____

_____

_____

_____

_____

_____

_____

_____

_____

_____

_____

_____

_____

_____

MEDICAL REPORT 6.5

HISTORY & PHYSICAL EXAMINATION

PATIENT:	Parks, Amy
MEDICAL RECORD #:	9999999
ADMITTED:	07/08
ROOM:	200

CHIEF COMPLAINT: Fever and vomiting since early today.

HISTORY OF PRESENT ILLNESS: This is a 7-month-old female who was brought to the Emergency Room by her mother for high fever and several episodes of vomiting since early today. Mother denies cough, congestion and rhinorrhea. There has been no diarrhea or irritability. She has been tolerating Pedialyte well since her arrival to the Emergency Room. Lumbar puncture for CSF culture performed in ER.

PAST MEDICAL HISTORY: Term delivery at this hospital on 12/07. She is currently followed by the County Health Department. According to the mother, her immunizations are up-to-date. She has not had any significant illnesses until today.

ALLERGIES: NKDA.

MEDICATIONS: Tylenol as needed for fever.

FAMILY HISTORY: Noncontributory.

REVIEW OF SYSTEMS: Infant has less p.o. intake today than usual. She tolerated liquids fairly well until early today when she had several episodes of vomiting. She had developed high fever at that time. She has had some mild fussiness but has been fairly easy to console today. She has not had any upper respiratory symptoms. She has not had any diarrhea.

PHYSICAL EXAM: Temperature 104.9, pulse 172, respiratory rate 26, weight 14 pounds 2 ounces.

GENERAL: Fussy but easily consoled infant, awake, alert, and interactive.

HEENT: Anterior fontanelle open only to the fingertip. TM are clear bilaterally. Red reflexes are seen bilaterally. Pupils are equal round and reactive to light. Oropharynx normal with moist mucous membranes.

LUNGS: Clear to auscultation bilaterally.

HEART: Regular rate without murmurs. Normal precordium.

ABDOMEN: Soft and benign.

GENITOURINARY: Remarkable for diffuse erythematous rash on the perineum with maceration.

MUSCULOSKELETAL: All exams were intact.

EXTREMITIES: Less than two second capillary refill.

LABORATORY: Metabolic panel Sodium 38, Potassium 4.4, Chloride 101, Bicarbonate 22, BUN 5, Creatinine 0.4, Glucose 24, Calcium 9.2, Serum Ketones 0. Urinalysis remarkable for trace Protein, 40 mg per deciliter of Ketones, CBC White Count 25,900 with 84 percent Neutrophils, 5 percent Bands, 10 percent Lymphocytes. Hemoglobin 11.2, Hematocrit 31, Platelet Count 693,000. Lumbar puncture shows cloudy fluid. CSF studies were pending at the time of dictation. Chest x-ray is clear.

IMPRESSION:

1. Fever, rule out sepsis, rule out meningitis.

2. Hypoglycemia.

PLAN: We will admit to Pediatrics for close cardiopulmonary monitoring. We will give IV Rocephin, Vancomycin and Decadron. We will await blood urine and CSF cultures. We will follow blood sugars. We will get patient's records from County Health Dept.

JANE SMITH, M.D.

DD: 07/08
DT: 07/09

MEDICAL REPORT 6.6

DOCTOR'S PROGRESS NOTES

DATE

7/17 S: Rested well.   Good p.o.   Afebrile.

6:40PM O: PHYSICAL EXAM: Temperature 97.6, Pulse 120, respiratory rate 20.

WEIGHT: 15 pounds, 0 ounces.

GENERAL: Sleepy but arousable.

HEENT: TMs clear, oropharynx clear.

LUNGS: CTA

HEART: Regular rate.

ABDOMEN: Soft and benign.

GENITOURINARY: Rash maceration improved.

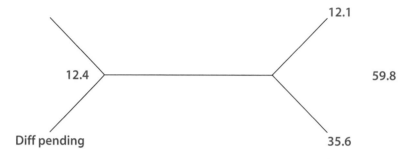

Diff pending.

A/P: Meningitis. Continue IV Rocephin and close observation today and tomorrow

7/17 Infant doing well. Afebrile. CSF Viral culture positive for Enterovirus.

Will D/C home. F/U with me 7/22.

_____

JANE SMITH, MD

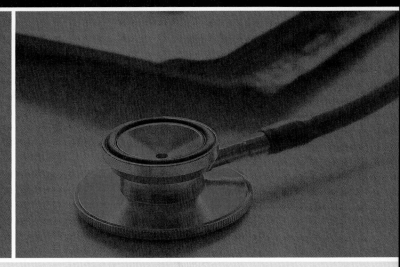

Coding for Digestive System Diseases

Chapter Outline

Diverticulosis

Gastrointestinal Ulcers

Gastrointestinal Bleeding

Esophagitis, Gastritis, and Duodenitis

Gastroesophageal Reflux Disease

Gallbladder and Biliary Duct Diseases

Cholecystitis

Pancreatitis

Bowel Obstructions

Inflammatory Bowel Diseases

Appendicitis

Hernias

Angiodysplasia (or Arteriovenous Malformations) of the
Gastrointestinal Tract

Diarrhea and Constipation

Testing Your Comprehension

Coding Practice I: Chapter Review Exercises

Coding Practice II: Medical Record Case Studies

Chapter Objectives

▶ Describe the pathology of common digestive system disorders.

▶ Recognize the typical manifestations, complications, and treatments of common digestive system disorders in terms of their implications for coding.

▶ Correctly code common digestive system disorders and related procedures by using the ICD-9-CM and medical records.

Digestive system diseases are included in code section 520 to 579 of chapter 9 in the Disease Tabular of the ICD-9-CM. This includes diseases of the stomach, intestines, gallbladder, pancreas, and esophagus (Figure 7.1). This textbook highlights some of the more common digestive system diseases that cause inpatient hospital admissions. These include diverticulosis, gastrointestinal (GI) ulcers, GI bleeding, esophagitis, gastritis, duodenitis, gastroesophageal reflux diseases (GERDs), gallbladder and biliary duct diseases, pancreatitis, bowel obstructions, inflammatory bowel diseases (IBDs), appendicitis, hernias, GI angiodysplasia or arteriovenous malformations, diarrhea, and constipation. To assist in your understanding, the Word Parts Box on page 149 reviews word parts and meanings of medical terms related to digestive system diseases.

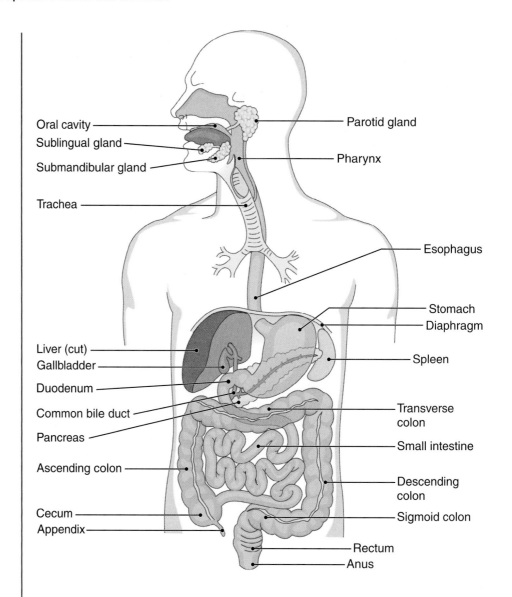

FIGURE 7.1 ■ Digestive System. (Reprinted with permission from Cohen BJ and Wood DL. Memmler's The Human Body in Health and Disease, 9th Ed. Philadelphia: Lippincott Williams & Wilkins, 2000.)

Diverticulosis

Diverticulosis is a condition that results in pockets along the GI tract (Figure 7.2). The most common site for diverticulosis is the colon (large intestine), and this disease more commonly occurs with middle age. When the small pockets in the wall of the colon fill with fecal material and become inflamed, the condition is called diverticulitis. Rarely, the pockets may cause obstruction, perforation, or bleeding.

Word Parts and Meanings of Digestive System Medical Terms

Word Part	Meaning	Example	Definition of Example
angi/o	vessel	angiodysplasia	Degenerative or congenital structural abnormality of the normally distributed vasculature
chol/e	bile, gall	cholangiogram	X-ray of bile vessels (ducts)
cholecyst/o	gallbladder	cholecystitis	Inflammation of the gallbladder
choledoch/o	common bile duct	choledochal	Pertaining to the common bile duct (CBD)
-ectomy	excision, surgical removal	appendectomy	Surgical removal of the appendix
esophag/o	esophagus	esophagus	The muscular tube that carries food from the pharynx to the stomach
gastr/o	stomach	gastroesophageal reflux disease	A syndrome of chronic or recurrent epigastric or retrosternal paindue to reflux of acid gastric lower esophagus juice into the
-itis	inflammation	duodenitis	Inflammation of the duodenum
lith/o	stones, calculus	cholelithiasis	Gallstones
nas/o	nose	nasogastric tube	A tube that is passed through the nose into the stomach
Pancreat/o	pancreas	pancreatitis	Inflammation of the pancreas
-sis	an abnormal condition	diverticulosis	The presence of diverticula (small pouches) in the wall of the digestive tract, especially in the colon

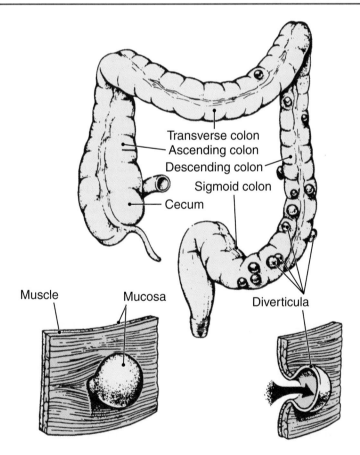

FIGURE 7.2 ■ Diverticula are most common in the sigmoid colon; they diminish in number and size as the colon approaches the cecum. Diverticula are rarely found in the rectum. (Reprinted with permission from Nettina, Sandra M., MSN, RN, CS, ANP, The Lippincott Manual of Nursing Practice, 7th ed. Lippincott, Williams & Wilkins, 2001.)

When you are locating the code for diverticulosis, carefully review the subterms (essential modifiers) for:

▶ the site of the inflamed sacs
▶ whether the diverticulosis is with or without diverticulitis
▶ whether it is associated with hemorrhage (bleeding)

When a physician documents diverticulosis without specifying the site, assume that it is the colon.

 TIP   If the physician documents diverticulosis with diverticulitis, code only the diverticulitis: diverticulitis assumes diverticulosis, and using both codes is unnecessary.

EXAMPLE

Diverticulosis of colon: 562.10
Diverticulosis with diverticulitis: 562.11
Diverticulosis with bleeding: 562.12
Diverticulosis with diverticulitis with bleeding: 562.13
Diverticulosis of esophagus, acquired: 530.6
Diverticulosis of esophagus, acquired, with hemorrhage: 530.6 + 530.82

Diverticulosis of the colon is commonly diagnosed through colonoscopy or barium enema. Conservative treatment for diverticulosis, with or without diverticulitis, routinely includes intravenous fluids, intravenous antibiotics (to prevent infection), and soft diet. Severe acute diverticulitis may include bleeding or perforation that could indicate the need for a colon resection and temporary colostomy to let the bowel rest and heal. After treatment, the physician would schedule an admission for a take-down (removal) colostomy (principal diagnosis code V55.3). You can locate the diagnosis code for take-down colostomy under "attention to" in the Disease Index (volume 2). The procedure code is located in the procedure index under "take-down, colostomy" (code 46.52).

Gastrointestinal Ulcers

An ulcer is an open sore on the skin or epithelial tissue that lines the internal organs (Figure 7.3). Gastric (stomach) and duodenal (first part of the small intestine) ulcers are common examples of GI ulcers and are often associated with GI bleeding. For gastric and duodenal ulcers (category codes 531 and 532, respectively), the fourth digit indicates whether the ulcer is acute or chronic and whether it has an associated bleed or perforation. The fifth digit indicates whether the ulcer is with or without obstruction.

EXAMPLE

Acute bleeding gastric ulcer with perforation and obstruction: 531.21
Acute bleeding duodenal ulcer with perforation and obstruction: 532.21

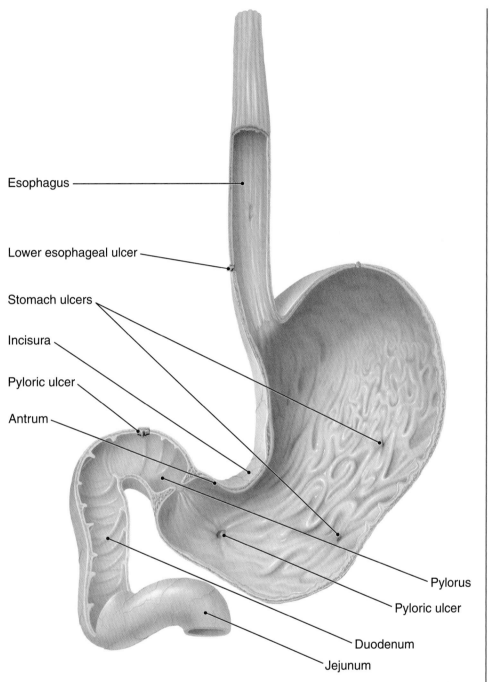

Esophagus

Lower esophageal ulcer

Stomach ulcers

Incisura

Pyloric ulcer

Antrum

Pylorus

Pyloric ulcer

Duodenum

Jejunum

FIGURE 7.3 ■ Common ulcer types and sites. (Reprinted with permission from Anatomical Chart Co.)

TIP

Gastric and duodenal ulcers are examples of types of peptic ulcers (category code 533). However, if the physician documents only peptic ulcer, this does not specify the site of the ulcer. With a diagnosis of peptic ulcer, a coder should review the complete record for a precise location of the ulcer.

Gastrointestinal Bleeding

If the specific site or cause of GI bleeding is undetermined, use code 578.9 (GI bleed, not otherwise specified [NOS]) as a principal or secondary diagnosis. If upon examination (e.g., lower or upper endoscopy or both) there is no current active bleeding but there is evidence of a recent site of GI bleed that is documented by the physician, you can still use the disease code specifying "with GI bleed," because this was the reason for examination (e.g., diverticulitis with recent bleed, 562.13).

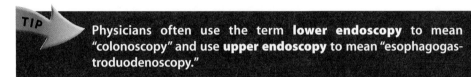

TIP Physicians often use the term **lower endoscopy** to mean "colonoscopy" and use **upper endoscopy** to mean "esophagogastroduodenoscopy."

Also, of clinical significance, dark blood in a stool (melena) is often associated with an upper GI bleed (e.g., older blood, possibly from a bleed above the duodenum), and bright red blood per rectum, or **hematochezia**, is often associated with a lower GI bleed (e.g., fresh blood, possibly from hemorrhoids). Stool hemoccult or guaiac test detects hidden (occult) blood in feces. Guaiac is a chemical that reacts with small traces of blood not readily seen in the stool.

If a diagnosis code does not include a combination code (single code) or subterm (essential modifier) that specifies "with bleeding," then use 578.9 as an additional (secondary diagnosis) code to provide more detail.

EXAMPLE   *GI bleeding secondary to colon polyps: 211.3 + 578.9*

Because there is no subterm, single combination code, or mandatory dual-coding rule that includes colon polyps with bleeding, add code 578.9 after the colon polyp code 211.3 to specify the bleed. When coding conditions associated with GI bleeding as a secondary diagnosis, be careful to review the medical record for the presence and treatment of blood-loss anemia, which is a common occurrence with GI bleeding. Treatment for acute or chronic blood-loss anemia (codes 285.1 and 280.0, respectively) can include packed red blood cell transfusions, increased monitoring of the patient's hemoglobin and hematocrit, and iron sulfate supplements.

TIP See the *Coding Clinic* 1990, fourth quarter; 1992, second quarter; and, 2005, third quarter for more information on GI hemorrhage.

Esophagitis, Gastritis, and Duodenitis

Esophagitis is an inflammation of the esophagus (a muscular tube connecting the throat to the stomach). Reflux esophagitis is a specific type of esophagitis commonly associated with GERD and/or hiatal hernias, in which the stomach protrudes through the esophageal opening in the diaphragm (a muscle that separates the abdominal and chest cavities and that aids in breathing). The ICD-9-CM classifies esophagitis (category 530) into the following types:

530.10—Esophagitis, unspecified
530.11—Reflux esophagitis
530.12—Acute esophagitis
530.19—Other esophagitis

Treatment for esophagitis usually includes gastric acid-suppression drugs and diet restrictions. For other causes of esophagitis, see the appropriate body system chapter (e.g., candidal esophagitis, 112.84, and tuberculous esophagitis, 017.8X, from ICD-9–CM chapter 1, on infectious diseases).

When locating the code for gastritis and duodenitis (inflammation of the stomach, duodenum, or both), found under category code 535, you must carefully review the fourth digits clarifying the subterms (essential modifiers) that specify the type of gastritis and whether it is acute or chronic. The fifth digits for gastritis and duodenitis indicate whether there is an associated hemorrhage (bleeding).

Acute gastritis with hemorrhage: 535.01
Duodenitis with hemorrhage: 535.61
Gastroduodenitis with hemorrhage: 535.51

EXAMPLE

Gastroesophageal Reflux Disease

In GERD (code 530.81), solid foods and liquids, along with hydrochloric/peptic acid, reflux (back up) from the stomach into the esophagus. (You will find the main term "reflux" in the Disease Index.) The main symptom that accompanies GERD is heartburn, which causes an epigastric (above the stomach) burning sensation. Over time, irritation of the esophagus can occur, causing reflux esophagitis (code 530.11). Treatment for GERD most often includes drugs that suppress gastric acid production. If GERDs progresses to reflux esophagitis, only assign the code for reflux esophagitis (530.11).

Gallbladder and Biliary Duct Diseases

The gallbladder is a reservoir for bile, a digestive enzyme that travels through biliary (bile) ducts to enter the duodenum (the first part of the small intestine), where it helps to break down and absorb fat (Figure 7.4). In the ICD-9-CM,

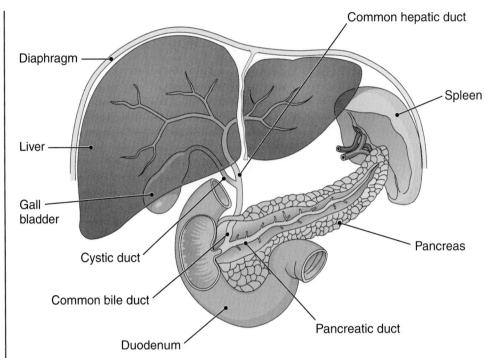

FIGURE 7.4 ■ Accessory organs of digestion. (Reprinted with permission from Cohen BJ and Wood DL. Memmler's The Human Body in Health and Disease, 9th Ed. Philadelphia: Lippincott Williams & Wilkins, 2000.)

many combination codes are used to describe gallbladder and biliary duct diseases. The key to coding them correctly is to understand the clinical meaning of each medical term (see Word Parts and Meaning Box on page 149).

Cholecystitis

The most commonly coded disease associated with the gallbladder is cholecystitis (inflammation of the gallbladder) with or without cholelithiasis (gallstones). Although many patients with gallstones do not have symptoms or require treatment, some experience sharp abdominal pain called **biliary colic**, for which treatment is required. Treatment usually includes cholecystectomy (excision of the gallbladder), choledocholithotomy (incision and exploration into the CBD to remove stones if present), or both. Cholecystectomies can be performed by open incision (code 51.22) or by a laparoscopic technique (code 51.23). Today, many more laparoscopic operations are being performed because they are less invasive and involve a shortened recovery time.

If what starts as a laparoscopic cholecystectomy is changed to an open procedure (usually because of poor visualization of the operative field or abnormal findings by the surgeon), then code the cholecystectomy to an open procedure (code 51.22) and add V64.41 as a secondary diagnosis code (look under the main term "laparoscopic surgical procedure converted to open procedure" in the Disease Index). This V code is used to describe another factor influencing the health status of the patient during the current episode of care.

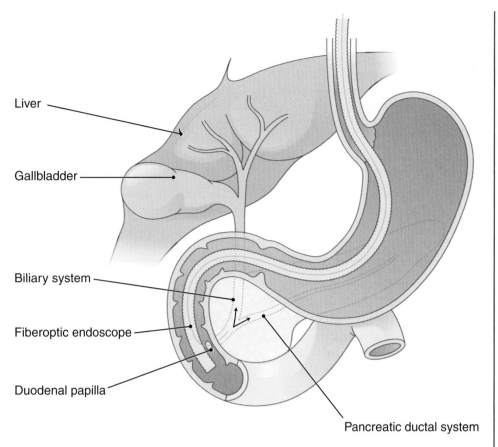

Liver

Gallbladder

Biliary system

Fiberoptic endoscope

Duodenal papilla

Pancreatic ductal system

FIGURE 7.5 ■ Endoscopic retro-grade cholangiopancreatogra-phy (ERCP). A contrast medium is injected into the pancreatic and bile ducts in preparation for radiography. (Reprinted with permission from Cohen BJ. Medical Terminology An Illustrated Guide, 4th Ed. Baltimore: Lippincott Williams & Wilkins, 2004.)

Code any associated open CBD exploration to 51.51 (without stone removal) or 51.41 (if stones or calculi are removed). **Calculus** (singular) and **calculi** (plural) are the medical terms for stones. Gallstones usually occur as hardened cholesterol from bile. An endoscopic retrograde cholangiopancreatography (code 51.10) is a radiograph that uses contrast dye to see whether the biliary ducts contain stones or other obstructions (Figure 7.5). An endoscopic retrograde cholangiopancreatography is sometimes followed by a laparoscopic removal of calculi of the bile duct, coded to 51.88 (locate the code under "removal, calculus, bile duct, laparoscopic or endoscopic" in the Procedure Index). Percutaneous (through the skin) removal of calculi from the CBD is coded to 51.96.

Often, an intraoperative (performed during the operation) cholangiogram radiograph with contrast dye (code 87.53) is performed to determine whether there is any biliary obstruction. A biliary (duct) obstruction can be caused by stones or tumor and can prevent bile (a substance from the liver that aids in digestion) from draining properly into the small intestine, where it is eliminated with feces. It is important to note that bile contains bilirubin (a substance that results from the death of worn-out red blood cells). If bile containing bilirubin cannot drain properly from the body, it will accumulate in the bloodstream as hyperbilirubinemia, and this will cause jaundice.

TIP Jaundice, or icterus, results in yellowing of the skin and sclerae (whites of the eyes). When coding for gallbladder and biliary diseases, carefully review the documentation of jaundice that may be an indication of a biliary obstruction. Then, review the medical record for documentation by the physician of biliary obstruction, because this can change the fifth digit subclassification. Even though jaundice is a clinical indication of an obstruction, the physician must still document the biliary obstruction for assignment of the fifth digit subclassification (e.g., cholecystitis with choledocholithiasis with obstruction: 574.4<u>1</u>).

Pancreatitis

Pancreatitis (category code 577) is an inflammation of the pancreas. Causes of pancreatitis can include drugs, alcohol, trauma, or an obstruction (e.g., biliary calculus) that causes pancreatic digestive enzymes to irritate the pancreatic tissue, causing inflammation. Symptoms of pancreatitis can include abdominal pain and swelling. Laboratory tests showing increased levels of amylase and lipase (pancreatic digestive enzymes) in the bloodstream also indicate the disease. The most common causes of pancreatitis are gallstones and alcoholism. A common diagnosis is gallstone pancreatitis, in which both diseases are coded.

EXAMPLE *The patient was admitted with acute gallstone pancreatitis and acute cholecystitis with choledocholithiasis and obstruction that was treated with open cholecystectomy with CBD exploration and removal of stones: 574.31, 577.0; 51.22, 51.41.*

Bowel Obstructions

A bowel obstruction results in a blockage of the intestines. There are many different types of bowel obstructions, but some of the most commonly coded include the following:

▶ bowel obstruction secondary to postoperative adhesions (code 560.81)
▶ volvulus (code 560.2), a kinking or twisting of the bowel (Figure 7.6)
▶ intussusception (code 560.0), a telescoping of the intestine seen most often in children (Figure 7.6)
▶ bowel obstruction secondary to fecal impaction (560.39)
▶ ileus (560.1), a mechanical bowel obstruction caused by tumors, overuse of laxatives, trauma, infection, or other reasons
▶ postoperative ileus (997.4 + 560.1), a mechanical bowel obstruction secondary to surgery

Some bowel obstructions, such as a postoperative ileus, can resolve by conservative treatment, such as placement of a nasogastric tube to drain fluids and decompress the bowel (Figure 7.7), restricted diet to provide bowel rest, intravenous fluids, or drugs to increase GI movement (i.e., motility or peristalsis). Medical emergency measures may include intestinal resections.

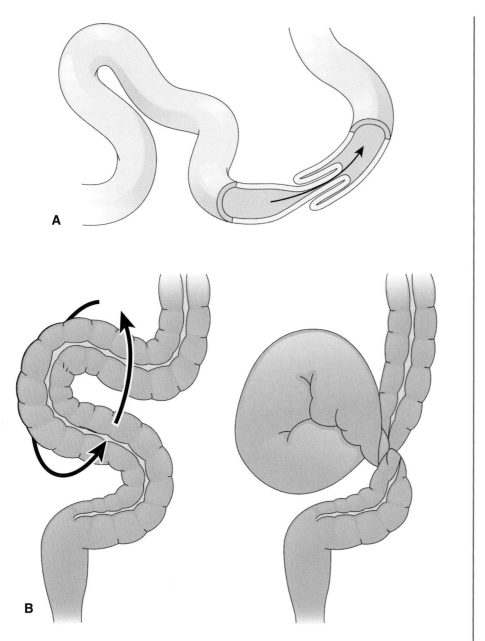

FIGURE 7.6 ■ Intestinal obstruction. **(A)** Intussusception. **(B)** Volvulus, showing counterclockwise twist. (Reprinted with permission from Cohen BJ. Medical Terminology, 4th ed. Philadelphia. Lippincott Williams & Wilkins 2003.)

Inflammatory Bowel Diseases

IBDs include ulcerative colitis (556.9) and Crohn's disease (555.9). The etiology (cause) of these diseases is often unknown. Symptoms include diarrhea and abdominal pain. IBDs are often characterized by relapses (an active disease state with symptoms) and remissions (an inactive disease state without symptoms). Conservative treatment includes diet restrictions, antidiarrheal drugs, and the use of corticosteroid drugs that reduce intestinal inflammation. However, severe IBD may require intestinal resection (surgical removal) of the diseased bowel with anastomosis (reconnection or creation of a new opening between nondiseased organ tissues). It is worth mentioning that

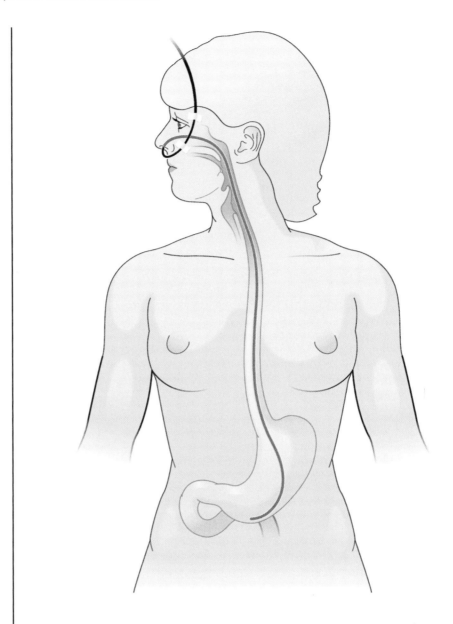

FIGURE 7.7 ■ A nasogastric (NG) tube in place. (Reprinted with permission from Cohen BJ. Medical Terminology: An Illustrated Guide, 4th Ed. Baltimore: Lippincott Williams & Wilkins, 2004.)

irritable bowel syndrome, or spastic colon (code 564.1), is a noninflammatory bowel disease. The etiology of this disease is related to stress, and symptoms include diarrhea or constipation, abdominal pain, and bloating. Treatment includes stress management and drugs to relieve diarrhea or constipation.

Appendicitis

Appendicitis is an inflammation of the appendix. The appendix is an appendage that hangs off the first part of the large bowel called the **cecum**. The appendix serves no useful function but can become inflamed, infected, and blocked with feces and can then rupture. Appendicitis is usually treated by surgical removal of the appendix (i.e., appendectomy). An incidental appendectomy (removal of a healthy appendix) may be performed in conjunction with other intra-abdominal surgery to prevent the need for future invasive surgery for appendiceal disease that may develop. Diagnosis and procedure codes for appendicitis include:

- ▶ acute appendicitis: code 540.9
- ▶ acute appendicitis with a perforation, peritonitis, or rupture: code 540.0 (with a peritoneal abscess, code 540.1)
- ▶ unspecified appendicitis: code 541 (be sure to review the medical record for a more specific diagnosis)
- ▶ open appendectomy: code 47.09
- ▶ laparoscopic appendectomy: code 47.01
- ▶ incidental appendectomy: code 47.19

Hernias

A hernia is an abnormal protrusion (bulging) of an organ through tissue. Although there are many different types of hernias, those commonly associated with the digestive system include inguinal hernias (groin area), ventral and incisional hernias (abdominal wall area), and hiatal hernias (gastroesophageal junction area).

Inguinal Hernias

Codes for inguinal hernia (category code 550) include five digits. The fourth digit specifies whether the hernia is gangrenous or obstructed. The fifth digit specifies whether the hernia is unilateral or bilateral and recurrent or unspecified. If an inguinal hernia is specified as obstructed, strangulated, or incarcerated, this means that because of the weakness in the inguinal wall, the bowel protrudes, causing an intestinal obstruction.

Recurrent left-sided incarcerated inguinal hernia: 550.11

EXAMPLE

To code for surgical repairs of inguinal hernias (category code 53), go to "repair, hernia, inguinal" in the Procedure Index. Watch for subterms that specify whether the repair is unilateral or bilateral, direct or indirect, and with prosthesis or graft (e.g., use of mesh), because this will change the third and fourth digit assignments. If a hernia is specified as direct, there is a protrusion directly through the abdominal wall. If a hernia is specified as indirect, there is a protrusion through the inguinal ring (a portion of the abdominal wall).

Pay particular attention if the diagnosis code specifies recurrent hernia. Surgical repair of a recurrent hernia may require the use of mesh (an artificial material such as Teflon™) because of the recurrent nature of the weakness of the inguinal wall tissues. Be sure to review the operative report carefully for the type of surgical repair. Depending on the severity of the hernia, initial hernias may also require mesh.

> **EXAMPLE**
>
> ► *The patient is admitted for an indirect right inguinal hernia. Right open repair of indirect inguinal hernia is performed (code 550.90; 53.02).*
> ► *The patient is admitted for a bilateral inguinal hernia repair: direct on right and indirect on left. Open bilateral inguinal hernia repair, one direct and one indirect is performed (code 550.92; 53.13).*
> ► *The patient is admitted for a repair of an incarcerated right direct inguinal hernia. Right open repair of direct inguinal hernia with mesh is performed (code 550.10; 53.03).*
> ► *The patient is admitted for a recurrent left direct inguinal hernia repair. Laparoscopic repair of direct inguinal hernia with mesh is performed (code 550.91; 17.11).*

Ventral and Incisional Hernias

A ventral hernia (category code 553) is an abdominal wall hernia, and the three-digit category code changes if there is mention of obstruction (category code 552) or gangrene (category code 551). You should code a recurrent ventral hernia as an incisional hernia. An incisional hernia is a ventral hernia in a previous surgical incision site. Sometimes physicians document ventral hernia NOS when they mean a recurrent ventral or incisional hernia, and this distinction changes the code assignment.

> **EXAMPLE**
>
> *Ventral hernia NOS: 553.20*
> *Recurrent ventral hernia: 553.21 (meaning incisional hernia)*
> *Incisional hernia: 553.21*
> *Ventral hernia in previous abdominal surgery site: 553.21*
> *Ventral hernia with obstruction: 552.20*
> *Ventral hernia with gangrene: 551.20*
> *Recurrent ventral hernia with obstruction: 552.21*
> *Recurrent ventral hernia with gangrene: 551.21*

> **TIP**   If a physician documents ventral hernia NOS, be sure to review the medical record (e.g., the operative report and the physical examination portion of the admission history and physical), which may reveal the hernia at the site of a previous surgical incision. This would be an incisional hernia and should not be coded to ventral hernia NOS.

The ventral and incisional hernia repair categories also provide a code for the use of a prosthesis or graft.

> **EXAMPLE**
>
> *Ventral hernia repair (without graft or prosthesis): 53.59*
> *Ventral hernia repair with graft or prosthesis: 53.69*
> *Other laparoscopic ventral hernia repair with graft or prosthesis: 53.63*
> *Incisional hernia repair (without graft or prosthesis): 53.51*
> *Other open incisional hernia repair with graft or prosthesis: 53.61*
> *Laparoscopic incisional hernia repair with graft or prosthesis: 53.62*

Hiatal Hernias

In hiatal hernias (code 553.3), also called **diaphragmatic hernias**, the stomach protrudes through the esophageal opening in the diaphragm at the gastroesophageal junction. A common complication of hiatal hernia occurs when food is swallowed and it refluxes back from the stomach, along with gastric acids that cause irritation to esophageal tissues and a burning sensation called **heartburn**. Chronic irritation of the esophageal lining from the gastric acids can cause reflux esophagitis. Hiatal hernias that cause reflux esophagitis are usually treated conservatively by using drugs that neutralize or suppress gastric acid production and by diet restrictions. However, in severe cases of reflux esophagitis caused by hiatal hernia, surgical correction may be necessary (located in the Procedure Index; see the main term "repair; hernia, esophageal hiatus"; laparoscopic repair with abdominal approach, code 53.71; other and open repair with abdominal approach, code 53.72; repair with abdominal approach, not otherwise specified, code 53.75; laparoscopic repair with thoracic approach, code 53.83; and, other and open repair with thoracic approach, code 53.84). In this case, the focus of care is directed at the hiatal hernia as the cause of the reflux esophagitis. Therefore, sequence the code for the hiatal hernia as the principal diagnosis, with the reflux esophagitis as an additional code (553.3 + 530.11).

Angiodysplasia (or Arteriovenous Malformations) of the Gastrointestinal Tract

Angiodysplasia, or arteriovenous malformations (AVMs), of the GI tract can result in bleeding from abnormal blood vessels that rupture in the stomach or intestine. The etiology is usually unknown, and symptoms of AVM include hematemesis (vomiting blood), melena (blood in stool), and secondary blood-loss anemia. An esophagogastroduodenoscopy or colonoscopy is often performed to diagnose the disease. Locate the diagnosis codes under the main term "angiodysplasia" in the Disease Index. There are codes that specify with and without bleeding.

EXAMPLE

Angiodysplasia of intestine: 569.84
Angiodysplasia of intestine with hemorrhage: 569.85
Angiodysplasia of stomach and (or) duodenum: 537.82
Angiodysplasia of stomach and (or) duodenum with hemorrhage: 537.83

Do not code AVMs of the GI tract as congenital (747.61) if they are acquired in an adult; this would be coded to the 569 or 537 category. This mistake is sometimes made when coders go to the main term "malformation" in the Disease Index that cross-references ("see also") to anomaly. "Anomaly, arteriovenous, gastrointestinal" will give you code 747.61, which is the code for congenital GI AVMs. Be sure to go to the main term "angiodysplasia" in the Disease Index when coding acquired AVMs.

> **TIP** *Coding Clinic* 1996, third quarter, describes more information regarding GI AVMs.

Diarrhea and Constipation

Depending on the etiology (cause) of diarrhea, it could be coded from chapter 9, "Diseases of the Digestive System"; chapter 1, "Infectious and Parasitic Diseases"; chapter 5, "Mental Disorders"; or chapter 16, "Symptoms, Signs, and Ill-Defined Conditions."

EXAMPLE

Chapter 1 (Infectious and Parasitic Diseases):
- ▶ *bacterial diarrhea, not elsewhere classified: 008.5*
- ▶ *infectious diarrhea: 009.2*

Chapter 5 (Mental Disorders):
- ▶ *psychogenic diarrhea: 306.4 (diarrhea resulting from a mental factor)*

Chapter 9 (Diseases of Digestive System):
- ▶ *functional diarrhea: 564.5 (diarrhea attributable to a GI tract dysfunction)*
- ▶ *postgastrectomy diarrhea: 564.4 (diarrhea after GI surgery)*

Chapter 16 (Symptoms, Signs, and Ill-Defined Conditions):
- ▶ *diarrhea, etiology unknown: 787.91*

You must pay careful attention to the subterms (essential modifiers) under the main term "diarrhea" in the Disease Index and notes within the Disease Tabular for correct code assignment. Do not assign the symptom code 787.91 for diarrhea NOS when "after study" a definitive diagnosis is determined to be the cause for the diarrhea (e.g., diarrhea attributable to clostridium difficile enteritis, code 008.45). Also, if there is a known cause for the diarrhea, do not assign the diarrhea NOS code 787.91 as an additional code if it is a symptom routinely associated with the disease (e.g., the physician documents diarrhea attributable to salmonella enteritis: code 003.0, not 003.0 + 787.91).

The diarrhea NOS code 787.91 would be questionable if assigned as the principal diagnosis for an inpatient stay. Unspecified diarrhea does not demonstrate the medical necessity for an inpatient admission. You should review the medical record for a more definitive diagnosis or query the physician to determine whether a more definitive diagnosis can be established and documented. 787.91 (diarrhea NOS) is a sign and symptom code and can be the principal diagnosis only if no related condition can be identified.

Constipation (category code 564) results in difficult defecation (i.e., elimination of stool). Treatments include drugs (laxatives or cathartics) to increase peristalsis (bowel movement). ICD-9-CM specifies different types of constipation:

- ▶ 564.00 unspecified constipation or constipation NOS
- ▶ 564.01 slow transit constipation (from smooth muscle dysfunction)

▶ 564.02 outlet dysfunction constipation (from pelvic floor muscle dysfunction)

▶ 564.09 other constipation

New codes have been added for constipation because physician specialists often request that the Centers for Medicare and Medicaid Services and the National Center for Vital Statistics increase code specificity (detail) to do research. However, although these new codes filter down to coders, physicians often do not document in sufficient detail for their use. If the patient's diagnosis is documented as "constipation," review the physician's orders for fecal disimpaction and radiographs to determine whether "constipation" may be further described as a fecal impaction. If there is evidence of fecal impaction, query the physician to confirm whether the constipation involves fecal impaction. If so, ask the physician to document an addendum of "fecal impaction" as the final diagnostic impression so you can assign the more precise code of 560.39. A patient is rarely admitted to an inpatient status for simple constipation; therefore, you should review the record further for a more precise diagnosis.

SUMMARY

You have now learned how to code common digestive system diseases, and you have had an opportunity to apply this new knowledge by locating correct digestive system disease codes in the ICD-9-CM codebook. The next chapter will address the subject of coding for respiratory diseases.

TESTING YOUR COMPREHENSION

1. What is the most common site for diverticulosis?

    _____

2. What medical procedures are most commonly used to diagnose diverticulosis?

    _____

3. What is an ulcer?

    _____

4. Gastric and duodenal ulcers are examples of what type of ulcer?

    _____

5. If a physician's diagnosis is peptic ulcer, what should the coder do?

    _____

6. Dark blood in a stool may be indicative of what occurrence?

    _____

7. An inflammation of the esophagus is referred to as what condition?

    _____

8. What is the acronym for gastroesophageal reflux disease?

    _____

9. Identify the digestive enzyme that travels from the liver through the biliary ducts to enter the duodenum.

    _____

10. When the suffix "-itis" is attached to a medical term, what condition does that refer to?

    _____

11. Identify the most common disease associated with the gallbladder.

    _____

12. Identify the condition associated with an inflammation of the pancreas.

    _____

13. What are the most common causes of pancreatitis?

    _____

14. What is an abnormal protrusion of an organ through tissue?

    _____

15. If an inguinal hernia is specified as obstructed, strangulated, or incarcerated, what does that signify?

    _____

16. With respect to a hiatal hernia, what happens to the stomach?

    _____

CODING PRACTICE I | Chapter Review Exercises

Directions

By using your ICD-9-CM codebook, code the following diagnoses and procedures:

	DIAGNOSIS/PROCEDURES	CODE
1	Diagnosis: Gallstone pancreatitis. Cholecystitis with cholelithiasis. Hypercholesterolemia. Morbid obesity. Procedure: Laparoscopic cholecystectomy changed to open procedure secondary to poor visual field. CBD exploration. Intraoperative cholangiogram.	
2	Diagnosis: Chronic duodenal ulcer with bleed. Blood-loss anemia. Procedure: Esophagogastroduodenoscopy.	
3	Antral gastritis with bleeding. Blood-loss anemia.	
4	Alcoholic gastritis. Alcohol dependence.	
5	Diagnosis: Recurrent right inguinal hernia, incarcerated. Procedure: Right herniorrhaphy, with mesh.	
6	GI bleeding, anemia, secondary diverticulosis with diverticulitis.	
7	GERDs with reflux esophagitis. Dehydration.	
8	Acute hemorrhagic gastric ulcer. Acute blood-loss anemia.	
9	Diagnosis: Ulcerative colitis. Procedure: Low anterior (rectosigmoid) resection.	
10	Diagnosis: Acute ruptured appendicitis. Postoperative ileus. Procedure: Laparoscopic appendectomy.	

	DIAGNOSIS/PROCEDURES	CODE
11	Diagnosis: Acute perforated gastric ulcer. Procedure: Suture of gastric ulcer.	
12	Diagnosis: Fecal impaction. Procedure: Manual removal of impacted feces.	
13	Arteriovenous malformations (angiodysplasia), stomach, with hemorrhage.	
14	Diagnosis: Right diverticulitis with bleeding. Acute blood-loss anemia. Procedure: Left hemicolectomy with temporary colostomy. Incidental appendectomy. Transfusion of packed red blood cells.	
15	Diagnosis: Admit for take-down colostomy, history of diverticular disease. Postoperative fever, etiology unknown, sepsis ruled out. Procedure: Closure of colostomy.	
16	Diagnosis: GERDs, hiatal hernia. Procedure: Nissen operation (fundoplication of stomach).	
17	Diagnosis: Acute gastric ulcer with hemorrhage and perforation. Procedure: Billroth II partial gastrectomy with gastrojejunostomy anastomosis.	
18	GI bleeding, etiology unknown.	
19	Diagnosis: Ventral hernia in previous incision line. Procedure: Repair ventral hernia with mesh.	
20	Crohn's disease of large intestine with abdominal pain and diarrhea.	

CODING PRACTICE II   Medical Record Case Studies

Instructions

1. Carefully review the medical reports provided for each case study.
2. Research any abbreviations and terms that are unfamiliar or unclear.
3. Identify as many diagnoses and procedures as possible.
4. Because only part of the patient's total record is available, determine what additional documentation you might need.
5. If appropriate, identify any questions you might ask the physician to code this case correctly and completely.
6. Complete the appropriate blanks below for each case study.

CHAPTER 7 CASE STUDIES

Case Study 7.1 (Coder/Abstract Summary Form)

Patient: **John Doe**

Patient documentation: **Review Medical Reports 7.1 and 7.2**

 1. Principal diagnosis:

 _____

 2. Secondary or other diagnoses:

 _____

 3. Principal procedure:

 _____

 4. Other procedures:

 _____

 5. Additional documentation needed:

 _____

 _____

 _____

 _____

Case Study 7.1 (Continued)

6. Questions for the physician:

_____

_____

_____

_____

_____

_____

MEDICAL REPORT 7.1

OPERATIVE REPORT

PATIENT:	Doe, John
MEDICAL RECORD #:	123456
DATE:	4/10
ROOM#:	200

PREOPERATIVE DIAGNOSIS: Reflux esophagitis, gastritis, bleeding prepyloric ulcer, diverticulosis.

SURGEON: John Jones, M.D.

OPERATION:

1. EGD with biopsies with injection of bleeding prepyloric ulcer.

2. Colonoscopy.

ANESTHESIA: Sedation

INDICATION FOR THE PROCEDURE: This 68-year-old gentleman presented with history of GI bleeding. Patient had been vomiting. Also, he had been passing some dark colored bowel movements and some bright red blood in the stools. It was decided to go ahead and do an EGD and colonoscopy to find the source of bleeding.

DESCRIPTION OF THE PROCEDURE:

1. EGD with biopsies with injection and cauterization of the bleeding ulcer. With the patient in the left lateral position, scope was introduced. Proximally, the esophagus was found to be normal. Distally, the patient had evidence of grade III reflux esophagitis. Scope was entered into the stomach. On entering the stomach, there was evidence of diffuse gastritis in the stomach. Multiple biopsies were taken and sent for histopathology and study for H. pylori. A J maneuver was done. A look at the fundus was made. Fundus had evidence of gastritis. Scope was then straightened up. At the level of the pylorus, there was a bleeding pyloric ulcer. The ulcer was injected with Epinephrine. Following this, the scope was introduced through the pylorus into the first and second parts of the duodenum. This was found to be normal. Scope was withdrawn. On withdrawing the scope, another close look at the stomach and the esophagus was made. With the exception of the reflux esophagitis, gastritis and bleeding prepyloric ulcer, no other lesion was found.

2. Colonoscopy. With the patient in the left lateral position, rectal examination was done. This was found to be normal. Scope was then advanced up the rectosigmoid into the sigmoid region. Patient had multiple diverticula extending throughout the sigmoid and the descending colon. The splenic flexure and transverse colon were entered. Transverse colon was relatively normal. There were few scattered diverticula. After negotiating the hepatic flexure, the ascending colon and cecum were entered. Ileocecal valve was visualized. Scope was withdrawn. On withdrawing the scope, another close look at the cecum, ascending colon, transverse colon, and sigmoid and rectum was performed. With the exception of the few scattered diverticula, no other lesion was found. Instrument and sponge count were correct after the procedure. Patient withstood the procedure well and there were no complications.

John Jones, M.D.

D: 4/10

T: 4/10

MEDICAL REPORT 7.2

INTERIM HISTORY & PHYSICAL

PATIENT:	Doe, John
MEDICAL RECORD #:	123456
DATE:	4/10
ROOM #:	200
PHYSICIAN:	Jane Smith, M.D.

INTERIM HISTORY: Mr. Doe underwent EGD this morning with findings of bleeding gastric ulcer. Hemostasis was achieved by Dr. Jones. He withstood the procedure very well. He was placed on Protonix and Carafate. This morning, he continues to complain of some abdominal cramping pain and the biggest complaint is back and leg pain.

PHYSICAL EXAMINATION: Temperature 98.4, pulse 63, respiration 20, blood pressure 145/69.

Intake: 6350 Output: 1800

GENERAL: Elderly male, weak, but alert.

CHEST: Good chest expansion, respirations even and unlabored, there are no rales or rhonchi.

CV: Regular rate and rhythm, grade 2/4 systolic murmur at the right second intercostal space which seems to radiate to the apex.

ABDOMEN: Soft. Complains of some mild cramping abdominal pain. There is no vomiting. No diarrhea. No rebound, guarding, or rigidity. No organomegaly. Mild gastric tenderness.

SKIN: Color is pink. Warm and dry. He has several scattered lesions over the extremities.

EXTREMITIES: No clubbing, cyanosis, or edema; no calf tenderness.

GU: Voiding without any dysuria, urgency, or frequency.

NEUROLOGIC: He does have some drooping to the left side of his mouth from an old CVA. He is alert and responsive, aware of surroundings. Able to move all extremities.

LABORATORY DATA: WBC 7.5, HGB 10.2, HCT 31.3, platelet count 137,000, SEGS 66, LYMPHS 22, MONOS 8, EOS 4, BASOS 0, glucose 88, BUN 27, CREAT 0.9, BUN/CREAT ration 30.0, sodium 139, potassium 3.9, chloride 110, CO_2 24, anion gap 9, calcium 8.1.

Lumbar spine x-ray: Degenerative changes. Acute abdominal series: No acute findings. CT of the abdomen: multiple hepatic lesions.

ASSESSMENT:
1. Anemia secondary to GI hemorrhage.
2. Bleeding gastric ulcer.
3. Osteoarthritis.
4. COPD.

PLAN: To treat with Protonix and Carafate. Will place on Mylanta liquid 15cc, every two hours. Will give Darvon 65 plain every four hours p.r.n. for pain and stop the Demerol. Will treat with Skelaxin 400 2 tabs t.i.d. Continue to monitor H&H. Possible discharge in the morning.

I have done a problem-focused history and physical examination. Medical decision-making is of high complexity. There are extensive diagnostic or management options. There is a high risk of morbidity or mortality.

Jane Smith, M.D.

D: 4/10

T: 4/10

Case Study 7.2 (Coder/Abstract Summary Form)

Patient: **Mike Smith**

Patient documentation: **Review Medical Reports 7.3, 7.4, and 7.5**

1. Principal diagnosis:

_____

2. Secondary or other diagnoses:

_____

3. Principal procedure:

_____

4. Other procedures:

_____

5. Additional documentation needed:

_____

_____

_____

_____

6. Questions for the physician:

_____

_____

_____

_____

_____

MEDICAL REPORT 7.3

HISTORY AND PHYSICAL

PATIENT: Smith, Mike

DATE: 07/14

MEDICAL RECORD #:   999999

PHYSICIAN: John Smith, M.D.

1. Acute and massive gastrointestinal hemorrhage with anemia, tachycardia, volume depletion. Although the nasogastric lavage was negative, I still think the highest likelihood is that he has a nonsteroidal and aspirin-induced ulcer, but certainly could have NSAID induced diverticula hemorrhage, angiodysplasia, and less likely malignancy or infection etiologies.

2. Stabilize him hemodynamically with blood transfusion, IV fluids, and plan diagnostic and possible therapeutic EGD and colonoscopy. Maintain hemoglobin above 9. Use oxygen. Begin proton pump inhibitor empirically and in view of the bleeding ulcer, we will use continuous infusion. He has lower abdominal pain likely due to the ulcer. I will review his old records in the office regarding other medical problems, but it seems as if his primary problems have been hypertension, arthritis, and allergies.

3. Mild renal insufficiency, probably prerenal.

4. Hyperglycemia, possible stress response.

DISCUSSION: Mr. Smith is an 86-year-old single, white male, retired 23 years ago from working in a hardware store with a past medical history of hypertension, arthritis, allergic rhinitis, status post cholecystectomy in 1996 who intakes 2 regular aspirin daily and 4 Aleve tablets daily for arthritis.

He presents with a several year history of chronic postprandial epigastric pain and bloating and acute onset of mild crampy lower abdominal pains and copious hematochezia this morning. He came to the ER at 7 A.M. and had noted dark red blood per rectum and passes dark blood in clots in the emergency room. Blood was running down his legs at home in the bathroom when he got up at 3 A.M. He had not been on any recent antibiotics or had any previous bleeding problems. There is no known history of ulcer disease, colitis or bleeding disorder. He denies any nausea, vomiting, heartburn, diarrhea problems, constipation, tenesmus. He feels mildly weak, light-headed, slowly orthostatic. In the ER, he was markedly tachycardic. He has no anorexia or weight loss at home.

PAST MEDICAL HISTORY: As detailed above. He has no history of angina, MI, diabetes, thyroid disease, etc.

ALLERGIES: No known drug allergies.

OUTPATIENT MEDICATIONS:

1. Aspirin 325 mg twice daily.

2. Aleve two tablets twice daily.

3. Diovan 80/12.5 mg daily.

4. Toprol XL 50 mg daily.

5. Clarinex 5 mg daily.

REVIEW OF SYSTEMS: He denies any history of CVA, TIA. He is mildly hard of hearing. He denies any dyspnea, palpitations, cough, chest pains. No sore throat, nosebleeds, or skin rashes. His arthritis is mostly in his lower extremities and controlled with his Aleve and aspirin.

SOCIAL HISTORY: He is single, non-smoker, denies alcohol use. He retired 23 years ago from working in a hardware store. His son, Joe Smith Jr. has power of attorney. Dr. John Smith is his primary care physician and Dr. Heart is his cardiologist.

FAMILY HISTORY: Negative for bleeding diathesis, ulcer disease, cancers, inflammatory bowel disease.

PHYSICAL EXAMINATION:

GENERAL APPEARANCE: Pleasant, elderly white male in no acute distress, slightly weak.

MEDICAL REPORT 7.3 (CONTINUED)

VITAL SIGNS: Height 6 feet 2 inches, weight 185 pounds. Blood pressure 135/85 with pulse of 107 initially, supine and standing 85/36 with pulse 120. Respiration 18. Temperature 99.

SKIN: Pale, nonicteric without rash or telangiectasias.

HEENT: Shows PERRLA, EOMI. Sclerae nonicteric. Throat clear, moist.

NECK: Supple, no lymphadenopathy, thyromegaly, or bruits.

LUNGS: Clear to auscultation and percussion.

CARDIAC: Regular rate and rhythm, no murmur or gallop.

ABDOMEN: Mildly obese, normal bowel sounds, soft with mild epigastric and left lower quadrant tenderness without guarding, mass, bruit, or hepatosplenomegaly.

RECTAL: In the ER, revealed gross blood, normal prostate and I will repeat it later when we do a colonoscopy.

EXTREMITIES: He has varicose veins, but no clubbing, cyanosis, or edema or palpable cords or calf tenderness.

NEUROLOGIC: He is alert and oriented. No focal deficits.

EKG reveals normal sinus rhythm with no ischemic changes. PT/PTT are normal. Initial hemoglobin 10.3 with MCV 89.6, white count 10 with no left shift, platelets 154. BUN 38, creatinine 1.6. Glucose 128.

_____

John Smith, M.D.

D: 07/14

T: 07/14

NOTES

MEDICAL REPORT 7.4

CONSULTATION REPORT

PATIENT:	Smith, Mike
MEDICAL RECORD #:	999999
CONSULTING PHYSICIAN:	Jane Smith, M.D.
ATTENDING PHYSICIAN:	John Smith, M.D.
CONSULTATION DATE:	07/15

HISTORY OF PRESENT ILLNESS: The patient is an 86-year-old gentleman who presented 7/14 with massive lower GI bleed with orthostasis, and tachycardia. He had multiple maroon colored stools. Colonoscopy and EGD revealed diverticula with blood in the right colon and just some antral gastritis. He does take aspirin and Aleve. He apparently has no history of lower GI bleed in the past.

ALLERGIES: None.

MEDICATIONS: Aspirin 325 mg b.i.d., Aleve two tablets twice daily, Diovan 80/12.5 q.d., Toprol XL 50 mg q. day, Clarinex 5 mg p.r.n.

PAST MEDICAL HISTORY: Hypertension, arthritis.

REVIEW OF SYSTEMS: He denies a history of heart disease, chest pain, shortness of breath, diabetes, deep vein thrombosis, pulmonary embolism.

PHYSICAL EXAMINATION:

VITAL SIGNS: Blood pressure 121/70, pulse 76, respiratory rate 12.

HEAD AND NECK: Supple. No cervical adenopathy. No bruits.

LUNGS: Clear.

CARDIOVASCULAR: Regular rate and rhythm with II/VI systolic ejection murmur.

ABDOMEN: Soft, nontender.

EXTREMITIES: Radial femoral pulses 2/3 bilaterally, pedal pulses 1/3 bilaterally. Calves soft, nontender.

LABORATORY VALUES: Hematocrit 28, sodium 140, potassium 4.2, chloride 109, CO2 26, BUN 33, creatinine 1.4, glucose 100.

IMPRESSION: An 86-year-old gentleman with lower GI bleed. It is stable with no active bleeding. He has currently received 3 units of packed red cells.

_____

Jane Smith, M.D.

D: 7/15

T: 7/15

MEDICAL REPORT 7.5

PROCEDURE REPORT

PATIENT:	Smith, Mike
PROCEDURE DATE:	07/14
MEDICAL RECORD #:	999999
PHYSICIAN:	John Smith, M.D.

PROCEDURE: Esophagogastroduodenoscopy with biopsy and colonoscopy with conscious sedation.

INDICATION: An 86-year-old gentleman with massive hematochezia, chronic postprandial epigastric pain on aspirin and Aleve regularly.

ENDOSCOPIST: Jane Smith, M.D.

INSTRUMENT: EG-2930K and EC-30LK.

MEDICATIONS: Fentanyl 75 mcg, Versed 2.5 mg, Levsin 0.25 mg.

SEDATION: Dr. Smith monitored conscious sedation throughout the procedure. See attached flow sheet for details. The procedure, risks, indications, and alternatives were reviewed with the patient.

Physical examination is unchanged today. Written consent was obtained. After adequate sedation and oral throat spray with 10% Xylocaine throat spray X1, the endoscope was passed under direct vision through the oropharynx into the esophagus.

The larynx and cords appeared normal. The mucosa reveals shallow erosions in the antrum and patchy erythema, but no active bleeding. There is some old bloody material scattered about. There are no ulcers, deformity, or tumor. Good flattening of the gastric rugae. Biopsy obtained of the gastritis, but this is likely due to the aspirin and Naprosyn.

The esophagus was normal through its course with no evidence of stricture, esophagitis, ulcer, varices, or Barrett's mucosa.

The scope was passed into the stomach. Gastric pool was aspirated. The gastric mucosa was normal on direct and retroflexed exam with good flattening of the gastric rugae and no evidence of ulcer, gastritis, or deformity.

PROCEDURE: Colonoscopy.

Preparation is fair with a large amount of bloody fluid and clots that we suctioned and washed most off.

There is severe sigmoid diverticulosis and mild diffuse diverticulosis. Suspect this is right colonic diverticula hemorrhage. There is bloody material throughout the colon beginning in the cecum. Could not get into the terminal ileum at this time. No evidence of angiodysplasia, cancers, or colitis. There is a small sessile polyp in the ascending colon which was not resected today to avoid bleeding complications and this will be done some time in the future. I washed the colon vigorously on withdrawal and do not see any diverticula that are bleeding or any visible vessels. Most of his diverticula are small in the right colon. The scope was withdrawn and the patient tolerated the procedure well with no complications.

ENDOSCOPIC DIAGNOSES:
1. Probable diverticular hemorrhage, suspect right colon source given blood throughout the colon. No active bleeding.
2. Severe sigmoid and mild diffuse diverticulosis.
3. Small mid ascending colon polyp—not removed today.
4. Mild antral erosive gastritis secondary to NSAID and aspirin.

Continued

MEDICAL REPORT 7.5 (CONTINUED)

RECOMMENDATIONS: Results reviewed with the patient and family members. He is receiving his second unit of blood and hopefully, if he has no further bleeding, we can discharge him in 48–73 hours. Remains mildly tachycardic and was transiently hypotensive with systolic blood pressure of 69 during his exam which responded to fluids. Will continue to watch serial hemoglobins. Long term—needs to avoid aspirin and nonsteroidals to avoid bleeding as 94% of diverticular hemorrhage attributed to aspirin and nonsteroidal use. If he needs surgery for massive repleting, I will contact Dr. Jones.

Jane Smith, M.D.

D: 7/14

T: 7/14

NOTES

Case Study 7.3 (Coder/Abstract Summary Form)

Patient: **Mark Jones**

Patient documentation: **Review Medical Reports 7.6 and 7.7**

1. Principal diagnosis:

   _____

2. Secondary or other diagnoses:

   _____

3. Principal procedure:

   _____

4. Other procedures:

   _____

5. Additional documentation needed:

   _____

   _____

   _____

6. Questions for the physician:

   _____

   _____

   _____

   _____

HISTORY AND PHYSICAL

PATIENT: Jones, Mark

PT ADMIT: 4/04

MED REC#: 123456

ATTENDING: Jane Smith, M.D.

CHIEF COMPLAINT: Weakness, rectal bleeding, and diarrhea.

HISTORY OF PRESENT ILLNESS: This is an 83-year-old male with a history of high blood pressure, exogenous obesity, prostate cancer, and cardiac arrhythmia. He refers that since Sunday he started having diarrhea, 4–5 × per day, very watery, and mild cramps. He does not remember what he ate that promoted all these symptoms. He has been taking over-the-counter medication without any improvement. Also, he refers mild abdominal discomfort and he has been bleeding rectally in small amounts. Denies fever or chills or vomiting.

CURRENT MEDICATIONS: Tiazac 240 p.o. b.i.d., Lisinopril 10 mg p.o. daily, Tricor 160 p.o. daily, aspirin one a day.

PAST SURGICAL HISTORY: TURP with 31 irradiation treatments. Colonoscopy, appendectomy, tonsillectomy, and right shoulder repair.

REVIEW OF SYSTEMS: No blurred vision, no double vision. No hearing difficulty. No gingival irritation. No epistaxis. No nasal congestion. No coughing spells, no wheezes. No chest pain, no shortness of breath at rest or exertion. No soreness in the muscles, no trauma.

GI: Low sodium diet. Has a lot of gas and burping. No constipation. Please see HPI. The diarrhea at the beginning was brownish and now is greenish, watery, and with foul odor.

GU: No frequent urination, no dysuria, no hematuria.

SKIN: No rashes. No frequent itching.

ALLERGIES: Valium, IVP dye.

SOCIAL HISTORY: He is retired. He drinks alcohol socially. He drinks 1–2 cups decaf coffee daily. No exercise. He only bowls. He quit smoking in 1965.

FAMILY HISTORY: Father died in a car accident, a brother has a history of lung cancer. Mother had a history of osteoporosis.

PHYSICAL EXAMINATION:

VITAL SIGNS: Blood pressure 140/80, heart rate 78, respiratory rate 16. He is oriented × 3, Afebrile. Obese.

SKIN: No jaundice. Good turgor.

LYMPHATICS: No cervical or axillary adenopathy.

HEENT: Head normocephalic. Conjunctivae clear. EOM's intact. Tympanic membranes clear. No bulging. No nasal obstruction. Mouth has dry lips. Thick saliva, posterior pharynx clear.

NECK: Supple.

LUNGS: Clear to auscultation.

HEART: Regular rate and rhythm. Systolic murmur, II/VI, heard in the mitral area.

ABDOMEN: Soft, depressible. No visceromegaly, no rebound. Increased peristalsis. Normal percussion.

MEDICAL REPORT 7.6 (CONTINUED)

RECTAL: Three external hemorrhoids, and one internal at 12 o'clock, no active bleeding. Hemoccult negative. Normal sphincter tone. No lesions or masses. No nodules felt in the prostate.

EXTREMITIES: Good dorsalis pedis and posterior tibial pulses. 1+ edema in both malleolar areas. Atrophic cutaneous changes in both legs.

NEUROLOGIC: Cranial nerves I-XII tested and intact. No gross motor deficit.

ASSESSMENT:
1. GENERALIZED WEAKNESS. DIARRHEA.
2. EXTERNAL HEMORRHOIDS, NO ACTIVE BLEEDING.
3. DEHYDRATION.

PLAN: The patient will be admitted for IV hydration. Please see orders.

Jane Smith, M.D.

D: 4/04

T: 4/04

NOTES

CONSULTATION REPORT

PATIENT:	Jones, Mark
PT ADMIT:	4/04
CONSULTING:	John Smith, M.D.
ATTENDING:	Jane Smith, M.D.

The patient is a very pleasant 83-year-old gentleman who approximately three days ago had an attack of "indigestion" characterized by burning discomfort in the epigastric area as well as eructation. The patient did treat himself with Pepcid and did have some improvement. Later that night, he developed "diarrhea" characterized by multiple liquid bowel movements with small amount of solid material. At first there was not any blood, but then the patient did notice bright red blood which he thought was due to his "hemorrhoids." The next day, the indigestion was much better, but the diarrhea persisted. This was then followed by vomiting undigested food without any blood in it. The patient has had no prior history of gallbladder disease, peptic ulcer disease, pancreatitis, diverticulitis, or renal stones. He has no history of any recent loss of weight or loss of appetite, denies any recent fever or chills, although two months ago he did have an episode of fever and chills.

PAST MEDICAL HISTORY: Does include history of transurethral resection of the prostate in 1993. This was then followed with diagnosis of cancer of his prostate for which he received "radium treatments." Also, he did undergo an appendectomy along with an exploratory laparotomy at the same time. He also had a tonsillectomy performed. He does have a history of arrhythmias and does have a history of hypertension as well as history of asthma as a child.

FAMILY HISTORY: Noncontributory.

ALLERGIES: Valium and IVP dye.

MEDICINES: Includes Tiazac, Lisinopril, Zocor, Motrin, and aspirin.

SOCIAL HISTORY: He stopped smoking in 1965. He is a social user in alcohol.

REVIEW OF SYSTEMS: He had a fever and chills two months ago. He denies any significant loss of weight or loss of appetite. He denies any hoarseness, dizziness or sudden loss of vision, chest pain, heart murmur. He does have a history of arrhythmias. He has some dyspnea on exertion. Denies any hemoptysis, seizure, stroke, bleeding diathesis.

PHYSICAL EXAMINATION: GENERAL:
Reveals a very pleasant 83-year-old gentleman in no acute distress. He is oriented $\times$ 3 with appropriate affect.

VITAL SIGNS: He is afebrile with normal vital signs.

SKIN: There is no obvious jaundice or scleral icterus.

LYMPHATIC SYSTEM: No significant cervical, supraclavicular, or axillary adenopathy.

BACK: There is no CVA tenderness.

LUNGS: Clear. No accessory muscles used.

NECK: Thyroid is not enlarged. No other neck masses.

HEART: S1, S2 are quite distant. No obvious murmurs. He does appear to be in a regular rhythm at this time.

ABDOMEN: Protuberant; however, he did say that he was "bloated" two or three days ago. Although his abdomen is protuberant now, he says that this is the way his abdomen normally is. He does not have any tenderness, spasm, guarding, mass, or organomegaly noted.

RECTAL: Just a small amount of brownish liquid on the examining finger. This is weakly Hematest positive. No rectal masses noted.

EXTREMITIES: He has some trace lower extremity edema bilaterally.

MEDICAL REPORT 7.7 (CONTINUED)

PULSES: Reveals his left dorsalis pedis pulse +2. No pulse felt on his right foot. I did review the patient's chest x-ray that is essentially negative. No acute change noted. His KUB yesterday does show a step-ladder pattern consistent with a small bowel obstruction and there was thought to be gas in his right colon. Today, after a nasogastric tube was placed, he has no significant small bowel dilatation. He does have gas in his transverse colon. Gastrografin enema was essentially negative. There is no obstruction. There is no reflux into the ileum. Pertinent aspects of the laboratory data: The patient's white count today is 11.5, hematocrit 42.3, platelet count 245,000. The patient's Comprehensive Metabolic Profile is essentially normal.

IMPRESSION: The patient appears to have resolving small bowel obstruction most likely adhesions from his previous appendectomy, although less likely from radiation therapy. He does not have any localized pain or fever, and he is not tachycardic. I think that the patient can be safely watched. His x-ray today is markedly improved. I have taken the liberty to order a KUB and upright of the abdomen tomorrow and if this is unchanged from today, then I would recommend his nasogastric tube be clamped for 24 hours and hopefully then it can be discontinued. Hopefully, we can avoid surgery on this patient. Thank you very much for this kind referral. I will be more than happy to follow this patient along with you.

John Smith, M.D.

D: 4/05

T: 4/05

NOTES

Case Study 7.4 (Coder/Abstract Summary Form)

Patient: **Jane Doe**

Patient documentation: **Review Medical Reports 7.8 and 7.9**

1. Principal diagnosis:

   _____

2. Secondary or other diagnoses:

   _____

3. Principal procedure:

   _____

4. Other procedures:

   _____

5. Additional documentation needed:

   _____

   _____

   _____

   _____

6. Questions for the physician:

   _____

   _____

   _____

   _____

   _____

   _____

MEDICAL REPORT 7.8

CONSULTATION REPORT

PATIENT: Doe, Jane

ROOM NUMBER: 300

PATIENT #: 123456

CONSULTING: Jane Smith, M.D.

MED REC#: 999999

ATTENDING: John Jones, M.D.

ADMIT DATE: 7/11

DISCHARGE DATE:

DATE: 7/11

REASON FOR CONSULT: Suspected gastrointestinal bleed.

HISTORY OF PRESENT ILLNESS: Ms. Doe is an 83-year-old nursing home resident at XYZ Manor who was just discharged earlier this week with urinary tract infection and a questionable TIA. During that admission, her hematocrit was noted to fall from 34 to 28% with stools documented positive for occult blood but never reported nausea and vomiting. On arrival, she is noted to have further fall in her hematocrit to 25%. She is on Plavix 75 mg daily and also was on aspirin earlier last week empirically for suspected TIA. She has a past history of GI bleed this past December 2001 with workup including upper and lower endoscopy revealing diverticulosis coli. She is alert and denies any abdominal pain or nausea at present. She has some stool in her diaper that is brown, with no gross blood present.

PAST HISTORY: The patient has no known drug allergies. Past medical history: Type 2 diabetes mellitus, hypertension, dementia, glaucoma, congestive heart failure. She has a known left hip dislocation. Medications include Tenormin, Glucovance, K-Dur, Lasix, Levaquin, Plavix 75 mg daily.

REVIEW OF SYSTEMS, SOCIAL HISTORY: Patient with no alcohol or tobacco use. This is essentially unobtainable from the patient. She does deny shortness of breath, chest pain.

PHYSICAL EXAMINATION: VITALS: Well developed, well nourished, elderly female, alert, in no acute distress. Temp. 99.0, blood pressure 138/50, pulse 60, respiratory rate 18.

HEENT: Anicteric. Conjunctiva pink. Oropharynx moist and without lesions.

NECK: Supple without adenopathy, goiter, JVD.

HEART: Regular rate and rhythm without gallop or rub.

ABDOMEN: Soft, non-distended, non-tender without mass, organomegaly. Bowel sounds normal.

EXTREMITIES: No clubbing, cyanosis, or edema.

RECTAL: Brown stool in rectal vault.

LABORATORY: White blood cell count 8,400. Hematocrit 25%. MCV 77. Platelet count 221,000. Urinalysis with too numerous to count (TNTC) white and red blood cells, 2+ bacteria. BUN 26, creatinine 0.8. Albumin 2.2. ALT 19. Total bilirubin 0.4.

IMPRESSION:

1. SUSPECTED GASTROINTESTINAL BLEED—HAS NO SIGNS OF ACTIVE BLEEDING BUT WITH DOCUMENTED OCCULT BLOOD IN STOOL PREVIOUSLY AND RECENT FALL IN HEMATOCRIT SUSPECT "OOZING" BLEED. THIS MAY BE RELATED TO HER ANTI-PLATELET THERAPY. WITH HER PREVIOUS BLEED LAST DECEMBER, I SUSPECT SHE PROBABLY HAS ENTERAL VASCULAR MALFORMATIONS.
2. URINARY TRACT INFECTION.
3. TYPE 2 DIABETES MELLITUS.

Continued

MEDICAL REPORT 7.8 (CONTINUED)

4. HYPERTENSION.

5. DEMENTIA.

RECOMMENDATIONS:

1. Agree with red blood cell transfusion, serial hematocrits, close observation.

2. Plan upper endoscopy tomorrow morning.

3. May continue Plavix for now but if continuation of significant bleeding, would hold this.

Thanks for allowing me to see this patient.

_____

Jane Smith, M.D.

D: 7/11

T: 7/12

NOTES

MEDICAL REPORT 7.9

PROCEDURE REPORT

PATIENT:	Doe, Jane
ROOM NUMBER:	300
PATIENT #:	123456
CONSULTING:	Jane Smith, M.D.
MED REC#:	999999
ATTENDING:	John Jones, M.D.
ADMIT DATE:	7/11
DISCHARGE DATE:	
DATE:	7/11

DATE OF OPERATION: 7/12

PREOPERATIVE DIAGNOSIS: GI bleed

POSTOPERATIVE DIAGNOSIS: Probable gastric malformations

PROCEDURE: Esophagogastroduodenoscopy

SURGEON: Jane Smith, M.D.

ANESTHESIA: Demerol 25, Versed 1 mgs

CLINICAL ABSTRACT: Ms. Doe is an 83-year-old woman who has had what appears to be a slow GI bleed over the last week or so with documented blood in her stool and significant drop in her hematocrit. History and physical exam were performed in consultation yesterday.

INDICATIONS FOR PROCEDURE: GI bleed, etiology undetermined.

FINDINGS AND PROCEDURE: Patient was placed in left decubitus position. Hurricaine spray was administered into her oral pharynx and posterior pharynx prior to the procedure. Video gastroscope was inserted into the upper esophagus under direct vision. No resistance was encountered. Esophageal mucosa appeared normal. Squamocolumnar junction sharply demarcated above a small hiatal hernia. The endoscope was advanced into the stomach which was carefully examined including retroflex view of the cardia and fundus and body of the stomach which appeared to be vascular mal-formations but these were not bleeding. There were at least 15–20 of these punctate areas and I elected not to coagulate them as they were not bleeding. The pyloric channel, duodenal bulb, second and third portion of the duodenum were carefully examined with no other abnormality seen. She tolerated the procedure well.

IMPRESSION:
1. SMALL HIATAL HERNIA.
2. RECENT GI BLEED SECONDARY TO PROBABLE MULTIPLE GASTRIC MALFORMATIONS.

RECOMMENDATIONS: If Plavix is needed, would continue for now but may have to discontinue if she has recurrent bleeding.

Jane Smith, M.D.

D: 7/12

T: 7/12

Case Study 7.5 (Coder/Abstract Summary Form)

Patient: **Mary Smith**

Patient documentation: **Review Medical Report 7.10**

1. Principal diagnosis:

   _____

2. Secondary or other diagnoses:

   _____

3. Principal procedure:

   _____

4. Other procedures:

   _____

5. Additional documentation needed:

   _____

   _____

   _____

   _____

6. Questions for the physician:

   _____

   _____

   _____

   _____

   _____

MEDICAL REPORT 7.10

OPERATIVE REPORT

PATIENT: Smith, Mary
AGE: 46
MED REC#:   123456
ROOM #:   100
ACCOUNT #:   9999999
DATE OF SURGERY: 7/17
DICTATED: 7/17
TRANSCRIBED: 7/17
SURGEON: John Smith, M.D.

PREOPERATIVE DIAGNOSES: Obstructive jaundice.

Common bile duct stones.

POSTOPERATIVE DIAGNOSES: Obstructive jaundice.

Multiple common bile duct stones.

Prior cholecystectomy.

OPERATION: Endoscopic retrograde cholangiopancreatography with sphincterotomy with balloon extraction of multiple common bile duct stones.

PREMEDICATIONS: Demerol and Versed titrated dosages, Glucagon; patient was on intravenous Fortaz prophylactically.

ENDOSCOPE: Olympus therapeutic duodenoscope and long nosed sphincterotome was used as well as multiple guide wires, balloons, and Isovue 61% diluted with saline about 50% was used.

PROCEDURE: Informed consent obtained prior to the procedure indicating the reason for doing this procedure. The alternatives were discussed, risks of bleeding, perforation, infection, adverse drug effect were discussed as well as the risk of death from the procedure or the anesthesia, the risk of cholangitis, bile duct injury and pancreatitis and the risk of bleeding were discussed—all of which might require emergency surgery or blood transfusion. She appeared to fully understand and comprehend. This was discussed prior to the procedure. She accepted all potential risks and benefits.

FINDINGS: The patient in the oblique position, the scope was advanced without difficulty. Retroflexing the scope in the stomach, a hiatal hernia was noted of moderate size. The scope was advanced to the antrum and pylorus which were unremarkable. The duodenal bulb, second portion of the duodenum appeared normal. The papilla was easily noted.

The tube was straightened in the straight position. A peri-ampullary diverticulum was noted. Bile was seen to come from the papilla which opened and closed quite nicely. The orifice opened and closed and it was clear. A standard catheter was used and initially I injected the pancreatic duct and filled it to its tail that was unremarkable. There was no filling of any secondary branches. No blush was seen.

The patient appeared to have a common channel between the pancreatic duct and the common bile duct so there was reflux of bile into the common bile duct. The scope and the catheter were re-oriented, guide wire was passed and at this point, I was able to cannulate freely the common bile duct. Multiple stones were noted, the largest I gathered was about 0.8 centimeters.

The common bile duct was dilated to about 12 millimeters or so and multiple stones were seen. There was intrahepatic biliary dilatation that was mild. The catheter was removed, the sphincterotome was passed over the guide wire and a cut was used using the cautery machine. Then, the sphincterotome was removed and over the guide wire, a standard 1.5 centimeter balloon was passed, inflated and stone material was removed.

Continued

MEDICAL REPORT 7.10 (CONTINUED)

Several sweeps were made, however, it was felt that the largest sphincterotomy would be helpful. So again, the sphincterotomy was performed in the usual way over an access wire and I made the sphincterotomy as wide as I could without impinging on the diverticulum. There was flow of bile with this maneuver. Several sweeps were made then with the inflated balloon and ultimately decided the stones were removed and that there was drainage of bile freely from the common bile duct after the last sweep.

It was felt that there might be residual small stones but at this point, the adequate sphincterotomy was felt should clear this. The plan will be NPO and then clear liquids later today. Continue the IV antibiotics. Repeat the labs tomorrow and see what the patient's clinical status is. The patient tolerated the procedure well.

_____

John Smith, M.D.

D: 7/17

T: 7/17

NOTES

Coding for Respiratory System Diseases

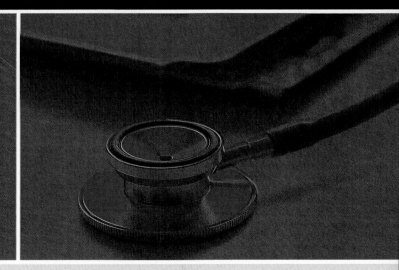

Chapter Outline

Chapter Objectives

- ▶ Describe the pathology of common respiratory system disorders.
- ▶ Recognize the typical manifestations, complications, and treatments of common respiratory system disorders in terms of their implications for coding.
- ▶ Correctly code common respiratory system disorders and related procedures by using the ICD-9-CM and medical records.

We usually think of respiration as an exchange of oxygen and carbon dioxide (a gaseous waste product of metabolism) between our lungs and the external atmosphere that occurs when we breathe. However, internal respiration also occurs in which there is an exchange of oxygen and carbon dioxide in body cells. To maintain health, body cells must take in oxygen and release carbon dioxide to do their special work (e.g., nerve cells conduct electricity, muscle cells contract, and skin cells protect).

189

Diagnosis Coding for Respiratory Diseases

The respiratory chapter of ICD-9-CM includes codes for diseases of the nose, pharynx (throat), larynx (voice box), trachea (windpipe), bronchial tubes, and lungs (where exchange of gases takes place) (Figure 8.1). Respiratory neoplasms (tumors) will be covered in Chapter 14 of this textbook. Respiratory diseases are included in code section 460 to 519 of chapter 8 of the Disease Tabular of the ICD-9-CM.

Common respiratory diseases and disorders covered in this chapter are pneumonia, chronic obstructive pulmonary disease (COPD), asthma, respiratory failure, pulmonary edema, atelectasis, pleural effusion, and adult (or acute) respiratory distress syndrome (ARDS).To assist in your understanding, the Word Parts Box on page 191 reviews word parts and meanings of medical terms related to respiratory system diseases.

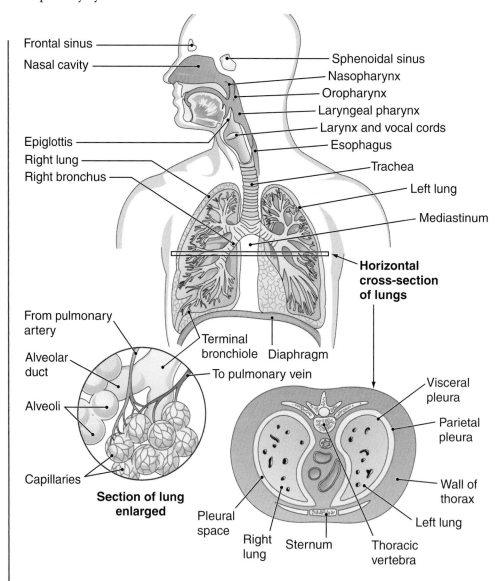

FIGURE 8.1 ■ Respiratory System. (Reprinted with permission from Cohen BJ and Wood DL. Memmler's The Human Body in Health and Disease, 9th Ed. Philadelphia: Lippincott Williams & Wilkins, 2000.)

Word Parts and Meanings of Respiratory System Medical Terms

Word Part	Meaning	Example	Definition of Example
bronch/o, bronch/i	Bronchus	bronchogenic	Originating in the bronchus
-centesis	puncture, tap	thoracentesis	Puncture of the chest
-ostomy	an opening into the body, usually created for elimination of body waste	tracheostomy	Incision of the trachea through the neck, usually to establish an airway in cases of tracheal obstruction
-pnea	Breathing	orthopnea	Difficulty in breathing except in an upright (ortho-) position
Pleur/o	Pleura	pleural effusion	Increased amounts of fluid within the pleural cavity, usually due to inflammation
Pneumon/o	Lung	pneumonectomy	Surgical removal of a lung or lung tissue
-sis	an abnormal condition	atelectasis	Incomplete expansion of a lung or part of a lung; lung collapse

Respiratory infections are usually noted through physicians' documentation, laboratory work (such as a culture and sensitivity report), and chest radiographs. In addition, physicians' orders and medication administration records reveal treatments for respiratory diseases, such as the administration of intravenous antibiotics. Be sure to review the patient's medical record to determine or substantiate a diagnosis of respiratory disease.

Pneumonia

Pneumonia, also called **pneumonitis,** is an inflammation of the lungs in which the lung sacs (alveoli) may fill with pus or other inflammatory debris. It is frequently caused by a bacterial infection. There are many different types of pneumonias, and some universal coding conventions (mentioned in Chapter 2)—such as (1) **mandatory dual coding,** in which two codes are required to describe the condition (e.g., pneumonia attributable to aspergillosis, 117.3 + *[484.5]*), or (2) **combination codes,** in which one code describes both the type of pneumonia and the organism (e.g., *Staphylococcus aureus* pneumonia, 482.41)—are often applied in this section.

Be particularly attentive when the physician documentation shows unspecified or community-acquired pneumonia without further documentation (e.g., pneumonia, not otherwise specified [NOS], 486). A reporting of pneumonia, unspecified, may not reveal the actual organism causing the infection or give an accurate clinical presentation of the patient. You should thoroughly review all laboratory work (especially culture and sensitivity reports) and query the physician if you need more information and additional supporting documentation to identify the specific type of pneumonia, if possible.

Always query the physician for the responsible organism (if known) in order to use the most precise pneumonia code. If the offending organism is unknown, use code 486 for unspecified pneumonia.

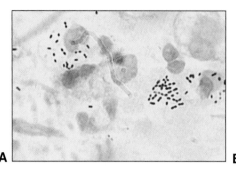
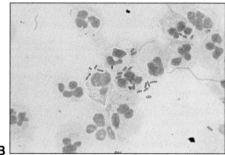

FIGURE 8.2 ■ Gram stained bacteria. (**A**) Gram positive diplococci. (**B**) Gram negative bacilli among white blood cells. (Reprinted with permission from Koneman EW, et al. Color Atlas and Textbook of Diagnostic Microbiology. 5th ed. Philadelphia: Lippincott Williams & Wilkins, 1997.)

Gram-Positive Versus Gram-Negative Pneumonia

Gram-positive and Gram-negative bacteria are types of microorganisms that can have pathogenic affects (cause harmful infections). They are typically identified through a laboratory culture of the tissue or substance from the suspected site or source of infection (e.g., sputum from the respiratory tract). When cultured (i.e., grown), bacteria can have particular staining qualities that allow them to be identified when viewed under a microscope (Figure 8.2). For example, staphylococci are berry-shaped bacteria that grow in clusters resembling grapes and are a type of Gram-positive bacteria. Unspecified Gram-positive pneumonia is classified 482.9 (bacterial pneumonia, unspecified), and unspecified Gram-negative pneumonia is classified 482.83 (Gram-negative pneumonia, NOS). When coding for pneumonia, you must thoroughly review all subterms (**essential modifiers** under the main term "pneumonia" in the Disease Index) and all **nonessential modifiers** (in parentheses after the main term "pneumonia" in the Disease Index). Then you must review the Disease Tabular to select the correct code.

For pneumonia coding, if a specific bacterial organism is identified but has not been assigned a unique code after your review of all subterms and nonessential modifiers, call the hospital's clinical laboratory department or review another resource (e.g., a medical dictionary) to correctly identify the organism as Gram-positive or Gram-negative before assigning a code.

As a rule, Gram-negative pneumonias are more aggressive and require more hospital resources to treat than Gram-positive pneumonias; therefore, Gram-negative pneumonias are generally reimbursed at a higher diagnosis-related group weight.

The Federal Office of the Inspector General has identified pneumonia coding as a high-risk area for **upcoding**, which can significantly change a hospital's reimbursement. Upcoding occurs when the codes reported are not representative of the patient's diseases and procedures and therefore cause the hospital or provider to be overpaid.

Sometimes, the early administration of broad-spectrum antibiotics in the emergency room or problems that can occur in laboratory testing prevent bacterial organisms from growing when cultured. A diagnosis of clinical Gram-negative pneumonia without a positive sputum culture does not prevent you from using this diagnosis; however, you must be able to support the diagnosis with physician documentation, clinical evidence (i.e., signs and symptoms), and treatment. These may include:

- high fever and chills
- tachycardia
- hypotension
- leukocytosis (e.g., increased white blood count or **shift to the left**)
- pus-filled (purulent) sputum
- use of broad-spectrum intravenous antibiotics
- presence in immunocompromised or elderly patients, who are more prone to aggressive Gram-negative pneumonias

Aspiration Pneumonia

Aspiration pneumonia is an extremely serious type of pneumonia that results from inhalation of food, liquid, vomit, or other substances into the respiratory tract (codes 507.0 and 507.8). Aspiration pneumonia can occur along with bacterial pneumonia. In this case, you should report both the code for the aspiration pneumonia and the code for the bacterial pneumonia.

TIP Be aware that patients transferred from nursing homes to acute care hospitals with pneumonia often have aspiration pneumonia. This happens because many nursing home residents have experienced previous strokes (cerebrovascular accidents; CVAs) and have residual deficits such as swallowing difficulties (i.e., dysphagia) and feeding disorders that put them at higher risk for aspiration pneumonia. Check the medical record for this information to help confirm the diagnosis.

Chronic Obstructive Pulmonary Disease

COPD (code 496) is a general term that denotes a chronic obstructive respiratory process (NOS). When the physician documentation shows COPD, review the medical record and the patient's old medical records or query the physician to see whether a more specific type of COPD diagnosis is present. If a more specific type of COPD has been documented, code only the more specific condition (e.g., if the physician has documented both COPD and emphysema in the record, only the code for emphysema would be assigned, because it is a specific type of COPD).

 EXAMPLE

Acute exacerbation of COPD: 491.21

COPD with emphysema: 492.8

Acute exacerbation of COPD with asthma: 493.22

COPD with chronic obstructive asthma: 493.20

COPD with chronic obstructive bronchitis: 491.20

COPD with acute bronchitis: 491.22

Physicians commonly use the term **acute exacerbation of COPD** to mean a severe attack or episode of what is usually a chronic, long-term disease. Acute exacerbation of COPD and acute bronchitis (inflammation of the bronchus) with COPD are coded to combination code 491.22. Codes for pulmonary insufficiency (518.82) or bronchospasms (519.11) with COPD are not assigned as separate codes because these symptoms are assumed in the COPD diagnosis.

Asthma

Asthma is "an inflammatory disease of the lungs characterized by reversible (in most cases) airway obstruction".[1] The airway obstruction results from narrowing and spasms of the bronchi that lead to the lung. This airway obstruction typically results in a high-pitched wheezing sound during respiration. Bronchodilator drugs (e.g., albuterol, epinephrine inhalants, and theophylline) that effectively widen the bronchi are typically used to relieve the obstructive process associated with an asthma attack. **Status asthmaticus** indicates an asthma attack that is not responding to conventional treatment and is difficult to control. There are different types of asthma (category code 493). The fourth digit within the code indicates the asthma type (e.g., allergic, childhood, intrinsic, or chronic obstructive), and the fifth digit indicates whether it is with or without status asthmaticus or whether there is an acute exacerbation of the disease.

TIP Status asthmaticus is a characterized by a prolonged asthmatic attack that does not respond effectively to conventional asthma treatments and is, therefore, difficult to control. Often, physicians do not document status asthmaticus, so you should review the medical record to see whether there is documented evidence of prolonged or intractable wheezing. Also, assess whether the asthma attack is refractory to treatment (i.e., not responding to treatment). Then query the physician to determine whether status asthmaticus exists and to add supporting documentation.

EXAMPLE

Allergic asthma: 493.90

Chronic obstructive asthma: 493.20

Acute exacerbation of allergic asthma: 493.92

Childhood asthma, refractory to treatment, status asthmaticus: 493.01

Respiratory Failure

Respiratory failure is a life-threatening situation. The causes of respiratory failure can include diseases such as end-stage COPD, severe decompensated congestive heart failure (CHF), acute myocardial infarction, or acute CVA. Respiratory failure can be used as a principal or secondary diagnosis, depending on the circumstances and conventional coding rules.

Table 8.1	Abnormal Arterial Blood Gas Laboratory Values	
Variable	**Abnormal Values**	**Description**
pH	<7.35, >7.45	the acidity or alkalinity of blood as measured on a scale of 0 to 14
P_{CO_2}	>50 mm Hg	the amount of carbon dioxide in arterial blood
P_{O_2}	<60 mm Hg	the amount of oxygen in arterial blood
Respiratory rate	>28 breaths/min	

Being aware of abnormal arterial blood gas laboratory values may guide you to query the physician in cases in which respiratory failure seems possible but has not been adequately documented by the attending physician. These abnormal values, explained below, would not be a sufficient indication of respiratory failure in patients with COPD, who are prone to abnormal arterial blood gas values. COPD patients may develop "hypoxic drive" in which the body adjusts to lower levels of oxygen (O_2) and higher levels of carbon dioxide (CO_2). However, abnormal values in other patients may indicate a need to query the physician for more information. To accurately code respiratory failure, supporting physician documentation would have to indicate at least two of the criteria found in Table 8.1.

As blood pH decreases, blood becomes more acidic. As blood pH increases, blood becomes alkaline or basic. Respiratory acidosis (caused by the retention of carbon dioxide in an abnormal exchange of gases) is a dangerous finding in a patient. At a pH of 7.0, the human body can no longer conduct the electricity necessary for contraction of muscles, including the heart.

On 4/20/05, the Central Office on ICD-9-CM provided updated guidelines for when to assign Respiratory Failure as a principal diagnosis. The guidelines describe that respiratory failure may be assigned as the principal diagnosis when it is the condition established after study to be chiefly responsible for occasioning the admission of the patient to the hospital for care. However, certain chapter specific coding guidelines (i.e.- obstetrics, poisonings, HIV, newborn, sepsis) will still take precedence in sequencing over respiratory failure. If a patient is admitted with respiratory failure associated with the above chapter specific codes, the respiratory failure would be sequenced as a secondary diagnosis; otherwise sequencing is dependent upon the circumstances of the admission.

If both acute respiratory failure and another acute condition are responsible for occasioning the admission to the hospital, the guideline that either may be sequenced as the principal diagnosis may be followed; unless the primary thrust of treatment is directed at one condition more than the other. In such a case, the condition that received the thrust of treatment should be sequenced first. If the documentation is unclear as to which diagnosis should be sequenced as the principal diagnosis, the coder should query the physician.

1. A patient with an exacerbation of end-stage COPD is admitted to the hospital for treatment of acute respiratory failure.

Principal diagnosis: *Respiratory failure, 518.81*
Secondary diagnosis: *COPD exacerbation, 491.21*

EXAMPLE

2. A patient is admitted to the cardiac intensive care unit of a hospital with an acute inferior wall MI with respiratory failure.

EXAMPLE	*Principal diagnosis:*	*Acute inferior wall myocardial infarction, 410.41*
	Secondary diagnosis:	*Respiratory failure, 518.81*

3. A patient was admitted to the hospital in acute respiratory failure and was intubated and put on a ventilator. The patient was also found to have congestive heart failure. The physician documents that the respiratory failure was the principal reason for admission.

EXAMPLE	*Principal diagnosis:*	*Acute respiratory failure, 518.81*
	Secondary diagnosis:	*Congestive heart failure, 428.0*

4. A patient is admitted to the hospital with acute respiratory failure and septic shock due to E-coli sepsis.

EXAMPLE	*Principal diagnosis:*	*E-coli sepsis, 038.42*
	Secondary diagnosis:	*Septic shock, 785.52*
		SIRS-sepsis with organ dysfunction, 995.92
		Respiratory failure, 518.81

5. A patient is admitted to the hospital for acute respiratory failure attributable to the progression of Duchenne's dystrophy

EXAMPLE	*Principal diagnosis:*	*Respiratory failure, 518.81*
	Secondary diagnosis:	*Duchenne's dystrophy, 359.1*

Because the principal diagnosis will not be the same in every situation, a careful medical record review is required if both acute respiratory failure and another acute condition are responsible for occasioning the admission (e.g. – acute myocardial infarction, acute cerebrovascular accident). Do not make it an automatic practice to assign acute respiratory failure as the principal diagnosis if a patient is placed on a ventilator in order to obtain a higher reimbursement under the Medicare MS-DRG system. The primary thrust of treatment must always be evaluated and clarified by the physician, if necessary. Prior to the onset of present-on-admission indicators in October 2007, when acute conditions were reported as secondary diagnoses, it was impossible to determine whether or not the acute conditions occurred on admission or after admission as a complication of care without a further review of the medical record (e.g., PDX = acute respiratory failure; SDX = acute cerebrovascular accident). The initiation of the POAs has resolved this issue; nonetheless, these records (i.e., with acute conditions reported as secondary diagnoses) may continue to be more closely scrutinized by insurance companies and targeted for internal and external quality-of-care reviews.

TIP   Coding Clinic 2005, first quarter, provides additional information regarding the sequencing of respiratory failure.

Pulmonary Edema

Most often, pulmonary edema (fluid in the lungs) is associated with a cardiac cause, usually CHF (code 428.0), which is also known as **biventricular heart failure** (i.e., meaning both left- and right-sided ventricular heart failure). The ICD-9-CM index specifies that edema, lung, acute, with mention of heart disease or failure should be coded to 428.1 (left heart failure) or, if CHF is present, 428.0. Whether documented as acute or not, pulmonary edema needs clarification and is a condition most often associated with CHF that results in the inability of the heart to pump blood. Blood then backs up or pools in the lungs, causing pulmonary edema (fluid from blood leaks from lung alveoli or air sacs into surrounding lung tissues).

Pulmonary edema with CHF: 428.0

Acute pulmonary edema with CHF: 428.0

Pulmonary edema, CHF, hypertensive cardiovascular disease: 402.91 + 428.0

EXAMPLE

Although not as common as cardiac-related pulmonary edema, noncardiac pulmonary edema can be coded as follows, depending on the circumstances:

Chronic pulmonary edema, NOS 514
Acute pulmonary edema (NOS) or postoperative pulmonary edema 518.4
Acute pulmonary edema caused by fumes and vapors (e.g., smoke
    inhalation) 506.1
Postradiation pulmonary edema 508.0
Pulmonary edema attributable to high altitude 993.2
Pulmonary edema attributable to nearly drowning (caused by the
    aspiration of water) 994.1

Physician documentation of pulmonary edema (code 514) or acute pulmonary edema (code 518.4) without any further specification is a red flag. To code correctly, you must first determine whether the pulmonary edema is of cardiac or noncardiac origin.

To clarify use of the correct code (i.e., cardiac versus noncardiac pulmonary edema), perform a complete review of the patient's record, with special attention to the physician's admitting and progress notes, review of the patient's chest x-ray report, and clinical interventions (documented in the physician's orders and medication administration records). Query the physician for additional documentation if necessary.

Clinical interventions for pulmonary edema can include the use of diuretics such as intravenous furosemide, cardiotonics such as digitalis (to make the heart pump more forcefully), oxygen therapy, a restriction on sodium (salt intake increases fluid retention), positioning the patient in a upright position (orthopnea) to decrease the venous return of blood to the heart, and use of vasodilators, which ease the work of the heart.

Atelectasis

Atelectasis (code 518.0) is a partial or complete collapse of a patient's lungs (Figure 8.3). Atelectasis can occur during the postoperative period because of a poor inspiration effort resulting from pain associated with surgery. Atelectasis can also be attributable to infections or trauma or can even occur spontaneously.

Postoperative atelectasis requires two codes to adequately describe the condition: Postoperative respiratory complications (code 997.39) and with atelectasis (code 518.0). Other atelectasis codes include:

Newborn atelectasis 770.5
Primary newborn atelectasis 770.4
Atelectasis attributable to tuberculosis 011.9X

Note that an incidental finding of atelectasis on a chest radiograph should not be coded. Atelectasis can be coded only if it meets the criteria for reportable diagnoses according to Uniform Hospital Discharge Data Set (UHDDS) definitions (i.e., it affects the patient's care) and has been adequately documented by the physician. Postoperative atelectasis should include adequate documentation from the physician and documented

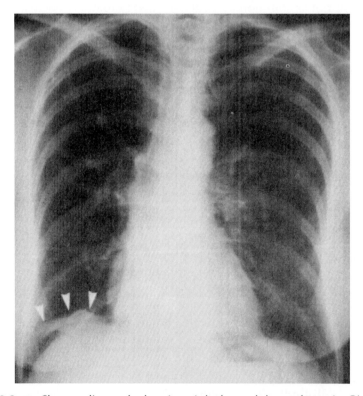

FIGURE 8.3 ■ Chest radiograph showing right lower lobe atelectasis. Right lower lobe atelectasis seen as area of density in right lung base behind right portion of the cardiac silhouette. Arrowheads highlight an area of linear atelectasis above the right hemidiaphragm, as well. (LifeART image copyright © (2008) Lippincott Williams & Wilkins. All rights reserved.)

signs, symptoms, and treatments for the disease (e.g., postoperative fever, physician's orders to increase the frequency of incentive spirometry [a device used to assist a patient in taking deeper breaths to expand the lungs], and administration of intravenous antibiotics).

Pleural Effusion

In a pleural effusion, there is an escape of fluid into the pleural cavity, the double-folded membrane surrounding and protecting the lungs (Figure 8.4). There are different types of pleural effusions, and correct coding requires adequate physician documentation of the cause. Attention to diagnostic thoracentesis (needle drainage) or insertion of a chest tube (i.e., tube thoracostomy) to drain the pleural effusion for analysis of pleural fluid (culture or cytologic examination) can help you establish the correct diagnosis for coding.

TIP
If drained, fluids contained in the pleural effusion can be examined and classified as transudates (clear serous fluid, as seen in CHF) or exudates (cloudy, pus-filled bacterial fluid, as seen in infections such as pneumonia). Fluids may even contain cancerous cells, as seen during cytologic examination (malignant pleural effusions). This can change the code assignments accordingly.

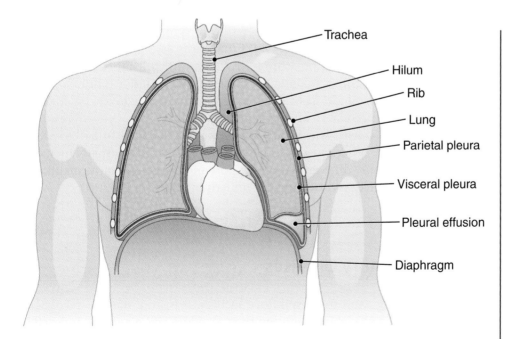

FIGURE 8.4 ■ Pleural effusion. An abnormal volume of fluid collects in the pleural space. (Reprinted with permission from Cohen BJ. Medical Terminology: An Illustrated Guide, 4th Ed. Baltimore: Lippincott Williams & Wilkins, 2004.)

Pleural effusions are commonly associated with CHF. Because pleural effusions are integral to the underlying disease of CHF, the effusions are not reported separately unless significant and separate treatment is directed toward the effusion (e.g., a thoracentesis was performed). If a patient was admitted with significant pleural effusion associated with CHF that received separate treatment, the code for CHF (428.0) would be sequenced as the principal diagnosis, with the code for the pleural effusion (511.9) sequenced second. With the exceptions noted previously for CHF, other types of pleural effusion can be designated as the principal or secondary diagnosis provided that this diagnosis conforms with UHDDS rules for principal or other reportable diagnosis assignments.

Codes for various pleural effusions include:

Pleural effusion, NOS 511.9
Bacterial pleural effusion 511.1
Malignant pleural effusion 511.81
Traumatic pleural effusion 862.29
Traumatic with open wound pleural effusion 862.39
Pleural effusion attributable to tuberculosis 012.0X
Pleural effusion attributable to CHF 428.0 (code the CHF only)
Pleural effusion attributable to CHF 428.0 + 511.9; 34.91 (thoracentesis procedure performed for significant effusion; significant pleural effusion is sequenced as a secondary diagnosis with CHF)

Adult Respiratory Distress Syndrome

A characteristic of syndromes is that a group of symptoms present together that point to a particular disease. ARDS manifests as a group of symptoms including tachypnea (rapid breathing), dyspnea (difficult breathing), tachycardia (rapid heartbeat), hypoxemia (insufficient oxygenation of blood), and cyanosis (bluish discoloration of skin caused by diminished oxygen content of blood) and often results in acute respiratory failure.

ARDS associated with shock, surgery, or trauma is coded to 518.5. ARDS associated with any other cause is coded to 518.82. Treatment usually includes providing the patient with ventilatory support and oxygen therapy, maintaining metabolic balance, and treating the underlying cause of the ARDS.

Procedure Coding for Respiratory Diseases

For correct coding from the respiratory section, it is important to recognize that there must be agreement between the procedure and diagnosis codes. If a significant procedure is performed, the medical necessity for the procedure must be reported through the assignment of diagnosis codes. Also keep in mind that procedures can be diagnostic (to help diagnose disease) or therapeutic (to treat or cure disease). UHDDS guidelines specify that definitive therapeutic procedures must be sequenced before diagnostic procedures.

Bronchial and Lung Biopsies

A biopsy is a diagnostic procedure. **Closed biopsies** (without incision) of the bronchus (code 33.24) include endoscopic biopsies (i.e., bronchoscopy with biopsies, washings, or brushings). An **open biopsy** (with incision) of the bronchus is coded to 33.25.

Closed biopsies of the lung include endoscopic or transbronchial lung biopsy (code 33.27), closed (endoscopic) brush biopsy of lung (33.24), percutaneous needle biopsy (33.26), and thoracoscopic lung biopsy (33.20). An open biopsy (with incision) of the lung is coded to 33.28.

TIP Sometimes it is difficult to determine from the physician's documentation in the operative report whether the closed-biopsy specimen came from lung or from bronchial tissue. This can have a significant effect on the provider's reimbursement. To clarify the location of the biopsy, perform a careful review of the pathologist's report, review where the initial lesion was located (lung or bronchus) from the physician's admitting diagnostic statement, and query the attending physician for more information and documentation regarding the biopsy location.

Thoracentesis

Thoracentesis (code 34.91) involves insertion of a needle through the skin into the pleural space to drain fluid from the pleural cavity and obtain fluid for analysis (e.g., treatment for pleural effusions) (Figure 8.5). This procedure can be diagnostic, therapeutic, or both. A new 2008 code is available for thorascopic drainage of pleural fluid cavity (34.06).

Chest Tube Insertion

Chest tube insertion, or thoracostomy tube placement (code 34.04), involves passing a chest tube through a small incision in the skin to drain pleural spaces, reinflate collapsed lungs (atelectasis), and drain pleural spaces after surgery (i.e., post-thoracotomy procedure [involving an incision into the chest]). This procedure can be diagnostic, therapeutic, or both.

Tracheostomy

A tracheostomy is a therapeutic procedure that creates an opening into the trachea (windpipe) through the neck to insert a tube to create a patent (open) airway (Figure 8.6). The tracheostomy placement may be permanent (code

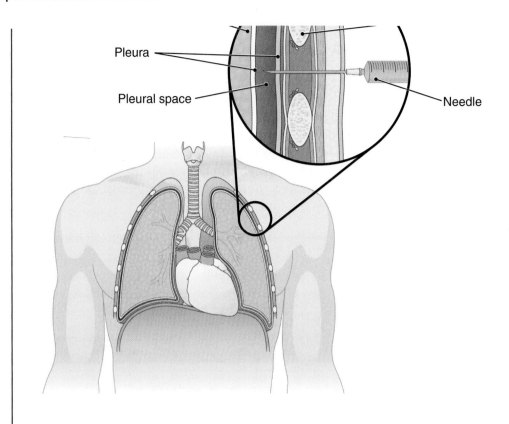

Pleura

Pleural space

Needle

FIGURE 8.5 ■ Thoracentesis. A needle is inserted into the pleural space. (Reprinted with permission from Cohen BJ. Medical Terminology: An Illustrated Guide, 4th Ed. Baltimore: Lippincott Williams & Wilkins, 2004.)

31.29)—for example, after laryngectomy for laryngeal cancer or for prolonged ventilation after a high spinal cord injury. The tracheostomy may be emergent and temporary (code 31.1) for cases such as a foreign body (e.g., food) lodged in a patient's airway which obstructs breathing.

Lung Resections, Lobectomy, or Complete Pneumonectomy

Pulmonary resections are therapeutic procedures that involve removal of localized areas of diseased lung tissue. They can include wedge resections (code 32.29), endoscopic lung resections (code 32.28), segmental lung resections (code 32.3), and lung volume reduction surgery (code 32.22).

Lobectomy is the removal of an entire lobe of the lung (open lobectomy is coded to 32.49; and, thorascopic lobectomy is coded to 32.41). The right lung is divided into three lobes, and the left lung is divided into two. Complete pneumonectomy is the removal of an entire lung, left or right (code 32.5).

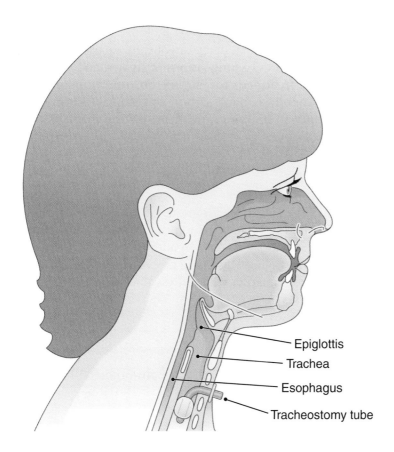

Epiglottis
Trachea
Esophagus
Tracheostomy tube

FIGURE 8.6 ■ A tracheostomy tube in place. (Reprinted with permission from Cohen BJ. Medical Terminology: An Illustrated Guide, 4th Ed. Baltimore: Lippincott Williams & Wilkins, 2004.)

Endotracheal Intubation and Mechanical Ventilation

To assist a patient in breathing (e.g., for a patient in acute respiratory failure), a tube is placed through the mouth or nose and positioned in the trachea (windpipe) to establish an airway and connect the patient to a ventilator (a machine that moves air in and out of the lungs). A patient can also be placed on a ventilator via a tracheostomy.

The code for the therapeutic placement of an endotracheal tube is 96.04. Codes for mechanical ventilation indicate whether the patient was on the ventilator for less than 96 hours (code 96.71) or longer than 96 consecutive hours (code 96.72). The count starts from the time of initiation of the ventilator (e.g., ventilation initiated in the emergency department or intensive care unit) or, for a patient received on a ventilator, the time of transfer to the hospital. The ventilator duration ends when patient is completely weaned from the device.

 Ventilatory assistance that is typically performed during surgery is not coded.

Respiratory procedure codes added in 2007 included 32.23–32.26 and 33.7X. Codes 32.23–32.26 describe open, percutaneous, thoracoscopic, or other ablation (destruction) procedures of lung lesions or tissues, and subcategory code 33.7X describes a new treatment for chronic obstructive pulmonary disease (COPD) that involves endoscopic insertion or removal of bronchial devices (i.e., valves) that reduce air trapping and hyperinflation that is associated with this disease.

SUMMARY

In this chapter, you have identified common pathologic conditions that affect the respiratory system. You have also identified the common clinical procedures related to the respiratory system. In addition, you have learned to correctly code respiratory system diseases and procedures by using the ICD-9-CM coding manual. The next chapter will address the subject of coding for genitourinary system diseases.

REFERENCE

1. Stedman's Medical Dictionary, 27th Ed. Baltimore: Williams & Wilkins, 2000.

TESTING YOUR COMPREHENSION

1. What is an inflammation of the lungs in which the lung sacs (alveoli) may fill with pus or other inflammatory debris, frequently attributable to a bacterial infection?

2. Which is considered more aggressive and requires more hospital re-sources to treat: Gram-positive pneumonia or Gram-negative pneumonia?

3. Identify a type of pneumonia that results from inhalation of foods, liquids, vomit, or other substances into the respiratory tract.

4. What is status asthmaticus?

5. What is pulmonary edema normally associated with?

6. What is the diagnosis for a partial or complete collapse of a patient's lung?

7. A pleural effusion is commonly associated with what diagnosis and is therefore not usually coded unless it receives separate treatment?

8. What does the acronym ARDS stand for?

9. What is thoracentesis? What is its purpose?

10. What is the purpose of a tracheostomy?

CODING PRACTICE I   Chapter Review Exercises

Directions

By using your ICD-9-CM codebook, code the following diagnoses and procedures:

	DIAGNOSIS/PROCEDURES	CODE
1	Acute pulmonary edema with congestive heart failure.	
2	Respiratory failure secondary to acute exacerbation of COPD. Endotracheal intubation with mechanical ventilation for less than 96 hours.	
3	*Pseudomonas* pneumonia with bacterial pleural effusion. Thoracentesis.	
4	Chronic obstructive asthma with acute exacerbation.	
5	Acute bronchitis. COPD. Fiberoptic bronchoscopy with bronchial biopsy.	
6	Aspiration pneumonia. Status post CVA with residual dysphagia and right-sided hemiplegia.	
7	Oat cell carcinoma of the lung. **Postoperative atelectasis.** Left upper lobe lobectomy, open.	
8	Respiratory failure secondary to acute subendocardial myocardial infarction.	
9	Postoperative ARDS.	
10	Congestive heart failure with large pleural effusion. Chest tube insertion for drainage.	
11	Bronchopneumonia secondary to typhoid.	
12	Acute respiratory failure secondary to embolic CVA with infarct.	
13	Admitted for Legionnaires pneumonia with respiratory failure.	

	DIAGNOSIS/PROCEDURES	CODE
14	Acute fracture to C2 vertebra. Quadriplegia. Respiratory failure. Fall from horse at riding school *(for practice, add E codes).* Permanent tracheostomy placement for prolonged ventilatory management.	
15	Deviated nasal septum. Chronic maxillary sinusitis. Submucous resection, nasal septum.	
16	End-stage COPD/emphysema with acute and chronic respiratory failure. Endotracheal intubation with mechanical ventilation for less than 96 hours.	
17	Childhood asthma with status asthmaticus.	
18	Post radiation pulmonary fibrosis. History of lung cancer. Status post radiation therapy *(for practice, add V and E codes).*	
19	Spontaneous tension pneumothorax. Thoracostomy tube placement.	
20	*Pneumocystis carinii* pneumonia. Acquired immune deficiency syndrome. Fiberoptic bronchoscopy with bronchial washings.	
21	Pulmonary edema attributable to chlorine fumes. Accidental inhalation of chlorine fumes by a hotel pool maintenance worker *(for practice, add E codes).*	

CODING PRACTICE II   Medical Record Case Studies

Instructions

1. Carefully review the medical reports provided for each case study.
2. Research any abbreviations and terms that are unfamiliar or unclear.
3. Identify as many diagnoses and procedures as possible.
4. Because only part of the patient's total record is available, determine what additional documentation you might need.
4. If appropriate, identify any questions you might ask the physician to code this case correctly and completely.
5. Complete the appropriate blanks below for each case study.

CHAPTER 8 CASE STUDIES

Case Study 8.1 (Coder/Abstract Summary Form)

Patient: **Jane Doe**

Patient documentation: **Review Medical Reports 8.1 and 8.2**

1. Principal diagnosis:

   _____

2. Secondary or other diagnoses:

   _____

3. Principal procedure:

   _____

4. Other procedures:

   _____

5. Additional documentation needed:

   _____

   _____

   _____

   _____

Case Study 8.1 (Continued)

6. Questions for the physician:

_____

_____

_____

_____

_____

HISTORY AND PHYSICAL

PATIENT NAME: DOE, JANE

RM #:   100-1

PHY: JONES

MR#   111111

ADMISSION DATE: 6/15

CHIEF COMPLAINT: FEVER, COUGH, LETHARGIC CONDITION FOR THE PAST 3 DAYS.

HISTORY OF PRESENT ILLNESS: This 92-year-old pleasant white female patient was admitted through the Emergency Room with the history of fever, coughing spells, increasing lethargic condition and weakness going on for about 3–4 days, much worse today. She was evaluated in the Emergency Room and was found to have pneumonia, electrolyte imbalance with dehydration. She was admitted for further treatment and management. She is running a fever with chills and rigors for the past 24 hours. She was having mostly a nonproductive cough and a little bit of a productive cough present. She was not having nausea, vomiting, or any diarrhea.

PAST HISTORY: She has the history of coronary artery disease, osteoarthritis, bilateral profound sensory neural hearing loss, hypertension, and hypothyroidism.

ALLERGIES: No known drug allergies.

MEDICATIONS: Paxil 10 milligrams once a day

Restoril 7.5 milligrams h.s. prn

Baby aspirin, once a day

Dyazide 50/25, once a day

Levothroid 0.075 milligrams, once a day

Oxygen as needed

Prinzide 20/25, once a day

Kaopectate 0.5 oz., every 6 hours prn

Imodium AD, I every 6 hours prn

Motrin 4000, every 6 hours prn

Vioxx 12.5 milligrams, once a day

Milk of Magnesia as needed

High protein diet

Megace suspension 40 milligrams/cc., 10 cc. b.i.d.

Tylenol, every 6 hours prn

Robitussin DM 2 teaspoons full t.i.d. prn

PAST SURGICAL HISTORY: Coronary artery bypass graft, 4 vessel bypass about 20 years ago.

FAMILY & SOCIAL HISTORY: The family history and social history was noncontributory.

PERSONAL HISTORY: She is widowed. She lives in XYZ Nursing Home. She is retired. She was mostly a housewife.

REVIEW OF SYSTEMS: Essentially negative.

PHYSICAL EXAMINATION

GENERAL: This patient is small and thin built. Looks pale and anemic. Appears to be in mild distress.

HEART: Rate rapid, 98 per minute, no murmurs

LUNGS: The patient has scattered rhonchi, coarse breathing, and a few rales at the right lung. The respirations are 24–26 per minute. Some nonproductive cough is present.

ABDOMEN: Slightly distended. Bowel sounds heard. No definite organomegaly.

EXTREMITIES & SPINE: Essentially negative, except for arthritis, arthralgia, and general weakness. She has a little rash in the perineal area.

EYES & PUPILS: Normal and reacting to light. Pupils are equal and symmetrical on both sides. Bilateral arcus senilis is present. Pupils are equal, symmetrical, and reaction to light is sluggish, but satisfactory.

ENT: Essentially negative, except for bilateral profound sensory neural hearing loss.

NECK: Supple, no thyromegaly, no lymphadenopathy, no carotid bruits.

CNS: The patient is slightly lethargic. All cranial nerves seem to be intact. Precise examination was not possible at this time.

GENITOURINARY: Negative.

RECTAL: Deferred at this time.

PELVIC: Deferred at this time.

IMPRESSION:
1. PROBABLE PNEUMONIA.
2. DEHYDRATION.
3. ELECTROLYTE IMBALANCE.
4. CORONARY ARTERY DISEASE.
5. HYPOTHYROIDISM.
6. OSTEOARTHRITIS.
7. SEVERE GENERALIZED OSTEOPOROSIS.
8. STATUS POST CORONARY ARTERY BYPASS GRAFT, 4 VESSEL AROUND 1980.

PLAN: The patient is admitted now. Please see orders.

John Jones, M.D.

cf

D: 06/15

T: 06/16

MEDICAL REPORT 8.2

PROGRESS NOTE

PATIENT NAME: DOE, JANE
RM #:   100-1
PHY: JONES
MR#:   111111

DATE: 6/19

S: Ms. Doe is resting comfortably in bed. She has difficulty hearing at times. She denies any problems at this time. She denies chest pain, shortness of breath, paroxysmal nocturnal dyspnea, orthopnea, nausea, or vomiting.

O: Temperature is 98.7, pulse 83, respirations 18, blood pressure 113/60. Over the last 24 hours, the patient had approximately 2600 cc in and 2400 cc out. Cardiac—irregular, irregular with controlled rate. Lungs—poor inspiratory effort is noted. Otherwise, the patient does have some scattered rhonchi and rales noted at the bases. Abdomen is soft, nontender to palpation. No guarding. Extremities—no clubbing, cyanosis, or edema.

A: Pneumonia with a sputum culture showing staph aureus, congestive heart failure, anemia, coronary artery disease, dementia, dehydration, malnutrition.

P: Continue to watch the patient very closely. She continues to be on IV antibiotics. Her lungs do sound like she still has some congestion. Will continue to encourage her nutritional status. Watch her temperature and nutritional status.

John Jones, M.D.
cf
D: 06/19
T: 06/19

NOTES

Case Study 8.2 (Coder/Abstract Summary Form)

Patient: **John Doe**

Patient documentation: **Review Medical Report 8.3**

1. Principal diagnosis:

   _____

2. Secondary or other diagnoses:

   _____

3. Principal procedure:

   _____

4. Other procedures:

   _____

5. Additional documentation needed:

   _____

   _____

   _____

   _____

6. Questions for the physician:

   _____

   _____

   _____

   _____

   _____

DISCHARGE SUMMARY

PATIENT NAME: DOE, JOHN
RM #: 102-1
PHY: SMITH
MR# 222222

ADMITTED: 6/16

DISCHARGED: 6/18

John Doe is a 64-year-old white male from Chicago who was admitted with gross hemoptysis. He also had acute worsening of his chronic hypoxemic respiratory failure caused by the hemoptysis.

HOSPITAL COURSE: The patient was admitted to the ICU and when he was settled in his ICU bed, he underwent emergency fiberoptic bronchoscopy. Bleeding was found coming from the apical segmental bronchus of the left upper lobe. No endobronchial lesions were seen and no biopsies were performed; however, bronchial washings were taken.

The bleeding ceased as suddenly as it had started and he had no further problems throughout the rest of the hospital stay. He had a CT of the chest done 6/17 which showed severe emphysematous changes and diffuse interstitial fibrosis. There were no lesions found in the left upper lobe.

The patient had transient hypotension which possibly could have been caused by the Lasix he was taking or he could have some mild adrenal insufficiency. He was given IV fluids and a serum Cortisol level was drawn. The hypotension resolved with IV fluids.

Throughout the hospital stay the patient was in a DNR status at his own request.

On the day of discharge 6/18, a CBC showed a hemoglobin of 16 with a hematocrit of 50.9% and a white count of 10,600. The platelets were 210,000. His oxygen saturation was running better than 90% on three liters per minute nasal cannula which is his usual oxygen dose.

FINAL DIAGNOSES:
1. Acute-on-chronic hypoxemic respiratory failure.
2. Gross hemoptysis from the apical segmental bronchus of the left upper lobe.
3. Hypotension.
4. Chronic obstructive pulmonary disease.
5. Secondary polycythemia.
6. Tobacco abuse.
7. Obesity.
8. Left anterior fascicular block on electrocardiogram.

SURGICAL AND DIAGNOSTIC PROCEDURES: Emergency fiberoptic bronchoscopy with bronchial washings on 6/17.

DISPOSITION: The patient was discharged home on a regular diet and normal activities. He is permanently and totally medically disabled secondary to his chronic lung disease.

The patient is to resume home aerosol therapy treatments at home oxygen at three liters per minute by nasal cannula continuously.

The patient is to resume medications taken prior to admission. In addition, he is placed on Levaquin 500 mg p.o. q.a.m. for seven days and vitamin C 500 mg p.o. q.i.d. for seven days.

MEDICAL REPORT 8.3 (CONTINUED)

The patient is to follow up with me in my office in one week at which time the results of the cytology from the bronchial washings should be available. It was not available at the time of discharge. Also the serum Cortisol values should be available.

_____

John Smith, M.D.

cf

D: 6/18

T: 6/19

Case Study 8.3 (Coder/Abstract Summary Form)

Patient: **Kathy Brown**

Patient documentation: **Review Medical Report 8.4**

1. Principal diagnosis:

   _____

2. Secondary or other diagnoses:

   _____

3. Principal procedure:

   _____

4. Other procedures:

   _____

5. Additional documentation needed:

   _____

   _____

   _____

   _____

Case Study 8.3 (Continued)

6. Questions for the physician:

_____

_____

_____

_____

_____

MEDICAL REPORT 8.4

HISTORY AND PHYSICAL

PATIENT NAME: BROWN, KATHY

RM #:   103-1

PHY: JONES

MR#   333333

ADMISSION DATE: 6/18

CHIEF COMPLAINT: SHORTNESS OF BREATH AND CHEST PAIN

HISTORY OF PRESENT ILLNESS: Ms. Brown is a 67-year-old white female with chronic obstructive pulmonary disease, atherosclerotic heart disease, and peripheral vascular disease, who presents with complaints of shortness of breath and chest pain. The patient states she has had increased cough and congestion for the past week. She called her family physician, Dr. Smith, and received an oral antibiotic which she has been taking for the last two days prior to admission. On the day of admission, she was having vague chest discomfort and increased shortness of breath and presented to the emergency room. Her initial electrocardiogram failed to show any acute changes. She was given a beta agonist nebulization for her breathing, and she subsequently developed ST depression on EKG. A nitroglycerin infusion was initiated as well as anti-coagulation with Lovenox. She was observed overnight in the emergency room. Her cardiac enzymes have returned negative × 3 sets.

This morning, the patient complains of a headache and shortness of breath. She is no longer having the chest discomfort. She describes it as a burning discomfort. She was not sure if it was indigestion. She did not try any medications for it at home.

PAST HISTORY: Her past history is significant for coronary artery disease, with her initial bypass surgery. She had subsequent angioplasty and then an inferior myocardial infarction. She underwent her second bypass procedure in June, receiving a left internal mammary artery to the first diagonal, and saphenous vein grafts to the ramus intermedius and the posterior descending artery. She also has a saphenous vein graft to the left anterior descending artery from her initial surgery, which was left in place. At the time of her catheterization preoperatively, her left ventriculogram revealed inferior wall hypokinesis with an ejection fraction of approximately 50%. A subsequent echocardiogram in August revealed inferoseptal and posterior hypokinesis with an ejection fraction of 45%, moderate to severe mitral regurgitation, and an estimated pulmonary artery pressure of approximately 50 mmHg.

The patient also has a history of hypertension, hyperlipidemia, and peripheral vascular disease with a history of aortobifemoral bypass. She has chronic obstructive pulmonary disease with frequent episodes of bronchitis. She is a lifelong smoker, and today she states that she quit smoking a month or so ago. She also has a history of hypothyroidism, and she is on thyroid replacement therapy. Her home medications listed include Xanax 0.25 mg t.i.d., aspirin 81 mg daily, Lasix 40 mg daily, K-Lor 25 mEq daily, Pravachol 20 mg daily, Premarin 0.625 mg daily, Thyroid 0.06 mg daily, and finally amiodarone 200 mg b.i.d. Her bottles are not with her. The patient is unsure if she is actually taking the amiodarone. She recalls that this was started by Dr. Smith, but she thinks she only took it for one month. Review of the old charts reveals that subsequent hospitalizations, including the most recent one on 4/1, failed to list amiodarone in her medications; and the patient did not receive the amiodarone, according to the MARs. The patient relates allergies to two antibiotics, and upon review of the chart, these appear to be Levaquin and Zithromax. She has been treated with cephalosporins in the past, uneventfully.

The patient also is on home oxygen therapy chronically. She is able to get around the house. She does cook but does very little cleaning. She may go to the grocery store, but takes her oxygen with her. She does not describe significant exertional chest discomfort and has not described any significant orthopnea or paroxysmal nocturnal dyspnea. She does have significant dyspnea on exertion.

Continued

PHYSICAL EXAMINATION

VITAL SIGNS: Her blood pressure is 140/70, heart rate in the 80s.

GENERAL: She is an elderly, chronically ill-appearing white female in no acute distress. She appears dyspneic with effort.

HEENT: Benign. There is no jugular venous distension. No carotid bruits are detected.

LUNGS: Reveal mild rhonchi and wheezes.

HEART: The cardiac rhythm is regular, with a 1 – 2/6 holosystolic murmur of mitral regurgitation at the apex. An extra heart sound is heard, probably S3.

ABDOMEN: Soft. The abdomen is tender in the epigastrium. There is no rebound tenderness and no mass.

EXTREMITIES: Reveal no edema.

DIAGNOSTIC TESTS: The EKG this morning is very close to normal. The ST pattern is significantly improved as compared to the EKG obtained yesterday after her breathing treatment.

LABORATORY: As stated earlier, the cardiac enzymes are negative X 3 sets. The white blood count is 11,500 with a hemoglobin of 12, hematocrit 35.9, platelets 191,000. Prothrombin time 12.3. International normalized ratio 0.98. Glucose is 98, sodium 140, potassium 4.6, chloride 105, bicarbonate 28, blood urea nitrogen 15, creatinine 1.1.

IMPRESSION:

1. Acute exacerbation of chronic bronchitis, chronic obstructive pulmonary disease.
2. Chest pain, noncardiac.
3. Atherosclerotic heart disease, status post coronary artery bypass graft.
4. Peripheral vascular disease.
5. Hypertension.

PLAN: The patient is admitted for further treatment of her bronchitis. We will employ beta agonist nebulizations and also cover her with empiric antibiotic therapy. Her epigastric discomfort may be due to gastritis, and we will therefore treat her with Prevacid and check her stool hemoccult. We will hydrate cautiously and be on the lookout for the development of congestive heart failure symptoms or signs.

Dr. John Jones, M.D.

cf

D: 6/18

T: 6/19

Case Study 8.4 (Coder/Abstract Summary Form)

Patient: **Sarah Jones**

Patient documentation: **Review Medical Report 8.5**

1. Principal diagnosis:

   _____

2. Secondary or other diagnoses:

   _____

3. Principal procedure:

   _____

4. Other procedures:

   _____

5. Additional documentation needed:

   _____

   _____

   _____

   _____

6. Questions for the physician:

   _____

   _____

   _____

   _____

   _____

MEDICAL REPORT 8.5

HISTORY AND PHYSICAL

PATIENT NAME:	JONES, SARAH
RM #:	104-1
PHY:	SMITH
MR#	444444

ADMITTED: 06/13

CHIEF COMPLAINT: FEVER, CONGESTION, AUDIBLE WHEEZING

HISTORY OF PRESENT ILLNESS: The patient is a 92-year-old Caucasian female with a history of Alzheimer's dementia and chronic asthma/COPD who was sent from XYZ Nursing Home for evaluation of fever, congestion, and audible wheezing. The patient is non-communicative and history of present illness is limited. At the nursing home, she was noted to be febrile to a temperature of 103 with audible wheezing on room air oxygen saturations of 91 percent. She was sent to the ER department for further evaluation and treatment.

PAST MEDICAL HISTORY:
1. Alzheimer's dementia.
2. Neurogenic bladder.
3. Asthma/reactive airways disease.
4. Status post CVA.
5. Chronic UTIs.
6. Status post right lower extremity DVT.
7. History of hip fracture.

ALLERGIES: No known allergies.

MEDICATIONS:
1. Zantac 150 mgs p.o. q.h.s.
2. Albuterol meter dose inhaler
3. Aspirin
4. Lasix 20 mgs p.o. q. day

SOCIAL HISTORY: She is a widow. She has been a resident of XYZ Nursing Home for over 5 years.

FAMILY HISTORY: Non-contributory.

REVIEW OF SYSTEMS: Unobtainable.

PHYSICAL EXAMINATION

VITAL SIGNS: Temperature 103.1. BP 150/80. Heart Rate 88. Respiratory rate 28.

Oxygen saturation is 91 percent on room air. It is 96 percent on 2 liters by nasal cannula.

HEENT: EOMI. No cervical or supraclavicular adenopathy. Dry mucous membranes.

HEART: Regular rate and rhythm.

CHEST: Bilateral expiratory wheezing with rhonchi.

ABDOMEN: Reveals slight distention but soft and non-tender.

MEDICAL REPORT 8.5 (CONTINUED)

EXTREMITIES: Reveal a trace of lower extremity edema.

LAB DATA: Sodium 142, Potassium 4.0, Chloride 106, Bicarb 85, BUN 23, Creatinine 1.0, Glucose 154, and Calcium 8.4. Urinalysis revealed a specific gravity of 1.02 with pH of 5, 1 to 4 white blood cells and 5 to 10 red blood cells. Hemoglobin 11.9, hematocrit 36.1, white blood cell 8.3 with 84 percent Segs., 4 percent Bands, 7 percent Lymph, and 5 percent Mono, with 183,000 platelets.

Chest x-ray reveals mild cephalization of flow and patchy densities bilaterally, right greater than the left.

IMPRESSION/PLAN:

1. This 92-year-old Caucasian female with Alzheimer's dementia, asthma/reactive airways disease, history of chronic urinary tract infections secondary to neurogenic bladder and a history of right lower extremity DVT presents for evaluation and treatment of pneumonia. Her pneumonia is likely secondary to aspiration.

PLAN:

1. IV Cefotaxime, Azithromycin, and Vancomycin to cover community acquired and aspiration organisms.
2. Albuterol and Atrovent neb treatment.
3. IV fluids.
4. Subcutaneous Heparin for DVT prophylaxis.
5. IV Zantac for GI prophylaxis.
6. Supplemental oxygen to maintain oxygen saturations greater than 92 percent.
7. Patient is a DNR, living will.

Dr. Jane Smith, M.D.

cf

D: 6/13

T: 6/13

NOTES

CODING PRACTICE III — Ethical Diagnosis-Related Group Assignment Optimization Case Study

To preserve the Medicare Trust Fund, in 1983 Congress mandated that a national hospital prospective payment system be implemented for all Medicare inpatients. From Chapter 1, remember that diagnosis-related groups (DRGs) are an inpatient prospective payment system that was developed by Centers for Medicare & Medicaid Services. This inpatient prospective payment system uses DRGs to determine hospital reimbursement rates that are determined in advance of the services rendered, primarily on the basis of the patient's diagnosis. The limits in provider reimbursement under DRGs provide incentives to hospitals to operate more efficiently and reduce unnecessary costs while providing quality patient care. For FY2008, the DRG system was changed to MS-DRG (Medicare Severity-DRG).

Instructions

1. Review the following case study and commentary.
2. Review the four coding summaries and associated MS-DRG groupings.
3. Answer the questions below.

Questions

1. Which coding summary do you believe is the correct, ethical, and optimal sequence of codes, and why?

_____

_____

_____

_____

_____

2. Do you believe you need to complete a physician query/clarification form? Why or why not?

_____

_____

_____

_____

SCENARIO: A 68-year-old woman is admitted from her home with acute shortness of breath attributable to exacerbated COPD, decompensated CHF, and pneumonia. Taken by the attending physician, her history reveals a 40-year smoking history, and she is status post stroke with residual dysphagia. During her hospital stay, the patient receives intravenous steroids for COPD exacerbation, intravenous diuretics for decompensated CHF, and intravenous antibiotics for acute pneumonia. Her sputum cultures are negative for bacterial growth.

COMMENTARY: If this patient were three separate patients (one with exacerbated COPD, one with decompensated CHF, and one with pneumonia), all three would need to be admitted to the hospital for care. Therefore, this woman is being admitted with three principal diagnoses on admission that all require treatment equally. Coding guidelines dictate that whenever a patient is admitted with more than one principal diagnosis, with all requiring treatment, you may sequence the most resource-intensive one as the principal diagnosis.

Coder Summary Form #1

MS-DRG 190—Chronic obstructive pulmonary disease w MCC
CMS wt. 1.3004
A/LOS 6.3
G/LOS 5.0

Medicare inpatient reimbursement
Total: $5,201.60

MDC 004 Diseases and disorders of the respiratory system

Principal diagnosis
491.21 Exacerbation COPD

Secondary diagnoses
Congestive heart failure 428.0
Pneumonia 486
Status post cerebrovascular accident with residual dysphagia, oral phase
438.82 + 787.21
History of smoking V15.82

Coder Summary Form #2

MS-DRG 291—Heart failure and shock w MCC
CMS wt. 1.4576
A/LOS 6.5
G/LOS 5.0

Medicare inpatient reimbursement
Total: $5,830.40

MDC 005 Diseases and disorders of the circulatory system

Principal diagnosis
Congestive heart failure 428.0

Secondary diagnoses
Pneumonia 486
Exacerbation COPD 491.21
Status post cerebrovascular accident with residual dysphagia, oral phase
438.82 + 787.21
History of smoking V15.82

Coder Summary Form #3

MS-DRG 194—Simple pneumonia and pleurisy w CC
CMS wt. 1.0041
A/LOS 6.8
G/LOS 5.4

Medicare inpatient reimbursement
Total: $4,016.40

MDC 004 Diseases and disorders of the respiratory system
Principal diagnosis
Pneumonia, organism unspecified 486

Secondary diagnoses
Congestive heart failure 428.0
Exacerbation COPD 491.21
Status post cerebrovascular accident with residual dysphagia, oral phase
438.82 + 787.21
History of smoking V15.82

Coder Summary Form #4

MS-DRG 178—Respiratory infections and inflammations w CC
CMS wt. 1.4979
A/LOS 7.4
G/LOS 6.0

Medicare inpatient reimbursement
Total: $5,991.60

MDC 004 Diseases and disorders of the respiratory system

Principal diagnosis
Pneumonitis attributable to inhalation of food or vomitus 507.0

Secondary diagnoses
Exacerbation COPD 491.21
Congestive heart failure 428.0
Status post cerebrovascular accident with residual dysphagia, oral phase
438.82 + 787.21
History of smoking V15.82

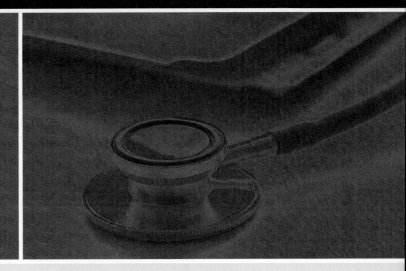

Coding for Genitourinary System Diseases

Chapter Outline

Genitourinary Symptoms
Genitourinary Infections and Inflammations
The Renal System and Associated Diseases
Female Genitourinary Conditions
Male Genitourinary Conditions
Testing Your Comprehension
Coding Practice I: Chapter Review Exercises
Coding Practice II: Medical Record Case Studies

Chapter Objectives

▶ Describe the pathology of common genitourinary system disorders.
▶ Recognize the typical manifestations, complications, and treatments of common genitourinary system disorders in terms of their implications for coding.
▶ Correctly code common genitourinary system disorders and related procedures by using the ICD-9-CM and medical records.

Genitourinary diseases are included in code section 580 to 629 of chapter 10, the Tabular List of Diseases *of the ICD-9-CM. This section includes diseases of the kidneys, urinary bladder, ureters (tubes from the kidneys to the bladder), urethra (tube from the bladder to the outside of the body), uterus, fallopian tubes, ovaries, breasts, and prostate gland. The most common genitourinary system diseases that result in hospital admissions include genitourinary symptoms, genitourinary infections and inflammations, renal failure, renal stones, and other specified renal diseases. Also classified in this chapter are common female genitourinary conditions, including endometriosis, cervical dysplasia, genital prolapse, dysfunctional uterine bleeding (DUB), and breast diseases. Common male genitourinary diseases involve disorders of the prostate gland. To assist in your understanding, the Word Parts Box on page 226 reviews word parts and meanings of medical terms related to digestive system diseases.*

Word Parts and Meanings of Genitourinary System Medical Terms

Word Part	Meaning	Example	Definition of Example
cyst/o	urinary bladder	cystocele	Hernia of the bladder, usually into the vagina and introitus
endo-	in; within	endometriosis	Ectopic occurrence of endometrial tissue (inner lining of uterus), frequently forming cysts containing altered blood
glomerul/o	glomerulus	glomerulonephritis	Renal disease characterized by inflammatory changes in glomeruli that are not the result of infection of the kidneys
hem/o	blood	hematuria	Any condition in which the urine contains blood or red blood cells
hypo-	under, below, abnormally low, decreased	hypocalcemia	Abnormally low levels of calcium in the circulating blood
-itis	inflammation	peritonitis	Inflammation of the peritoneum
nephr/o	kidney	nephrosis	Any noninflammatory disease of the kidney
-pathy	any disease of	obstructive uropathy	Any pathologic condition, anatomic or functional, of the urinary tract caused by obstruction
trans-	through	transurethral resection	Endoscopic (through the urethra) removal of the prostate gland or bladder lesions, usually for relief of prostatic obstruction or treatment of bladder malignancies
ur/o	urine, urinary tract	uremia	An excess of urea and other nitrogenous waste in the blood

Genitourinary Symptoms

Before assigning a symptom code as a principal diagnosis in the inpatient setting, always review the medical record for a more definitive diagnosis. Remember, if you find an underlying diagnosis causing the symptom(s), assign the diagnosis code, not the symptom code. However, as noted in Chapter 4 of this textbook, there are some exceptions to this rule (e.g., a symptom is followed by contrasting conditions or the etiology is unknown).

Often, genitourinary symptoms routinely associated with a disease are included as nonessential modifiers (in parentheses) after the main term for the definitive disease within the *Alphabetic Index to Diseases* or are presented within the *Tabular List of Diseases* within "includes notes" under the code. Unless noted otherwise, symptoms given within nonessential modifiers or includes notes should not be coded in addition to the definitive disease code. As a coder, you must learn to recognize whether a symptom is a routine part of the defined disease or not, and to apply discretion regarding whether symptom coding is appropriate for each case. Symptoms presented as nonessential modifiers or within includes notes are provided to assist the coder in making that distinction.

Some genitourinary symptoms are coded from chapter 16 of the ICD-9-CM, "Symptoms, Signs, and Ill-Defined Conditions" (section 780 to 799), whereas others are coded from chapter 10 of the ICD-9-CM, "Diseases of the Genitourinary System" (section 580 to 629). Some common examples of genitourinary symptoms include the following:

- hematuria, unspecified (599.70)—blood in the urine
- gross hematuria (599.71)—blood in the urine that cannot be seen be seen by the naked eye but can be seen under microscopic analysis
- microscopic hematuria (599.72)—blood in the urine that cannot be seen be seen by the naked eye but can be seen under microscopic analysis
- urinary incontinence (788.3X)—the inability to hold one's urine
- nocturia (788.43)—excessive urination at night
- urinary urgency (788.63)—sudden urges to urinate
- painful urination (788.9)—painful urination, not otherwise specified
- obstructive uropathy (599.60)—urinary blockage, not otherwise specified
- bladder hemorrhage (596.8)—bladder bleeding, not elsewhere classified
- renal colic (788.0)—sharp flank pain (between pelvis and ribs) commonly associated with renal (kidney) stones

Examples of the correct application of symptom coding from the genitourinary chapter (chapter 10), section 580 to 629, include the following:

EXAMPLE

Hemorrhagic cystitis: 595.9 (code only the cystitis because "hemorrhagic" is included as a nonessential modifier within the parentheses after the main term "cystitis" in the Alphabetic Index to Diseases).

Renal colic attributable to ureteral stones: 592.1 (code only the ureteral stones because renal colic is sharp flank pain that is routinely associated with ureteral stones).

Urinary tract infection (UTI) with hematuria: 599.0 + 599.70 (sequence the UTI first and hematuria as an additional diagnosis; hematuria is not listed as a nonessential modifier or in the includes notes for the UTI code because it is not routinely associated with all UTIs).

Bladder cancer with gross hematuria: 188.9 + 599.71 (sequence the bladder cancer first and gross hematuria as an additional diagnosis; gross hematuria is not included as a nonessential modifier or in the includes notes for the bladder cancer code and is not routinely associated with all bladder cancers).

Genitourinary gonorrhea with painful urination: 098.0 (code only the genitourinary gonorrhea because painful urination is routinely associated with this disease).

Hematuria secondary to renal calculus: 592.0 (code only the renal calculus because hematuria is routinely associated with renal stones)

When coding for genitourinary symptoms, do not code symptoms routinely associated with a disease; assign additional symptom codes as secondary diagnoses only if they are not routinely associated with the underlying disease.

Genitourinary Infections and Inflammations

Genitourinary infections and inflammations can include such diseases as UTI, cystitis (inflammation of the urinary bladder), urethritis (inflammation of the urethra), nephritis (inflammation of the kidney), and pyelonephritis (inflammation of the renal pelvis portion of the kidney) (Figure 9.1). Often these diseases are caused by specific bacterial organisms. A single code (i.e., combination code) or dual codes may be required to indicate the specific bacterial organism responsible for the infection.

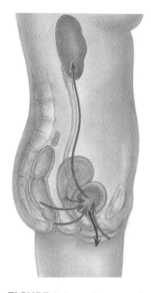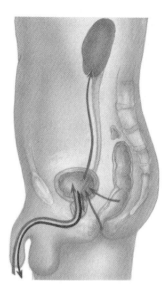

1. Ascending from bladder to kidney (reflux)

2. Ascending from urethra to bladder

3. Descending from bladder to urethra

4. From rectum, cervix, or prostate to bladder

5. From bowel to bladder

FIGURE 9.1 ■ Routes of infection in the urinary tract. (Reprinted with permission from Anatomical Chart Co.)

Locate the main term for the disease in the Alphabetic Index and then carefully review the indented subterms (i.e., essential modifiers) for a combination code (i.e., single code) that describes the disease and the responsible organism. Generally, if a combination code or mandatory dual coding (two codes) is not provided, you must add an additional code from category 041 to indicate the precise bacterial organism responsible for the disease.

EXAMPLE

Escherichia coli UTI: 599.0 (indicates UTI) + 041.4 (additional code indicates Escherichia coli as the responsible bacterial organism).

Chlamydial cystitis: 099.53 + 595.4 (mandatory dual coding). For some conditions, a single combination code is not available to describe the etiology and manifestation of a condition. In these cases, the etiology and manifestation are coded individually. It is important to report these codes in the exact sequence provided in the Alphabetic Index to Diseases. In this case, code 099.53 describes the chlamydial infection, which is the etiology or cause of the condition, and code 595.4 describes cystitis, which is the manifestation of the chlamydial infection.

Enterobacter cystitis: 595.9 + 041.85 (additional code for bacterial organism needed).

Monilial cystitis: 112.2 (single combination code).

Syphilitic pyelonephritis: 095.4 (single combination code).

Gonococcal urethritis: 098.0 (single combination code).

The Renal System and Associated Diseases

As explained in Chapter 5, cells throughout the body must receive nutrients (e.g., proteins and sugars) in the presence of oxygen to do their work (e.g., muscle cells contract, nerve cells transmit electrical impulses, and fat cells insulate and protect deeper tissues). However, in the process of human metabolism, cells also produce waste products (i.e., nitrogenous waste, which we excrete in urine, and carbon dioxide, which we exhale from the lungs). An accumulation of nitrogenous waste and carbon dioxide is harmful (toxic) to the human body. For example, progressive renal failure resulting in an accumulation of nitrogenous waste in the

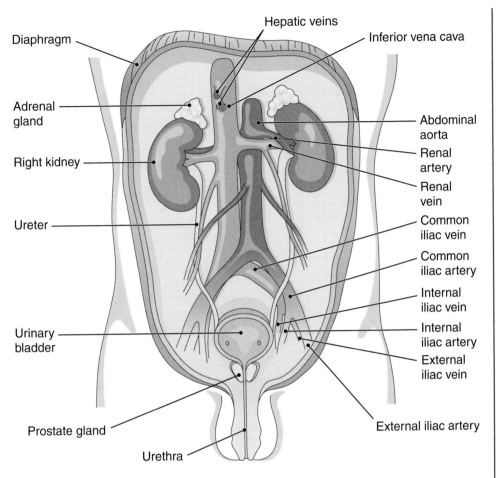

FIGURE 9.2 ■ Urinary system, with blood vessels. (Reprinted with permission from Cohen BJ and Wood DL. Memmler's The Human Body in Health and Disease, 9th Ed. Philadelphia: Lippincott Williams & Wilkins, 2000.)

body can cause metabolic acidosis, and certain progressive lung diseases (e.g., COPD) result in an accumulation of carbon dioxide in the body causing respiratory acidosis. Acidosis, regardless of its cause, increases the acidity of the blood (lowers the pH acid-base balance), which can have life-threatening consequences unless compensated. The urinary, or renal (kidney), system (Figure 9.2) works primarily to rid the body of excess nitrogenous waste and thereby helps in maintaining homeostasis (an internal constancy necessary for healthy life). The main functions of the urinary system are filtration, reabsorption, and elimination.

How the Renal System Works

From the circulating bloodstream, nitrogenous wastes (urea and creatinine) are filtered by the kidneys through the glomeruli, thousands of tight bundles of blood capillaries that act like a coffee filter. Unless there is damage to the glomeruli (such as from glomerulonephritis), blood cells and proteins (with large particles) will not normally filter through the glomerulus but are held back in the bloodstream while nitrogenous wastes, sodium, and potassium (with small particles) are filtered through.

Surrounding the glomeruli within the kidneys, the Bowman's capsule acts as a catcher's mitt that leads the filtered solution to the renal tubules (small tubes), where reabsorption of certain substances occurs. Reabsorption within the renal tubules holds back substances the body needs (e.g., water, sugar, and

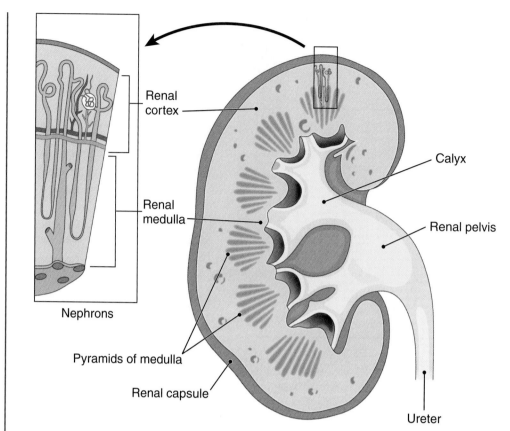

FIGURE 9.3 ■ Longitudinal section through the kidney showing its internal structure, and an enlarged diagram of a nephron. (Reprinted with permission from Cohen BJ and Wood DL. Memmler's The Human Body in Health and Disease, 9th Ed. Philadelphia: Lippincott Williams & Wilkins, 2000.)

sodium) while eliminating nitrogenous waste (e.g., urea) and other excess substances (e.g., excess potassium, acids, and water). The renal tubules then lead to collecting cups called **renal calyces** that lead to the renal pelvis within the kidney (Figure 9.3). Urine travels from the renal pelvis to the ureters, bladder, and urethra, and this provides for the elimination of urine (carrying nitrogenous waste to the outside of the body).

The documentation of azotemia (code 790.6) by a physician is a nonspecific abnormal laboratory finding, which means that increased nitrogenous wastes are present in the patient's bloodstream. Carefully review the patient's record to determine whether the physician really meant uremia, another common term for renal failure that would change the coding. Also, you should be aware that uremic encephalopathy (code 293.0) is commonly associated with renal failure (i.e., uremia) and describes an acute confusional state associated with an endocrine, metabolic, or cerebrovascular disorder. Coders sometimes fail to recognize the connection of confusion to renal failure if it is not clearly documented in the medical record. This condition is sometimes incorrectly coded to confusion not otherwise specified (NOS; code 298.9) when it is confusion attributable to a metabolic imbalance associated with the renal failure which would be coded to 293.0.

Renal Hormones

Although the kidneys function primarily to rid the body of excess nitrogenous waste, these vital organs also produce certain hormones that enable the body to maintain homeostasis. Erythropoietin is a hormone produced by the kidneys that helps one produce red blood cells. That is why people who have chronic renal disease sometimes develop a secondary anemia (deficiency of red blood cells). Anemia in chronic kidney disease is coded to 285.21.

The kidneys require a constant supply of blood to do their work; therefore, they also produce a hormone called renin, which increases blood pressure and flow. Secondary hypertension can develop from renal artery stenosis (narrowing), wherein the kidney increases its production of renin in order to increase blood pressure to maintain its supply of blood.

Hypertension secondary to renal artery stenosis: 440.1 + 405.91	**EXAMPLE**

The kidneys also secrete vitamin D, which is necessary for the absorption of calcium from the small intestine. In chronic renal disease, hypocalcemia (deficiency of calcium in the bloodstream) can lead to symptomatic bone diseases such as osteomalacia (softening of bone) and osteopenia (decreased bone density).

Renal Failure: Acute Versus Chronic

Renal failure NOS (code 586) involves a failure of the kidneys to produce and eliminate urine. Acute renal failure (ARF) is coded to 584.9. Severe and sometimes reversible, ARF can be caused by trauma, drugs or chemicals, or severe dehydration. Clinically, ARF (code 584.9) is different from chronic renal failure (CRF) or end-stage renal disease (ESRD), which are both coded within category 585. CRF or ESRD can develop from the progressive long-term or secondary complications of diabetes, hypertension, polycystic kidney disease, or systemic lupus erythematosus (systemic lupus erythematosus is a connective tissue disease that can affect many organs, including the kidneys).

Starting October 1, 2005, new codes were added for **chronic kidney disease** (CKD - category 585), which has been revised from the previous chronic kidney failure, often documented as chronic renal failure (CRF). CKD has five stages based on the glomerular filtration rate. CKD, category 585 has been expanded to a fourth digit level and includes:

Stage	Code	Kidney function remaining
CKD, Stage I	585.1	>90%
CKD, Stage II (mild)	585.2	60–90%
CKD, Stage III (moderate)	585.3	30–60%
CKD, Stage IV (severe)	585.4	15–30%
CKD, Stage V	585.5	<15%
End-stage-renal-disease (ESRD)	585.6	Requiring dialysis or kidney transplantation
CKD, unspecified	585.9	Describes chronic renal disease, chronic renal failure NOS, and chronic renal insufficiency

> **TIP** When a patient has a diagnosis of CRF or ESRD, thoroughly review the record for the presence of secondary anemia in ESRD (code 285.21) or secondary anemia NOS (code 285.9) if the physician does not document the connection.

Laboratory tests routinely performed to determine renal function include blood urea nitrogen and creatinine, which reveal the amount of nitrogenous waste in the bloodstream. Hyperkalemia (excessive potassium in the bloodstream) may also be noted in patients with renal problems. High values in these tests can indicate renal disease or renal compromise; however, only a physician can establish the diagnosis of renal failure. If a patient has both ARF and CRF, code both conditions, sequencing the ARF first (584.9 + 585.9).

> **TIP** If a patient is admitted to the hospital in ARF secondary to dehydration and the main treatment is intravenous hydration, with which the blood urea nitrogen and creatinine laboratory values return to normal ranges, sequence ARF (code 584.9) as the principal diagnosis, with dehydration as an additional secondary code. ARF remains the chief reason for admission.

Renal Failure With Hypertension

ARF and hypertension are coded separately. However, renal failure NOS (code 586), or CKD (category 585) associated with hypertension (category code 401) is automatically coded to 403.9X (hypertensive chronic kidney disease) with the fifth digit assigned according to specific stage of renal disease. Excluding ARF, ICD-9-CM assumes a relationship between CKD or unspecified renal failure/disease and hypertension and provides a combination code because the combined conditions present a complicated clinical situation. In renal failure, the kidneys cannot eliminate excess water and sodium, and high blood pressure (hypertension) often develops. This in turn can lead to heart failure. If untreated, renal failure that progresses to ESRD is a fatal condition. Treatment involves dialysis or kidney transplantation to maintain life. Hypertension with documentation of CKD, Stages I–V, require an additional code to specify the CKD stage or ESRD (e.g., HTN with ESRD = 403.91 + 585.6; HTN with CKD Stage IV = 403.90 + 585.4).

As of October 2006, official changes were made at the fifth-digit subclassification level for categories 403 (hypertensive renal/kidney disease) and 404 (hypertensive heart and renal/kidney disease) that correspond with category 585 (used as an additional code) to describe the various stages of chronic kidney disease (CKD) that include the following:

For use with category 403 (hypertensive renal/kidney disease):

▶ fifth digit "0" describes that the CKD is in stage I through stage IV (or unspecified)

▶ fifth digit "1" describes that the CKD is in stage V or end-stage renal disease (ESRD)

For use with category 404 (hypertensive heart and renal disease):

- fifth digit "0" is assigned for hypertensive heart and renal disease *without* heart failure and with chronic renal/kidney disease stage I through stage IV, or unspecified
- fifth digit of "1" is assigned for hypertensive heart/renal disease *with* heart failure and with chronic kidney disease stage I through stage IV, or unspecified
- fifth digit "2" is assigned for hypertensive/renal disease *without* heart failure and with chronic renal/kidney disease stage V or end-stage renal disease
- fifth digit of "3" is assigned for hypertensive heart/renal disease *with* heart failure and with chronic renal/kidney disease stage V or end-stage renal disease

Remember, when using codes from category 403 or 404, an additional code is always assigned to specify the stage of chronic kidney disease (CKD) present, and with category 404 an additional code from category 428 is used to identify the type of heart failure, if present.

Renal Dialysis and Transplantation

There are two different types of dialysis: hemodialysis and peritoneal dialysis (Figure 9.4).

HEMODIALYSIS

Hemodialysis (code 39.95) uses an artificial kidney machine to filter nitrogenous waste from the bloodstream (Figure 9.5). For hemodialysis to occur, there must be venous access (i.e., access to the patient's bloodstream via a vein). Venous catheterization (code 38.95) can be used for short-term or emergent vascular access for hemodialysis; however, repeated vascular insult (from repeated puncture of veins) can cause venous trauma or injury, collapse or "blow-out" of the vein, and infection; therefore, a venous catheter is insufficient for long-term dialysis.

ESRD requires long-term vascular access, often through placement of a vascular access device (code 86.07) or formation of an arteriovenous shunt or fistula (code 39.27). An arteriovenous fistula is the anastomosis (surgical connection) of an artery to a vein, usually in an arm. When an artery (with high blood pressure) is connected to a vein (with low blood pressure), an aneurysmal (dilated or widened) vessel results. In addition, a synthetic graft material (e.g., Gore-Tex™) is routinely placed that allows repeated vascular access through this enlarged vessel with a large-bore needle for hemodialysis. This permits repeated vascular access without subsequent injury to the vessel, as well as faster access and reduced patient hemodialysis time.

PERITONEAL DIALYSIS

Peritoneal dialysis (code 54.98) uses a solution that is infused into the patient's peritoneal cavity from a plastic bag through a catheter (i.e., Tenckhoff catheter placement; code 54.94) (Figure 9.6). The peritoneal tissue acts as a semipermeable membrane through which nitrogenous waste is drawn into the solution (via osmosis), returned to the plastic bag, and then disposed of. This procedure is referred to as chronic ambulatory peritoneal dialysis. It is more often used in patients who are active and can provide for their own

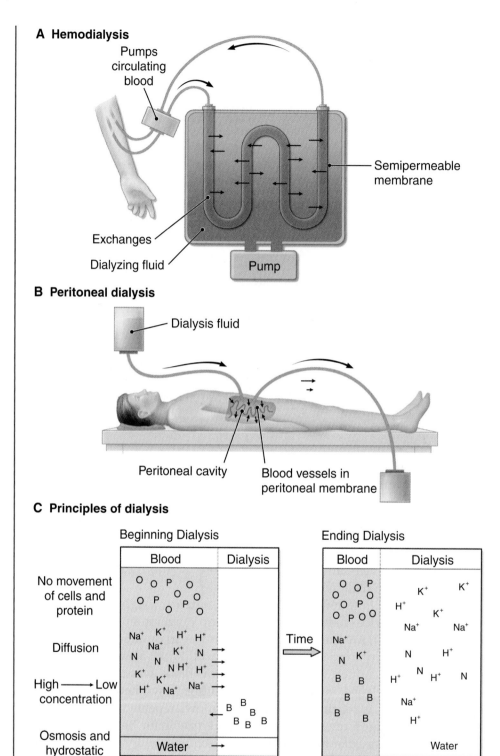

FIGURE 9.4 ■ **(A)** Hemodialysis; **(B)** Peritoneal dialysis; **(C)** Principles of dialysis. (Reprinted with permission from Premkumar K. The Massage Connection Anatomy and Physiology. Baltimore: Lippincott Williams & Wilkins 2004.)

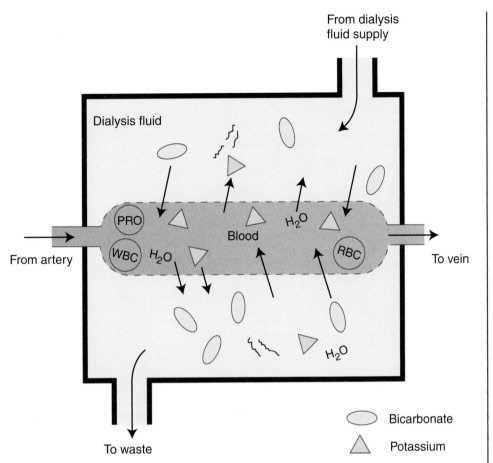

FIGURE 9.5 ▪ Schematic diagram of a hemodialysis system. A cellophane membrane separates the blood compartment and dialysis solution compartment. This membrane is porous enough to allow all of the constituents except the plasma proteins and blood cells to diffuse between the two compartments. (Reprinted with permission from Porth CM. Pathophysiology: Concepts in Altered Health States. 6th Ed. Philadelphia: Lippincott Williams & Wilkins, 2002.)

personal care, because chronic ambulatory peritoneal dialysis is usually self-administered.

Depending on their health history and the availability of organs, some ESRD patients may qualify as candidates for renal transplantation. A kidney can be transplanted into the patient from another individual donor (allograft) or, for a closer match, from a relative.

▸ *Kidney recipient: admission for kidney transplantation for ESRD*

Primary diagnosis: 585.6 ESRD

Procedure: 55.69 kidney transplantation

▸ *Kidney donor: admission kidney donor*

Primary diagnosis: V59.4 kidney donor

Procedure: 55.51 nephrectomy

EXAMPLE

If the only purpose of the patient admission or encounter is to have dialysis or if the patient is admitted for dialysis catheter or shunt placement and dialysis is performed during that same encounter, code 56.X (admit for dialysis) is

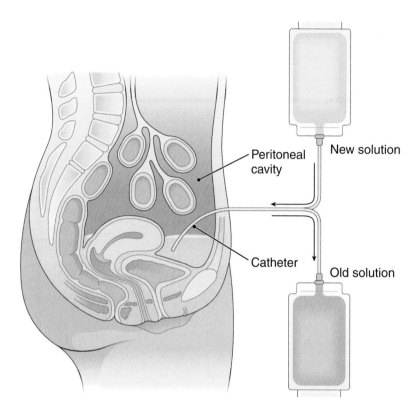

FIGURE 9.6 ■ Peritoneal dialysis. A semipermeable membrane richly supplied with small blood vessels lines the peritoneal cavity. With dialysate dwelling in the peritoneal cavity, waste products diffuse from the network of blood vessels into the dialysate. (Reprinted with permission from Cohen BJ. Medical Terminology: An Illustrated Guide, 4th Ed. Baltimore: Lippincott Williams & Wilkins, 2004.)

sequenced as the principal diagnosis. You can locate extracorporeal dialysis or hemodialysis (code V56.0) or peritoneal dialysis (code V56.8) under the main term "dialysis" or "admission for" dialysis in the *Alphabetic Index to Diseases*.

If patients are admitted for the purpose of having a dialysis catheter or shunt placed and if dialysis is not performed during the same encounter, then sequence the condition of CKD or ESRD as the principal diagnosis.

COMPLICATIONS OF HEMODIALYSIS AND PERITONEAL DIALYSIS

Complications that can result from hemodialysis include dialysis dementia NOS, dialysis dementia attributable to aluminum overloading (a "poisoning" resulting from the filtration therapy), and dialysis disequilibrium. These conditions are not readily located in the *Alphabetic Index to Diseases*, and examples for the correct coding for these conditions are given below. For these cases, be sure to include the condition of CKD or ESRD as a secondary diagnosis.

Dialysis dementia is located in the *Alphabetic Index to Diseases* under the main term "dementia, dialysis." Dialysis dementia attributable to aluminum overloading is coded to "poisoning, metals, NEC [not elsewhere classified]" from the Table of Drugs and Chemicals, and E879.1 (an E code used in all the examples given below) is located in the External Cause of Injury Index under the main term "reaction, abnormal to or following [medical or surgical procedure], dialysis").

EXAMPLE

▶ *Dialysis dementia: 294.8 (chronic or unspecified); or 293.9 (if the dementia is specified as transient)*

ESRD: 585.6, E879.1

▶ *Dialysis dementia attributable to aluminum overloading: 985.8 (coded to "poisoning, metals, NEC"); 294.8 or 293.9 (if transient)*

CKD Stage V: 585.5, E879.1

▶ *Dialysis disequilibrium: 276.9 (electrolyte imbalance NEC—chemical equilibrium disturbance)*

CRF: 585.9, E879.1

A potential complication of peritoneal dialysis is peritonitis (inflammation or infection of the peritoneum). The attending physician may need to be queried about the underlying cause of the peritonitis. If the peritonitis is attributable to infection of the peritoneal catheter itself, codes 996.68 and 567.29 (suppurative peritonitis) are assigned (infection secondary to peritoneal dialysis catheter). If, however, the infection was secondary to the infusion process and not attributable to the catheter, codes 999.3 and 567.29 are assigned.

Other Specified Renal Diseases

Acute renal insufficiency (code 593.9) describes insufficient urinary production by the kidneys of a nonspecific origin. Hypertensive renal disease (code 403.9X) indicates that renal disease is secondary to or associated with hypertension. Diabetic nephropathy (code 250.4X + 583.81) represents renal disease that is secondary to the long-term effects of diabetes.

Nephrotic syndrome (category code 581) can result from damage to the kidney glomeruli from glomerulonephritis (inflammation of the glomeruli), the harmful effects of drugs or chemicals, or the long-term effects of diabetes. (The term **syndrome** is a key word meaning a group of symptoms that point to a particular disease.) The combined symptoms of edema (fluid in the tissues), proteinuria (excess protein in the urine), hypoalbuminemia (reduced protein in the bloodstream), and hypercholesterolemia (excess cholesterol in the bloodstream) may indicate the diagnosis of nephrotic syndrome.

TIP Recently, physicians have been documenting the term "acute kidney (or renal) injury" when it is not intended to mean an injury due to trauma. This non-traumatic acute kidney injury is now being coded to acute renal failure, code 584.9.

Renal Stones

Urine contains salts, and urinary stones (also referred to as **calculi**) often are composed of uric acid or calcium salts (Figure 9.7). As a general rule, the location of stones in the body indicates their composition (e.g., renal stones are often composed of salts, whereas gallstones are composed of cholesterol). Renal stones (calculi; **urolithiasis** is the condition of urinary stones) can get lodged in the kidney pelvis, ureters, bladder, or urethra. Often, stones are associated with a sharp flank pain called **renal colic.**

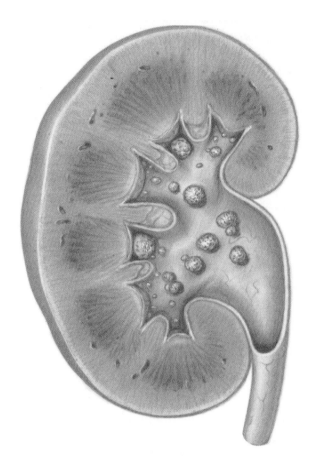

FIGURE 9.7 ■ The urinary tract, calcium stones (gravel). (Reprinted with permission from Anatomical Chart Co.)

Renal colic and hematuria associated with renal calculus are not coded as additional diagnoses because these symptoms are commonly associated with the disease. Renal calculi can also be associated with urinary retention attributable to urinary obstruction (obstructive uropathy) caused by the stones. Sometimes this condition can lead to hydronephrosis (backup of fluid in the kidney) (Figure 9.8). Renal calculus can be associated with hyperuricemia (excess uric acid in the blood), hypercalcinuria (excess calcium in urine), and UTIs.

If the stones are small, treatment can help the patient pass them during urination. Conservative (noninvasive) treatment often consists of intravenous hydration, diuretics to increase urination, analgesics to relieve pain, drugs to reduce uric acid production (e.g., allopurinol), and diet restrictions of foods that are high in uric acid (e.g., red meat, cheese, and alcohol).

If the renal stones are large and will not pass during urination, noninvasive procedures (without incision) or invasive surgery (with incision) may be used to remove them or break them down. Extracorporeal shockwave lithotripsy (ESWL), for example, is a noninvasive procedure to remove stones by fragmenting them. Under x-ray visualization, a physician directs ultrasonic (sound) shock waves, focused at the stone, through the patient's body. The shock waves pulverize the stone, which is then passed during urination. This procedure can be located in the Procedure Index under the main terms "ESWL" or "lithotripsy" (code 98.51). Transurethral procedures use an endoscope (a scoped instrument that is passed through the urethra) to remove stones without an incision.

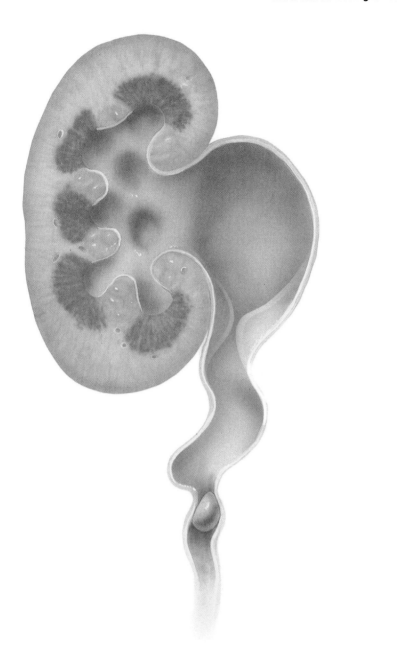

FIGURE 9.8 ■ Diseases of the urinary tract, hydronephrosis, kidney stone. (Reprinted with permission from Anatomical Chart Co.)

Because hematuria often results from ESWL or transurethral endoscopic procedures to remove renal stones, it is not coded as a postprocedural complication.

TIP Generally, all removals (noninvasive or invasive) of renal or other stones can be located in the *Alphabetic Index to Procedures* under the main terms "removal, calculus," "lithotripsy" ("litho-" means *stones*, and "-tripsy" means *to crush*), or "ESWL." Under these main terms, you will find various subterms that indicate urinary tract sites and techniques used to remove urinary calculi.

Refer to the Procedure Index to locate the following procedures, and always verify your code assignments in the Procedure Tabular.

REMOVAL
    Calculus
        bladder (without incision) 57.0
            (with incision) 57.19
        kidney (by incision) 55.01
            (without incision) 56.0
            percutaneous 55.03
            (with fragmentation nephrostomy) 55.04
            transurethral 56.0
        ureter (by incision) 56.2
            (without incision) 56.0
        urethra (by incision) 58.0
            (without incision) 58.6

LITHOTRIPSY
    bladder 57.0
        extracorporeal shock wave (ESWL) 98.51
        with ultrasonic fragmentation 57.0 [59.95]
    kidney 56.0
        extracorporeal shock wave (ESWL) 98.51
        percutaneous nephrostomy with fragmentation 55.04
    renal pelvis
        extracorporeal shock wave (ESWL) 98.51
        percutaneous nephrostomy with fragmentation 55.04
    ureter
        extracorporeal shock wave (ESWL) 98.51
        percutaneous nephrostomy with fragmentation 55.04

ESWL
    bile duct 98.52
    bladder 98.51
    gallbladder 98.52
    kidney 98.51
    Kock pouch (urinary diversion) 98.51
    renal pelvis 98.51
    specified site NEC 98.59
    ureter 98.5

Following are examples of procedure coding for removal of renal stones:

Transurethral removal of ureteral calculus (without incision): 56.0

Transurethral removal of bladder calculus (without incision): 57.0

Nephrotomy (incision into kidney) to remove calculus: 55.01

Ultrasonic lithotripsy, bladder calculus: 57.0 + 59.95

Lithotripsy, extracorporeal shock wave, renal pelvis: 98.51

Basket manipulation using double-J (ureteral) stent and percutaneous nephrostomy with fragmentation to remove ureteral stone: 55.04 + 59.8 (the placement of a ureteral catheter or stent for manipulation can be located in the Procedure Index under "catheterization," "manipulation," or "insertion, ureteral stent")

Female Genitourinary Conditions

Common female genitourinary conditions include endometriosis, cervical dysplasia, genital prolapse, DUB, and breast diseases. Please note that ICD-9-CM's chapter 11 codes for complications of pregnancy, childbirth, puerperium, and abortion take precedence (are sequenced first) over its chapter 10 codes for genitourinary system diseases and will be discussed in Chapter 15 of this textbook.

Endometriosis

The uterus is made up of three layers that include the endometrium ("endo-," *inner lining*), myometrium ("myo-," *middle muscle layer*), and perimetrium ("peri-," *surrounding outer layer*). Endometriosis ("metri/o," *uterus*) is a condition in which the inner endometrial layer of the uterus is found in abnormal locations outside of the uterus (code 617.X). This **ectopic** ("ecto-" means *outside of*) endometrial tissue can be found in the fallopian tubes, ovaries, and pelvis, causing severe pelvic pain, dysmenorrhea (painful menstruation), and infertility. Treatments can include symptomatic pain relief with drugs or surgical interventions such as excision or ablation (destruction) of endometrial tissue (code 68.2X) or hysterectomy (codes 68.3 to 68.9).

Cervical Dysplasia

After a diagnostic Papanicolaou smear (a pathologic examination that uses a microscope to view cervical epithelial cells that have been scraped from the uterine cervix), atypical cervical cells may be present that can represent cervical dysplasia (code 622.1). A pathology report with a diagnosis of cervical intraepithelial neoplasia I or II identifies cervical dysplasia. Cervical intraepithelial neoplasia III represents carcinoma in situ (a noninvasive superficial localized cancer), which will be covered in Chapter 14 of this textbook, "Coding for Neoplasms and Oncology."

Genital Prolapse

The physical stress of childbirth and the progressive loss of estrogen that occurs as women age can cause weakening of tissues and supporting structures and may result in genital prolapse (e.g., drooping or sagging) disorders. These disorders, which are often coded incorrectly, include uterine, vaginal, or uterovaginal prolapse.

If a patient is diagnosed as having vaginal prolapse, carefully review the medical record—especially the history and physical report—to determine whether the patient has a history of hysterectomy. Vaginal prolapse in such a patient is coded to 618.5.

Common symptoms of genital prolapse disorders can include stress incontinence (urinary) and dyspareunia (painful intercourse). Patients often describe a feeling of the "bladder falling out" or pelvic pressure.

Female genital prolapse codes (category code 618) include the following:

EXAMPLE	*Vaginal prolapse without uterine prolapse: 618.00* *Uterine prolapse without mention of vaginal wall prolapse: 618.1* *Uterovaginal prolapse, incomplete: 618.2* *Uterovaginal prolapse, complete: 618.3* *Uterovaginal prolapse, unspecified: 618.4* *Prolapse of vaginal vault after hysterectomy: 618.5* *Vaginal enterocele, congenital or acquired: 618.6*

In uterovaginal prolapse described as incomplete, the uterus droops into the uterovaginal opening (i.e., introitus). Complete uterovaginal prolapse means the uterus droops down beyond the uterovaginal opening. Uterine prolapse can be described as first, second, or third degree or complete, with each higher degree denoting a worsening descensus (protrusion and falling).

The suffix "-cele" means a herniation or an abnormal bulging forth of an organ. Many of the includes notes under the 618 category code from the *Tabular List of Diseases* section describe conditions ending in the suffix "-cele," such as cystocele, cystourethrocele, proctocele, rectocele, urethrocele, and enterocele. Common procedures to treat female genital prolapse disorders include the following:

- ▶ Marshall-Marchetti-Krantz urethral suspension 59.5
- ▶ Urethrocele, enterocele repair 70.92
- ▶ Cystocele repairs 70.51
- ▶ Combined cystocele and rectocele repair 70.50
- ▶ Vaginal suspension and fixation 70.77
- ▶ Hysterectomy
  - ▶ Total abdominal hysterectomy 68.49
  - ▶ Vaginal hysterectomy 68.59
- ▶ Laparoscopic assisted vaginal hysterectomy 68.51
- ▶ Laparoscopic total abdominal hysterectomy 68.41

Dysfunctional Uterine Bleeding

DUB, code 626.8, most often occurs because of hormonal changes. DUB can be prolonged, heavy, and irregular and can occur near the time of a woman's first menstrual cycle (menarche) or near the time of menopause. In DUB menstrual cycles, most often a woman does not ovulate (release an ovum or egg), and this results in a deficiency of the hormone progesterone. Without progesterone, the endometrial uterine lining overgrows and breaks down incompletely or irregularly, with excessive bleeding. DUB can be treated with hormone therapy (birth control pills or progesterone replacement), by uterine dilation and curettage, by endometrial ablation (destruction of endometrial tissue), or by hysterectomy if the disease fails to respond to more conservative treatment.

Breast Diseases

Most often, breast cancer is a cause for inpatient admissions, and this will be covered in Chapter 14 of this textbook. Breast diseases specifically covered in the genitourinary chapter (category codes 610 to 611) of the ICD-9-CM include such diseases as solitary breast cysts (code 610.0), fibrocystic disease of the breast (code 610.1), mastitis (611.0), breast hypertrophy (611.1), or symptoms such as a lump or mass in the breast (code 611.72). These breast diseases are more often diagnosed and treated on an outpatient basis.

Coded to 611.1, breast hypertrophy (enlargement) in females or males (in which case it is called **gynecomastia**) can cause significant back pain and physical discomfort, and patients may wish to reduce their breast size. Patients with this condition may elect to reduce their breast size for cosmetic reasons as well. For breast hypertrophy, a reduction mammoplasty (85.3X) is performed to reduce breast size. In contrast, breast augmentation (enlargement) or enhancement for cosmetic purposes is coded to 85.5X with a principal diagnosis of V50.1: admission (encounter) for plastic surgery, cosmetic.

Admission for breast reconstruction (procedure codes 85.7X) after mastectomy for cancer is coded to the principal diagnosis V51.0 (located under the main term "Admission for" followed by the subterm "plastic surgery; following healed injury or operation"), with V10.3 (personal history of breast cancer) as an additional diagnosis. These breast procedures are routinely performed on an outpatient basis and, therefore, are coded by using the Current Procedural Terminology 4th Ed. (CPT-4) procedural coding system for reporting and reimbursement purposes. However, diagnoses will continue to be reported with ICD-9-CM.

Diagnostic procedures such as mammograms and breast biopsies are usually performed on an outpatient basis as well. However, a pathology report revealing breast cancer warrants, at least initially, an inpatient admission for definitive surgery. Breast biopsies can be coded to open (85.12) or closed (85.11). Open biopsies involve an incision into the breast, whereas closed biopsies are performed percutaneously (through the skin) by using a needle. An excisional biopsy of the breast is coded to excision, lesion, breast (85.21), because it involves the excision of the entire lesion or lump. This procedure is also referred to as a **lumpectomy**.

Male Genitourinary Conditions

Common male genitourinary conditions are classified in chapter 10 of the ICD-9-CM and include disorders of the prostate. Although many of these procedures are performed in an outpatient setting, some are handled as inpatient admissions if the patient has preexisting comorbid conditions (e.g., emphysema or coronary artery disease) that prevent the procedure from being safely performed during an outpatient encounter (i.e., patients require more care or monitoring than is routinely available in the outpatient surgery setting). Inpatient admission for those prostate procedures performed in the outpatient setting often requires precertification through the patient's insurer (prior approval for coverage).

Prostate disorders, excluding prostate cancer, are located within category codes 600 to 602 in the *Tabular List of Diseases*. One of the most common prostate diseases is benign prostatic hyperplasia (BPH). BPH frequently occurs in men older than 60 years. Sometimes physicians call this disorder **benign prostatic hypertrophy**, although that is a misnomer because BPH causes the gland to enlarge from an increased number of cells (hyperplasia), whereas hypertrophy causes enlargement of an organ from the enlargement of the cells themselves (e.g., muscle hypertrophy occurs from weight lifting).

Symptoms routinely associated with BPH are urinary retention (788.20) and postvoid residual (788.21 - retention of urine in the bladder after urination). Although routine symptoms associated with a disease are not commonly coded, the instructional notes under code category 600 for hyperplasia of the prostate have been revised and now direct the coder to "use additional code to identify symptoms," if present. Bladder neck obstruction sometimes occurs as the enlarged prostate gland encircles and compresses the male urethra, causing a urinary obstruction. With the use of fourth digits, category code 600 for hyperplasia of the prostate can be further broken down to add more detail to the diagnosis and includes 600.0X hypertrophy (benign) of prostate, 600.1X nodular prostate, 600.2X benign localized hyperplasia of the prostate, and 660.3 cyst of the prostate. Fifth digits added to subcategories 600.0X, 600.1X, and 600.2X further describe if the condition is with or without urinary obstruction and other lower urinary tract symptoms (e.g., 600.01 = benign hypertrophy of prostate with urinary obstruction and other urinary tract symptoms). Unfortunately, it is rare for physicians to give that level of specificity within the diagnosis. Pathology report findings may help to clarify a more precise diagnosis. However, the attending physician will have to be queried to add supporting documentation to the patient's medical record.

Conservative medical management for BPH can include the use of drugs such as finasteride (Proscar) as a means of reducing the size of the prostate.

A common surgical procedure to relieve the symptoms of BPH is a transurethral resection (removal) of the prostate (TURP), code 60.29. In this procedure, a resectoscope is inserted into the male urethra, and prostate tissue is resected to relieve the flow of urine for the patient. This procedure, obviously, removes urethral tissue as well; however, the patient has a Foley catheter (indwelling urinary catheter) inserted after the operation within the lumen (opening) through the urethra, which quickly heals. Do not code a cystoscopy performed with a TURP, because this is considered an operative approach (i.e., transurethral). Post-TURP patients often experience hematuria, which is often associated with surgery. Therefore, for a post-TURP patient, do not code hematuria as a secondary diagnosis or as a postoperative complication.

Other types of prostatectomies (to remove prostatic tissue) in category 60.X include the following:

▶ Transurethral guided laser induced prostatectomy (TULIP) 60.21
▶ Transurethral microwave thermotherapy (TUMT) 60.96
▶ Transurethral needle ablation of the prostate (TUNA) 60.97

▶ Cryoablation of the prostate (destruction of prostate tissue by freezing) 60.62

▶ Radical prostatectomy (an open excision of the prostate gland by any approach) 60.5

Other techniques that specify operative approaches include:

▶ Suprapubic prostatectomy (an open prostatectomy procedure that removes prostate tissue through a lower abdominal incision through the bladder) 60.3

▶ Retropubic prostatectomy (an open prostatectomy procedure that removes prostate tissue through a lower abdominal incision without an opening through the bladder) 60.4

The open radical, suprapubic, and retropubic prostatectomy procedures can require a longer stay in the hospital than the newer or less invasive (transurethral) operations noted previously. The specific type of prostate disorder (e.g., cancer or BPH), the size of the prostate gland, or both usually determine the type of prostatectomy to be performed. Radical prostatectomy procedures are more often associated with prostate cancer and will be discussed in Chapter 14, "Coding for Neoplasms and Oncology."

Another common prostate disorder is prostatitis (inflammation of the prostate). If both acute and chronic prostatitis are present, code both conditions, sequencing the acute condition first according to coding rules (601.0 + 601.1). Use an additional code to identify a bacterial agent such as staphylococcus (041.1) if it is present. This disorder is often treated medically, including intravenous antibiotics, bed rest, and analgesics for pain control.

SUMMARY

This chapter has addressed the subject of coding for genitourinary system diseases. Genitourinary symptoms, infections, and inflammations have been discussed in the context of common coding principles. The chapter has included a discussion of pathologic conditions that affect the genitourinary system, as well as of other conditions that may be caused by these disorders. Also included are diagnoses and common procedures related to this system. Chapter 10 addresses skin and subcutaneous tissue diseases.

TESTING YOUR COMPREHENSION

1. Genitourinary diseases address problems affecting several different organs. Name at least four commonly affected organs.

   _____

2. Name five common female genitourinary conditions that require treatment.

   _____

3. Identify the most common male genitourinary disease that requires treatment.

   _____

4. Identify five common examples of genitourinary symptoms.

   _____

5. Identify the three main functions of the urinary system.

   _____

6. Identify the hormone produced by the kidneys that assists in producing red blood cells.

   _____

7. If the kidneys fail to produce and eliminate urine, what occurs?

   _____

8. Why does high blood pressure frequently develop as a consequence of renal failure?

   _____

9. What can result from high blood pressure?

   _____

10. Identify the two different types of renal dialysis.

    _____

11. Common in hemodialysis is the need for access to the circulatory system of the patient. Identify the procedure required to accomplish that end.

    _____

12. How does peritoneal dialysis work?

    _____

13. Ultimately every renal dialysis patient seeks a more permanent solution to the disease. What procedure can facilitate that goal?

    _____

14. Identify a common manifestation of renal stones.

    _____

15. If renal stones do not pass, there are several common methods of dealing with this problem. One is invasive surgery. Others are noninvasive or less-invasive procedures. Identify them.

    _____

16. Surrounding the glomeruli within the kidneys is a capsule that acts as a catcher's mitt. It leads the filtered solution to the renal tubules, where reabsorption of certain substances occurs. What name is attached to the capsule that acts as a catcher's mitt?

_____

17. Identify the laboratory tests used to determine renal function. These tests reveal the amount of nitrogenous waste in the bloodstream.

_____

18. What surgical procedure is often performed to remove the symptoms of BPH (benign prostatic hyperplasia)?

_____

CODING PRACTICE I   Chapter Review Exercises

Directions

By using your ICD-9-CM codebook, code the following diagnoses and procedures:

	DIAGNOSIS/PROCEDURES	CODE
1	Benign nodular hyperplasia of the prostate. Bladder neck obstruction. Urinary retention. Transurethral resection of the prostate.	
2	Ureteral calculus with hematuria and hydronephrosis. Ureteral lithotripsy.	
3	Acute and chronic renal failure. Hyperkalemia. Insertion of a venous catheter for hemodialysis. Hemodialysis.	
4	Urinary tract infection attributable to enterococcus.	
5	Admission for arteriovenous shunt insertion for end-stage renal disease. Hypertension. Creation of an arteriovenous fistula. Hemodialysis.	
6	Vaginal prolapse, status post hysterectomy. Marshall-Marchetti-Krantz operation.	
7	Dysfunctional uterine bleeding. Family history of cervical cancer. Dilation and curettage.	
8	Endometriosis. Cervical dysplasia. Dilation and curettage; endometrial ablation. Conization of cervix.	
9	Urinary retention.	

	DIAGNOSIS/PROCEDURES	CODE
10	Urethral stenosis. Prostatitis. Cystoscopy with urethral dilation.	
11	Stress urinary incontinence. Cystocele and rectocele. Cystocele/rectocele repair.	
12	Acute pyelonephritis. Hematuria secondary to above.	
13	Chronic renal insufficiency and urinary retention secondary to benign prostatic hypertrophy. Cystoscopy.	
14	Ovarian adenoma. Pelvic adhesions. Ovarian cystectomy. Lysis of adhesions.	
15	Intramural leiomyoma. Pelvic pain. Pelvic adhesions. Stress incontinence. Total abdominal hysterectomy, bilateral salpingo-oophorectomy, Burch procedure.	
16	Cervical polyps. Vaginal hysterectomy.	
17	Orchitis with scrotal swelling. Intravenous antibiotics.	
18	Organic impotence. Hypertension. Penile implant, inflatable.	
19	Acute renal failure with dehydration.	
20	Acute renal failure attributable to obstructive uropathy.	

CODING PRACTICE II | Medical Record Case Studies

Instructions

1. Carefully review the medical reports provided for each case study.

2. Research any abbreviations and terms that are unfamiliar or unclear.

3. Identify as many diagnoses and procedures as possible.

4. Because only part of the patient's total record is available, determine what additional documentation you might need.

5. If appropriate, identify any questions you might ask the physician to code this case correctly and completely.

6. Complete the appropriate blanks below for each case study.

CHAPTER 9 CASE STUDIES

Case Study 9.1 (Coder/Abstract Summary Form)

Patient: **Jane Doe**

Patient documentation: **Review Medical Report 9.1**

1. Principal diagnosis:

   _____

2. Secondary or other diagnoses:

   _____

3. Principal procedure:

   _____

4. Other procedures:

   _____

5. Additional documentation needed:

   _____

   _____

   _____

Case Study 9.1 (Continued)

6. Questions for the physician:

_____

_____

_____

_____

_____

MEDICAL REPORT 9.1

CONSULTATION

NAME: JANE DOE

NUMBER:

SEX: F

AGE: 67

ADMIT:

TYPE:

ROOM:

ATTENDING PHYSICIAN: DR. SMITH

CONSULTANT: DR. JONES

DATE OF CONSULTATION:

ADDRESS:

PHONE:

BIRTHDATE:

AGE:

MEDICARE:

MEDICAID:

HISTORY OF PRESENT ILLNESS: She is a 67-year-old, white female admitted last night by Dr. Smith with a diagnosis of acute renal failure and hyperkalemia.

She was in the hospital with a diagnosis of acute renal failure with severe hyperkalemia, sinoatrial block, paroxysmal atrial fibrillation, hypertension, history of coronary artery disease with coronary artery bypass graft surgery in 1994, history of cerebrovascular accident with mild right hemiparesis, history of depression, mild pancytopenia, osteoarthritis, history of right hip fracture, history of pain syndrome on opioid and analgesic dependency, and history of chronic obstructive pulmonary disease.

On that admission, she had a BUN of 60, creatinine 2.4, potassium 6.3, which were all corrected to a value of 19 and 0.9 and the potassium was normal.

On the actual admission the digoxin level was 1.9. The drug screen was negative. The CPK was 807. The hemoglobin was 10.3. The white blood count was 4400. The platelet count was 94,000. The metabolic profile revealed a sodium of 129, potassium 7.6, CO_2 4, BUN 114, creatinine 6.7, chloride 111, glucose 61, bilirubin 1.0, albumin 3.8, calcium 8.7, alkaline phosphatase 108, protein 6.9, SGOT 37 and SGPT 21. ABGs revealed a pH of 7.063, PCO_2 17.6, PO_2 99.4 and bicarbonate of 4.8. The urinalysis showed a dark, yellow, turbid color with ketones and bile negative, specific gravity 1.020, protein 100 mg/dl, nitrite negative, white blood cells 8-15, red blood cells 4-8 and a large amount of bacteria. The repeated CBC today shows a white blood count partial thromboplastin time normal. Yesterday evening, the BUN was 111, creatinine 7.0, CO_2 9, sodium up to 133, potassium 5.7, calcium 8.6, CPK down to 728. Today's metabolic profile reveals a sodium of 135, potassium 6.1, CO_2 9, chloride 113, BUN 109, creatinine 6.5, glucose 108, bilirubin 0.8, albumin 3.1, calcium 8.1, alkaline phosphatase 89, protein 5.8, SGOT 32 and SGPT 20. The phosphorus is 6.3 and the magnesium is 2.5. Today's CBC reveals a hemoglobin of 7.9, hematocrit 3.1, white blood count 2800 and a platelet count of 66,000. The urine culture revealed no growth for 24 hours. The chest x-ray shows cardiomegaly with no definite evidence of pneumonia or pulmonary edema. The CAT scan of the brain shows a very small right caudate nuclear lacunar infarct of uncertain age, minimal bilateral cerebral white matter ischemic disease, and brain atrophy compatible with age.

PHYSICAL EXAMINATION

GENERAL: She is awake, alert, and asking for water. She is n.p.o. now because of insertion of dialysis catheter soon.

VITAL SIGNS: Temperature: On admission, 99.9. It is down to 98.2 now. **Pulse:** 100. **Respirations:** 16. **Blood pressure:** 170/82. Intake and output were about 1040 cc in and 175 cc out in the last 16 hours.

HEAD, EYES, EARS, NOSE, AND THROAT: Normal.

NECK: Supple. The neck veins are not distended to a horizontal degree. Carotids present and equal.

CHEST: Symmetrical.

LUNGS: Clear.

HEART: Regular. No gallop. No rub. No murmur. There is no sign of fluid overload.

ABDOMEN: Supple. No organomegaly. No ascites. Bowel sounds present.

EXTREMITIES: No edema. Skin turgor is slightly depleted.

NEUROLOGICAL: No localized deficits.

IMPRESSION: Acute renal failure related to hypovolemia, mild rhabdomyolysis, possible overdose on pain medications, history of addiction to pain medications in the past, previous history of renal insufficiency on previous admission which was reverted previously with IV fluids.

PLAN FOR TREATMENT: Urine sodium osmolality was sent to rule out the possibility of prerenal uremia. Venous dialysis catheter will be placed for starting dialysis considering the hyperkalemia recurrent after treatment and the severe metabolic acidosis and the severe uremia and elevated creatinine.

_____

Dr. Jones

D:

T:

NOTES

Case Study 9.2 (Coder/Abstract Summary Form)

Patient: **Mary Smith**

Patient documentation: **Review Medical Report 9.2**

1. Principal diagnosis:

   _____

2. Secondary or other diagnoses:

   _____

3. Principal procedure:

   _____

4. Other procedures:

   _____

5. Additional documentation needed:

   _____

   _____

   _____

6. Questions for the physician:

   _____

   _____

   _____

   _____

OPERATIVE REPORT

NAME: MARY SMITH

ROOM NUMBER:

PATIENT #:

ATTENDING: JONES

MR #:

ADMIT DATE:

DISCHARGE DATE:

DATE OF OPERATION:

PRE-OPERATIVE DIAGNOSIS:
1. MENORRHAGIA, UNRESPONSIVE TO HORMONAL THERAPY IN THE PAST
2. SICKLE CELL DISEASE

POST-OPERATIVE DIAGNOSIS:
1. MENORRHAGIA, UNRESPONSIVE TO HORMONAL THERAPY IN THE PAST
2. SICKLE CELL DISEASE

PROCEDURE: LAPAROSCOPIC ASSISTED VAGINAL HYSTERECTOMY

SURGEON:

ASSISTANT:

ANESTHESIA: GENERAL ENDOTRACHEAL

COMPLICATIONS: NONE

ESTIMATED BLOOD LOSS: 300 CC'S

URINE OUTPUT: 200 CC'S CLEAR URINE

IV FLUIDS: 1800 CC'S

FINDINGS: NORMAL OVARIES BILATERALLY, HISTORY OF TUBAL LIGATION, AT PRESENT UTERUS 8 X 5 CENTIMETERS AND GROSSLY NORMAL. THE PATIENT DID HAVE PELVIC RELAXATION.

INDICATIONS: Patient is a 37-year-old female with history of sickle cell disease, undesired fertility. Has had a tubal in the past, who has had menorrhagia and she has been unresponsive to Depo Provera in the past. She was counseled on options of oral contraceptives and declined secondary to sickle cell disease and the fact that she could have problems related to clotting. Patient discussed alternatives with the doctor who agreed that a hysterectomy would be in the patient's best interest and she underwent exchange transfusion with hemoglobin up to 13 prior to surgery.

PROCEDURE: Patient was taken to the operating room where general anesthesia was obtained without difficulty. The patient was placed in dorsal lithotomy position, prepped and draped in normal sterile fashion. A weighted speculum was placed in the patient's vagina. Anterior lip of the cervix was grasped with a single tooth tenaculum. Attention was then turned to the patient's abdomen where infraumbilical skin incision was made with scalpel. Veress needle placed intra-abdominally without difficulty. Pneumo-peritoneum was obtained with CO2 gas and 5mm. Trocar in sleeve placed intra-abdominally without difficulty. Two lateral trocars were placed under direct visualization without difficulty using scalpel to make skin incisions. Bipolar forceps with cutting was then used to perform the intra-abdominal part of hysterectomy bilaterally. The utero-ovarian ligament was clamped, electrocoagulated and cut. This was carried down though the utero-ovarian ligament to the broad ligaments which was carried down through the round ligament. This was done in a step-wise fashion, first on the left, then on the right and hemostasis was assured with each pedicle. Patient had adhesions of the

Continued

MEDICAL REPORT 9.2 (CONTINUED)

ovary to the uterus on the left and this was slightly more difficult and some bleeding was noted. This was coagulated with the bipolar forceps without difficulty. Once down below the round ligaments reach on each side, the bladder flap was elevated and anterior broad ligament incised with scissors without difficulty. At this point, attention was then turned back to patient's vagina.

A weighted speculum was placed in the patient's vagina and cervix grasped with Lahey clamps. Cervix was circumferentially injected with saline for hydrodissection. Incision was made circumferentially around the cervix and the bladder was pushed off anteriorly and the peritoneal cavity entered without difficulty. Posteriorly, the cul-de-sac was entered using scissors without difficulty. Posterior vaginal cuff was sutured with 0 Vicryl in a running locking fashion. Haney clamps were then used to bilaterally clamp the uterosacral ligament, transected them and then ligated with 0 Vicryl Haney fixation suture. The uterine arteries were then clamped bilaterally with curved Haney clamp, transected and ligated with 0 Vicryl in a fixation suture. The remainder of the broad ligament was step-wise clamped, cut and ligated with 0 Vicryl and Haney fixation sutures. Step-wise, up the uterus, the uterus was then flipped after sufficient relaxation was noted and the uterus was flipped posteriorly and delivered through the vagina. Remaining pedicles were ligated with 0 Vicryl fore and aft stitch and hemostasis noted. All pedicles were inspected and noted to be hemostatic. Peritoneum was then grasped anteriorly and modified cul-de-plasty performed starting anteriorly, incorporating the uterosacral and then the posterior peritoneum and then tying down. The vaginal cuff was closed with 0 Vicryl in a running locking fashion, anterior to posterior without difficulty. All pedicles were noted to be hemostatic prior to final closure. No bleeding was noted from vaginal cuff and therefore packing was not used. Foley was left in for drainage.

Attention was then turned back to patient's abdomen where insufflation was again obtained and all pedicles inspected intra-abdominally and noted to be hemostatic. Pelvis was irrigated copiously with saline and again irrigated and suctioned with copious amounts of saline and again, all pedicles noted to be hemostatic. Instruments were removed from the patient's abdomen. Subcutaneous sutures of 4-0 Vicryl were then placed and then the skin was closed with Dermabond without difficulty.

Patient tolerated the procedure well. Sponge, lap, needle, instrument counts correct times 2. Patient was taken to recovery room in stable condition.

_____

Dr. Jones

DD:

DT:

cc:

NOTES

Case Study 9.3 (Coder/Abstract Summary Form)

Patient: **John Doe**

Patient documentation: **Review Medical Reports 9.3, 9.4, and 9.5**

1. Principal diagnosis:

   _____

2. Secondary or other diagnoses:

   _____

3. Principal procedure:

   _____

4. Other procedures:

   _____

5. Additional documentation needed:

   _____

   _____

   _____

   _____

6. Questions for the physician:

   _____

   _____

   _____

   _____

   _____

MEDICAL REPORT 9.3

HISTORY AND PHYSICAL

NAME: JOHN DOE

ROOM NUMBER:

PATIENT #:

ATTENDING: SMITH

MR #:

ADMIT DATE:

DISCHARGE DATE:

IDENTIFICATION: Patient is a 76-year-old male that lives with his wife.

CURRENT PROBLEM: Left renal mass.

HISTORY OF PROBLEM: He has had a history of gross hematuria in the past. We worked him up initially with an IVP five years ago. Now more recently he is noted to have an enhancing cystic mass in the upper pole of the left kidney. We did a follow-up study and found that it had actually enlarged a little bit. We did an MRI scan with and without contrast that showed an abnormal enhancing cystic mass in the upper pole highly concerning for cystic renal neoplasm. We discussed options for treatment. He has elected for nephrectomy and presents at this time for removal of his left kidney.

PAST HISTORY:

Medical
- Positive for hypertension and hyperlipidemia.
- He also has a history of DVT.

Medical Allergies
- No known medication allergies.

Current Medications
- He ordinarily takes Coumadin 5 mg three days a week and 2.5 mg four days a week.
- Procardia 90 mg daily.
- Lescol 20 mg daily.

Previous Surgery
- None.

REVIEW OF SYSTEMS:
- Denies chest pain, shortness of breath, hemoptysis.
- GI—denies diarrhea, constipation, melena, hematochezia.

PHYSICAL EXAMINATION:

GENERAL: Well-developed, well-nourished male who appears younger than stated age.

Ht: 5'10" (1.7 m)   **Wt:** 197 (89 kg)

VITAL SIGNS:

P: 64   **BP:** 104/70   **RR:** 16

HEENT: WNL.

HEART: Regular with occasional skipped beat.

MEDICAL REPORT 9.3 (CONTINUED)

LUNGS: Clear.

ABDOMEN: Benign.

PROSTATE: Smooth without induration of nodule. There is no rectal mass.

EXTREMITIES: No cyanosis, clubbing, or edema.

IMPRESSION:

- Left renal mass consistent with cystic hypernephroma.

PLAN:

- Will proceed with laparoscopic nephrectomy. Consent form has been signed.

ANTICIPATED ADMISSION:

DD: Electronically Signed
TD: Dr. Smith

NOTES

MEDICAL REPORT 9.4

OPERATIVE REPORT

PATIENT NAME: JOHN DOE

DATE OF PROCEDURE:

PREOPERATIVE DIAGNOSIS: LEFT RENAL MASS

POSTOPERATIVE DIAGNOSIS: SAME

OPERATION PERFORMED: CYSTOSCOPY, URETERAL CATHETER PLACEMENT, PARTIAL LEFT NEPHRECTOMY (SUBCOSTAL)

SURGEON: SMITH

ASSISTANTS: JONES

ANESTHESIA: GENERAL

INDICATIONS FOR PROCEDURE: Left renal mass, progressive, consistent with cystic hypernephroma noted on preoperative CT scans and MRI. Because of this, his kidney was explored.

FINDINGS: Reveal a cystic lesion involving the upper pole of the kidney. However, pathologic frozen section did not reveal malignancy; therefore a segmental polar nephrectomy was completed.

PROCEDURE IN DETAIL: After informed consent was obtained in my office, the patient was identified and brought into the operative suite, placed under an excellent general anesthetic in the supine position. At this point his genitalia were sterilely prepped and draped. A 15.5-French flexible Olympus cystoscope was passed through the urethra into the bladder and the left ureteral orifice was identified. A 0.8 Zebra guide wire was passed into the kidney and the cystoscope was then removed. A 16-French two-way Foley catheter was placed. The ureteral access catheter was taped to the Foley catheter. The Foley was placed to gravity drainage. An IV extension tubing was attached to the ureteral catheter so that we could inject retrograde indigo carmine. Once this was completed, a standard left subcostal incision was made and carried down through skin and subcutaneous tissue. The two abdominal wall layers were divided. The peritoneum was identified. An extraperitoneal approach was completed by dissecting the peritoneum away from the abdominal wall with blunt finger dissection and counter traction. Once this was completed, the plane between the posterior parietal peritoneum and Gerota's fascia was developed. The entire peritoneum was dissected away from Gerota's fascia. At this point, Gerota's fascia was opened and extended toward the upper pole of the kidney at the level of the renal vessels. At this point, we elected to put vascular loops around the artery and the vein, so that we had adequate proximal control.

At this point, the superior pole of the kidney was dissected out, a cyst was identified. Utilizing the back blade of the surgical knife, the plane of the kidney was developed at the level of the segmental polar vessel; approximately one-third of the parenchyma was excised. The calices were tied off with #2-0 Vicryl. Bleeders were suture ligated with figure of eight #3-0 Chromic sutures. At this point, there was no significant bleeding renal parenchyma. We injected retrograde indigo carmine 5ccs. The infundibulum of the upper pole leaked the dye material and therefore was over sewn with #3-0 Vicryl. At this point, there was no bleeding and no further leakage of urine. Avitene was placed on the raw edge of the kidney and then Gerota's fascia was closed and buttressed over the top of the cut surface of the kidney. Once this was completed, no active bleeding or leak was identified. The peritoneum was then allowed to lay on top of Gerota's fascia. The abdominal wall was closed in two layers with #0-0 PDS running sutures. The skin was closed with skin staples, an indwelling Foley catheter was left in place and a sterile dressing was applied. The patient appeared to tolerate the procedure well.

Estimated blood loss: 800, one unit of packed cells transfused. No drains.

_____

Dr. Smith

D:

T:

Electronically Signed

MEDICAL REPORT 9.5

PATHOLOGY RESULTS

ACCT#:

PATIENT: JOHN DOE

DOB:

ATTN: SMITH

Received: Collected:

Spec #:   Subm Practitioner:

CLINICAL INFORMATION

PREOP DIAGNOSIS: (L) Renal Mass

POSTOP DIAGNOSIS: Same—see pathology report

SPECIMEN: (I) upper pole of left kidney for FS

GROSS DESCRIPTION: Received is a single pole of one kidney, presenting as a brown soft tissue structure with diameters of 50 and 55 mm, and a dimension between the cut surface and pole of 40 mm. A number of metal clips are seen on the surgical margin. The specimen is sectioned sagittally, revealing a 7 mm diameter simple cyst near the surgical margin on the anterior surface. Hilar fat is found in the center sections, which is surrounded by the usual-appearing medullary and cortical renal tissue. Representative sections are submitted.

TISSUE CODE: 8   4

PATHOLOGIC IMPRESSION

1. SMALL SIMPLE CYST, BENIGN, OF A KIDNEY SEGMENT, CLINICALLY THE LEFT UPPER POLE.

2. MILD ARTERIAL NEPHROSCLEROSIS, SAME BIOPSY MATERIAL.

Electronically Signed:

NOTES

Case Study 9.4 (Coder/Abstract Summary Form)

Patient: **Frank Parker**

Patient documentation: **Review Medical Reports 9.6 and 9.7**

1. Principal diagnosis:

   _____

2. Secondary or other diagnoses:

   _____

3. Principal procedure:

   _____

4. Other procedures:

   _____

5. Additional documentation needed:

   _____

   _____

   _____

   _____

6. Questions for the physician:

   _____

   _____

   _____

   _____

MEDICAL REPORT 9.6

HISTORY AND PHYSICAL

PATIENT: Frank Parker

ROOM NUMBER:

PATIENT #:

MR #:

ATTENDING: JONES

DISCHARGE DATE:

ADMIT DATE:

REASON FOR ADMISSION: Acute uremic pericarditis

OTHER SIGNIFICANT DIAGNOSES:
1. End-stage renal disease; AV shunt status.
2. Peripheral vascular disease.
3. Perforating folliculitis.
4. History of past atrial fibrillation.
5. Sick sinus syndrome.
6. Severe low back pain for which he uses Lortab chronically.
7. Anxiety with depression.
8. History of noncompliance with medications and treatment regimens including dialysis.

This is a 46-year-old male who missed at least three dialysis sessions resulting in severe volume overload. He did receive dialysis on the outpatient setting, but then subsequently presented to the emergency room with increasing-ongoing chest discomfort. On evaluation he was also found to have a cardiac rub and tachycardia-bradycardia syndrome. He is admitted to the hospital for what appears to be uremic pericarditis.

MEDICATIONS: Unclear, but receiving Epogen and Hectorol in the dialysis unit. He receives Lortab 10 q.i.d. p.r.n. for severe ongoing chronic low back pain and Metoprolol 25 mg p.o. b.i.d. for hypertension.

He is supposed to also be using phosphate binders including PhosLo 667 2 p.o. t.i.d. with meals, but states he has not done so.

SOCIAL HISTORY: He smokes cigarettes. He does not use alcohol or illicit medications. He denies the use of OTC medications including nonsteroidals.

FAMILY HISTORY: There are no other family members with renal disease.

REVIEW OF SYSTEMS: He denies bleeding from any site. He notes palpitations. He has some vague chest discomforts, but no overt pain. His appetite is reduced. He has a sense of puffiness. There is no new focal joint discomfort, but he complains of malaise.

PHYSICAL EXAMINATION: This is a 46-year-old man in mild-to-moderate distress with a blood pressure of 184/103, a temperature of 96.9, a pulse of 88 respiratory rate of 24. Room air oxygen saturation is 98%. His pain intensity is 6/10.

LUNGS: There are basilar crackles and occasional scattered wheezing. There is no stridor.

NECK: The neck is supple with no jugular venous distention. The thyroid exam is normal.

HEART: Tachycardia. A positive cardiac rub is present.

ABDOMEN: Soft, nontender with no abdominal bruit.

Continued

MEDICAL REPORT 9.6 (CONTINUED)

EXTREMITIES: There is 2 + pitting edema. Perforating folliculitis is noted throughout. There are no focal neurological deficits. There has been no recent change in vision.

LABORATORIES: Sedimentation rate is 42. The CPK is 0.55 with a normal total CPK. The INR is 1.4. The white blood cell count is 6.8, a hemoglobin of 11 with a hematocrit of 34. The mean cell volume is 95. The mean cell hemoglobin is 31. The mean cell hemoglobin concentration is 32. The platelets of 260,000 with 86% neutrophils. The sodium is 137, a potassium of 5.8, a chloride of 95, a CO_2 of 27, a glucose of 111, a BUN of 76 with a creatinine of 15. The calcium is 9.6. The CK is 71.

EKG reveals sinus rhythm with left ventricular hypertrophy changes.

IMPRESSION AND PLAN: The patient apparently has uremic pericarditis. We will arrange for hemodialysis on a daily basis and consult Dr. Smith cardiology for further evaluation and treatment for tachy-brady syndrome. Emphasis in need of dialysis compliance is emphasized with initiation of other medications needed for probable coronary artery disease, hyperlipidemia, renal failure, and hypertension.

See orders for details.

TIME OF DICTATION:

TIME OF TRANSCRIPTION:

Electronically signed:

_____

Dr. Jones

NOTES

MEDICAL REPORT 9.7

OPERATIVE REPORT

PATIENT NAME: FRANK PARKER

DATE OF PROCEDURE:

PREOPERATIVE DIAGNOSIS: TACHY/BRADY SYNDROME, SINUS PAUSES, AND CHRONOTROPIC INCOMPETENCE

POSTOPERATIVE DIAGNOSIS: SAME

OPERATION PERFORMED: DUAL CHAMBER PERMANENT CARDIAC PACEMAKER IMPLANTATION

SURGEON: SMITH

ANESTHESIA: The patient gave consent to pacemaker implantation after discussion of risks, benefits, and alternatives to the procedure.

PROCEDURE: In the operating room he was sterilely prepped and draped. The subcutaneous tissue below the left clavicle was infiltrated with 1% lidocaine with epinephrine for local anesthesia. The left subclavian vein was then cannulated with a needle and an introducer was placed over a guide wire, which was done under fluoroscopy. Using guide wire and introducer technique, both atrial and ventricular leads were placed into the right atrium via the SVC. Pacemaker pulse generator pocket was dissected using blunt dissection. The ventricular lead was placed under fluoroscopic guidance in the apex of the right ventricle with initial impedance 656 ohms, sensing R-waves at greater than 10 millivolts and ventricular pacing threshold of 0.7 volts at 0.5 milliseconds. As the patient was in atrial fibrillation I attempted to cardiovert him out of atrial fibrillation and into sinus rhythm unsuccessfully with synchronous cardioversion attempted at 50, 100, 200, and 300 joules. After unsuccessful attempts at cardioversion the atrial lead was placed with initial impedance 560 ohms, P-wave sensing at greater than 2 millivolts. Atrial pacing threshold was not tested as patient was in atrial fibrillation. We attempted to overdrive pace the atrium to convert him to sinus rhythm at a rate of 300 per minute, which was unsuccessful. Both leads were actively fixated. Pacing at 10 volts through both leads resulted in no diaphragmatic stimulation. The leads were attached to the pacemaker pulse generator and sewn into the underlying connective tissue, as was the pacemaker pulse generator, and the pulse generator pocket was closed with interrupted deep sutures and running subcuticular sutures with good hemostasis. Follow up chest x-ray reveals no pneumo or hemothorax and good lead position with a minimal amount of lead slack in both the atrial and ventricular leads.

Pacemaker pulse generator is an Identity XL DR, Serial Number 999999. The atrial lead is a Tendril SDX 46cm, Model Number 9999TC, Serial Number NA99999. The ventricular lead is a Tendril SDX, Model Number 9999TC, Serial Number NB99999.

Final pacemaker interrogation and setting parameters are: DD DR mode with a base rate of 60, max track 110, auto capture is off. Ventricular pulse amplitude is set at 3.50 volts at 0.4 milliseconds, bipolar configuration. Atrial pulse amplitude is set at 3.50 volts at 0.4 milliseconds, bipolar configuration. Auto mode switch is on with an atrial tachycardia detection rate of 180 beats per minute. AF suppression is on. Lower rate overdrive of 10, upper rate overdrive of 5 and 15 overdrive pacing cycles. Pacemaker media tachycardia option is on auto detect with a rate of 110.

Patient tolerated the procedure well without any detected complications. He will be observed on telemetry today and may be discharged home if he has no tachycardia, has good pain control, is able to take p.o. and ambulate independently. His primary care provider might opt to attempt cardioversion at a later date with the patient on antiarrhythmic therapy. He will be discharged home on Coumadin. He is given instructions not to raise his elbow above his shoulder for the next two weeks. He should not drive for the next two weeks. He needs to see me in two weeks time for suture removal and will be following up in six weeks time for initial pacemaker interrogation and programming post implant. If he has any signs or symptoms of arrhythmias or infection or bleeding, he should contact either his primary care provider or myself immediately. He will also be discharged home with a prescription for Vicodin, one to two p.o. q6h as needed for pain control.

_____

Dr. Smith

DD:

DT:

Electronically signed:

Coding for Skin and Subcutaneous Tissue Diseases

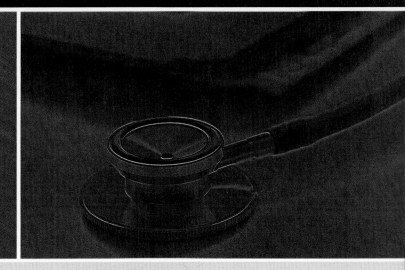

Chapter Outline

Cellulitis

Skin Ulcers

Dermatitis

Erythematous Conditions

Debridement Procedures

Biopsies and Excisions of Skin Lesions

Repairs of the Skin

Testing Your Comprehension

Coding Practice I: Chapter Review Exercises

Coding Practice II: Medical Record Case Studies

Chapter Objectives

▶ Describe the pathology of common skin and subcutaneous tissue disorders.

▶ Recognize the typical manifestations, complications, and treatments of common skin and subcutaneous tissue disorders in terms of their implications for coding.

▶ Correctly code common skin and subcutaneous tissue disorders and related procedures by using the ICD-9-CM and medical records.

Diseases of the skin and subcutaneous tissue are classified in code section 680 to 709 of chapter 12 in the Tabular List of Diseases of ICD-9-CM. This relatively short chapter includes diseases of the integumentary system, which consists of the skin and its accessory organs, which include specialized glands (sweat and sebaceous), hair, and nails (Figure 10.1). The skin serves as a protective covering for the body; sebaceous glands produce sebum, which helps keep the skin lubricated; and sweat glands produce sweat, which helps to cool the body, thus aiding in thermoregulation.

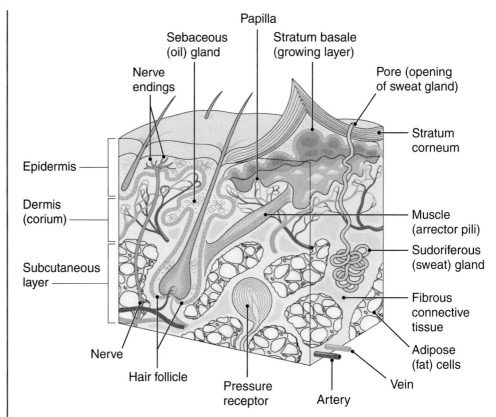

FIGURE 10.1 ■ Cross-section of the skin. (Reprinted with permission from Cohen BJ and Wood DL. Memmler's The Human Body in Health and Disease, 9th Ed. Philadelphia: Lippincott Williams & Wilkins, 2000.)

Some of the more common skin diseases that are coded with ICD-9-CM and cause hospital inpatient admissions include cellulitis, ulcers, gangrene, dermatitis, and certain erythematous conditions. Many other common skin diseases, such as eczema, psoriasis, seborrhea, actinic keratosis, and keloid scars, are sometimes seen as secondary diagnoses during an inpatient stay because they affect the overall care given to the patient. However, these conditions would rarely be the principal cause for inpatient admission because they are routinely treated on an outpatient basis.

Cellulitis

Cellulitis is a bacterial infection that spreads in the skin, causing a severe inflammation of the underlying soft tissues. The affected area appears swollen and red and feels tender and hot (Figure 10.2). Cellulitis usually occurs as a result of an open wound, an injury, or an ulcer. Often the offending bacterial agent is streptococcus, but many other types of bacteria can also cause cellulitis. Cellulitis is a serious medical condition, because the infection can spread from the skin to lymph nodes (presenting as red streaks) and the bloodstream, resulting in a life-threatening sepsis (systemic blood infection).

TIP After the cellulitis code, list an additional code to identify the organism, if it is known. You should carefully review the culture and sensitivity report, as well as the physician's progress notes.

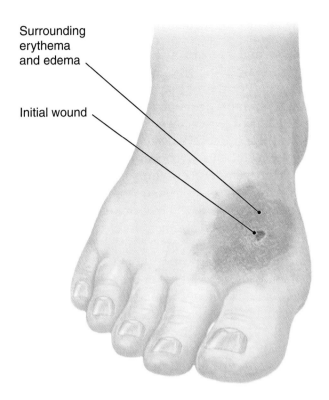

Surrounding
erythema
and edema

Initial wound

FIGURE 10.2 ■ Recognizing cellulitis. (Reprinted with permission by Anatomical Chart Co.)

Word Parts and Meanings of Medical Terms Related to the Skin and Subcutaneous Tissue

Word Part	Meaning	Example	Definition of Example
cutane/o	Skin	subcutaneous tissue	The layer of tissue beneath the skin
De-	down, without, removal of	debridement	Removal of dead or damaged tissue, as from a wound
derm/o, dermato/o	Skin	dermatitis	Inflammation of the skin, often associated with redness and itching
Epi-	Above	epidermis	The upper (outermost) layer of the skin
erythr/o, erythem/o	red, redness	erythematous	Characterized by erythema (redness of the skin)
hetero-	other, different, unequal	heterograft	A graft of tissue transplanted between animals of different species (also called xenograft)
hypo-	under, below, abnormally low, decreased	hypodermic	Pertaining to under the skin
-itis	Inflammation	cellulitis	A spreading inflammation of tissue due to a bacterial infection
Sub-	under, below	subdermal	Beneath the skin

Following are five general rules for sequencing codes for cellulitis:

1. If the cellulitis is secondary to an open wound, injury, or ulcer, the correct sequencing of codes depends on the principal reason for the admission and whether the primary treatment or treatments were directed toward the complicated open wound, cellulitis, or ulcer.

2. If the primary treatment is directed at the wound, sequence "wound, open, complicated" for the specified site as the principal diagnosis, and list the code for the cellulitis as a secondary diagnosis. Located in the Disease Index under the main term "wound, open" is a box with italicized notes. ICD-9-CM defines "complicated wound" as one with delayed healing, delayed treatment, foreign body, or primary infection. Cellulitis within the wound constitutes a primary infection, and you should use the subentry under the main term for the open wound site with complication. Treatments directed at wounds include excisional or nonexcisional debridements, suturing, grafts, or other repairs. However, minor cleansing of the wound would not require an inpatient admission.

3. If the primary treatment is directed at the cellulitis, sequence cellulitis as the principal diagnosis, and list the code for the "open wound, complicated" second. Treatments directed at the cellulitis include intravenous antibiotics, analgesics for pain, elevation of the affected area, and wet dressings to reduce swelling. You should note that cellulitis can occur from a minor wound (e.g., puncture wound from a thorn or needlestick) that does not receive separate medical attention. In that case, code only the cellulitis, because the wound did not affect the care given.

4. If the cellulitis is associated with a skin ulcer, two codes are required. Code both the skin ulcer (707.X) and cellulitis (681 to 682), because cellulitis is not routinely associated with all ulcers. Whether the admission treatment is directed toward the ulcer or the cellulitis determines which condition you should sequence as the principal diagnosis.

5. Cellulitis with gangrene is coded only to gangrene (785.4). Locating the main term "gangrene" in the *Alphabetic Index to Diseases*, you will note that the nonessential modifiers after the main term gangrene include the term "cellulitis." However, gangrene is rarely given as a principal diagnosis for an inpatient admission because the 785.4 code for gangrene comes from chapter 16, "Symptoms, Signs, and Ill-Defined Conditions." Usually, you would code the underlying cause for the gangrene (e.g., diabetes, ulcer, or injury) first and then gangrene second as a manifestation of the condition.

EXAMPLE

1. *A woman punctured her index finger on a rose thorn while working in her garden. Her finger became red and swollen with developing cellulitis. She was admitted to the hospital and given intravenous antibiotics. Attention to the puncture wound was not necessary.*

   Code: *681.00—cellulitis of finger*

2. *A man lacerated his hand while working on his car. The wound became infected, and cellulitis developed. He presented to the hospital and underwent nonexcisional debridement of the infected wound with simple suturing of the hand. He also was given intravenous antibiotics and underwent multiple dressing changes.*

   Codes: *882.1—laceration hand, complicated*
                 682.4—cellulitis, hand

86.59—suture, hand
86.28—nonexcisional debridement

3. *A woman was scratched on the wrist while playing with her cat and developed cellulitis. The patient's wound was cleaned, and antibiotic ointment and a bandage were applied to the minor wound. She was admitted and placed on intravenous antibiotics for the cellulitis.*

    Codes: *682.4—cellulitis, wrist*
                 881.12—open wound, wrist, complicated (with primary infection)

4. *A patient presented with cellulitis and an ulcerated great toe. The patient underwent excisional debridement of the ulcer and was given intravenous antibiotics.*

    Codes: *707.15—ulcer, toe*
                 681.10—cellulitis, toe
                 86.22—excisional debridement

5. *A patient presented with diabetic gangrene with cellulitis of the right foot. The patient had a known history of insulin-dependent diabetes mellitus. The patient underwent transmetatarsal amputation of the right foot and was placed on intravenous antibiotics.*

    Codes: *250.71—insulin-dependent diabetes mellitus, Type I, with peripheral vascular disorder*
                 785.4—gangrene
                 84.12—transmetatarsal amputation, foot

6. *A patient presented with cellulitis, with an ulcer and gangrene of the right foot. The patient underwent excisional debridement of the right foot and was given intravenous antibiotics.*

    Codes: *707.15—ulcer, foot*
                 785.4—gangrene, foot (nonessential modifier for gangrene includes cellulitis)
                 86.22—excisional debridement

Skin Ulcers

A skin ulcer involves an open sore or erosion of the skin. Skin ulcers are coded to category 707. Pressure ulcers (707.0X), also called decubitus ulcers or bedsores, are problematic for hospitals and long-term health-care facilities such as nursing homes. They are the result of skin damage associated with pressure from lying or sitting in one position for an extended period of time. Reddened areas can signify a breakdown of the skin and an impending ulcer for bedridden patients or wheelchair-bound patients. Preventive care through frequent repositioning of patients and the use of "egg-crate" mattresses help to relieve pressure on the areas most often affected (e.g., sacrum or tailbone and heels of the feet). Elderly bedridden patients are also more predisposed to pressure ulcers caused by a thinning of the skin that comes with age. Health-care personnel work diligently to prevent pressure ulcers through careful examination of residents of long-term nursing or rehabilitation facilities and hospital inpatients.

Pressure ulcers can be classified into stages. As of October 1, 2008, new codes (707.2X) are available to describe the stage (degree of severity) that include the following:

▶ Stage I—intact skin with redness (erythema) or other color changes that usually occur over a bony prominence (e.g., tailbone, heels, elbows); code 707.21

> ▶ Stage II—partial thickness loss of dermis (skin) without slough (necrosed tissue); code 707.22
> ▶ Stage III—full thickness tissue loss without visible bone, muscle or tendon; 707.23
> ▶ Stage IV—full thickness tissue loss with exposed bone, muscle, ot tendon; code 707.24

Starting October 1, 2008, hospital's will not receive additional reimbursement for any stage III or IV hospital acquired pressure ulcer (i.e., a stage III or IV ulcer that was not present-on-admission [POA]). That is, the facility will be financially penalized for the occurrence of this hospital-acquired condition (HAC). As these ulcers are classified as Major CCs under the MS-DRG payment system and can significantly impact the reimbursement to the facility, it is imperative for physicians, during the initial patient assessment at admission, to document the presence and site of any pressure ulcer.

Ulcers can also represent a long-term or secondary complication associated with diabetes mellitus. In such cases, you would sequence the diabetes code as the etiology or cause for the ulcer first, and then list the ulcer code second as the manifestation of the disease (e.g., diabetic heel ulcer—250.80 + 707.14). Because the fourth digit (8) on the diabetes code means diabetes with "other specified complication," review the record to see whether a more precise fourth digit can be used with the diabetes code in place of the 8 (e.g., diabetic peripheral vascular disease with heel ulcer—250.70 + 707.14).

In atherosclerosis, arteries can become clogged with fatty deposits and slow the circulation of blood, which can result in ulcers of the extremities. Atherosclerosis of the extremities associated with ulcer is coded to 440.23. Code 440.23 first, with an additional code to identify the precise ulcer site (e.g., right ankle ulcer attributable to atherosclerotic peripheral vascular disease—440.23 + 707.13). A single combination code is provided to describe atherosclerotic ulcerations of the extremities with gangrene (code 440.24), and an additional code for gangrene is not needed (e.g., right ankle ulcer with gangrene attributable to atherosclerotic peripheral vascular disease—440.24 + 707.13).

In nonatherosclerotic ulcers, if ulcers include gangrene, assign an additional code for the gangrene, because gangrene is not routinely associated with ulcers (e.g., foot ulcer with gangrene—707.15 + 785.4).

Dermatitis

Dermatitis is an inflammation of the skin. There are various types of dermatitis that are attributable to either external or internal causes.

Dermatitis can be attributable to external causes, such as contact with poison ivy (code 692.6). It can also be a reaction to topical drugs (code 692.3) or the result of contact with some allergen such as dust, detergents, cosmetics, or jewelry. Even sunburn (code 692.71) and diaper rash (code 691.0) are examples of dermatitis attributable to external causes.

Dermatitis can also be attributable to agents taken internally, such as foods eaten (code 693.1) or medications ingested or injected (Figure 10.3). When coding dermatitis attributable to a drug, you must determine whether the drug was taken correctly as prescribed or was taken incorrectly, because this significantly changes the manner in which it is coded.

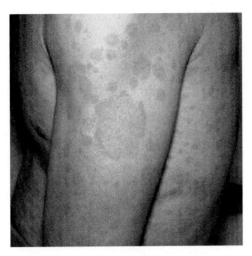

FIGURE 10.3 ■ Urticarial drug eruption. Note the bizarre shapes of the urticarial plaques. (Reprinted with permission from Goodheart HP, MD. Goodheart's Photoguide of Common Skin Disorders, 2nd Edition. Philadelphia: Lippincott Williams & Wilkins, 2003.)

If a patient develops dermatitis from a drug taken correctly as prescribed, the dermatitis is considered an adverse effect (of the drug) and not a poisoning episode. According to coding guidelines, sequence the adverse effect first, and then list an additional E code from the Table of Drugs and Chemicals that specifies the drug causing adverse effects in therapeutic use (e.g., dermatitis secondary to penicillin, taken as prescribed—693.0 + E930.0). If the drug was not taken as prescribed, it is considered a poisoning. From the Table of Drugs and Chemicals, sequence the poisoning code first, and then list an additional code to describe the manifestation. Then assign an E code to describe the external cause of the poisoning.

Dermatitis secondary to accidental overdose of penicillin tablets: 960.0 + 693.0 + E856. **EXAMPLE**

Erythematous Conditions

Conditions that cause redness of the skin are described as erythematous. Certain erythematous conditions, such as forms of erythema multiforme, produce hypersensitivity reactions serious enough to warrant inpatient admission. Erythema multiforme (code 695.1X) includes toxic epidermal necrolysis and Stevens-Johnson syndrome.

Toxic epidermal necrolysis (code 695.15), also called "scalded skin syndrome," can be a life-threatening form of erythema multiforme in which the skin peels off in sheets. Many cases are attributable to an extreme allergic (hypersensitivity) reaction to a drug such as penicillin or a complication of another disease. In other cases, the etiology may be unknown. As is sometimes seen in burn patients, the extreme loss of skin because of toxic epidermal necrolysis can be life threatening because fluids seep from the patient, who then becomes more susceptible to infection. Treatment includes discontinuation of any drugs suspected of causing the reaction, intravenous replacement of fluids, covering the patients with protective bandages, and strict isolation to prevent secondary infections.

Stevens-Johnson syndrome (code 695.13) is another serious and sometimes fatal form of erythema multiforme in which the patient breaks out in red patches and blisters that can cover the mouth, throat, genitals, and eyes. This syndrome may result from a drug reaction or an infectious disease, such as herpes simplex. Treatment includes intravenous fluids and nutrition, as well as the administration of antibiotics to prevent or treat any possible secondary infections.

As of October 1, 2008, new codes (695.5X) have been added to describe the degree of exfoliation (shedding, peeling of skin) attributable to these erythematous conditions. For example, 695.51 describes exfoliation due to an erythematous condition involving 10-19 percent of body surface; and, 695.59 describes exfoliation due to an erythematous condition involving 90 percent or more of body surface.

Debridement Procedures

Debridement involves the removal of devitalized (unhealthy) tissue and foreign matter from a wound to allow healthy tissue a better chance of healing the wound.

 Coders must cue in to diagnoses such as ulcers or gangrene and thoroughly search the medical record for debridement procedures that are routinely performed for these conditions.

Depending on the medical staff policies of the hospital, a debridement procedure may not require a separate dictated operative report. Therefore, you should carefully review the medical record to determine whether a procedure note was written in the physician's progress notes, consultant's notes, or therapist's notes. Debridements can be performed in operating or special procedures rooms, as well as on the nursing unit at the patient's bedside or in the emergency room.

It is important that coders determine and validate (through appropriate provider documentation) whether an excisional or a nonexcisional debridement was performed. Look for key terms such as "sharp" or "surgical" that indicate that an excisional debridement (code 86.22) was performed in which the devitalized tissue was cut back. As physicians must document "excisional," when in doubt, always query the responsible physician. Have the physician document any clarification through an addendum, if necessary. Excisional debridement is an operative procedure that can change the diagnosis-related group and affect reimbursement; therefore, incorrect coding of debridements can result in overpayment or underpayment to the facility. Nonexcisional debridement (code 86.28) is a nonoperative procedure in which the devitalized tissue is usually scrubbed away.

Incorrectly coding nonexcisional debridements to excisional debridements results in a higher payment to the facility and is an example of *upcoding*—an unethical and fraudulent practice.

According to *Coding Clinic* guidelines, physicians—as well as nonphysicians such as physical therapists, physician assistants, nurses, and therapists—may perform excisional debridements. The coding is the same regardless of the person who performs the debridement.

The extent and depth of the debridement are also important factors in ensuring correct code assignment. If the debridement of same site includes skin and subcutaneous tissue but also goes to deeper muscle tissue, code only debridement of muscle. If debridement of the same site includes skin and subcutaneous tissue and muscle down to and including bone, code only debridement of bone. In other words, code debridements to the deepest tissue involved. If the debridements are of multiple sites, including skin/subcutaneous tissue of one site and muscle of another site, then code for debridement of both the subcutaneous tissue and the muscle for each different site.

Biopsies and Excisions of Skin Lesions

Biopsy of the skin is coded to 86.11 (e.g., a "punch" skin biopsy uses a surgical tool to remove a core of tissue). In skin biopsies, skin lesions that are abnormal areas of skin tissue are removed and sent to the pathologist, who examines the tissue cells to provide a definitive diagnosis (e.g., cancer or a benign mole). A simple excision of a skin lesion is coded to 86.3 and can be located in the *Alphabetic Index to Procedures* section under the main term "excision, lesion, skin." A radical excision of a skin lesion is coded to 86.4, and this includes a wide excision of the skin lesion involving underlying tissues with a flap (adjacent tissue transfer) closure of the defect area. If the surgeon describes the procedure as an "excisional biopsy" of the skin lesion, assign code 86.3. Excisional biopsies denote that the entire lesion was removed.

Repairs of the Skin

A simple repair (sutures, staples, or surgical or tissue adhesives) of a laceration or wound of the skin and subcutaneous tissue is coded to 86.59; a plastic (i.e., reconstructive) repair of the skin without a graft is coded to 86.89. You should be careful to note that a diagnosis of jagged wounds may indicate the need for more than a simple skin repair. Perform a thorough index search, because repairs of skin wounds of more specific sites may require more precise coding (e.g., repair lip laceration—27.51; repair nose laceration—21.81). Also, code wound repairs to the deepest tissue affected (e.g., suture repair of skin, subcutaneous tissue, and muscle of the same site is coded to a muscle suture repair—83.65).

Various skin graft codes can be located in the *Alphabetic Index to Procedures* section under the main term "graft, skin." There are skin graft codes that specify the precise site for the graft (e.g., hand, ear, or nose) and whether the graft is split thickness (partial) or full thickness. Also included are adjacent tissue transfer–type grafts (pedicle flap, rotation flap, and so on) or free grafts (detached from the donor site and transferred to a defect area on the same patient).

Heterografts use animal skin, and homografts use human skin from a donor. Dermal regenerative graft code 86.67 describes new biologic skin substitutes (e.g., neodermis) or artificial skin not otherwise specified. This procedure may be indicated for patients with extensive loss of skin attributable to burns, ulcers, or injuries or for patients who do not have sufficient donor skin available for grafting.

SUMMARY

This chapter has identified the common pathologic conditions that affect the skin and subcutaneous tissue. Use of the ICD-9-CM to identify proper diagnoses and procedures that are often performed to treat these conditions has been addressed. In addition, medical reports and clinical records that promote the identification of diagnoses and procedures for correct coding have been further explained. Chapter 11 addresses diseases of the musculoskeletal system and connective tissue.

TESTING YOUR COMPREHENSION

1. What purpose is served by skin?

2. What purpose is served by sebaceous glands?

3. What is the purpose of sweat glands?

4. What skin conditions often result in hospital admissions?

5. Why is cellulitis considered so serious as a medical condition?

6. Why are pressure ulcers considered to be a problematic condition?

7. What serious ailments can ulcers be associated with?

8. What external causes may result in dermatitis?

9. What internal agents may cause dermatitis?

10. What condition resulting in redness of the skin, known as erythema, can be life threatening?

11. If a patient breaks out in red patches and/or blisters that cover the mouth, throat, genitals, and eyes, what diagnosis may be applied?

12. The removal of devitalized (unhealthy) tissue from a wound is referred to as what?

13. What does a skin biopsy involve?

14. Are all skin grafts assigned the same code?

CODING PRACTICE I   Chapter Review Exercises

Directions

By using your ICD-9-CM codebook, code the following diagnoses and procedures:

	DIAGNOSIS/PROCEDURES	CODE
1	Pressure ulcer, right buttock, Stage IV. Chronic obstructive pulmonary disease. Alzheimer's dementia. Chronic congestive heart failure. Acute renal insufficiency. Rotation flap graft closure, right buttock defect.	
2	Ulcer, left elbow with cellulitis. Excisional debridement, intravenous antibiotics.	
3	Diffuse rash secondary to Bactrim (sulfamethoxazole). Bactrim taken as prescribed for current urinary tract infection.	
4	Chronic actinic dermatitis. History of smoking. Quit 9 months ago.	
5	Hypertrophic keloid scarring, right cheek, from previous laceration. Scar excision.	
6	Infected stasis ulcer, left leg.	
7	Atherosclerotic ulcer with gangrene, left leg. Left below-the-knee amputation.	
8	Cellulitis, right arm secondary to spider bite (use E code). Admitted for intravenous antibiotics.	
9	Dermatitis, hands, secondary to latex gloves.	
10	Erythema multiforme. Admitted for intravenous steroids.	

	DIAGNOSIS/PROCEDURES	CODE
11	Actinic keratosis. Cryosurgery for three facial lesions.	
12	Allergic urticaria secondary to eating shellfish.	
13	Hives and dizziness secondary to omeprazole (Prilosec; antiulcerative) with alcohol ingestion. Patient had consumed several Manhattan cocktails with medication. Alcohol abuse.	
14	Graves' disease. Non-insulin-dependent diabetes mellitus. Vitiligo.	
15	Paronychia of great toe, left. Debridement of nail.	
16	Erythematosus pemphigus with bullae.	
17	Sebaceous cyst, right cheek. Incision and drainage, sebaceous cyst.	
18	Psoriasis, back. Phototherapy to back.	
19	Impetigo with streptococcus infection. Intravenous antibiotics.	
20	Acute lymphadenitis secondary to staphylococcus infection. Intravenous antibiotics.	
21	Ulcer of right foot. Diabetes mellitus, uncontrolled. Essential hypertension. Whirlpool debridement. Intravenous antibiotics.	

CODING PRACTICE II   Medical Record Case Studies

Instructions

1. Carefully review the medical reports provided for each case study.
2. Research any abbreviations and terms that are unfamiliar or unclear.
3. Identify as many diagnoses and procedures as possible.
4. Because only part of the patient's total record is available, determine what additional documentation you might need.
5. If appropriate, identify any questions you might ask the physician to code this case correctly and completely.
6. Complete the appropriate blanks below for each case study.

CHAPTER 10 CASE STUDIES

Case Study 10.1 (Coder/Abstract Summary Form)

Patient: **John Doe**

Patient documentation: **Review Medical Reports 10.1 and 10.2**

1. Principal diagnosis:

   _____

2. Secondary or other diagnoses:

   _____

3. Principal procedure:

   _____

4. Other procedures:

   _____

5. Additional documentation needed:

   _____

   _____

   _____

   _____

Case Study 10.1 (Continued)

6. Questions for the physician:

_____

_____

_____

_____

_____

MEDICAL REPORT 10.1

DISCHARGE SUMMARY

PATIENT NAME: JOHN DOE

MR#:

ATTENDING PHYSICIAN: SMITH

ADMISSION DATE: DISCHARGE DATE:

This 82-year-old white male came to our office with severe marked cellulitis and ulcer in the external malleolus. Clinically he is much better. He significantly improved. His cellulitis improved and the ulcer is much more improved. In my impression, there is better granulation and there is no evidence of worsening or osteomyelitis. We will do an x-ray prior to discharge. Our suggestion is to continue antibiotics such as Levaquin 250 mg q.d. and wash with peroxide b.i.d. and continue Bactroban and keep open. Leg elevation will help. From the cardiovascular and respiratory point of view, he is stable. He was on Coumadin because there is history of deep venous thrombosis in the remote past. Clinically he is stable. His ABI showed 1.78 and 1.78 in both legs. Arterial flow seems okay. In addition, pulses are reasonable. With this instruction, we plan to discharge the patient.

DIAGNOSTIC IMPRESSION

1. Cellulitis and leg ulcer, right foot, improving.
2. Pseudo testicular hypogonadism, unchanged, on therapy.
3. Hypercholesterolemia.
4. Peripheral vascular disease.
5. Peripheral neuropathy.
6. Urethral stenosis controlled.
7. Severe peripheral neuropathy with old cerebrovascular accident.

PLAN FOR DISCHARGE: As outlined above.

_____

Dr. Smith

DATE DICTATED:

DATE TRANSCRIBED:

NOTES

HISTORY AND PHYSICAL

PATIENT: JOHN DOE

MR NO.:

DOB:

CHIEF COMPLAINTS: Cellulitis right foot, ankle ulcer. Right ankle open wound draining.

HISTORY OF PRESENT ILLNESS: He is an 82-year-old male patient presenting with a new found severe cellulitis of the right foot and open draining ulcer of the right ankle.

MEDICATIONS HISTORY: Current medications prescribed to the patient are:

1. Allegra 180 mg, 1 PO QD prn
2. Ambien 10 mg, 1 PO QHS
3. Aspirin 81 mg, 1 PO QD
4. Captopril 25 mg, 1 PO TID
5. Celebrex 200 mg, 1 PO BID
6. Depo-testosterone Cypionate 200 mg/ml, 1 ml Monthly
7. Diflucan 150 mg, 1 today then 1 in 2 days
8. Neurontin 300 mg, 1 PO QHS
9. Ultracet 37.5-325, 1 PO QID
10. Coumadin 2 mg daily

Patient is also taking Effexor 25 mg.

ALLERGIES: codeine

REVIEW OF SYSTEMS:

GENERAL—fever and chills

SKIN—unremarkable

EYES—Denies blurred vision, or change in visual acuity

EARS—Denies ear pain, or difficulty hearing

MOUTH—unremarkable

NECK—Denies pain or swelling

RESPIRATORY—Denies shortness of breath, cough, wheezing

CARDIOVASCULAR—Denies palpitations, chest pain, orthopnea, PND, peripheral edema, syncope or claudication

GASTROINTESTINAL—Denies nausea, vomiting, diarrhea, constipation, abdominal pain, melena, or bright red blood

GENITOURINARY—frequency of urination

MUSCULOSKELETAL—joint pain

NEUROLOGICAL—numbness, tingling sensations, weakness, and paralysis

PSYCHIATRIC—energy level decreased

ENDOCRINE—unremarkable

PAST HISTORY: Thrombophlebitis of popliteal vein and long-term (current) use of anticoagulants; Illnesses—peripheral ischemic disease, hypercholesterolemia, DVT, CVA; Surgeries—Rt. Hip × 2, low back, and thyroid.

Continued

MEDICAL REPORT 10.2 (CONTINUED)

FAMILY HISTORY: Father—deceased and TB; Mother—deceased; Son—alive and well; Daughter—alive and well;

SOCIAL HISTORY: Alcohol Use—rare; Smoking—denies smoking; Occupation—auto worker; Spouse's Occupation—married;

EXAMINATION:

VITAL SIGNS: B/P—115/71, Pulse—98, Temperature—98.5, Weight—158 lbs

CONSTITUTIONAL—well developed and in no distress

SKIN—dry and pale

HEAD—no trauma, normocephalic

EYE—PERRLA and EOMI with normal external exam

ENT—TM's intact, no injection, uvula midline and normal tongue movement

NECK—no nodes, no nuchal rigidity, thyroid normal size and texture and JVD not raised

CHEST—basilar crackles

CARDIAC—normal s1, normal s2, no s3

ABDOMEN—normal bowel sounds, no masses, no tenderness, no bruits and liver & spleen not palpable, no tenderness

GENITALIA—no inguinal hernia or adenopathy

RECTAL—deferred

EXTREMITIES—cellulitis right foot, ankle ulcer

NEUROLOGICAL—DTR equal and symmetrical, alert, oriented, no focal signs and weakness

PSYCHIATRIC—anxious and depressed

IMMUNOLOGIC—no lymphadenopathy

ASSESSMENT:

1. Cellulitis, Foot, New
2. Ulcer of Ankle, New
3. Testicular Hypogonadism, Unchanged
4. Hypercholesterolemia, Unchanged
5. Peripheral Vascular Disease, Unspecified, Worsening
6. Peripheral Neuropathy, Stable
7. Urethral Stenosis, Improving
8. Edema, Resolved

DRUG RX: The following drugs were stopped: Diflucan 150 mg

PLAN DISCUSSION: admit for IV antibiotics, today and daily.

DD:

DT:

_____

Dr. Smith

Case Study 10.2 (Coder/Abstract Summary Form)

Patient: **Mark Jones**

Patient documentation: **Review Medical Reports 10.3 and 10.4**

1. Principal diagnosis:

   _____

2. Secondary or other diagnoses:

   _____

3. Principal procedure:

   _____

4. Other procedures:

   _____

5. Additional documentation needed:

   _____

   _____

   _____

   _____

6. Questions for the physician:

   _____

   _____

   _____

   _____

   _____

MEDICAL REPORT 10.3

HISTORY AND PHYSICAL

PATIENT: MARK JONES

DOB:

MED REC:

PT ADMN:

PHYSICIAN:

ADMN DTE:

LOCATION:

DATE OF ADMISSION:

HISTORY OF PRESENT ILLNESS: He is an 80-year-old male who presented to the office today with the complaint of cellulitis to the left lower leg, x approximately 1 week, getting worse. The patient denied any fevers, nausea, vomiting, diarrhea, shortness of breath, or chest pain.

PAST MEDICAL HISTORY: Significant for peripheral vascular disease, chronic cellulitis, osteoporosis, osteoarthritis, hypertension, Parkinson's disease, chronic congestive heart failure. Coronary artery disease. Chronic obstructive pulmonary disease.

ALLERGIES: No known allergies.

HABITS: Denies ever smoking. Denies drinking or drug abuse. The patient lives at home with his son.

REVIEW OF SYSTEMS: As above. Vital signs stable at this present moment.

PHYSICAL EXAM

GENERAL: This is a somewhat lethargic male in no acute distress. Opens his eyes to name called.

HEENT: Neck no lymphadenopathy, no bruits.

HEART: Regular rate and rhythm, S1, S2, with loud systolic murmur, grade IV, VI.

LUNGS: Bibasilar crackles, fine respirations even and unlabored without wheezes or rhonchi.

ABDOMEN: Soft and nontender, without distention. Bowel sounds are positive × 4 quadrants.

EXTREMITIES: 4+ pitting edema, both ankles and feet which the son says is not new for the patient. Right lower and left lower leg have chronic dermatologic changes. Left lower leg is red and weeping with numerous vesicular areas.

PLAN: Admit the patient with cellulitis, the medical floor, whirlpools b.i.d., wound care, Levaquin 500 IV piggyback q.day. Wound culture and sensitivity. Sinemet 5/200, 7 times a day. Lasix 40 q. day. Zocor 20 q.p.m., Valium 5 q.h.s., Nitro .4 q. day, Prinivil 10 mg p.o. mg h.s. Continue to monitor the patient. Eventually discharge to home with daughter.

_____

Signed:

DD:

DT:

MICROBIOLOGY

PATIENT: MARK JONES

MRN:

BILLING#:

DOB:

AGE:

SEX:

WARD:

ORDERED BY:

SOURCE: Leg left lower extremity

COLLECTED:

ORDER#:

RECEIVED:

ANTIBIOTICS AT COLLECTION:

WOUND CULTURE OF LLE

CULTURE WOUND
- Reincubating for more growth.
- Moderate growth of Staph species, coagulase POSITIVE.
- Identification and sensitivity to follow.
- Light growth of gram negative rods.
- Identification and sensitivity to follow.

Isolate 1 Staphylococcus aureus
Isolate 2 Acinetobacter lwoffii

Isolate ANTIBIOTICS	Iso# 01 mcg/ml	Intrp	Iso# 02 mcg/mg	Intrp	Relative Cost
Trimeth/Sulfa	<2/38	S	<2/38	S	$
Erythromycin	0.5	S			$
Cefazolin	<8	S			$
Clindamycin	0.5	S			$$
Levofloxacin	<2	S	<1	S	$$
Ampicillin/Sulbact			<8/4	S	$$$
Ceftazidime			8	S	$$$
Cefotaxime			>32	R	$$$
Ticar/K Clavate			<16	S	$$$$$
Imipenem			<1	S	$$$$$$$$
Aztreonam			>16	R	$$$$$$$$

Relative Cost Key—($ = approx. $1–$10)

S = Susceptible   I = Intermediate   R = Resistant   Blac = beta-lactamase Positive
MS = Moderately Susceptible   Blank = Drug not tested or advisable Gentamicin Synergy: S = synergy exists between Aminoglycosides and Beta Lactam Drugs, for the treatment of serious infections. Gentamicin Synergy: R = synergy DOES NOT EXIST between Aminoglyconides and Beta Lactam drugs. Interpretations based on NCCLS most recent recommendations.

GRAM STAIN   - PLATED   Bite = B

Case Study 10.3 (Coder/Abstract Summary Form)

Patient: **Jane Doe**

Patient documentation: **Review Medical Report 10.5**

1. Principal diagnosis:

   _____

2. Secondary or other diagnoses:

   _____

3. Principal procedure:

   _____

4. Other procedures:

   _____

5. Additional documentation needed:

   _____

   _____

   _____

   _____

6. Questions for the physician:

   _____

   _____

   _____

   _____

   _____

MEDICAL REPORT 10.5

HISTORY AND PHYSICAL

NAME: JANE DOE

ROOM NUMBER:

PATIENT #:

ATTENDING:

MR #:

DISCHARGE DATE:

ADMIT DATE:

CHIEF COMPLAINT: FULMINATING RASH—UNRESPONSIVE TO OUTPATIENT MANAGEMENT.

PRESENT ILLNESS: This 87-year-old white female is admitted to the hospital today after progressively deteriorating with fulminate rash over her body. This patient has Parkinsonism, atrial fibrillation, insulin- dependent diabetes mellitus, and hyperlipidemia as well as diffuse osteoarthritis. She is on multiple medications including the following: 1. Parlodel 2.5 mgs _ tablet b.i.d., 2. Inderal 20 mgs b.i.d., 3. Ultram 50 mgs q.i.d. prn, 4. Meclizine 25 mgs t.i.d, 5. Sinemet 25/100 one q.i.d., 6. Centrum Silver one daily, 7. Excedrin ES prn and Excedrin PM prn, 8. Coumadin 6 mgs daily, 9. Humulin 70/30 30 units in the am and 13 units in the pm. This rash started several weeks ago although the exact time of evolution is not well known as she tended to ignore this. About two weeks ago, she presented to my office and this appeared initially to be an allergic type dermatitis. She was given a dose of Decadron that did not help. Subsequent to that, I have seen her again and we treated her with Atarax. She felt at that time about one week ago that the rash was gradually improving to some degree but returned today with rash now encompassing her chest, abdomen, arms, back, hips and beginning to involve the thighs. This has become intensely itching. She lives by herself at home with a dog and can really not manage. Her home situation is rather deplorable and we have in the past tried to place her in a tertiary care facility but she adamantly refuses. I am going to admit her at this time for hospital management and will have a second doctor see her with me, as at this point, I am not sure of the precise diagnosis of this advancing dermatitis.

PAST HISTORY:

ILLNESSES: Parkinsonism, Type I, insulin-dependent diabetes mellitus, degenerative arthritis, previous fractures.

SURGERY: Hysterectomy secondary to apparent uterine cancer. Also a right mastectomy secondary to previous CA of breast. Cataract surgery and LASIK surgery.

ALLERGIES: NONE KNOWN.

REVIEW OF SYSTEMS:

HEENT: Bilateral cataract surgery. Occasional respiratory infection but otherwise unremarkable.

RESPIRATORY: Patient is a non-smoker and has no significant lung disease.

CARDIOVASCULAR: History of vasovagal reactions and atrial fibrillation. Presently relatively stable.

GASTROINTESTINAL: No significant history of reflux or ulcers or GI bleed.

GENITOURINARY: Unremarkable except for occasional urinary tract infections. She has had previous hysterectomy.

NEUROLOGICAL: Parkinsonism.

FAMILY HISTORY: Noncontributory for this admission although there is a remote history of diabetes.

Continued

PHYSICAL EXAMINATION

GENERAL: This is a well-developed, well-nourished white female who is in acute distress with fulminating rash.

Vital signs: pulse rate 83 per minute, respirations 20 per minute, blood pressure 179/64, temperature 98 degrees. Weight 77.1 kilograms. Height 5'5".

SKIN: Grossly intact but there is a diffuse macular and occasionally pustular rash diffusely oriented over the neck and very heavily over the chest and back. It extends onto the arms to the buttocks and over the thighs at this time. This rash has progressively worsened.

LYMPHATICS: No lymphadenopathy.

HEENT: Intact. The patient wears dentures.

NECK: Supple without masses or tenderness or noticeable bruits.

CHEST: Normal AP diameter. Right mastectomy. No chest wall tenderness.

HEART: Regular rhythm on auscultation.

LUNGS: Clear to auscultation and percussion.

ABDOMEN: Flat and free of masses, tenderness or evidence of organomegaly. The bowel sounds are normal. There is diffusely noted dispersed rash.

PELVIC/RECTAL: Not done.

EXTREMITIES: Long bones intact. All joints freely movable. The joints are arthritic.
Her feet have deformities but no open ulcers at this time.

NEUROLOGICAL: Slight cogwheel rigidity of extremities. She has when she is fatigued a slight Parkinsonian tremor. Cranial nerves 2–12 intact. Sensory and motor function grossly intact. Patient well oriented to time, person, and place.

IMPRESSION:
1. ACUTE PROGRESSIVE DERMATITIS—ETIOLOGY UNCERTAIN.
2. INSULIN-DEPENDENT DIABETES MELLITUS.
3. PARKINSONISM.
4. HYPERTENSION.
5. DEGENERATIVE ARTHRITIS.
6. OSTEOPOROSIS.
7. STATUS POST CARCINOMA OF RIGHT BREAST AND UTERUS.
8. PREVIOUS EPISODES OF SYNCOPE RELATED TO ATRIAL FIBRILLATION.
9. PREVIOUS HISTORY OF HUMERAL NECK FRACTURES OF RIGHT ARM AND HIP FRACTURES.
10. HISTORY OF COMPRESSION FRACTURES OF SPINE.

_____

DD:
DT:

Case Study 10.4 (Coder/Abstract Summary Form)

Patient: **Susan Jones**

Patient documentation: **Review Medical Reports 10.6 and 10.7**

1. Principal diagnosis:

   _____

2. Secondary or other diagnoses:

   _____

3. Principal procedure:

   _____

4. Other procedures:

   _____

5. Additional documentation needed:

   _____

   _____

   _____

   _____

6. Questions for the physician:

   _____

   _____

   _____

   _____

   _____

MEDICAL REPORT 10.6

DISCHARGE SUMMARY

PT NO:

PT NAME: SUSAN JONES

PHYSICIAN: SMITH

This 82-year-old white female was admitted to the hospital with cellulitis associated with a hematoma of the anterior tibial area. For details, please see the dictated admission history and physical examination.

HOSPITAL COURSE: Her admission laboratory showed renal insufficiency with BUN of 28 and creatinine of 1.5. Lanoxin level was 2.6. We stopped her Maxzide and gave her IV fluids and her BUN and creatinine dropped down but creatinine never dropped to normal. She also had her Lanoxin held due to toxicity. INR was elevated at 3.2 and we held her Coumadin. However, the following day her INR was up to 3.6. She will hold Coumadin for an additional three days and then restart it at home. For her cellulitis, she was started on IV Ancef and when she failed to improve, she was started on Dicloxacillin. With this, she had started improving and I felt that she was well enough to go home and return to my office next week.

DISCHARGE MEDICATIONS: Discharge medications are the following: Lanoxin 0.125 mg daily, Dicloxacillin 500 mg p.o. q.i.d., Maxzide 25 one every day, Coumadin 2 mg daily except 1 mg on Sunday and she is not to start her Coumadin until next week and will get a protime in two weeks, Norpace 150 mg two p.o. b.i.d.

FOLLOW-UP: She will follow-up in my clinic next month.

DISCHARGE DIAGNOSES:

1. Cellulitis of right lower extremity with associated hematoma.

2. Lanoxin toxicity.

3. Anticoagulation with Coumadin.

4. Acute renal insufficiency secondary to dehydration.

DISCHARGE DIET: Low sodium.

DISCHARGE ACTIVITY: Ad lib and keep feet elevated when she is sitting or lying and never to stand too long in one place.

DD:

DT:

_____

Dr. Smith

MEDICAL REPORT 10.7

HISTORY AND PHYSICAL

PT NO:

PT NAME: SUSAN JONES

PHYSICIAN: SMITH

This 82-year-old white female called the office on the morning of admission stating that she had leg pain associated with a bruise on her right lower extremity. She had been using ice on it without success. She is on Coumadin. When seen in the office, she had cellulitis of the right lower extremity and was admitted to the hospital.

PAST MEDICAL HISTORY: Past medical history is significant for ovarian and endometrial carcinoma; strokes; chronic atrial fibrillation; degenerative joint disease; venous insufficiency; squamous cell carcinoma of the face; osteoporosis; and previous small bowel obstruction which was partial and resolved without surgery.

REVIEW OF SYSTEMS:

CARDIOVASCULAR: She has had a cardiac stress test in the past that was negative. She also has atrial fibrillation as stated above that is controlled with Norpace and Lanoxin.

MUSCULOSKELETAL: She has been having pain in her triceps muscle on the left and hammer toe deformities of the right foot and has had steroid injections to her shoulder and prescription shoes for her feet. She has frequent urination due to past surgery.

ENDOCRINE: She does have osteoporosis and her last T-score was −2.5. She does take calcium and Actonel.

PAST SURGICAL HISTORY: She had a Cesarean section, hernia repair, cholecystectomy, complete abdominal hysterectomy, removal of ovarian cancer, and right cataract extraction and lens insertion.

FAMILY HISTORY: Pertinent for cardiac disease.

SOCIAL HISTORY: Active with her church. No alcohol or tobacco abuse.

MEDICATIONS: Lanoxin 0.125 mg alternating with two daily, Norpace 150 mg two p.o. b.i.d., Maxzide 25 every day, Kay Ciel 20 mEq daily, Coumadin 2 mg daily, calcium 500 mg b.i.d., Actonel 35 mg q. every week, Muco-Fen q. six hours p.r.n. for cough.

PHYSICAL EXAMINATION:

VITAL SIGNS: Weight 125, blood pressure 180/83, pulse 68.

GENERAL: Well-developed, well-nourished white female who is in no acute distress.

HEENT: Pupils are equal, round and reactive to light. Extraocular eye movements are intact. Oropharynx is without lesions.

NECK: Supple. Good carotid upstroke without bruit. No lymphadenopathy ot thyroid enlargement. There is no jugular venous distention.

LUNGS: Clear to auscultation and percussion.

HEART: Point of maximal pulse not displaced. Irregularly irregular rhythm. No murmur or gallop.

BREASTS: Without masses.

ABDOMEN: Soft. No organ enlargement, masses or tenderness and bowel sounds are normal.

RECTAL: Deferred

PELVIC: Deferred

Continued

MEDICAL REPORT 10.7 (CONTINUED)

EXTREMITIES: With a trace of edema in the left leg; 3+ in the right leg. The right leg is swollen with erythema, warmth and tenderness and a purpura area on the anterior tibial lower 1/3 of the leg. She has good peripheral pulses. No cyanosis or clubbing.

IMPRESSION:
1. Cellulitis, right lower extremity.
2. Chronic atrial fibrillation.

PLAN OF CARE: Bed rest. Elevation. Rule out deep venous thrombosis with duplex venous scan. IV antibiotics after blood cultures.

DD:

DT:

_____

Dr. Smith

NOTES

Coding for Musculoskeletal System and Connective Tissue Diseases

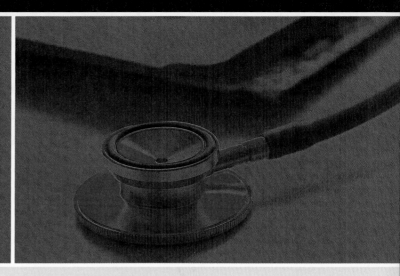

Chapter Outline

Musculoskeletal Disorders
Connective Tissue Diseases
Testing Your Comprehension
Coding Practice I: Chapter Review Exercises
Coding Practice II: Medical Record Case Studies

Chapter Objectives

▶ Describe the pathology of common musculoskeletal and connective tissue diseases.

▶ Recognize the typical manifestations, complications, and treatments of common musculoskeletal and connective tissue diseases in terms of their implications for coding.

▶ Correctly code common musculoskeletal and connective tissue diseases by using the ICD-9-CM and medical reports.

Musculoskeletal and connective tissue diseases are classified in code section 710 to 739 of chapter 13 of the Disease Tabular of the ICD-9-CM, which includes diseases of the bones, muscles, joints, soft tissues, ligaments, tendons, and cartilage. To assist in your understanding, the Word Parts Box on page 296 reviews word parts and meanings of medical terms related to common musculoskeletal and connective tissue diseases.

Word Parts and Meanings of Musculoskeletal and Connective Tissue Terms

Word Part	Meaning	Example	Definition of Example
arthr/o	Joint	arthritis	Inflammation of a joint
oste/o	Bone	osteoarthritis	Inflammation of a bone and joint
my/o	Muscle	fibromyalgia	Pain of fibrous connective tissue and muscle
cost/o	Rib	costochondritis	Inflammation of rib and cartilage
Spondyl/o	vertebra (singular), vertebrae (plural)	spondylosis	An abnormal condition of the vertebrae
myel/o	bone marrow; spinal cord	osteomyelitis; myelogram	Inflammation of bone and bone marrow; radiograph of the spinal cord
fasci/o	fibrous tissue covering and separating muscle	fasciitis	Inflammation of fascia (fibrous tissue surrounding muscle)
chondr/o	cartilage	costochondral	Referring to ribs and cartilage
lamin/o	lamina (part of vertebral bone called *vertebral arch*)	laminectomy	Removal of lamina to relieve compression on spinal cord
-malacia	softening	osteomalacia	Softening of bone
-porosis	porous; containing pores	osteoporosis	Increased porosity of bone (results in a loss of density and weakening of the bone)
-penia	deficiency	osteopenia	Deficiency or decrease in bone density

Musculoskeletal Disorders

Some of the more common musculoskeletal diseases that result in hospital admissions and are coded with ICD-9-CM include arthritic disorders, chronic joint derangements, pathologic bone fractures, osteomyelitis, necrotizing fasciitis, costochondritis, and back and spine disorders.

Arthritic Disorders

Arthritis is inflammation of the joints (Figure 11.1). Some common types of arthritis that give rise to inpatient admissions include osteoarthritis (OA), rheumatoid arthritis, and gouty arthritis. Symptoms associated with these common forms of arthritis include joint pain, swelling, and stiffening.

OSTEOARTHRITIS

OA (715.0–9X), also called **degenerative joint disease**, causes a loss of joint cartilage with a subsequent thickening (hypertrophy) of bones of the affected joint and results in severe joint pain and swelling (Figure 11.2). Joint cartilage, also called articular cartilage, acts as a cushion where two bones come together, or articulate, at a joint structure (union of two bones).

OA can be classified as **primary** (not caused by injury) or **secondary** (caused by injury or another disease process). Primary OA results from stress on joints over time (wear and tear of joints that occurs with age), and it can affect one joint (localized) or many joints (generalized). Primary OA commonly occurs in the knees, hips, lower vertebrae (spine), and finger joints of elderly people. Secondary OA usually results from an injury or trauma to a

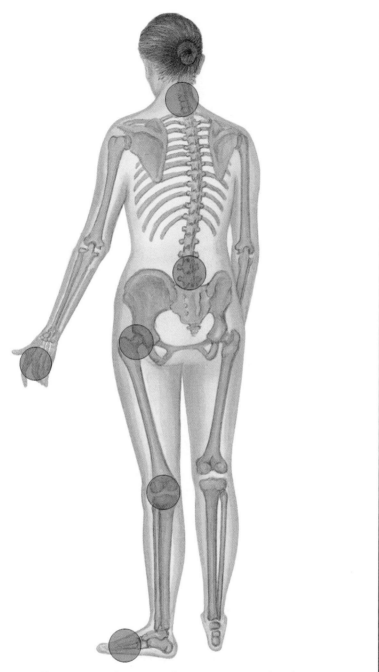

FIGURE 11.1 ■ Joints affected by arthritic conditions. (Reprinted with permission from Anatomical Chart Co.)

joint and is typically localized (i.e., it affects one or few joints). The fourth digit for OA disorders depends on the physician's documentation of the specific type (i.e., primary, secondary, generalized, or localized). However, physician documentation may be nonspecific, and the fourth digit of 9 (OA, not otherwise specified regarding type) is often assigned. It is important for you to recognize that the fifth digit assignment adds detail by specifying the specific joint affected (e.g., hip, knee, or shoulder).

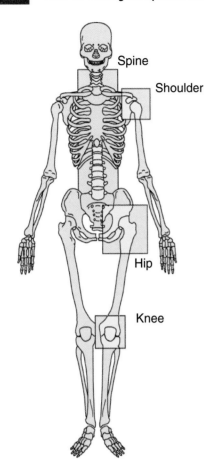

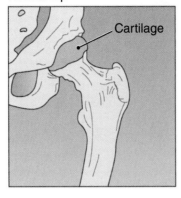

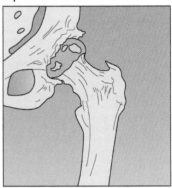

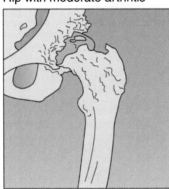

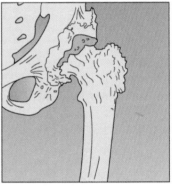

FIGURE 11.2 ■ Osteoarthritis. A. Common sites of osteoarthritis. B. How osteoarthritis affects the hip. (Reprinted with permission from Willis MC. Medical Terminology: A Programmed Learning Approach to the Language of Health Care. Baltimore: Lippincott Williams & Wilkins, 2002.)

EXAMPLE

Osteoarthritis, left hip: 715.95

Osteoarthritis, generalized: 715.00

Secondary osteoarthritis, right knee, attributable to old football tackle sprain injury: 715.26 + 905.7 + E929.3

Primary osteoarthritis of both knees: 715.16

Medical treatments (conservative and nonsurgical) for OA include the use of nonsteroidal anti-inflammatory drugs (NSAIDs), analgesics to reduce associated joint pain (e.g., aspirin), exercise, and physical therapy. However, OA may also require joint-replacement surgery, which necessitates an inpatient admission.

Joint replacement for the hips, knees, and shoulders can be total or partial. These are freely moving synovial "ball and socket" and "hinge" type joints. Freely moving synovial joints have a joint capsule, articular cartilage where bones join together, and a synovial membrane and cavity that contain a lubricating synovial fluid to reduce friction within the joint. Freely moving joints are often affected by increased wear over time, and joint-replacement surgery is often indicated. In total hip replacement surgery (code 81.51), both the femoral head (ball of the long bone in the thigh) and the acetabular cup (the hollow or socket within the pelvis) are replaced. The commonly performed bipolar endoprosthesis (code 81.52; e.g., Austin-Moore hemiarthroplasty) is a partial hip replacement. You should be aware that hip-replacement surgery often involves a significant amount of blood loss that is replaced by transfusion. If the physician documents postoperative blood loss anemia, code it to 285.1 (acute posthemorrhagic anemia). Do not code it as a complication of surgery.

Starting October 1, 2005, new codes were added to provide more detail to hip and knee replacement and revision surgery. For **total hip replacement** (81.51) or **partial hip replacement** surgery (81.52), an additional code 00.74-00.76 can be used to specify the type of bearing surface, if known (e.g.- total hip replacement with bearing surface type, metal on polyethylene = 81.51 + 00.74). Rather than coding **hip revision, not otherwise specified (NOS)** (81.53) and **knee revision, not otherwise specified (NOS)** (81.55) surgery, codes have been added to describe the precise component revised, if known. Codes 00.70-00.73 describe the component of the hip being revised (e.g.- acetabular, femoral, or both), and codes 00.80-00.84 describe the component of the knee being revised (e.g.- femoral, tibial, patellar, or all), which would be used in place of the NOS code. For hip replacements or revisions, an additional code is used to specify the type of bearing surface, if known (00.74-00.76). Also, for both hip and knee revisions, there is an additional code that can be used for the removal of a joint (cement) spacer (84.57).

EXAMPLE

Primary osteoarthritis of hip with Austin-Moore endoprosthesis placement; postoperative (blood loss) anemia: 715.15 + 285.1 + 81.52

Degenerative joint disease of both knees with bilateral total knee replacement: 715.96 + 81.54 + 81.54

Status post hip replacement with recurrent hip dislocation admitted for total hip-replacement revision: 996.42 + 00.70

Osteoarthritis of shoulder with total shoulder replacement: 715.91 + 81.80

Post-traumatic osteoarthritis, left femoral head in 20 y.o. admitted for left femoral head resurfacing: 715.25 + 908.6 + 00.86

There is no single combination code in the ICD-9-CM to express bilateral joint-replacement surgery. Therefore, you must code the joint-replacement procedure twice for bilateral joint replacements (e.g., bilateral knee replacement: 81.54 + 81.54). This can have a profound effect on the reimbursement and case-mix reporting for the hospital (see MS-DRG 470 versus MS-DRG 462 reporting). Remember that MS-DRGs use the ICD-9-CM classification system to describe the type of patients a hospital treats (case mix). MS-DRGs were developed by the Federal government to categorize patients into clinically similar groups that use similar resources. Through MS-DRGs, the federal government can establish prospective payment rates to hospitals for inpatient services on the basis of the patient's diagnosis. Thus, MS-DRGs are an inpatient prospective payment system.

<table>
<tr><td>**EXAMPLE**</td><td>

MS-DRG 470: Major joint and limb reattachment procedures of lower extremity w/o MCC

MDC: 008 Diseases and disorders of the musculoskeletal system and connective tissue

CMS wt.: 2.0144

A/LOS: 3.9

G/LOS: 3.6

Principal diagnosis: 715.96 Osteoarthritis, lower leg

Principal procedure: 81.54 Total knee replacement

Medicare inpatient reimbursement: $8,057.60

MS-DRG 462: Bilateral or multiple major joint procedures of the lower extremity w/o MCC

MDC: 008 Diseases and disorders of the musculoskeletal system and connective tissue

CMS wt.: 3.1564

A/LOS: 4.2

G/LOS: 3.9

Principal diagnosis: 715.96 Osteoarthritis, lower leg

Principal procedure: 81.54 Total knee replacement

Other procedures: 81.54 Total knee replacement

Medicare inpatient reimbursement: $12,625.60

</td></tr>
</table>

RHEUMATOID ARTHRITIS

Rheumatoid arthritis (714.0) is an autoimmune disease in which a person produces abnormal antibodies that attack his or her own normal joint tissues and structures. This produces joint swelling, joint pain, fever, and joint deformity (Figure 11.3). Rheumatoid arthritis is a progressive disease that affects the smaller joints of the hands and feet, as well as larger joints (Figure 11.4). Treatment includes the use of anti-inflammatory drugs such as steroids or NSAIDs,

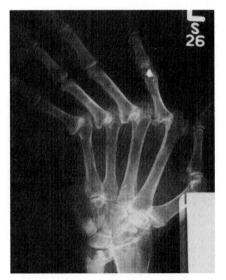

FIGURE 11.3 ■ Rheumatoid arthritis. (Reprinted with permission from Harris JH Jr, Harris, WH, Novelline RA. The Radiology of Emergency Medicine. 3rd ed. Baltimore, MD: Williams & Wilkins; 1993:440.)

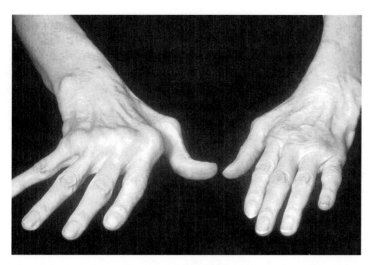

FIGURE 11.4 ■ Ulnar deviation with volar subluxation of the MCP joints of the fingers in an individual with rheumatoid arthritis occurs when swelling destabilizes the joints and the tendons of the fingers migrate and exert a deforming force. (Reprinted from the AHPA Teaching Slide Collection Second Edition now known as the ARHP Assessment and Management of the Rheumatic Diseases: The Teaching Slide Collection for Clinicians and Educators. Copyright 1997. Used by permission of the American College of Rheumatology.)

gold compounds, analgesics to reduce pain, physical therapy, and joint-replacement surgery.

GOUTY ARTHRITIS

Gouty arthritis (274.0) produces excessive uric acid-containing salt crystals that damage the (articular) cartilage of the joint and cause inflammation. Podagra (painful big toe) is a classic symptom associated with gout; however, many joints can be affected. Treatment consists of drugs to reduce hyper-uricemia (excess uric acid in the blood), such as allopurinol or colchicine; NSAIDs; and a diet that restricts consumption of foods high in uric acid (e.g., red meat, cheese, and alcohol).

Chronic versus Traumatic Joint Derangements

Joint derangements coded from chapter 13 of the ICD-9-CM on the musculoskeletal system and connective tissue represent chronic or old injuries and are coded to category 717.0–717.9. You should not confuse chronic (recurrent or old) joint derangements (category 717.0–717.9) with acute traumatic (current or new) joint derangements coded to category 836.0–836.6X (from chapter 17 of the ICD-9-CM on injury and poisoning).

For precise coding of a joint derangement, first determine whether the injury is chronic (recurrent or old) or acute traumatic (current or new). For example, if a person fell while ice-skating 10 years ago and has had problems with knee derangement since then, the injury would be considered chronic or old (codes 717.0–717.9). However, if a person was playing football today and received a sudden, traumatic derangement injury to the knee, the injury would be considered acute and current (codes 836.0–836.6X).

TIP To avoid mistakenly coding an old derangement of the knee to a current injury, remember that current injury codes are easy to recognize (i.e. have an 800–999 appearance). Double-check for coding accuracy on the basis of the history of the present illness in the patient's history and physical report to distinguish chronic old injuries from current traumatic injuries.

EXAMPLE

Chronic anterior cruciate ligament tear/derangement, right knee, from old twisting injury while playing soccer in high school: 717.83 + 905.7 + E929.8

Acute anterior cruciate ligament tear/derangement, right knee, from twisting injury while playing soccer earlier this afternoon: 844.2 + E927

Pathologic Versus Traumatic Bone Fractures

There are critical differences between pathologic fractures and traumatic fractures of bone. Pathologic (spontaneous) fractures are classified in the musculoskeletal and connective tissue chapter of ICD-9-CM (section 710 to 739), and traumatic fractures are classified in the injury and poisoning chapter of ICD-9-CM (section 800 to 999). Unlike traumatic fractures, which are caused by an external injury, pathologic fractures occur spontaneously in bones that are weakened by diseases such as osteoporosis, osteomalacia, osteopenia, aseptic necrosis, and bone cancer. In other words, pathologic fractures are secondary to a diseased or weakened bone and are not attributable to an external injury or trauma. Common sites for pathologic fractures are the vertebrae (back bones and spinal column) and hip (i.e., femoral head or neck).

A leading cause of pathologic fractures is osteoporosis (733.0X), which causes bones to become porous, lose density (mass), and become weak. Pathologic fractures of the spine (733.1X) are common causes of inpatient admissions in elderly women. These fractures tend to occur in the lumbar (weight-bearing) region of the spine as a result of postmenopausal osteoporosis (733.01). Postmenopausal osteoporosis occurs when a loss of estrogen weakens bones, especially of the spine. This condition can lead to pathologic vertebral compression fractures, sometimes referred to as **spontaneous fractures.**

If a patient admission is the result of a pathologic fracture attributable to osteoporosis, assign the pathologic fracture code as the principal diagnosis, because that was the chief reason for admission; sequence the osteoporosis code as a secondary diagnosis. Coders can mistakenly code pathologic fractures to traumatic fractures when the physician has not provided sufficient documentation of osteoporosis.

Spontaneous pathologic fractures are often associated with a fall; this could mistakenly lead you to believe that it is a traumatic fracture. However, if the patient's history indicates weakened bones attributable to osteoporosis or another weakened bone state and if the fall or injury is minor or does not seem significant enough to cause a healthy bone to fracture, query the physician to determine whether the fracture was attributable to trauma or pathologic disease. As a final check, review your final code selection to ensure that what was intended to be reported as a pathologic fracture (code 733.1X) has not been mistakenly coded as a traumatic fracture (codes 800–829).

> *An elderly woman slipped from wheelchair to floor with minor trauma. However, the patient did sustain a femoral neck fracture. The patient has a history of severe osteoporosis, and the physician has classified the fracture as pathologic: 733.14 + 733.00.*
>
> *An elderly woman slipped on ice on the front porch and fell down three stairs, landing hard on her right hip. The fall resulted in right femoral neck fracture: 820.8 + E880.9.*

EXAMPLE

Stress Fractures

Overuse or repetitive jarring of the bone causes stress fractures. In contrast to acute traumatic injuries, stress fractures are the result of unaccustomed strenuous activity such as running or marching long distances. Stress fractures can also be caused by increasing the intensity of an activity too quickly, or from increased physical stress on an unfamiliar surface or when using improper equipment; and therefore, are coded to 733.93–733.98 within Chapter 11: Coding for Musculoskeletal and Connective Tissue Diseases rather than the Injury Chapter (800–899).

Osteomyelitis

Osteomyelitis (730.XX) is bone and bone marrow inflammation caused by a bacterial infection. It commonly occurs in the extremities (legs and arms) and is caused by bacteria that enter through an open wound or fracture. If the responsible bacterial organism is known, assign an additional code. Treatments include the administration of intravenous antibiotics, incision and drainage of any abscess, excisional debridement of the bone and surrounding tissues, and, in some cases, amputation of the affected limb.

> *Osteomyelitis, right great toe, with skin ulcer. The patient underwent debridement of the ulcers down to and including the bone: 730.27 + 707.15 + 77.69 (code debridement to the deepest layer of the same site only).*

EXAMPLE

Necrotizing Fasciitis

Necrotizing fasciitis (728.86) is a severe infection of the fascia (fibrous membrane that surrounds muscle) and subcutaneous tissues. When coding necrotizing fasciitis, assign additional codes to convey the presence of gangrene (785.4) or any responsible bacterial organism (see category 041).

> *Necrotizing fasciitis, right thigh, with gangrene. Culture grew staphylococci: 728.86 + 785.4 + 041.10.*

EXAMPLE

Costochondritis

Costochondritis (733.6) is an inflammation of the costochondral junction between the sternum (breastbone) and the ribs that can sometimes result from an injury or strain to the chest muscles. The etiology can also be unknown. Symptoms include a sharp anterior wall chest pain that can sometimes be similarly described in patients with coronary artery disease. This confusion of the symptoms of costochondritis with those of heart disease can sometimes result in patient admission. However, diagnostic studies such as chest radiograph, electrocardiogram, and blood chemistry (e.g., troponin and creatine kinase-myocardial band are laboratory tests that can identify myocardial damage) typically rule out the possibility of serious cardiac disorders in these cases. Costochondritis is a self-limiting condition. Medical treatment includes NSAIDs, and the pain usually resolves within a short time.

Back and Spine Disorders

Back pain not otherwise specified is coded to 724.5, and low back pain is coded to 724.2. These conditions, although nonspecific, can cause severe pain, which can sometimes result in an inpatient admission and be sequenced as the principal diagnosis. However, after study, a more definitive diagnosis is usually listed as the principal diagnosis (e.g., low back pain attributable to a slipped lumbar disk: 722.10). More often, back pain not otherwise specified or low back pain may not be the principal reason a person was admitted to the hospital but is sequenced as a secondary diagnosis if its occurrence affects a patient's course of care.

Figure 11.5 illustrates the vertebral column. Some spinal (vertebral) disorders commonly result in inpatient admissions for treatment, such as for displacement of an intervertebral disk—also referred to as a **herniated disk**, **slipped disk**, **ruptured disk**, or **herniated nucleus pulposus** (Figure 11.6). Between the bones of the spine (vertebrae) are disks of cartilage that cushion the vertebrae. These intervertebral disks consist of an outer annulus and inner nucleus pulposus. Sometimes degenerative changes or physical stress can cause these cartilaginous disks to slip (i.e., the nucleus ruptures or herniates), which can then put pressure on the root nerves of the spinal cord. This pressure can result in symptoms including severe back pain, causalgia (burning pain usually associated with damage to the nerves), sciatica (pain traveling down a leg), and radiculitis (pain from inflammation of the spinal nerve roots).

Disk herniation often leads to a hospital admission for definitive (corrective) surgical intervention. This may include a (decompression) laminectomy (03.09) in which a portion of a vertebral bone (the vertebral arch) is removed to relieve compression on the nerves of the spinal cord. If a laminectomy is performed with diskectomy (removal of the intervertebral disk), the laminectomy is considered an operative approach, and you code only the diskectomy (80.51). This may be followed by a spinal fusion procedure (81.0X), in which adjacent vertebrae may be surgically immobilized (fused) together. If a spinal fusion occurs, an additional code is assigned to indicate the number of vertebrae fused (e.g., fusion of two to three vertebrae: 81.62).

Other less invasive procedures to surgically repair a herniated disk include a percutaneous diskectomy (80.59), which removes the disk by aspirating it through a tube inserted through the skin, and chemonucleolysis (80.52), in which a surgeon injects an enzyme that dissolves the herniated portion of the intervertebral disk.

EXAMPLE

Diagnosis: Sciatica attributable to herniated L2-3 lumbar disk

Procedures: Laminectomy with L2-3 diskectomy and spinal fusion; posterior technique with iliac crest bone graft: 722.10 + 80.51 + 81.08 + 77.79 + 81.62

Another common back and spine disorder is spondylosis (degenerative joint disease of the spine), which is the result of a degeneration of the intervertebral disks of the spine. Spondylosis, as well as herniation of intervertebral disks of the cervical, thoracic, or lumbar spine, can occur with or without

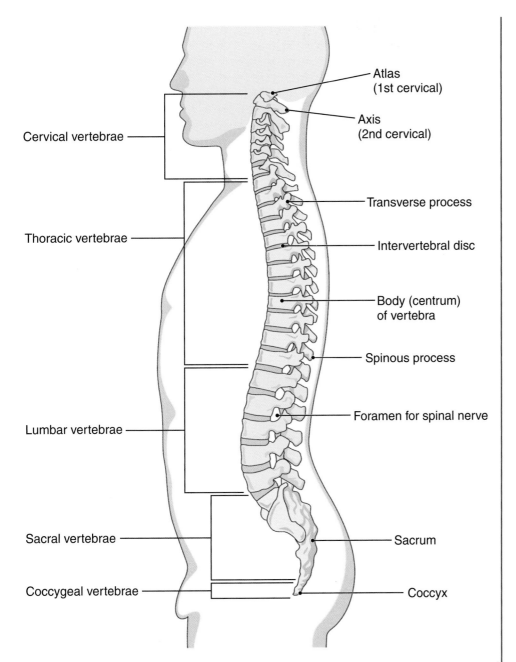

Atlas
(1st cervical)

Axis
(2nd cervical)

Cervical vertebrae

Transverse process

Thoracic vertebrae

Intervertebral disc

Body (centrum)
of vertebra

Spinous process

Foramen for spinal nerve

Lumbar vertebrae

Sacral vertebrae

Sacrum

Coccygeal vertebrae

Coccyx

FIGURE 11.5 ■ Vertebral column from the side. (Reprinted with permission from Cohen BJ and Wood DL. Memmler's The Human Body in Health and Disease, 9th Ed. Philadelphia: Lippincott Williams & Wilkins, 2000.)

myelopathy. Documentation of "myelopathy" by the physician, which describes a functional impairment of the spinal cord, changes the fourth-digit subcategory for these conditions.

Other common back and spine disorders include kyphosis, scoliosis, and lordosis (Figure 11.7). *Kyphosis* results in a "humpback," and this condition is often caused by a weakening of the vertebral bones due to osteoporosis (also called osteopenia). Kyphosis causes reduced height that can lead to excessive pressure on the spinal cord, peripheral nerves, and internal organs (viscera). Another spinal condition, *scoliosis*, causes a lateral curvature of the spine (i.e., the spine bends abnormally to the side), and it occurs more frequently in

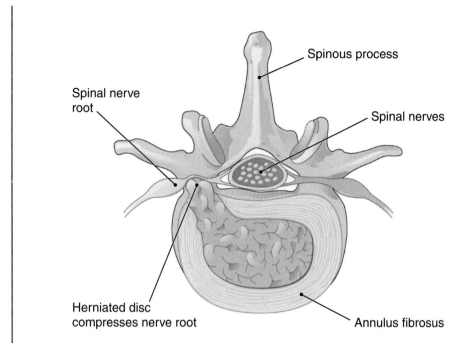

FIGURE 11.6 ■ Herniated Disk. (Reprinted with permission from Cohen BJ. Medical Terminology: An Illustrated Guide, 4th Ed. Baltimore: Lippincott Williams & Wilkins, 2004.)

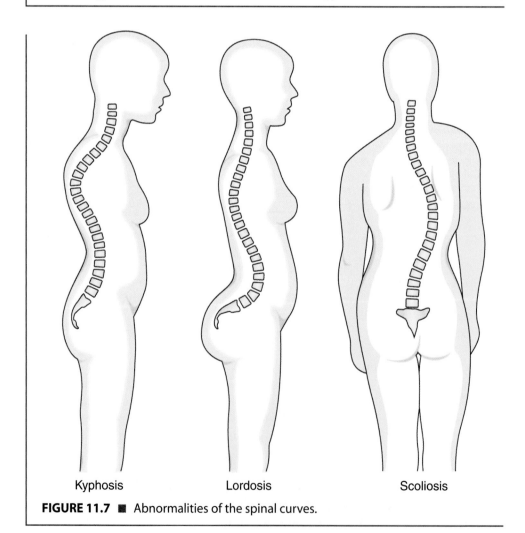

Kyphosis   Lordosis   Scoliosis

FIGURE 11.7 ■ Abnormalities of the spinal curves.

adolescent girls. Lastly, *lordosis* (swayback) results in an exaggerated anterior curvature of the lumbar (lower) spine, which causes the person to lean heavily backwards, in what appears to be, a "lordly" fashion. Depending on the circumstances of the admission, these spinal conditions can be assigned as the principal or secondary diagnosis; however, they are more commonly assigned as secondary diagnoses when their occurrence affects the overall care of the patient (e.g., affects the ability to ambulate).

Connective Tissue Diseases

The most common connective tissue diseases that result in hospital admissions and are coded with ICD-9-CM include systemic lupus erythematosus and systemic scleroderma.

Systemic Lupus Erythematosus

Systemic lupus erythematosus (710.0) is a crippling disease that can affect the joint structures in the musculoskeletal system and many other organs, such as the skin, heart, lungs, and kidneys. It is believed to be an autoimmune disorder in which abnormal antibodies attack normal connective tissue throughout the body.

Symptoms commonly associated with systematic lupus erythematosus include joint pain, fever, and skin rash. Treatment includes steroids to reduce inflammation and resulting tissue damage, immunosuppressive drugs, and physical therapy.

ICD-9-CM uses a mandatory dual-coding mechanism that requires you to assign an additional code to identify any secondary manifestation(s) of the disease.

Chronic nephritis secondary to systematic lupus erythematosus: 710.0 + 582.81 **EXAMPLE**

Systemic Sclerosis

Systemic sclerosis, or scleroderma (710.1), results in the hardening and shrinking of connective tissue which can progress throughout the body. It can affect the skin, heart, lungs, kidneys, and esophagus. The etiology of this disease is unknown. Treatment can include steroids to reduce inflammation, immunosuppressive drugs, and physical therapy. Often, patients with systemic sclerosis have a resultant esophageal disorder (hardening of esophageal tissues) that requires hyperalimentation (tube feeding) or parenteral (intravenous) feeding.

SUMMARY

This chapter has addressed musculoskeletal system and connective tissue diseases. Common conditions affecting the musculoskeletal system and connective tissue have been described. Proper coding of the procedures used to treat these conditions has been presented and discussed, and this has been extended to include the assignment of correct codes from medical reports and records. Also emphasized in this chapter is the application of this new knowledge to assign a correct DRG. Chapter 12 will deal with diseases of the nervous system and sense organs.

TESTING YOUR COMPREHENSION

1. What is another name for osteoarthritis?

_____

2. Which digit specifies the affected joint for osteoarthritis?

_____

3. In extremely severe cases of osteoarthritis, what type of surgical intervention may be required?

_____

4. If a bilateral joint replacement procedure is undertaken, how will that affect the coder's responsibilities?

_____

5. Hip-replacement surgery often is accompanied by a significant amount of blood loss. Should this be coded as a complication of surgery?

_____

6. Identify the common treatment protocols for rheumatoid arthritis.

_____

7. Identify a classic symptom of gout.

_____

8. What is the first step in ensuring proper coding of joint derangement?

_____

9. What is a common cause of a traumatic fracture?

_____

10. What is a common cause of a pathologic (spontaneous) fracture?

_____

11. What are the most common sites for a pathologic fracture?

_____

12. Identify the treatment regimens that may be considered for osteomyelitis.

_____

13. What is the diagnostic term for a severe infection of the fibrous membrane surrounding muscle?

_____

14. Identify a common cause of costochondritis.

_____

15. What is a common result of disk herniation?

_____

16. What are the most common connective tissue diseases that result in hospital admissions?

_____

17. What symptoms are commonly associated with systemic lupus erythematosus?

18. What are the common treatment regimens for systemic sclerosis or scleroderma?

19. What is a diagnosis for a hardening and shrinkage of connective tissue?

CODING PRACTICE I   Chapter Review Exercises

Directions

By using your ICD-9-CM codebook, code the following diagnoses and procedures:

	DIAGNOSIS/PROCEDURES	CODE
1	Osteoarthritis, left hip. Postoperative anemia due to acute blood loss. Bipolar endoprosthesis, femoral head.	
2	Nonunion, fibular fracture. Open reduction, internal fixation, fibular fracture.	
3	Sciatica attributable to herniated L4-5 disk. Decompressive laminectomy, L4-5.	
4	Nontraumatic compression fracture, L4. Spondylosis, lumbar.	
5	Encephalitis secondary to systemic lupus erythematosus.	
6	Necrotizing fasciitis, right thigh. Right thigh fasciectomy.	
7	Degenerative rotator cuff tear. Rotator cuff repair.	
8	Anterior cruciate ligament tear, chronic. Repair anterior cruciate ligament.	
9	Septic arthritis, right shoulder. Intravenous antibiotics.	
10	Chest wall pain secondary to costochondritis.	
11	Aseptic necrosis, right hip. Total hip replacement, right. Bearing surface, metal on polyethylene.	

	DIAGNOSIS/PROCEDURES	CODE
12	Acute osteomyelitis, right great toe, secondary to insulin-dependent (type 1) diabetes mellitus. Amputation, right great toe.	
13	Spinal stenosis, L3-4. L3-4 diskectomy with spinal fusion using an iliac crest donor graft.	
14	Calcinosis cutis, Raynaud phenomenon, sclerodactyly, and telangiectasia syndrome. Esophageal dyskinesia. PEG.	
15	Left knee joint effusion. Arthrocentesis, left knee.	
16	Rheumatoid arthritis with deformity, right thumb. IP joint arthroplasty with prosthetic implant, right thumb.	
17	Bone spur, left calcaneus. Excision, bone spur, left heel.	
18	Lower back pain and radiculitis attributable to herniated lumbar disk with myelopathy. L2-3 laminectomy with diskectomy.	
19	Degenerative disk disease, thoracic spine.	
20	Pathologic fractures, T11 and T12. Postmenopausal osteoporosis.	

CODING PRACTICE II　Medical Record Case Studies

Instructions

1. Carefully review the medical reports provided for each case study.
2. Research any abbreviations and terms that are unfamiliar or unclear.
3. Identify as many diagnoses and procedures as possible.
4. Because only part of the patient's total record is available, determine what additional documentation you might need.
5. If appropriate, identify any questions you might ask the physician to code this case correctly and completely.
6. Complete the appropriate blanks below for each case study.

CHAPTER 11 CASE STUDIES

Case Study 11.1 (Coder/Abstract Summary Form)

Patient: **Jane Doe**

Patient documentation: **Review Medical Reports 11.1, 11.2, and 11.3**

1. Principal diagnosis:

_____

2. Secondary or other diagnoses:

_____

3. Principal procedure:

_____

4. Other procedures:

_____

5. Additional documentation needed:

_____

_____

_____

_____

Case Study 11.1 (Continued)

6. Questions for the physician:

_____

_____

_____

_____

_____

MEDICAL REPORT 11.1

DISCHARGE SUMMARY

PATIENT: Jane Doe

MEDICAL RECORD #:

ATTN PHYSICIAN: Smith, M.D.

FINAL DIAGNOSES:

1. Compression fractures of T11-T12, L1-L2 secondary to osteoporosis.
2. Hypertension.
3. Renal insufficiency, acute.
4. Anemia.
5. Osteoarthritis.
6. Hiatal hernia.
7. Please look at list of problems with history and physical.

CONSULTATIONS: Orthopedic consult.

PROCEDURES: None.

PERTINENT PATIENT ASSESSMENT INFORMATION/ PHYSICAL EXAM: Please see Admission History and Physical.

HOSPITAL COURSE AND LABORATORY DATA: Ms. Doe is an 87-year-old, white female who presented with severe low back pain. The patient was found to have compression fracture. The patient was treated conservatively. There was no neuro deficit. The patient was seen by Orthopedics. The patient was also found to have renal insufficiency. The patient was given Normal Saline, her creatinine was trending down. In the last couple of days of hospitalization, the patient refused lab work which made it difficult to further evaluate her renal function. The patient was discharged to the nursing home.

DISCHARGE CONDITION:

DISPOSITION: ABC Manor.

DIET: Continue current.

ACTIVITIES: As tolerated.

FOLLOW-UP APPOINTMENT: With me in one week.

DISCHARGE MEDICATIONS: Please see list of discharge medications.

FAMILY INVOLVEMENT: Involved.

CONTROL OF CARE: Patient and family. The nursing home was instructed to d/c Celebrex, HCTZ, Toradol because they can be contributing to her renal insufficiency.

WOUND CARE: N/A

PAIN MANAGEMENT: As outlined.

D:

T:

_____

Smith, M.D.

MEDICAL REPORT 11.2

HISTORY AND PHYSICAL

PATIENT: Jane Doe

MEDICAL RECORD #:

ATTN PHYSICIAN: Dr. Smith, M.D.

IDENTIFICATION, CHIEF COMPLAINT AND PRESENT ILLNESS: Ms. Doe is an 87-year-old white female who presented to the Emergency Room with severe low back pain. Patient was seen and evaluated. She was found to have compression fracture of T11, T12, L1, and L2. Patient has history of severe osteoporosis. Patient was also found to have renal insufficiency. Patient was admitted to the hospital for further evaluation.

Patient denies any chest pain, palpitations, pedal edema, orthopnea, PND, dyspnea on exertion, cough, wheezing, pleuritic chest pain, syncope or hemoptysis. Patient denies any nausea, vomiting, abdominal pain, diarrhea, constipation, heartburn or epigastric pain. Patient denies any hematemesis, coffee ground emesis, melena or bright red blood per rectum. Patient has no dysuria, frequency, urgency, hematuria or polyuria. Patient has no diplopia or visual field cuts, facial weakness, facial droop, dysarthria, dysphagia, no focal weakness, altered level of consciousness, neck stiffness, urinary incontinence, or fecal incontinence. Patient has no fever or chills. Patient has no other symptoms or complaints at the present time.

PAST HISTORY:

1. Osteoporosis
2. Osteoarthritis
3. Hiatal Hernia
4. GERD
5. HTN

**** ALLERGIC TO MINIPRESS ****

HOME MEDICATIONS: Please look at list of home medications.

SOCIAL HISTORY: Patient is a widow; denies any tobacco, alcohol or illicit drugs.

FAMILY HISTORY: Positive for HTN.

REVIEW OF SYSTEMS: Otherwise unremarkable.

PHYSICAL EXAMINATION: Well developed white female in no acute distress.

VITAL SIGNS: Afebrile, BP 151/69; Pulse 70; RR 20.

SKIN: No new lesions.

HEENT: Pupils are equal, reactive to direct and consensual light.

NECK: Supple.

LUNGS: Clear to auscultation.

HEART: Regular rhythm; no S3 or murmur.

ABDOMEN: Bowel sounds present; soft; non tender.

KUB: Costovertebral angle tenderness is negative bilaterally.

EXTREMITIES: Pulses are adequate; no edema, clubbing, or cyanosis.

Continued

Medical Report 11.2 (Continued)

NEUROLOGIC: Alert and oriented x3; no apparent focal deficit.

LAB DATA: Reviewed.

ASSESSMENT & PLAN OF TREATMENT:

1. Low back pain secondary to compression fracture of T11, T12, L1, and L2. No neuro deficit at the present time. Will consult Orthopedics. Treatment will be conservative.
2. Renal insufficiency, most likely secondary to prerenal azotemia. Will hold on HCTZ at the present time and re-evaluate.
3. HTN: continue current anti-hypertensive medications.
4. Hiatal hernia.
5. Osteoporosis: continue current treatment.
6. Osteoarthritis: continue Celebrex 200 mgs PO every day.
7. Anemia: anemia work-up will be done as an out-patient.

PROGNOSIS: Guarded.

LEVEL OF CARE NEEDED: Four.

ADVANCE DIRECTIVE: Has not been executed.

D:

T:

_____

Smith, M.D.

NOTES

MEDICAL REPORT 11.3

CONSULTATION

PATIENT: Jane Doe

MEDICAL RECORD #:

ATTN PHYSICIAN: Dr. Smith, M.D.

CONSULTING PHYSICIAN: Dr. Jones, M.D.

DIAGNOSIS:
1. L1 and L2 vertebral body compression fractures, age indeterminate.
2. Question of a sacral fracture, volar surface, minimal angulation, nondisplaced.

HISTORY: The patient is an 87-year-old, white female who previously worked as an instructor. She doesn't look her stated age. She gives a history of having had progressive problems with back pain which has been of recent onset. She has had no antecedent trauma.

PAST MEDICAL HISTORY: This patient had a stroke that has left her with right hemiplegia. She walks with a walker. She is able to ambulate up and down 5 flights of steps at her home.

PHYSICAL EXAMINATION: Shows an alert, oriented, white female who does not appear to be her stated age. Examination of both feet demonstrate that she has deep tendon reflexes in the ankles that were symmetrical and equal. She has normal sensation in her lower extremities. Internal and external rotation of the hips does not cause pain in her back. The patient is resting comfortably in bed.

IMPRESSION/PLAN: I have reviewed the x-rays and the CT reconstructions of her lumbar spine. She has severe degenerative changes with osteopenia, vertebral body compression fractures of L1 and L2, age indeterminate. The patient has a possible fracture of the sacrum on the volar surface of the S2 level. It is angulated, but not displaced.

I would opt for conservative modalities. I will speak with Dr. Smith about fitting this lady with an extension brace or a lumbosacral corset for comfort purposes. I think she should be out of bed and mobilized as quickly as possible. Surgery is not indicated. She is neurologically intact. Her primary problem is that she has osteopenia from old age and has had vertebral body compression fractures.

If I can be of further assistance, please fell free to call me; I will follow the patient with you.

D:

T:

_____

Dr. Jones, M.D.

Case Study 11.2 (Coder/Abstract Summary Form)

Patient: **Anne Brown**

Patient documentation: **Review Medical Report 11.4**

1. Principal diagnosis:

   _____

2. Secondary or other diagnoses:

   _____

3. Principal procedure:

   _____

4. Other procedures:

   _____

5. Additional documentation needed:

   _____

   _____

   _____

6. Questions for the physician:

   _____

   _____

   _____

   _____

   _____

MEDICAL REPORT 11.4

REPORT OF OPERATION

PT NAME: Anne Brown

MED REC NO:

ATTN MD: Smith

DATE OR OPERATION:

SURGEON: SMITH

ANESTHESIOLOGIST:

PRE-OP DIAGNOSIS: Osteoarthritis, right knee, with associated valgus deformity.

POST-OP DIAGNOSIS: Same.

ANESTHESIA: Spinal.

PROCEDURE: Right total knee replacement.

ESTIMATED BLOOD LOSS: Less than 20 cc.

DRAINS: OrthoPak to autotransfusion unit.

COMPLICATIONS: None.

DESCRIPTION OF PROCEDURE: The patient was taken to the operating room, placed in the right lateral decubitus position, left hip up. Spinal anesthetic was initiated. The patient was then placed in the supine position. Right lower extremity was then prepped and draped in the usual sterile fashion. Using a #10 blade, a 16-cm midline incision was made. Using a combination of sharp and blunt dissection technique, the subcutaneous tissue was incised and explored. The medial and lateral full thickness flaps were elevated and reflected in a medial and lateral direction.

A second #10 blade was used to make a medial parapatellar incision, retinaculum incised. The patella was then flipped. The patient was noted to have marked degenerative arthritis, particularly of the lateral compartment of the knee. The patient was noted to have osteophytic spurring. Using the Zimmer step drill, an intermedullary guide hole was drilled. The patient was sized to a size E femoral component. After sizing, the patient intermedually guide was placed and the cutting jig was placed and the femoral cuts were made, according to the Zimmer cutting jig.

The patella recess was then cut and peg holes for the femoral components were drilled. A size E femoral component was then tried and this was found to be acceptable. Having completed the cutting of the femoral component, the medial and lateral compartments were debrided of residual meniscal tissue. A standard step drill was then used to drill the intermedullary hole for the femur. 10 mm of proximal tibial surface was resected using the medial compartment as a reference. The patient was then sized to a #5 tray. The thinned guides were drilled and the patient was tried. It was found that the patient would accept a 10-mm insert. The patient was stable in all planes of motion.

The patient was demonstrated at this point to be ready to perform a lateral retinacular release. The patient's patella was resected of a mm of bone and the 35-mm patella resection component was tried. A lateral retinacular release was completed and the patient's patella was noted to track well. The patient's wound was irrigated copiously with normal saline. The tibial component and patellar components were cemented. The femoral component was press-fit. The patient's knee was reduced. The medial retinacular incision was repaired using interrupted sutures of #1 Ethibond. Subcutaneous tissue was approximated with staples. A large-bore drain was placed in the substance of the wound prior to wound closure. The drain was connected to the OrthoPak autotransfusion unit. The patient was dressed and she was transferred to the recovery room in stable and satisfactory condition.

D:

T:

_____

Dr. Smith

Case Study 11.3 (Coder/Abstract Summary Form)

Patient: **Mike Thompson**

Patient documentation: **Review Medical Reports 11.5 and 11.6**

1. Principal diagnosis:

   _____

2. Secondary or other diagnoses:

   _____

3. Principal procedure:

   _____

4. Other procedures:

   _____

5. Additional documentation needed:

   _____

   _____

   _____

   _____

6. Questions for the physician:

   _____

   _____

   _____

   _____

   _____

MEDICAL REPORT 11.5

DISCHARGE SUMMARY

PATIENT: Mike Thompson

MEDICAL RECORD #:

ATTN PHYSICIAN: Smith, M.D.

FINAL DIAGNOSES:

1. Rheumatoid arthritis flare and exacerbation.
2. Delirium, probably secondary to corticosteroids.
3. Dementia, senile.

HOSPITAL: The patient was discharged to SNU. The patient was admitted for IV fluids at 75 an hour. Sed. Rate, CH50, C3 and C4 obtained. Bone scan to rule out occult fracture was ordered. The patient was typed and screened two units of packed cells. CBC, iron and retic and Ferritin ordered. This was for anemia of chronic disease. The patient was started on IV Rocephin for possible CNS infection also given his febrile illness. Regular diet was initiated. The history and physical dictated. The patient ambulated. Rocephin was decreased to 1 gram q 24 hours. Percocet was given 1 to 2 tabs q. 4 hours p.r.n. pain. OxyContin initiated 10 mgs twice daily. The patient had a serum H. pylori level and the results are pending at this time. This was to evaluate abdominal pain. The delirium persisted. This was thought to be due to corticoid steroids. This was being given for the patient's rheumatoid arthritis flare. He was given Haldol IV and Ativan IV. The Haldol was given routinely b.i.d. Posey vest was ordered temporarily to protect the patient from injury or pulling out the IVs. IV SoluMedrol was changed to p.o. 30 mgs daily. Zyprexa ordered, 5 mgs daily. Prednisone was ordered, 30 mgs daily. IV corticosteroids initiated. Ativan was given q. 8 hours, p.r.n. p.o. Valium was given IV x1. Haldol, as well. The patient was given influenza pneumococcal vaccine. Zyprexa was increased to 10 mgs daily. Prednisone was increased to 20 mgs daily. Plaquenil was ordered 20 mgs b.i.d. The patient's Zyprexa was increased to 10 mgs q.h.s. Given that the family is unable to care for him for his current debilitated condition, he was placed in a skilled care facility. Medications were given to resolve his dementia that will probably persist.

DISCHARGED LABS: Serum iron of 13, TIBC 228, Saturation of 6 percent. Creatinine .8, BUN 15 and Sodium 140. Potassium 4.3, Chloride and Bicarb of 30, Calcium 8.3 and Albumin 2.8. Sed rate of 94. White count 20,000 and hemoglobin 9 and hematocrit of 28, platelet count 324. Cultures negative.

The patient will be seen by me on a monthly or p.r.n. basis.

D:

T:

_____

Smith, M.D.

MEDICAL REPORT 11.6

HISTORY AND PHYSICAL

PATIENT: Mike Thompson

MEDICAL RECORD #:

ATTN PHYSICIAN: Smith, M.D.

HISTORY OF PRESENT ILLNESS: This is an elderly 76-year-old male with a chief complaint of malaise, weakness, and lethargy.

PAST MEDICAL HISTORY: Significant for rheumatoid arthritis, hypertension, esophagitis, pneumonia recently released from the hospital.

SOCIAL HISTORY: Recently widowed. No history of tobacco abuse. Several adult children.

REVIEW OF SYSTEMS: Negative for headaches. Positive for malaise. Negative for diplopia. Negative for nosebleed. Negative for tinnitus. Negative for dysphagia. Negative for abdominal pain. Negative for shortness of breath. Negative for chest pain or palpitation. Negative for intermittent claudication. Negative for bowel or bladder incontinence. Negative for thalassemias, hepatitis. Negative for hemolytic anemia.

MEDICATIONS: Prednisone 10 mg a day. Elavil 25 mg q.h.s. Percocet for pain p.r.n.

PHYSICAL: An elderly, frail, male who is lying in bed alert and oriented at the time of my examination.

HEENT: Normocephalic. Atraumatic. Pupils equal, round, and reactive to light. Dentition fair. Cushingoid face due to corticosteroids for which the patient is on long term.

NECK: Supple. Carotid upstroke brisk. No carotid bruits.

EXTREMITIES: DTRs equivocal.

Neuromuscular and neurosensory examination intact.

Skeletal exam revealed bony enlargement, ulna deviation, atrophic musculature, limited range of motion of neck all due to rheumatoid arthritis.

IMPRESSION AND PLAN: Malaise, weakness, lethargy, poor p.o. intake.

Will admit. Rule out dehydration. Continue corticosteroids for rheumatoid arthritis. Check sed rate. Check inflammation flare of rheumatoid arthritis.

D:

T:

_____

Smith, M.D.

Case Study 11.4 (Coder/Abstract Summary Form)

Patient: **Susan Jones**

Patient documentation: **Review Medical Reports 11.7, 11.8, and 11.9**

1. Principal diagnosis:

   _____

2. Secondary or other diagnoses:

   _____

3. Principal procedure:

   _____

4. Other procedures:

   _____

5. Additional documentation needed:

   _____

   _____

   _____

   _____

6. Questions for the physician:

   _____

   _____

   _____

   _____

DISCHARGE SUMMARY

PT NAME: Susan Jones

MED REC NO:

ATTN PHYSICIAN: Smith, M.D.

DATE OF ADMISSION:

DATE OF DISCHARGE:

DIAGNOSIS: Aseptic necrosis of the left hip.

Ms. Jones underwent a total hip replacement. Postoperatively, she had exceptional bleeding with acute blood loss postop anemia. It was discovered that she had taken an aspirin-containing medication preoperatively under the false impression that she was not taking aspirin. It was a brand name that she misunderstood. At any rate, after blood replacement and careful monitoring, she recovered nicely and then went on to have an uneventful recovery with ambulation. On discharge, she was sent home with a walker, instructed to see me in one week. She was given a commode seat and abduction pillow, regular diet. She was placed on no pain medication or aspirin. The wound was healing nicely. She had no other medical problems or complications. She was in good health postoperatively and no problems were noted at the time of discharge.

D:

T:

_____

Smith, M.D.

NOTES

MEDICAL REPORT 11.8

HISTORY AND PHYSICAL

PT NAME: Susan Jones

MED REC NO:

ATTN PHYSICIAN: Smith, M.D.

DATE OF ADMISSION:

This 72-year-old female is admitted for total left hip replacement. She has severe rheumatoid arthritis. She injured her hips in an automobile accident two years ago and the left hip has been progressively getting more painful. She has no known cardiopulmonary history or history of hypertension. Her only medication is Feldene.

Physical examination shows blood pressure 150/80, pulse 72 and regular, afebrile. Skin is without lesions. HEENT examination shows head without signs of trauma. Neck is supple. No pharyngeal lesions. No thyromegaly. Pupils equal and reactive to light and accommodation. Full extra-ocular movements. No scleral icterus. Chest is clear bilaterally. Breasts are without masses. Cardiac examination shows normal S1 and S2 without S3 or S4. Grade 1/6 early systolic murmur at the apex is noted bilaterally. No carotid bruits. Abdomen is soft and nontender without masses or organomegaly. Pelvic and rectal examinations deferred. Musculoskeletal examination shows deforming arthritic changes both hands, chronic arthritic mild changes in both knees, decreased range of motion of hip secondary to pain without pedal edema. Neurologically, the patient is alert and oriented x3 without focal deficits.

Electrocardiogram shows normal sinus rhythm without acute changes.

ASSESSMENT: Basically healthy 72-year-old female with the exception of severe rheumatoid arthritis, rule out aseptic necrosis, left hip.

PLAN OF CARE: Admit for total hip replacement on left.

D:

T:

_____

Smith, M.D.

NOTES

OPERATIVE REPORT

PT NAME: Susan Jones

MED REC NO:

PREOPERATIVE DIAGNOSIS: Avascular necrosis of the left hip.

POSTOPERATIVE DIAGNOSIS: Same

OPERATION: Total hip replacement.

SURGEON: Smith, M.D.

ASSISTANT:

ANESTHESIA:

PROCEDURE: Ms. Jones was placed on her side; left hip was prepped and draped in the usual fashion. A paralateral incision was made cutting the tensor fascia lata. External rotators were defined and detached. The capsule was excised. She had a fulminating synovitis which bled. All this was excised. Then I went anteriorly and incised the inferior capsule. The hip was dislocated. The head was quite distorted as one would expect from the advanced necrosis. The head and neck were amputated at its base. The acetabulum was reamed with a truncated reamer down to 50 mm. We then made our appropriate slot and drove the 50 mm porous coated cup. It went in solidly. Next, we went to the femoral shaft, reamed out a canal. She bled profusely from the canal. Used a standard head. The hip was quite stable in all directions.

The wound was closed in layers over a Hemovac drain. Blood loss was about 800 ccs.

She left the operating room in excellent condition with an abduction pillow.

D:

T:

_____

Smith, M.D.

NOTES

Case Study 11.5 (Coder/Abstract Summary Form)

Patient: **Joe Brown**

Patient documentation: **Review Medical Report 11.10**

1. Principal diagnosis:

2. Secondary or other diagnoses:

3. Principal procedure:

4. Other procedures:

5. Additional documentation needed:

6. Questions for the physician:

MEDICAL REPORT 11.10

DISCHARGE SUMMARY

PT NAME: Joe Brown

MED REC NO:

ATTN PHYSICIAN: Smith, M.D.

DATE OF ADMISSION:

CHIEF COMPLAINT: Weakness and atrophy, right leg.

HISTORY: This is a 40-year-old male with a six-week history of progressive weakness and atrophy in the right leg. A CT scan of the lumbosacral spine recently performed demonstrated a disk herniation probably at two levels and some anatomical abnormality of the spine itself. Nerve conduction studies showed multiple level involvement from L3 to L5. The patient was admitted and neurosurgical consultation was requested. His past history showed that the patient had been markedly overweight and hypertensive and had lost about 150 lbs. three years ago. Since that time, he has been in relatively good health until now. Neurological history showed that the patient in the last two weeks had been experiencing increasing amounts of pain in his right leg and back that radiated to the groin. There was no obvious history of numbness. No sphincter disturbance.

PHYSICAL EXAMINATION: He was alert and oriented. His general physical exam was normal with a blood pressure of 120/70. He had flabby abdominal skin from weight loss. On neurological exam of the lower extremities, he had selective weakness of his quadriceps muscle with quite a bit of palpable atrophy. He also had some weakness of the abductors. Distally, he was strong. Sensory exam showed no abnormalities. His right knee jerk, surprisingly, showed no significant abnormalities. There was a spondylolysis present on the CT scan. The patient was admitted. Myelography was recommended.

LABORATORY: White count 5600, hemoglobin 15.2, hematocrit normal. Platelet count was 251,000. CSF neg, Urogram was negative. BUN was 11, creatinine .9. SMA-12 profile showed no abnormalities. X-ray examination of the chest was normal. Lumbar myelogram showed a large ruptured disk at the L3-4 level causing almost a complete block. Central bulging at L4-5 level was found as well as a CT scan verified these findings seen on the myelogram. Flexion/extension films were obtained during myelography but no slippage or instability could be diagnosed. The CT scan at the L3-4 level showed no evidence of dye in the subarachnoid space.

HOSPITAL COURSE: The patient was counseled regarding surgery. The pros, cons of surgery and alternatives were discussed with him. In spite of the fact that his pain pattern was quite atypical, it was felt that the patient could benefit from being operated on to relieve neurological symptoms. He was taken to the Operating Room and lumbar laminectomy at L3-4 level was done with bilateral diskectomy with laser. A large amount of disk material was removed. The L4-5 level was explored but no herniation was found. The patient did extremely well postoperatively and his pain subsided. He was ambulating well. He was requesting to go home on the second postoperative day. On the third postoperative day he was discharged. He will be seen in my office for suture removal in one week. He was advised to get plenty of rest and not wet the incision.

FINAL DIAGNOSIS:
1. Ruptured L3-4 disk.
2. Hypertension.

D:

T:

_____

Smith, M.D.

Coding for Diseases of the Nervous System and Sense Organs

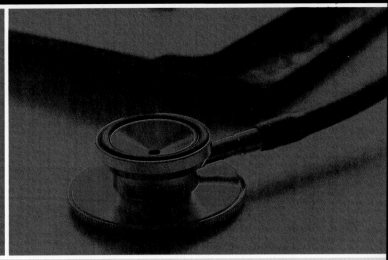

Chapter Outline

Chapter Objectives

▶ Describe the pathology of common disorders of the nervous system and sense organs.

▶ Recognize the typical manifestations, complications, and treatments of common disorders of the nervous system and sense organs in terms of their implications for coding.

▶ Correctly code disorders and procedures related to the nervous system and sense organs by using the ICD-9-CM and medical records.

Diseases of the nervous system and sense organs are classified in code section 320 to 389 of chapter 6 of the Disease Tabular of ICD-9-CM. This chapter is subdivided into disorders of the central nervous system (CNS), disorders of the peripheral nervous system (PNS), and disorders of the sensory organs (eyes and ears). To assist in your understanding, see Figure 12.1, an illustration of the anatomic divisions of the nervous system, and the Word Parts Box on page 331, which lists word parts and meanings of medical terms related to the nervous system and sense organs.

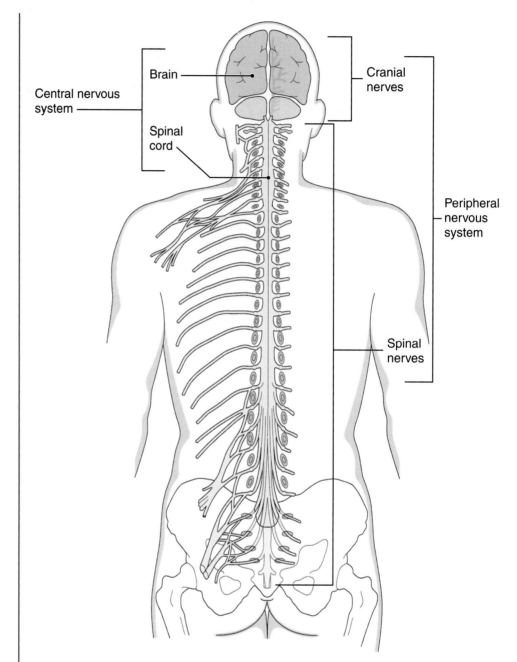

FIGURE 12.1 ■ Anatomic divisions of the nervous system. (Reprinted with permission from Cohen BJ. Medical Terminology: An Illustrated Guide, 4th Ed. Baltimore: Lippincott Williams & Wilkins, 2004.)

Word Parts and Meanings of the Nervous System and Sense Organs

Word Part	Meaning	Example	Definition of Example
menin/o- meningi/o-	meninges; Membranes	Meningitis	Inflammation of the meninges
neur/o-	nerves	neuropathy	Disease condition of nerves
-lepsy	seizure	Epilepsy	A chronic seizure disorder
-paresis -plegia	paralysis	hemiparesis; hemiplegia	Paralyzed on one side (half) of the body
encephal/o-	brain	encephalitis	Inflammation of the brain
-sclerosis	hardening	multiple sclerosis	Disease that results in hardening (plaquing) of the myelin sheath that covers nerves of the central nervous system
oto-	ear	otosclerosis	Hardening of small bones in the ear, causing conduction deafness
hemi-	half	hemianopsia	Loss of vision in half of the visual field
retin/o-	retina	Retinitis	Inflammation of the retina (nerve tissue) of the eye
-opia	vision	myopia; hyperopia	Near-sightedness; far-sightedness
glauc/o-	gray	Glaucoma	Clouding or "graying" of the lens of the eye
myring/o- tympan/o-	eardrum	myringotomy; tympanoplasty	Incision into the eardrum; surgical repair of the eardrum
presby/o-	old age	Presbyopia	Poor vision attributable to old age
-plasty	surgical repair	neuroplasty	Surgical repair of a nerve
-pathy	disease	encephalopathy; polyneuropathy	Disease of the brain; disease of many nerves

Disorders of the Central Nervous System (CNS)

Category code range 320 to 349 includes diseases of the CNS, which is composed of the brain and spinal cord. Common CNS diseases that can cause hospital admissions include inflammatory disorders, degenerative disorders, and other disorders such as demyelinating and paralytic disorders.

Inflammatory Disorders

Meningitis and encephalitis are common inflammatory disorders of the CNS.

MENINGITIS

The meninges are three membranes (dura, arachnoid, and pia) that surround and protect the CNS. Meningitis (category code range 320 to 322) is an inflammation of the meninges that can be caused by bacteria (e.g., streptococci and staphylococci), viruses (e.g., Enterovirus and herpes simplex), or fungi (e.g., candidiasis and histoplasmosis). Meningitis can be classified with a single combination code from chapter 1 of the Disease Tabular of the ICD-9-CM codebook, "Infectious and Parasitic Diseases" (category 001 to 139), or with a single combination code from chapter 6, "Diseases of the Nervous System and Sense Organs" (category 320 to 389). Alternatively, meningitis can be described with dual coding from chapters 1 and 6.

EXAMPLE	*Adenoviral meningitis: 049.1 (single combination code from chapter 1)*
	Escherichia coli meningitis: 320.82 (single combination code from chapter 6)
	Meningitis attributable to Lyme disease: 088.81 + 320.7 (dual coding from chapters 1 and 6)

Symptoms commonly associated with meningitis are stiff neck, headache, fever, and hypersensitivity to light (photophobia). Antibiotics are used to treat the bacterial forms of meningitis, antifungal drugs are used to treat fungal forms, and viral forms are treated symptomatically. Antibiotics are not effective for treating viral forms of the disease.

To confirm a diagnosis of meningitis, a procedure called a **lumbar puncture**, also called a **spinal tap**, is routinely performed to withdraw cerebrospinal fluid (CSF) for laboratory analysis. CSF is a normally clear liquid that contains water, glucose (sugar), protein, sodium (salt), and chloride and that circulates in the CNS. CSF helps to cushion and protect the brain and spinal cord. A laboratory analysis of CSF can include a culture, cytologic (cell) examination, and cell counts to determine whether any abnormalities are present (e.g., bacterial growth, cancer cells, other abnormal substances, or cell concentrations). A lumbar puncture is often indicated for infants who present to the emergency department crying or lethargic and with a fever, apparent stiff neck, and rigidity. In a lumbar puncture, the physician inserts a needle between two lower lumbar vertebrae just beyond the distant end of the spinal cord to withdraw CSF without incurring damage to the spinal cord itself.

A lumbar puncture is an important test for diagnosing meningitis and other diseases. Normal CSF is clear. If the CSF is turbid (cloudy), it may indicate bacterial growth; if the fluid contains blood, it may indicate a hemorrhagic stroke or brain injury. Cytologic analysis may reveal cancer cells in cases of CNS malignancy.

EXAMPLE	*Meningitis attributable to group B streptococcus, lumbar puncture (spinal tap) with CSF culture positive for group B streptococcus: 320.2; 03.31*
	Cryptococcal meningitis, lumbar puncture with CSF culture positive for cryptococci: 117.5 + 321.0; 03.31

ENCEPHALITIS

Encephalitis (category code 323) is an inflammation of the brain that is often caused by a virus (e.g., herpes simplex, measles, influenza, or arboviruses carried by mosquitoes and ticks). Other types of encephalitis can result from protozoal diseases (e.g., malaria) or the toxic effects of chemicals or metals (e.g., lead or mercury).

Dual coding is often required. The underlying disease is expressed first, and the manifestation of encephalitis is sequenced as an additional code.

EXAMPLE	*Encephalitis attributable to cat-scratch disease: 078.3 + 323.0*
	Encephalitis attributable to infectious mononucleosis: 075 + 323.0
	Postinfectious mononucleosis: 136.9 + 323.6

Symptoms of encephalitis can include headache and stiff neck, fever, sensitivity to light, seizures, lethargy, and confusion. Young children and people who are immunocompromised, such as the elderly or those with acquired immunodeficiency syndrome (AIDS), are at a higher risk for contracting encephalitis from an infection. Most people recover within a few weeks, but encephalitis is a serious disease that can, in some cases, be fatal.

Important tests to diagnose encephalitis include a spinal tap to obtain CSF or a blood culture that may reveal the virus. Some forms of viral encephalitis respond to antiviral drugs. However, other forms may be treated only symptomatically. Analgesics (e.g., aspirin) can be used to reduce fever, and antiseizure medications (e.g., phenobarbital or phenytoin) can be used if needed.

Degenerative Diseases

Common degenerative diseases of the CNS include Parkinson's disease, Alzheimer's disease, and amyotrophic lateral sclerosis (ALS; also known as Lou Gehrig's disease).

PARKINSON'S DISEASE

Parkinson's disease (code 332.0) usually occurs in the elderly and results in progressive degeneration of the nerves in the brain. It can result in hand tremors, a shuffling gait (sometimes referred to as **cogwheel rigidity**), and muscle weakness. Parkinson's disease is caused by a deficiency of dopamine, a chemical (i.e., neurotransmitter) that is required to transmit nerve impulses in the brain. The symptoms of Parkinson's disease can be alleviated with drugs such as levodopa or dopamine agonists (drugs that increase the reception of dopamine in the brain); however, such drugs do not cure the disease. Secondary parkinsonism (code 332.1) is a form of Parkinson's disease that is secondary to another underlying disease (e.g., Huntington's disease or syphilis) or that occurs as an adverse effect of the therapeutic use of a drug (e.g., antipsychotic drugs). In the case of an adverse effect, you should use an additional E code from the Table of Drugs and Chemicals to identify the responsible drug.

Primary parkinsonism: 332.0

Parkinson's disease secondary to haloperidol (Haldol) prescribed for chronic schizophrenia:
   332.1 + E939.2 + 295.62

Parkinsonism in Huntington's disease: 333.4

EXAMPLE

ALZHEIMER'S DISEASE

Alzheimer's disease (code 331.0) is a progressive, degenerative brain disorder that can occur in elderly people. It is characterized by progressive memory loss, loss of intellectual abilities, confusion and dementia, emotional disturbances such as anxiety and/or depression, and wandering. Alzheimer's disease results in a progressive destruction of brain cells. Certain pathogenic (disease-causing) changes also occur in the brain, such as atrophy (shrinkage of parts of the brain), neural plaques (deposits) and tangles (bundles) that contain a protein (amyloid) that degenerates brain cells, and a loss of substances called **neurotransmitters.** Neurotransmitters are chemicals that help to carry messages between nerve cells (neurons) in the brain. Alzheimer's patients often lose their sense of person, place, and time, and they often wander away from safety; as such, they are sometimes cared for in locked medical units. There is no known cure for Alzheimer's disease. However, medications are available—tacrine (Cognex), donepezil (Aricept), rivastigmine (Exelon), and galantamine (Reminyl). How these drugs work is not fully understood, but it is believed that they increase the level of a neurotransmitter (acetylcholine) in the brain. These drugs will not cure the disease; however, they may help to slow symptom progression (e.g., memory loss) and control behavioral disturbances.

ICD-9-CM allows an additional code for reporting Alzheimer's dementia (senile) with or without behavioral disturbances. This information is required for health-care providers to assess the patient's individual needs and establish the appropriate plan of care, because Alzheimer's patients with behavioral disturbances may become demanding, disruptive, combative, and overly suspicious of others.

EXAMPLE	*Alzheimer's dementia with behavioral disturbance: 331.0 + 294.11*
	Alzheimer's dementia without behavioral disturbance: 331.0 + 294.10

AMYOTROPHIC LATERAL SCLEROSIS

ALS (code 335.20) is a progressive CNS disease of unknown etiology that causes a degeneration of motor nerves from the brain and spinal cord. Motor nerves carry impulses from the CNS to internal organs and muscles. ALS is also known as Lou Gehrig's disease (named after the famous major-league baseball player who died from the disease).

With ALS, progressive skeletal muscle weakness results in paralysis, shortness of breath, difficulty speaking and swallowing, and increasing respiratory depression as the diaphragm (the muscle that aids in respiration) becomes increasingly affected. Eventually, respiratory paralysis occurs. There is no known cure for ALS. Palliative (not curative) treatment is directed at controlling symptoms, providing comfort, and alleviating pain.

Other Disorders of the CNS

Other common disorders of the CNS include multiple sclerosis, hemiplegia, hemiparesis, and epilepsy.

MULTIPLE SCLEROSIS

Multiple sclerosis (code 340) is suspected to be an autoimmune disorder in which abnormal antibodies attack and destroy normal myelin tissues. Like the covering over an electrical wire, a myelin sheath (white matter) insulates nerves. However, in multiple sclerosis, the myelin sheath is destroyed and replaced by a hard plaque in a process called **demyelinization**. Demyelinization prevents the proper conduction of nerve impulses in the body, and this can cause muscle weakness, numbness, and paralysis and can result in difficulty walking (i.e., gait disorders). Speech and vision can also be affected. Multiple sclerosis is a chronic disease marked by periods of remission (no symptoms) and relapses (exacerbation of symptoms). Some drugs are available that can shorten exacerbations of the disease (e.g., steroids and interferon-β); however, there is no specific treatment for the disease.

Hemiplegia and Hemiparesis

Both **hemiplegia** and **hemiparesis** (code 342.XX) refer to paralysis of one side of the body. This can result from a cerebrovascular accident (CVA; stroke) (Figure 12.2), traumatic brain injury, or tumor. The fourth-digit subcategory conveys the type of hemiplegia. For example, 342.0X classifies flaccid hemiplegia, which is characterized by the loss of muscle tone (atrophy) and tendon reflexes of the affected (paralyzed) side. Spastic hemiplegia (code 342.1X) is characterized by increased muscle spasms and tendon reflexes of the affected

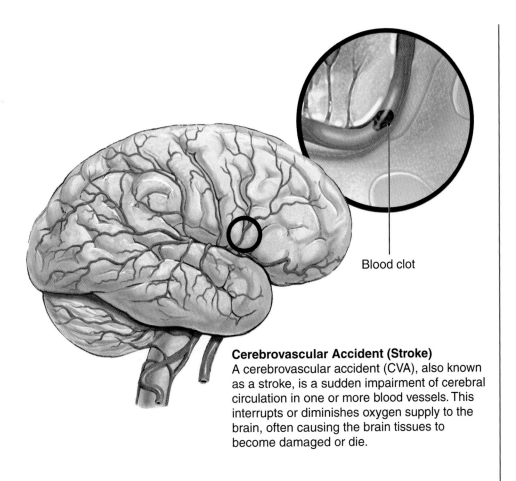

Blood clot

Cerebrovascular Accident (Stroke)
A cerebrovascular accident (CVA), also known as a stroke, is a sudden impairment of cerebral circulation in one or more blood vessels. This interrupts or diminishes oxygen supply to the brain, often causing the brain tissues to become damaged or die.

FIGURE 12.2 ■ A cerebrovascular accident (CVA), also known as a stroke, is a sudden impairment of cerebral circulation in one or more blood vessels. This interrupts or diminishes oxygen supply to the brain, often causing the brain tissues to become damaged or die. (Reprinted with permission from Anatomical Chart Co.)

(paralyzed) side. The fifth-digit subclassification conveys whether the side affected is dominant, nondominant, or unspecified.

If an individual who is right-hand dominant experiences a stroke that results in paralysis of the right side of his or her body, the course of rehabilitation is greatly affected. This fact points to the importance of accurately and completely reporting this information through coding.

EXAMPLE	*Acute left-sided CVA with infarct resulting in hemiplegia, right side. Patient is right-hand dominant: 434.91, 342.91*

If an individual has a stroke affecting the right side of the brain, a left-sided paralysis may manifest; conversely, if an individual has a stroke affecting the left side of the brain, a right-sided paralysis may occur. Hemiplegia will be contralateral, or opposite, the brain lesion because nerve fibers cross over to the opposite side in the medulla oblongata. The medulla oblongata is part of brain stem and helps to connect the spinal cord to the brain.

Category code 342 is used exclusively to describe hemiplegia or hemiparesis for the current admission or episode of care. It is used as a secondary diagnosis; the underlying reason for the hemiplegia (e.g., CVA with infarction) is sequenced as the principal diagnosis. Once a patient is discharged from acute care to a rehabilitation facility or is readmitted to the hospital, you should code hemiplegia as a "late effect" of cerebrovascular disease (code 438.2X).

Unfortunately, patients who have CVAs may have repeated or new CVAs. Coding hemiplegia (342.9X) or other symptoms as current with the new CVA while coding residual conditions or symptoms associated with old CVAs to late effects (438.XX) enables a coder to report which residual conditions or symptoms are attributed to the new acute CVA versus symptoms that are residual conditions of the old CVAs.

EXAMPLE	*Acute left-sided CVA with infarct and right-sided hemiplegia: 434.91, 342.90*
	Patient had a CVA 5 years ago with residual aphasia: 438.11

If a patient experiences a CVA with hemiplegia or other residuals, such as aphasia (i.e., speech impairment), that are transient and that clear before hospital discharge, do not assign a code for the hemiplegia or other residuals because it will not affect the patient's future course of care. If a patient has a CVA with hemiplegia or other residual conditions that are present at hospital discharge, add these as additional or secondary diagnosis codes, because the hemiplegia or other residuals will require continuing care (i.e., rehabilitation).

EXAMPLE	*Acute CVA with infarction with left-sided hemiplegia, aphasia, and dysphagia (all present on discharge to a rehabilitation facility): 434.91, 342.90, 784.3, 787.20*
	Acute CVA with infarction with left-sided hemiplegia, aphasia, and dysphagia (hemiplegia and dysphagia cleared before discharge; only aphasia was present at discharge to rehabilitation): 434.91, 784.3

EPILEPSY

Epilepsy (345.XX) is a chronic (recurrent) seizure disorder characterized by sudden abnormal electrical activity in the brain that can cause seizures. Epilepsy is classified into two major categories: **generalized** epilepsy, which involves abnormal electrical discharges that affect the entire brain, and **partial** epilepsy, which involves abnormal electrical discharges that affect only a part of the brain. The major categories of generalized or partial epilepsy are further divided into different types of epilepsy: grand mal, petit mal, focal, and temporal lobe.

Grand mal epilepsy (generalized convulsive; code 345.1X) is characterized by a loss of consciousness with convulsive seizures that can include **tonic** stiffening and contractions of muscles and **clonic** jerking and twitching movements of the extremities. **Petit mal epilepsy** (generalized nonconvulsive; code 345.0X) is characterized by a momentary loss of awareness and surroundings, but no loss of consciousness or convulsive seizures. In **focal epilepsy** (partial epilepsy; code 345.5X), one part of the body will jerk and twitch (convulsive seizures), but there is no impairment of consciousness (loss of awareness). In **temporal lobe epilepsy** (partial epilepsy; code 345.4X), there is abnormal brain activity in the temporal lobe of the brain (near the ears) with an impairment of consciousness (loss of awareness).

Never automatically code a diagnosis of seizures or convulsions to epilepsy. Epilepsy or recurrent seizures must be documented by the physician.

Some seizures, such as tonic/clonic (grand mal) seizures, can occur without a diagnosis of epilepsy. A diagnosis of epilepsy can be made only by a physician who has assessed that a pattern of repeated brain seizures is attributed to epilepsy. Convulsions and seizures can often occur as a temporary result of an infection or fever (febrile seizure, 780.31; seizure not otherwise specified, 780.39) and should not be coded to epilepsy. If a physician documents a diagnosis of seizures or convulsions, carefully review the patient's record for a documented history of epilepsy, review the patient's current medications and old medical records, and then query the physician before assigning the code for epilepsy, recurrent seizures, or seizure disorder. As of October 2006, if the diagnosis is "recurrent seizures" or "seizure disorder" (even in the absence of term "epilepsy"), a code from category 345 (epilepsy and recurrent seizures) is assigned. However, if the diagnosis is that of a **single**, isolated seizure or that of convulsions, the code assigned remains 780.39.

The fifth-digit assignment in the epilepsy code describes whether the epilepsy is intractable. Intractable epilepsy means that it is difficult to control by conventional treatments, such with the drugs phenytoin or phenobarbital (anticonvulsant medications). Physicians rarely document intractable epilepsy. Therefore, you should review the medical record for epileptic seizures described as prolonged or refractory to treatment and then query the physician as appropriate.

EXAMPLE

A patient with a known history of grand mal epilepsy was admitted with uncontrolled seizures that were refractory to outpatient treatment. The physician described the seizures as "intractable": 345.11

A patient was admitted secondary to a breakthrough seizure. The patient's medications were adjusted, and the patient did not have any further seizures while in the hospital: 780.39

TIP It is important to remember that physicians are not always aware of the Uniform Hospital Discharge Data Set rules for reporting inpatient diagnoses. According to Uniform Hospital Discharge Data Set rules, if an inpatient diagnosis is documented as possible, probable, suspected, questionable, or rule out, then it would be coded as if the condition were established. However, as an exception to these rules, if epilepsy is documented as possible, probable, suspected, questionable, or rule out, then query the physician for clarification before assigning the code for epilepsy. This is because of the social and work-related consequences that might affect the patient (e.g., patients diagnosed with epilepsy must report their condition to the Department of Motor Vehicles and may be denied a driver's license). Such care should also be taken for suspected human immunodeficiency virus and cancer diagnoses. For these conditions, do not assign the definitive code unless they are specifically documented or clarified by the physician.

Disorders of the Peripheral Nervous System (PNS)

Category code range 350 to 359 includes disorders of the peripheral nervous system, which are classified according to the nerves involved. The **cranial nerves** carry nerve impulses to and from the brain, head, and neck. The **spinal nerves** carry impulses to and from the brain, trunk, and extremities.

Also part of the peripheral nervous system, the autonomic nervous system is further subdivided into sympathetic and parasympathetic systems. The sympathetic nervous system stimulates the body in times of crisis by inducing the "fight or flight" response: heart rate, blood pressure, and respiration increase; the body increases the production of epinephrine (adrenaline); pupils widen; and digestion slows (e.g., a sympathetic nervous response may be stimulated in a student getting an unannounced pop quiz in class). After the crisis has passed, the parasympathetic nervous system counters the sympathetic system and returns the person to a more relaxed state (e.g., heart rate, blood pressure, and respiration slow).

Common peripheral nervous system disorders include peripheral nerve lesions, palsies, mononeuropathies and polyneuropathies, inflammatory and toxic neuropathies, and myoneural disorders. Many peripheral nervous system disorders are the manifestation of an underlying disease, which you would code first.

EXAMPLE

Diabetic polyneuropathy: 250.60 + 357.2

Polyneuropathy in disseminated lupus erythematosus: 710.0 + 357.1

Polyneuropathy in rheumatoid arthritis: 714.0 + 357.1

Acute Infective Polyneuritis (Guillain-Barré Syndrome)

A significant disease in this code range that often causes hospital admission is acute infective polyneuritis. Also known as Guillain-Barré syndrome (code 357.0), acute infective polyneuritis is an autoimmune disorder in which the body's immune system attacks the peripheral nervous system. The etiology of this disorder is unknown; however, it can sometimes follow a viral illness. Guillain-Barré syndrome results in a sudden, acute, and progressive motor nerve (voluntary muscle) paralysis. Symptoms include rapidly progressive weakness and paresthesias (abnormal sensations such as tingling or numbness in the extremities) that begin in the legs and move to the upper body. Ultimately, the individual can experience incapacitating paralysis with subsequent respiratory paralysis and respiratory failure.

Because there is no specific treatment for Guillain-Barré syndrome, the symptoms are treated. The primary focus is to keep patients alive and functioning and to prevent them from succumbing to secondary complications (e.g., pneumonia) until the paralysis resolves. This usually occurs within a few weeks. Patients with Guillain-Barré syndrome often require many inpatient resources because of profound respiratory difficulties that can necessitate placement in the intensive care unit and treatments such as endotracheal intubation with mechanical ventilation and emergent tracheostomy placement.

Developed by the federal government, MS–DRGs use coded data to establish prospective payment rates to hospitals for inpatient services under Medicare (see Appendix 1: MS Diagnosis-Related Groups (DRG) List). The coding of procedures makes the difference in DRG assignment and, therefore, reimbursement (see below diagnosis-related group MS–DRG 094 versus MS–DRG 004 reporting).

TIP *Coding Clinic* 1991, second quarter, describes more information about Guillain-Barré syndrome with respiratory failure.

EXAMPLE

MS-DRG 094: Bacterial & tuberculous infections of nervous system w MCC
MDC: 001 Diseases and disorders of the nervous system
CMS wt: 3.3477
A/LOS 11.9
G/LOS 9.2
Principal diagnosis: 357.0 Acute infective polyneuritis (Guillain-Barré syndrome)
Secondary diagnosis: 518.81 Acute respiratory failure
Principal procedure: 96.71 Continuous mechanical ventilation (96 hours)
Other procedure: 96.04 Insert endotracheal tube
Medicare inpatient reimbursement: $13,390.80

MS-DRG 004: Tracheostomy with mechanical ventilation 96 + hours or PDX except face/mouth/neck without major OR procedure
MDC: Pre-MDC—surgical
CMS wt: 11.1684
A/LOS 28.8
G/LOS 23.5
Principal diagnosis: 357.0 Acute infective polyneuritis (Guillain-Barré syndrome)

Secondary diagnosis: 518.81 Acute respiratory failure
Principal procedure: 31.1 Temporary tracheostomy
Other procedures: 96.71 Continuous mechanical ventilation (96 hours)
96.04 Insert endotracheal tube
Medicare inpatient reimbursement: $44,673.60

Disorders of the Eye and Adnexa

Category code range 360 to 379 includes disorders of the eye and adnexa (tissues surrounding the eye), including blindness, cataracts, glaucoma, strabismus, macular degeneration, and retinal detachment.

Anatomy and Physiology

Understanding the anatomy (structure) and physiology (function) of the eye can lead to a better understanding of the pathologies (dysfunctions) that affect the eyes and can enable you to code more precisely (Figure 12.3).

The eyes transmit sensory impulses that provide pictures to the brain. Primarily, an eye consists of three layers. The outer layer consists of the following:

▶ Cornea—an outer clear lens in front of the pupil (dark opening in the eye).
▶ Sclera—the white of the eye.
▶ Conjunctiva—a clear covering over the front sclera and lining the eyelids.

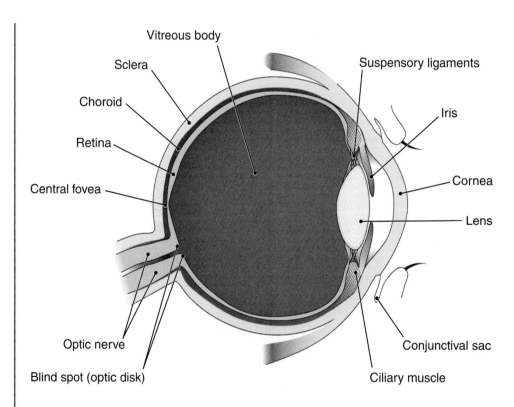

FIGURE 12.3 ■ The eye. (Reprinted with permission from Cohen BJ and Wood DL. Memmler's The Human Body in Health and Disease, 9th Ed. Philadelphia: Lippincott Williams & Wilkins, 2000.)

The middle layer (uveal tract) consists of the following:

▶ Choroid—a membrane containing blood vessels that nourish the eye.
▶ Ciliary body—muscle tissue that surrounds and applies tension to inner lens of the eye so that the lens can thicken for close vision and thin for distance vision. *Presbyopia* (far-sightedness associated with old age) occurs when the inner lens loses flexibility and can no longer thicken for close vision, resulting in the need for reading glasses (bifocals).
▶ Iris—the colored part of the eye surrounding the pupil. The iris contains circular and radial muscles that widen or constrict to control the amount of light entering through the pupil. The iris constricts in bright light as a protective mechanism to prevent damage to the retina (nervous tissue of the eye), and it widens to let in more light in dim lighting.

The inner layer consists of the following:

▶ Retina—the nervous tissue of the eye, consisting of nerve cells called **rods** and **cones**. Rods aid in peripheral vision and seeing in the dark; cones assist in central vision and seeing color. The retina includes an area called the **macula** that contains the fovea centralis (i.e., central macula). When light rays coming into the eye are focused on this area, it produces the sharpest vision.
▶ Optic nerve—a cranial nerve that communicates with the optic disc to send impulses to the brain for visual interpretation. Optic nerve fibers leading to the brain cross over in an area called the **optic chiasm** that allows each eye to communicate with both sides of the brain, thus producing three-dimensional vision (height, width, and depth). Without three-dimensional vision, the world would look flat.

The outer cornea, inner lens, aqueous humor (fluid behind the cornea), and vitreous humor (fluid behind the inner lens) combine to direct and bend light (refraction) to focus on the fovea centralis for the sharpest vision. In **myopia** (near-sightedness), the eye shape is too long, and the rays being refracted do not reach the fovea. In **hyperopia** (far-sightedness), the eye shape is too short, and the rays being refracted overshoot the fovea (Figure 12.4). These refraction errors can be corrected with glasses (biconcave for near-sightedness and biconvex for far-sightedness), contact lenses, and refractive operations, such as laser-assisted stromal in situ keratomileusis (LASIK), or radial keratotomy, that reshape the cornea.

The **Snellen chart** is an important visual acuity test. Standing at a distance of 20 feet away, a patient will read large black letters on the top of a white chart that gradually decrease in size toward the bottom. If you have 20/20 vision, this means that at 20 feet away from the chart, you can see every letter clearly. OD (oculus dexter) is an abbreviation for the right eye, OS (oculus sinister) is an abbreviation for the left eye, and OU (oculus uterque) is an abbreviation for both eyes. If a person has 20/20 OD and 20/800 OS vision, that would indicate that vision is normal in one eye but profoundly impaired in the other eye. (A person with 20/20 vision standing 800 feet away can see what the person with 20/800 vision sees at 20 feet away.)

Blindness

Blindness and low vision not otherwise specified are coded to category 369 of ICD-9-CM. Under category 369, the ICD-9-CM codebook includes a table to describe the level of visual impairment based on the recommendations of the

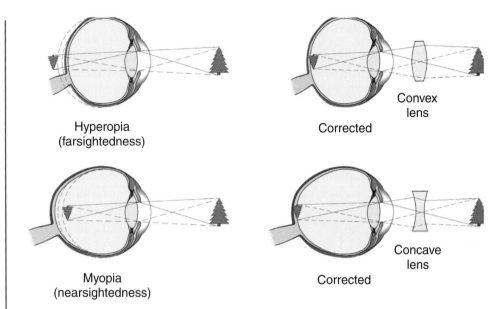

Hyperopia
(farsightedness)

Corrected

Convex
lens

Myopia
(nearsightedness)

Corrected

Concave
lens

FIGURE 12.4 ■ Errors of refraction. (Reprinted with permission from Cohen BJ and Wood DL. Memmler's The Human Body in Health and Disease, 9th Ed. Philadelphia: Lippincott Williams & Wilkins, 2000.)

World Health Organization. A person with 20/20 OD and 20/800 OS vision would be coded to 369.69 (one eye, profound impairment; other eye, normal vision).

 Often, physicians document the diagnosis of blindness inadequately, and the condition is coded to blindness without further specificity (code 369.00). However, ICD-9-CM provides more detailed coding of visual impairment, which may, in turn, refine the assignment of future MS-DRGs. Good documentation facilitates more precise coding and provides a more accurate description of the patient's visual impairment.

Blindness is not often listed as the principal diagnosis or the reason for inpatient admission. However, blindness is sometimes reported as a secondary diagnosis that affects the patient's episode of care because of the need for increased patient assistance. Although it is generally accepted that blindness is a reportable condition that affects patient care, the Centers for Medicare and Medicaid Services do not recognize blindness as a comorbid condition that significantly affects the health-care services provided such that it would increase the reimbursement to the provider. A lack of documentation and inadequate specificity in the reporting of blindness provide insufficient data for the government to determine its true effect on patient care, health-care resource use, and provider reimbursement.

EXAMPLE

Profound legal blindness in both eyes: 369.08
Nearly total blindness in the right eye with normal vision in the left eye: 369.66
Total blindness, both eyes: 369.01

Cataracts

Cataracts (category code 366) result in a cloudiness of the inner lens of the eye that leads to a loss of vision. Some cataracts are associated with age (senile), others may be congenital (present at birth), secondary to trauma, or related to the long-term affects of diabetes.

You should never assume a senile cataract if the patient is elderly or a diabetic cataract if the patient has diabetes. Only a physician can document the exact nature of a cataract.

Cataracts are routinely removed by operation on an outpatient basis. An intracapsular cataract extraction (13.1X) involves the removal of the entire inner lens. In an extracapsular cataract extraction (13.2-5X), the lens is removed, leaving the posterior (back) portion of the lens capsule in place (Figure 12.5). Whichever technique is used, these cataract-extraction procedures are routinely accompanied by the insertion of an intraocular lens implant, which requires an additional procedure code (13.71).

Glaucoma

Glaucoma (category code 365) is "a disease of the eye characterized by increased intraocular pressure, excavation, and atrophy of the optic nerve that produces defects in the field of vision"[1]. Glaucoma can be specified as acute, chronic, angle-closure, open-angle, or other ways. You can think of

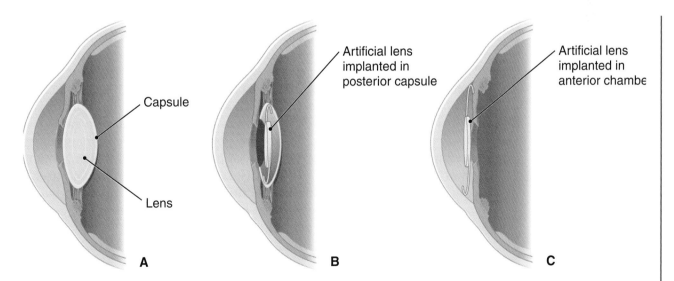

FIGURE 12.5 ■ Cataract extraction surgeries. **A.** Cross-section of normal eye anatomy. **B.** Extracapsular lens extraction involves removing the lens but leaving the posterior capsule intact to receive a synthetic intraocular lens. **C.** Intracapsular lens extraction involves removing the lens and lens capsule and implanting a synthetic intraocular lens in the anterior chamber. (Reprinted with permission from Cohen BJ. Medical Terminology: An Illustrated Guide, 4th Ed. Baltimore: Lippincott Williams & Wilkins, 2004.)

glaucoma as hypertension of the eye caused by the buildup of aqueous humor in the anterior (front) chamber of the eye that cannot drain properly. Tonometry, a common test to diagnose glaucoma, measures intraocular pressure. Glaucoma is often refractory to treatment. However, eyedrops (e.g., pilocarpine) can sometimes be used effectively to decrease intraocular pressure, and surgical procedures including trabeculectomy, trabeculotomy, or iridectomy with scleral fistulization may offer some relief. These surgical procedures use a laser to create a hole in the iris or sclera to facilitate intraocular circulation.

Strabismus

Strabismus is the inability of the eyes to remain balanced or parallel when looking in the same direction (e.g., cross-eyed). Different forms of strabismus include exotropia (378.1X), in which one eye is deviated outward, and esotropia (378.0X), in which one eye is deviated inward. Some forms of strabismus can result in visual impairments such as diplopia (double vision). Often corrective surgery is performed on the extraocular muscles (the muscles surrounding the eye). Such operations may involve recession procedures that lengthen the extraocular eye muscles (15.11 and 15.3) or resection procedures that shorten the extraocular muscles to bring the eyes into proper balance (15.13 and 15.3).

Macular Degeneration

Age-related macular degeneration (code 362.5X) results in degeneration of the macular area of the retina and leads to a loss of central vision (i.e., cannot see straight ahead). It is a leading cause of blindness for elderly people in the United States. Peripheral vision is usually maintained. There are two forms of the disease: the wet form, which results from leaky blood vessels beneath the retina, is not as common as the dry (atrophic) form, which results from retinal thinning and degeneration. Generally, there are few treatments available for the dry form; however, a new procedure (code 13.91) involves implanting a miniature telescopic lens prosthesis for patients with moderate to profound visual impairment due to end-stage age-related macular degeneration (AMD). This allows the patients to maintain peripheral vision in the untreated affected (untreated) eye and to gain central vision in the treated eye. For the wet form, laser photocoagulation can sometimes be used to destroy the damaged blood vessels, but this only manages or slows the progression of the disease. A newer procedure, photodynamic therapy, with a photosensitive drug called verteporfin (Visudyne), can selectively destroy leaking vessels in the retina with the use of a laser. There is no cure for macular degeneration.

Retinal Detachment

Retinal detachment (361.0X, 361.9) results in a retinal tear. This condition can be preceded by numerous **floaters** (floating dark spots), the perception of flashes of light, and a blind spot in the field of vision. Surgery is required to restore vision. A scleral buckling procedure with a silicone implant is used to suture the separated sections of retinal tissue back together (code 14.41).

Disorders of the Ear

Category code range 380 to 389 includes disorders of the ear and mastoid process that include various outer, middle, and inner ear disorders and deafness attributable to conductive, neural, and mixed hearing dysfunction.

Anatomy and Physiology

The primary function of the ears is to transmit sensory impulses to the brain that enable one to perceive sounds. The ear has three sections (Figure 12.6):

▶ The outer section consists of the auricle or pinna (external flap of the ear) and the external auditory canal. A membrane called the eardrum (tympanic membrane) separates the outer ear from the middle ear. It vibrates to conduct sound to the middle ear.

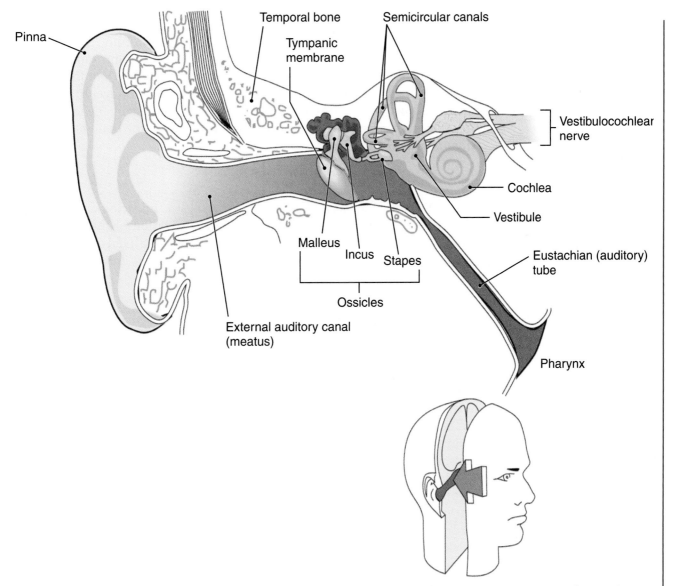

FIGURE 12.6 ■ The ear, showing the outer, middle, and inner subdivisions. (Reprinted with permission from Cohen BJ and Wood DL. Memmler's The Human Body in Health and Disease, 9th Ed. Philadelphia: Lippincott Williams & Wilkins, 2000.)

▶ The middle section consists of three small bones (ossicles) called the malleus, the incus, and the stapes. The ossicles transfer sound through vibrations to the oval window, which separates the middle ear from the inner ear.

▶ The inner section is a mazelike structure called the labyrinth, which contains the snail-shaped cochlea, the organ of Corti, vestibular and semicircular canals, auditory fluids (perilymph and endolymph), and small hairs (cilia). In the inner ear, the auditory fluids and specialized tiny hairs carry vibrations to the auditory nerves, which, in turn, transmit nerve impulses to the brain, where sound is perceived. In addition, the fluids and tiny hairs of the semicircular canals give one a sense of balance or spatial sense in response to body movement. This is why when a child rapidly spins in circles, he or she feels dizzy: the inner-ear apparatus sends mixed spatial messages to the brain. Classic symptoms associated with labyrinthitis or inner ear inflammation or infection include vertigo (dizziness) with accompanying nausea.

Sound is received by the external ear (auricle) and travels through the external auditory canal, where it vibrates against the eardrum. The vibration of the eardrum is relayed to the ossicles (malleus, incus, and stapes) of the middle ear, which, in turn, transmit the vibration to the oval window leading to the inner ear. The vibrations of the oval window then travel through the fluids and tiny hairs of the cochlea until they are picked up by the receptors of the auditory nerves, which send the sound impulses to the brain for auditory interpretation.

External Ear Conditions

A condition often associated with the external ear is impacted cerumen (earwax) (380.4), which can be removed through irrigation of the ear (96.52). Although impacted cerumen would not be a cause for hospital admission, it is frequently a secondary diagnosis that requires attention during the current episode of patient care.

Middle Ear Conditions

Conditions associated with the middle ear include otosclerosis and otitis media. **Otosclerosis** (387.X) is a hardening of bone tissue around the oval window. Conduction deafness occurs, because the ossicles in the middle ear cannot pass along vibrations through the oval window to the acoustic nerves of the inner ear. Stapedectomy with a prosthetic incus replacement (19.11) can be performed to restore hearing. **Otitis media** is an inflammation of the middle ear. It can be described as acute or chronic and as suppurative (infectious with pus formation) or serous (noninfectious with clear fluid).

Unique to the middle ear is the eustachian, or pharyngoeustachian, tube, an opening that allows the middle ear to communicate with the pharynx (throat). This is an important protective mechanism that prevents the eardrum from being perforated (ruptured). For example, when you ascend quickly in an airplane, where the atmosphere is thin and the external air pressure is low, the air pressure in the middle ear remains high and the eardrum bulges outward. The eustachian (pharyngoeustachian) tube responds by opening to allow the pressure of the middle and external ear to equalize, to prevent perforation of the eardrum.

Children often experience recurrent or chronic middle ear inflammations or infections called **chronic otitis media** that are attributable to dysfunction of the eustachian tube, which provides drainage from the middle ear to the pharynx. A tympanotomy or myringotomy (incision into the eardrum) with intubation (pharyngoeustachian tube insertion: 20.01) can be performed to keep the eustachian tube open for drainage.

Inner Ear Conditions

Conditions associated with the inner ear include labyrinthitis and Ménière's disease. Labyrinthitis (otitis interna; code 386.3X) is an inflammation of the inner-ear labyrinth. The fifth digit describes the type or form of labyrinthitis (serous or diffuse, circumscribed or focal, suppurative or purulent, toxic or attributable to chemicals, and viral).

Ménière's disease (code 386.0X) is a disorder of the inner ear labyrinth that results from an excess accumulation of fluid pressure (endolymph) in the cochlea and semicircular canals. Symptoms include vertigo (dizziness), tinnitus (ringing in the ears), headache, and nausea and vomiting.

Conductive deafness (code 389.0X) usually results from a transmission disorder of the ossicles of the middle ear, tympanic membrane, or oval window. Sensorineural deafness (code 389.1X) occurs when there is a dysfunction involving the cochlea or acoustic nerves of the inner ear. Mixed hearing loss involves both conductive and sensorineural hearing loss (code 389.2X).

TIP The type of deafness indicated (i.e., conductive, sensorineural, or mixed conductive and sensorineural) is key to understanding and assigning the correct procedure codes for the various hearing devices available.

Conductive hearing loss is treated with external (battery-powered) hearing aids (95.49), implantation of an electromagnetic bone-conduction device (20.95), or a stapedectomy with prosthetic incus replacement (19.11) for otosclerosis. Sensorineural hearing loss can be treated with a cochlear implant device (single or multiple channels with electrodes) that stimulates the auditory nerve (20.9X).

SUMMARY

This chapter has reviewed the pathology of common disorders of the nervous system and sensory organs. The discussion has been subdivided into the following topical areas: disorders of the CNS, disorders of the peripheral nervous system, and disorders of the sensory organs. The chapter has focused on recognizing manifestations of these disorders and on the complications one might encounter and the treatments commonly used. This has been presented along with an in-depth review of the implications for coding. Proper coding with the ICD-9-CM and medical records has been emphasized throughout the chapter. Chapter 13 addresses the subject of diseases of the circulatory system, blood, and blood-forming organs.

REFERENCES

1. Stedman's Medical Dictionary, 27th Ed. Baltimore: Williams & Wilkins, 2000.

TESTING YOUR COMPREHENSION

1. What are the causes of meningitis?

2. What procedure is performed to confirm a diagnosis of meningitis?

3. What is a common diagnosis for an inflammation of the brain?

4. What tests are performed to confirm a diagnosis of encephalitis?

5. What drug may be used to relieve the symptoms of Parkinson's disease?

6. Alzheimer's patients lose three senses. Please identify them.

7. What are the symptoms associated with multiple sclerosis?

8. Coding hemiplegia or other symptoms as current with a new CVA while coding residual conditions or symptoms associated with old CVAs to late effects enables the coder to accomplish what objective?

9. A sudden loss of consciousness associated with a fall, stiffening of muscles, and clonic movements may characterize what ailment?

10. What does the fifth digit in the epilepsy code describe?

11. What does the outer layer of the eye consist of?

12. What does the middle layer of the eye consist of?

13. What does the inner layer of the eye consist of?

14. Lack of documentation and inadequate specificity in reporting blindness creates what problems?

15. Glaucoma produces defects in the field of vision. How is this condition manifested?

16. What is the cause of glaucoma?

17. What is strabismus?

_____

18. What does macular degeneration lead to?

_____

19. What are the components of the outer section of the ear?

_____

20. What are the parts of the middle ear?

_____

21. What are the parts of the inner ear?

_____

22. What is otosclerosis?

_____

23. What is labyrinthitis?

_____

CODING PRACTICE I   Chapter Review Exercises

Directions

By using your ICD-9-CM codebook, code the following diagnoses and procedures:

	DIAGNOSIS/PROCEDURES	CODE
1	Monocular esotropia, nonaccommodative, OD. Recession of medial rectus muscle, OD.	
2	Conductive and sensorineural deafness. Multiple-channel cochlear implantation.	
3	Senile dementia with Alzheimer's disease with disturbance of behavior.	
4	Recurrent seizure disorder, controlled with phenobarbital.	
5	Keratoconjunctivitis with corneal ulcer.	
6	Retinal detachment with giant tear. Retinal repair with cryotherapy. Scleral buckle.	
7	Leg pain, secondary phantom-limb syndrome. Status post right below-the-knee amputation.	
8	Grand mal epilepsy.	
9	Normal pressure hydrocephalus with dementia and behavior disorder.	
10	Restless-leg syndrome.	
11	Spinal cord infarction.	
12	Dizziness secondary to Ménière's disease.	
13	Brain abscess.	
14	Senile cataract. Extracapsular cataract extraction with intraocular lens insertion.	
15	Acute glaucoma.	

	DIAGNOSIS/PROCEDURES	CODE
16	Spinal headache. Fever. Status post recent spinal tap.	
17	Carpal tunnel syndrome. Carpal tunnel release.	
18	Chronic otitis media. Tube (myringotomy) insertion.	
19	Multiple sclerosis exacerbation.	
20	Classic intractable migraine.	
21	Severe head and jaw pain secondary to trigeminal neuralgia.	
22	Staphylococcal meningitis. Spinal tap.	

CODING PRACTICE II | Medical Record Case Studies

Instructions

1. Carefully review the medical reports provided for each case study.
2. Research any abbreviations and terms that are unfamiliar or unclear.
3. Identify as many diagnoses and procedures as possible.
4. Because only part of the patient's total record is available, determine what additional documentation you might need.
5. If appropriate, identify any questions you might ask the physician to code this case correctly and completely.
6. Complete the appropriate blanks below for each case study.

CHAPTER 12 CASE STUDIES

Case Study 12.1 (Coder/Abstract Summary Form)

Patient: **Jane Doe**

Patient documentation: **Review Medical Reports 12.1 and 12.2**

1. Principal diagnosis:

   _____

2. Secondary or other diagnoses:

   _____

3. Principal procedure:

   _____

4. Other procedures:

   _____

5. Additional documentation needed:

   _____

   _____

   _____

Case Study 12.1 (Continued)

6. Questions for the physician:

_____

_____

_____

_____

_____

MEDICAL REPORT 12.1

DISCHARGE SUMMARY

PATIENT: JANE DOE

MED REC NO.:

DATE OF ADMISSION:

DATE OF DISCHARGE:

ATTENDING PHYSICIAN: SMITH, M.D.

REASON FOR ADMISSION: This 51-year-old white woman with a history of multiple sclerosis passed out while sitting and taking a shower at home. The patient was taken to the emergency room where she was found to have a blood pressure of 108/80 lying and 80/50 sitting. She was admitted to PCU (progressive care unit) for full evaluation of this syncopal-type episode.

HOSPITAL COURSE: On admission the potassium was found to be 3.2 and this was corrected with IV (intravenous) potassium replacement. Neurologic consultation was obtained and EEG (electroencephalogram) performed. This was found to be within normal limits. The patient continued to complain of some right upper extremity weakness and numbness. The remainder of her physical examination was unchanged from what had been her previous examination. The neurology evaluation by Dr. Nerve confirmed the already known diagnosis of multiple sclerosis and felt that this may be an exacerbation of the same. An MRI (magnetic resonance imaging) of the brain and the C-spine was obtained which did show mild cervical cord degeneration. The patient's condition remained approximately the same. She continued to have lightheaded spells when changing position from lying to sitting. A cardiology consultation was obtained to rule out the possibility of any significant pathologic problem. Dr. Heart's evaluation felt that this was most probably due to autonomic dysfunction in the large extremity secondary to multiple sclerosis. Several recommendations were made to try and correct the situation and these were implemented. The episodes seemed to somewhat improve but continued to happen. Routine chest x-ray revealed a retrocardiac mass. This was evaluated with CT (computerized tomography) scan and the possibility of a tumor could not be excluded. Subsequently, Dr. Lung performed a bronchoscopy and there was no mass or endobronchial lesions seen. The patient remained on a steady course with no other significant problems. As there was nothing further that we could offer and as the patient was stable, she was discharged.

FINAL DIAGNOSIS:

1. Hypokalemia.
2. Exacerbation of multiple sclerosis.
3. Urinary tract infection.
4. Orthostatic hypotension due to autonomic dyskinetic syndrome of multiple sclerosis.
5. Syncope due to hypotension.
6. Solitary coin lesion of the lung.

DISCHARGE MEDICATIONS: Florinef 0.1 mg q.d. Will continue Prednisone 20 mg b.i.d. Thigh-high TED hose. Ativan 1 mg q.h.s. Fioricet 1 q.6.h. p.r.n. pain. Darvocet-N 100 1 q.6.h. p.r.n. pain.

The patient is instructed to change positions from lying to sitting very slowly. She was informed that these episodes, in all likelihood, will continue. Her urinary tract infection had been adequately treated throughout her hospital stay with Floxin 200 mg b.i.d. Due to her inability to get around she was sent home with the Foley catheter in place. Arrangements were made for visiting home nurse and physical therapy if possible. The patient will follow-up in my office in approximately one week or sooner if there is a problem.

DD:

DT:

JOHN SMITH, M.D.

MEDICAL REPORT 12.2

HISTORY AND PHYSICAL

PATIENT: JANE DOE

MED REC NO.:

DATE OF ADMISSION:

ATTENDING PHYSICIAN: SMITH, M.D.

CHIEF COMPLAINT: Complaint of fainting.

HISTORY OF PRESENT ILLNESS: This is a 51-year-old Caucasian female, who fainted at her home today as she was sitting, taking a shower. Paramedics were called and the patient revived by the time they arrived but they did go ahead and give her some glucose solution. At the emergency room, she was found to be orthostatically hypotensive with a blood pressure of 108/80 lying and 80/50 sitting. The patient is an excellent historian and has had MS (multiple sclerosis) since 1980s. She has had occasional relapses that have usually responded to Cortisone; most recently severe was in 1990s. She developed progressive weakness over the past 6 months and took a 3-week Cortisone regimen near Thanksgiving of this year, discontinuing the medication a week ago. She again resumed, a few days ago, due to progressive weakness. She is wheelchair bound but normally can do most of her household activities such as fixing meals for the family, tending to her bodily needs, and transferring quite well. She has not walked in quite some time.

She has been under the care of Dr. Muscle, physical medicine specialist, and Dr. Nerve, neurologist. She is bothered by chronic back pain for which she was thoroughly evaluated at the Clinic earlier this year with conclusion being some type of "central pain disorder." She is bothered by headaches for which she takes Fioricet and is unable to sleep at night for which she has been taking Ativan. The Cortisone makes her feel quite nervous which also seems helped by Ativan. She has had depression over the past year with feeling blue much of the time and has tried various types of antidepressant drugs without much improvement. She has had an unexplained loss of appetite the past 6 months with associated 10 lb. weight loss.

PAST MEDICAL HISTORY: Denies diabetes, hypertension or heart disease. She has had a hysterectomy, lumbar spinal fusion and debridement and closure of a sacral ulcer.

ALLERGIES: SULFA, CODEINE, URECHOLINE.

SOCIAL HISTORY: She is married, does not smoke or use alcohol. Drinks 5-6 glasses of tea daily.

FAMILY HISTORY: Unremarkable.

REVIEW OF SYSTEMS: General: Progressive weakness, feels cold much of the time recently. Weight loss. HEENT: Legally blind in the right eye, occasional loss of vision in the left when she has relapses of MS. Cardiorespiratory: Denies chest pain, shortness of breath or cough. GI: Loss of appetite. Forces herself to eat. Denies abdominal pain, constipation or diarrhea. GU: Incontinence with Foley catheter indwelling at this time. Musculoskeletal: As in history of present illness. Neuro: Frequent headaches, feels depressed and blue much of the time. Unable to move her legs. Occasional numbness and tingling in the right upper extremity which is patchy and diffuse.

PHYSICAL EXAM: Reveals a Caucasian female, age 51, well-developed, well-nourished.

BP: 110/80.

PULSE: 72.

RESPIRATIONS: 16.

TEMP: 98.

Continued

MEDICAL REPORT 12.2 (CONTINUED)

HEENT: Eyes reveal mildly asymmetric right pupil, mid-sized, reacts poorly to light with absence of consensual reflex in left eye. Left pupil reacts briskly to light and a consensual reflex is present in the right eye. Ears clear. Mouth and throat: Permanent teeth. Tongue midline with pharynx clear. Mild dryness.

NECK: Is supple. Carotid pulsations are brisk without bruits. No adenopathy or thyroid enlargement.

LUNGS: Equal breath sounds.

HEART: Regular rhythm without murmur or gallop.

BREASTS: Not done.

BACK: Some prominence of the dorsal spine due to muscle atrophy. In the lumbar region, a well-healed lumbar surgical scar.

ABDOMEN: Soft, nontender, no organomegaly. A well-healed surgical lower abdominal midline scar. Femoral pulses are 1+ and symmetrical.

EXTREMITIES: Reveal atrophy of the musculature of the thighs and calves with mild flexion contractures at the knee. Pedal pulses are a trace bilaterally. There is no edema.

NEURO: The patient is alert, coherent with mildly depressed affect. She is oriented x 3. She holds her arms, upper extremities well. Unable to move the lower extremities at all.

SKIN: Is warm and dry and pale.

LAB: Serum potassium of 3.2. Electrocardiogram shows sinus rhythm, multiple atrial premature complexes.

IMPRESSION:
  1. Syncopal episode.
  2. Multiple sclerosis.
  3. Hypokalemia.

PLAN: Admission to the progressive care unit for intravenous fluids, adequately rehydrate, correct the potassium deficiency, further evaluate the cause of her syndrome.

DD:

DT:

_____

SMITH, M.D.

Case Study 12.2 (Coder/Abstract Summary Form)

Patient: **Frank Smith**

Patient documentation: **Review Medical Report 12.3**

1. Principal diagnosis:

   _____

2. Secondary or other diagnoses:

   _____

3. Principal procedure:

   _____

4. Other procedures:

   _____

5. Additional documentation needed:

   _____

   _____

   _____

   _____

6. Questions for the physician:

   _____

   _____

   _____

   _____

MEDICAL REPORT 12.3

XYZ REGIONAL HOSPITAL

PATIENT NAME: SMITH, Frank

MEDICAL RECORD NUMBER:

ACCOUNT NUMBER:

ADMISSION DATE:

DISCHARGE DATE:

CLINICAL RESUME

FINAL DIAGNOSIS:
1. Intracranial hemorrhage.
2. Diabetes.

ATTENDING PHYSICIAN: Dr. Jones

RESIDENT PHYSICIAN: Dr. Smith

CONSULTANTS: Dr. Nerve of neurosurgery

ADMITTING DIAGNOSIS:
1. Intracranial hemorrhage
2. Diabetes

INITIAL FINDINGS: This is an 82-year-old white male with multiple past medical history who presents from XYZ Hospital with intracranial hemorrhage. According to Dr. Nerve, there are no surgical options for this patient. According to family, patient got up today from a chair and fell hitting his head against the floor. The patient was conscious after the fall but was weak on the right side. Mental functioning as per family has decreased progressively since then. Normally patient is active, oriented x2, ambulatory with cane and has only mild signs of dementia. Review of systems as per family: Patient denies fever and chills, chest pain, shortness of breath, nausea, vomiting, abdominal pain, or change in bowel movements. Patient does complain of chronic weakness. While at XYZ Hospital, the patient was given 1 unit of FFP and 10 mg of vitamin K.

PAST MEDICAL HISTORY:
1. Atrial fibrillation, on (long-term) Coumadin.
2. Alzheimer's dementia, mild symptoms only as per family.
3. Hypertension.
4. GERD.
5. CVA.
6. Diabetes, diet controlled.

PAST SURGICAL HISTORY:

Case Study 12.3 (Coder/Abstract Summary Form)

Patient: **Ann Johnson**

Patient documentation: **Review Medical Reports 12.4 and 12.5**

1. Principal diagnosis:

   _____

2. Secondary or other diagnoses:

   _____

3. Principal procedure:

   _____

4. Other procedures:

   _____

5. Additional documentation needed:

   _____

   _____

   _____

6. Questions for the physician:

   _____

   _____

   _____

   _____

MEDICAL REPORT 12.4

DISCHARGE SUMMARY

PATIENT NAME: JOHNSON, ANN

DATE OF ADMISSION:

DATE OF DISCHARGE:

ATTENDING PHYSICIAN: SMITH, M.D.

DISCHARGE DIAGNOSIS:

1. Acute renal failure, etiology uncertain.
2. History of paroxysmal atrial fibrillation, controlled on meds.
3. Grand mal epilepsy, on Dilantin and Phenobarbital.

This is a 51-year-old female admitted through the Emergency Room because of 48 hours of abdominal pain with low-grade fever, nausea and vomiting. She was admitted for further observation. On examination her chest was clear to auscultation and percussion. Cardiac examination showed regular sinus rhythm. The abdomen was benign. There was some decrease in bowel sounds. No organomegaly, no masses, no tenderness noted although earlier in the Emergency Room apparently there was some discomfort in the left lower quadrant. She was admitted with the diagnosis of gastroenteritis; however, this was ruled out.

I was asked to see the patient in consultation. It was apparent that she had an episode of acute renal failure seemingly related to her congenital solitary kidney. She had mild cardiomegaly. She underwent acute hemodialyses in the Intensive Care Unit. These were uncomplicated. Electrocardiogram demonstrated sinus bradycardia, question of an old anteroseptal defect and nonspecific S-T-T wave changes. Electrocardiogram was essentially negative for significant lesions. There was a minimal sized pericardial effusion. No evidence of a thrombus and there was evidence of the old mitral valve prolapse. Laboratory data was remarkable for the following findings. The electrolytes demonstrated hyponatremia consistent with her acute renal failure. Her urinary electrolytes demonstrated a serum sodium of 35 and subsequently rose to 111 at the time of her maximum defect. Initially her urinalysis demonstrated +4 protein. There was still +4 protein 6 days later and there were 10-20 white cells, reached its peak at 53. The patient was undergoing dialysis through this period of time. Her creatinine similarly had risen to a peak of 8.1. However, the patient subsequently had a spontaneous increase in infiltration rate. By the time of discharge she was vastly improved with a spontaneously decreasing creatinine of 4.4. The cardiac profile suggested an elevated CPK with positive LDH isoenzymes consistent with renal ischemia, perhaps infarction. The patient's course continued to be benign and she was released to be followed up in the office. All other studies were negative. Urine for myoglobin was negative but this was done approximately five days after admission. The patient was sent home on controlled salt diet with follow up in one week to see me.

DD:

DT:

_____

SMITH, M.D.

MEDICAL REPORT 12.5

HISTORY AND PHYSICAL

PATIENT: JOHNSON, ANN

DATE OF ADMISSION:

ATTENDING PHYSICIAN: SMITH, M.D.

CHIEF COMPLAINT: Abdominal pain.

PRESENT ILLNESS: The patient is a 51-year-old white female being admitted from the emergency room to the floor for observation. She presented to the emergency room earlier this afternoon with a 24-hour history of generalized abdominal pain associated with multiple episodes of nausea and vomiting. She has noted in the last 6–12 hours a localization of the pain more in the left lower quadrant of the abdomen.

The patient was visiting the area and saw a physician there who recommended hospitalization. She came back here for evaluation. The patient has had no fever or chills. She has had no diarrhea or rectal bleeding. She has not consumed alcohol recently, has not been taking Aspirin products. She has had no gastrointestinal tract history.

The patient has had a history of grand mal epilepsy since the 1980s with her last seizure occurring in 1990s. She takes Dilantin 200 mg daily and Phenobarbital 30 mg daily. Additionally, the patient has a history of mitral valvular prolapse with paroxysmal atrial fibrillation, and takes Lanoxin .25 mg daily and Inderal long acting 80 mg per day.

PAST HISTORY: Current medications; see above. Allergies; none claimed. Infections/disease; none. Previous hospitalizations; paroxysmal atrial flutter, seizure work-up in the early 1980s. The patient was hospitalized twice for childbirth, and was hospitalized many years go for a tonsillectomy.

SOCIAL HISTORY: The patient is married with two children. She is a former smoker, but not recently. She does not drink alcohol.

FAMILY HISTORY: Notable for cardiovascular disease.

REVIEW OF SYSTEMS:

GENERAL: Stable weight, no chills, fevers or night sweats.

SKIN: Negative.

HEENT: Presbyopic with glasses, otherwise benign.

RESPIRATORY: No pulmonary disease.

CARDIOVASCULAR: No chest pain or dyspnea, but periodic palpitations have been present. The patient was recently seen in the office the past week with a brief episode of paroxysmal atrial fibrillation.

GASTROINTESTINAL: See above.

GENITOURINARY: Solitary congenital kidney per history.

MUSCULOSKELETAL: No amputation or arthritis.

CNS: Negative.

PHYSICAL EXAMINATION

VITALS: Temperature 96.9, heart rate 58, blood pressure 100/60, respiratory rate 16.

GENERAL: The patient is a pleasant white female who is weak, but in no acute distress.

SKIN: Dry with diminished turgor across all four extremities.

HEAD: Normocephalic without signs or trauma.

Continued

MEDICAL REPORT 12.5 (CONTINUED)

EYES: Reveal symmetrical eye movements with reactive pupils. Fundi are benign.

ENT: Unremarkable.

NECK: Carotids are symmetrical, there are no bruits. There is no jugular venous distention.

CHEST: Clear to percussion and auscultation.

CARDIAC: Rhythm is regular. I can hear a mid-systolic click with an apical systolic murmur. There is no rub or gallop rhythm.

ABDOMEN: Notable for diminished bowel sounds. There is no hepatosplenomegaly, no mass and no tenderness; however, in the Emergency Room earlier left lower quadrant tenderness was noted.

RECTAL: The ampulla is empty, but there is some stool on the glove that is occult negative.

PELVIC: Not performed.

EXTREMITIES: Free of cyanosis, clubbing or edema.

IMPRESSION: Probable gastroenteritis with dehydration.

PLAN: Admit for observation and symptom relief, as well as hydration.

DD:

DT:

SMITH, M.D.

NOTES

Case Study 12.4 (Coder/Abstract Summary Form)

Patient: **Sarah Hanson**

Patient documentation: **Review Medical Report 12.6**

1. Principal diagnosis:

   _____

2. Secondary or other diagnoses:

   _____

3. Principal procedure:

   _____

4. Other procedures:

   _____

5. Additional documentation needed:

   _____

   _____

   _____

   _____

6. Questions for the physician:

   _____

   _____

   _____

   _____

   _____

MEDICAL REPORT 12.6

HISTORY AND PHYSICAL EXAMINATION

PATIENT NAME: HANSON, SARAH

ROOM#:

MED REC NO.:

ADMIT DATE:

ATTENDING PHYSICIAN: SMITH, M.D.

CHIEF COMPLAINT: Weakness, ataxia, confusion.

HISTORY OF PRESENT ILLNESS: This 86-year-old female with weakness, difficulty walking or standing, and pain in her right foot and leg that has been progressive for the last several weeks. Also, she has been having increasing confusion, especially over the last 3–4 days. No other modifying factors or associated signs or symptoms.

PAST MEDICAL HISTORY: Remarkable for CHF, hypertension, type 2 diabetes mellitus, CAD, back pain with radiculopathy, severe PVD, chronic renal failure, hyperlipidemia, hypokalemia, allergic rhinitis, diabetic retinopathy, OA. Surgeries: CABG, cholecystectomy, C-section, right arm and shoulder surgery, tumor removed from her neck in 1990, also had bilateral cataract surgery.

ALLERGIES: Penicillin and questionable pain medication.

CURRENT MEDICATIONS: Humulin 70/30, 55 units subcu q. a.m. and 25 units subcu q.p.m., tramadol 50 mg one to two q.6.h. p.r.n. pain, hydroxyzine 25 mg t.i.d. p.r.n., Neurontin 400 mg, two t.i.d., enteric coated aspirin 325 mg q.d., Lasix 40 mg q.d., Lanoxin .125 mg q.d., liquid antacid 2–4 teaspoons a.c. and q.h.s. p.r.n., Pletal 100 mg p.o. b.i.d. a.c., Lipitor 10 mg q. h.s., Coreg 3.125 mg b.i.d., lorazepam .5 mg b.i.d. p.r.n., Advil 200 mg one to two q.6.h. p.r.n.

FAMILY HISTORY: Remarkable for ulcers and cancer.

PSYCHOSOCIAL HISTORY: She resides with her family. They have electric heat, city water. No pets, no smokers. Patient denies nicotine, alcohol or drug use. She taught Sunday school for many years. No difficulty reading or writing.

REVIEW OF SYSTEMS:

EYES: Bilateral cataract surgery. Wears reading glasses.

EARS, NOSE, MOUTH AND THROAT: Edentulous with dentures.

CARDIOVASCULAR: CAD, status post CABG.

RESPIRATORY: No complaints of shortness of breath, dyspnea on exertion, cough, sputum production, hemoptysis or orthopnea.

GASTROINTESTINAL: No complaints of dysphagia, abdominal pain, diarrhea, constipation, nausea, vomiting or hematemesis, melena, hematochezia, hemorrhoids or fecal incontinence.

GENITOURINARY: No complaints of burning, urinary frequency, urgency, vaginal discharge, irregular menses, dyspareunia, hematuria, nocturia, hesitancy or oliguria.

MUSCULOSKELETAL: History of generalized pain and joint stiffness with OA with difficulty standing.

INTEGUMENTARY: No complaints of itching, rashes, flaking or history of skin CA.

NEUROLOGICAL: Profound weakness with difficulty walking and ataxia.

PSYCHIATRIC: History of anxiety with confusion.

ENDOCRINE: Type 2 diabetes mellitus, insulin requiring.

HEMATOLOGICAL/LYMPHATIC: No history of anemia, blood disorders, free bleeding or easy bruising.

MEDICAL REPORT 12.6 (CONTINUED)

ALLERGY/IMMUNOLOGICAL: Penicillin and questionable pain pills.

PHYSICAL EXAM: Admission vital signs are as follows: Temp. 98.4, pulse 80, BP 142/86.

GENERAL APPEARANCE: This is a well developed elderly female in no acute distress.

HEENT: Head is normal cephalic and atraumatic. Eyes PERRLA. Extraocular movements intact. Tympanic membranes patent. Posterior pharynx and oral mucosa moist and clear.

NECK: Supple without masses or lymphadenopathy. No jugular vein distension.

RESPIRATORY: Respiratory effort is even and non-labored with all fields clear to auscultation.

CARDIAC: Regular rate and rhythm without murmur, rub, or gallop.

ABDOMEN: Soft and nontender. No masses or hepatosplenomegaly.

GENITOURINARY: Deferred.

MUSCULOSKELETAL/EXTREMITIES: Tenderness in the heel of the foot. Diminished pulses bilaterally.

NEUROLOGICAL: The patient does walk with an ataxic gait. She is also confused. Otherwise, no gross neurosensory deficits.

ASSESSMENT:
1. Confusion, probable OBS of Alzheimer's type.
2. Dyspnea/bronchitis.
3. PVD.
4. Compensated CHF.
5. CAD, status post CABG.
6. Chronic renal failure.
7. Hypertension.
8. Type 2 diabetes mellitus, insulin requiring.
9. Diabetic retinopathy.
10. Osteoarthritis.

PLAN: We will admit, continue medications, do CT, carotids, RPR, sed rate, B-12, thyroids, x-ray right foot, we will monitor closely, Accucheck and await studies.

DD:

DT:

_____

Smith, M.D.

Case Study 12.5 (Coder/Abstract Summary Form)

Patient: **Betty Jones**

Patient documentation: **Review Medical Reports 12.7 and 12.8**

1. Principal diagnosis:

   _____

2. Secondary or other diagnoses:

   _____

3. Principal procedure:

   _____

4. Other procedures:

   _____

5. Additional documentation needed:

   _____

   _____

   _____

   _____

6. Questions for the physician:

   _____

   _____

   _____

   _____

   _____

MEDICAL REPORT 12.7

DISCHARGE SUMMARY

PATIENT: JONES, BETTY

DISCHARGE DATE:

ADMISSION DATE:

ATTENDING PHYSICIAN: SMITH, M.D.

DISCHARGE DIAGNOSES:

1. MIGRAINE VARIANT
2. LEFT HEMIPLEGIA
3. VISION LOSS
4. DIABETES
5. OSTEOPOROSIS

HPI/HOSPITAL COURSE: Ms. Jones is a 53-year-old female with past medical history of atypical migraines who was admitted to XYZ Hospital after she presented with one-sided weakness.

Ms. Jones has had problems with vision loss in the past. This usually involves the left eye. It is then followed by return of her vision and with unilateral throbbing headache. This is often associated with nausea. The day of admission, she had some weakness in the left side of her body. She had difficulty walking. She also had some problems with her equilibrium and felt somewhat dizzy.

Workup in the Emergency Room including CAT scan of the brain that was unremarkable. She was followed with serial neural checks during her hospitalization. Her symptoms improved. However, slight hemiplegia on the day of discharge. She still had persistent occasional dizziness but overall was doing better. She had no problems with vision loss.

Carotid ultrasound and echocardiogram were obtained. These were without significant abnormalities. MRI of the brain was obtained and this was pending on the day of discharge.

She did well during her hospitalization. CBC and profile were unremarkable.

LABORATORY DATA: Please refer to chart.

DISCHARGE INSTRUCTIONS: DIET: Low fat. Low salt. No alcohol. No nicotine. No stimulants. No chocolate.

MEDICATIONS ON DISCHARGE:

Depakote 250 mg p.o. b.i.d.
Aspirin 1 p.o. q.d.
Antivert 25 mg p.o. q.6.h. p.r.n., for dizziness.

FOLLOW-UP:

1. She is to follow-up with her primary care physician. She is to call or return if she has any worsening of her symptoms or neurological deficit.
2. She was started back on Depakote 250 mg p.o. b.i.d. as this seemed to help her previously with decreased problems with migraine headache.
3. She was counseled extensively regarding lifestyle and dietary intervention. She is to avoid caffeine, stress, keep regular hours, incorporate exercise, and avoid any precipitants such as MSG, chocolates, cheeses, etc.
4. She should consider additional neurological follow-up. Consideration could be given to obtaining an angiogram.
5. Risks and side-effects of Depakote were reviewed with the patient.

DD:

DT:

Smith, M.D.

MEDICAL REPORT 12.8

PATIENT ASSESSMENT/ EMERGENCY ROOM ADMISSION

PATIENT: JONES, BETTY

ADMISSION DATE:

PHYSICIAN: SMITH, M.D.

DEPARTMENT OF EMERGENCY MEDICINE

REASON FOR HOSPITALIZATION: This 53-year-old female brought to the ER via ambulance with a chief complaint of left facial droop, weakness left side (both arm and leg) along with headache and sore throat. Patient described "aura" onset the other day with onset of headache that remains on top of her head and left side. Patient also claims pain behind left eye. She has an unsteady gait. She describes dizziness, with whirling movement of the walls and room.

Pain? Pain scale (1-10) #8

Mode of Arrival: Stretcher

Loss of Consciousness: No

Complete GCS, if applicable.

Eye Opening 1-4 4; Motor function 1-6 5; Verbal response 1-5 4; TOTAL (3-15): 13

Corrective Lenses/Contacts? N

Psychosocial: Patient requests or needs: N Spiritual Assistance/Pastoral Care: N

Family Support Present: N Live Alone: Y Homeless: No

Does patient exhibit any S/S of abuse? N

Patient comfortable in present environment? Y

Patient feels safe to go home? Y

Patient afraid of being hurt? N

Patient has been hit or injured by someone? N

PAST MEDICAL HISTORY

PAST MEDICAL HISTORY? Y

Afib:

Angina:

Arthritis:

Asthma: Y

Cancer: Y

CAD:

CHF:

Colitis:

COPD:

CVA/TIA:

Dementia:

Diverticulitis:

Diverticulosis:

MEDICAL REPORT 12.8 (CONTINUED)

Drug/alcohol:

FTT:

GERD:

Gout:

Hepatitis:

Hyperthyroid:

Hypothyroid

Hiatal Hernia:

HTN:

IDDM:

Kidney stones:

Lupus:

Major Fracture:

Mental illness:

MI:

Migraine: Y

NIDDM: Y

Osteoporosis: Y

Pacemaker:

Phlebitis:

Pneumonia:

PVD:

Renal Failure:

Rheumatism:

Seizure:

TB:

Ulcers:

UTI:

Comment/Other PMH:

PAST SURGICAL HISTORY? Y

Appendectomy:

Bowel: Y

Cancer:

CABG:

Cataracts:

Cholecystectomy:

Colostomy/ileostomy:

C-section:

Cysto:

EGD:

Continued

MEDICAL REPORT 12.8 (CONTINUED)

Hernia:
Hysterectomy: Y
Mastectomy:
Orthopedic:
Tonsillectomy:
Transplant:
Tubal Ligation:
TURP:
Valve replaced:
Other:

MEDICATION?

Xanax
Nose Spray
For Osteoporosis

ALLERGIES?

Codeine
Sulfa

VITAL SIGNS:

Temp: 97.5
Pulse: 68
Resp: 18
BP: 150/90
Pulse Ox: 97 RA
Weight: 160
LMP: Hyster
G: P: AB: L:
Height: Ft: 5 In: 5

VACCINATION HISTORY:

Date of Pneumococcal Vaccination:
Date of last Influenza Vaccination:
Immunizations Up To Date?
Last Tetanus: Unknown

Priority Code: URGENT

RN Review: Smith, RN

Coding for Diseases of the Circulatory System, Blood, and Blood-Forming Organs

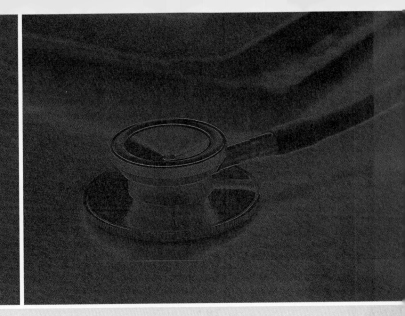

Chapter Outline

The Circulatory System
Diseases of the Circulatory System
Blood and Blood-Forming Organ Diseases
Testing Your Comprehension
Coding Practice I: Chapter Review Exercises
Coding Practice II: Medical Record Case Studies

Chapter Objectives

▶ Describe the pathology of common circulatory system, blood, and blood-forming organ disorders.

▶ Recognize the typical manifestations, complications, and treatments of common circulatory system, blood, and blood-forming organ disorders in terms of their implications for coding.

▶ Correctly code common circulatory system, blood, and blood-forming organ disorders and related procedures by using the ICD-9-CM and medical records.

Circulatory system diseases are included in chapter 7, code section 390 to 459, and blood and blood-forming organ diseases are included in chapter 4, code section 280 to 289, of the Disease Tabular of the ICD-9-CM. Because the circulatory system is essential to transporting blood and because blood is essential to transporting important substances to and from all cells of the body, the two systems are presented together in this chapter. To assist in your understanding, the Word Parts Box on page 372 reviews word parts and meanings of terms related to the circulatory system, blood, and blood-forming organs.

Word Parts and Meanings for the Circulatory System, Blood, and Blood-Forming Organs

Word Part	Meaning	Example	Definition of Example
cardi/o-	heart	cardiomyopathy	Disease of heart muscle
angi/o-	blood vessel	angioplasty	Surgical repair of artery
arter/o- arteri/o-	artery	arteriosclerosis	Hardening of the arteries
ather/o-	fatty plaque (deposits)	atherosclerosis	Condition of fatty plaque within the lining of an artery
phleb/o- ven/o-	vein	phlebitis	Inflammation of a vein
thromb/o-	clot	thrombocyte; thrombus	A clotting cell (platelet); a clot
-plasty	surgical repair	arterioplasty	Surgical repair of an artery
brady-	slow	bradycardia	Slow heartbeat
tachy-	fast	tachycardia	Fast heartbeat
aort/o-	aorta (largest artery in the body)	aortic	Pertaining to the aorta
-sclerosis	hardening	aortic sclerosis	Hardening of the aorta (largest artery in the body)
-osis	abnormal condition	thrombosis	Condition of blood clot
a- an-	no; without; low; deficient	anemia	A condition of deficient red blood cells
cyt/o-	cell	cytology	The study of cells
-emia	blood condition	hypoglycemia	A condition of low blood sugar
ventricul/o-	ventricle (within the heart or brain)	ventricular	Pertaining to a ventricle
-ole -ule	small; little	arteriole; venule	Smallest artery; smallest vein
cerebr/o-	cerebrum (largest part of brain)	cerebral	Pertaining to cerebrum
erythr/o-	red	erythrocyte	Red blood cell
leuk/o-	white	leukocyte	White blood cell
-penia	deficiency	thrombocytopenia	Deficiency of clotting cells
pan-	all	pancytopenia	Deficiency of all three of the formed elements of the blood (red blood cells, white blood cells, and platelets)

The Circulatory System

The circulatory system is composed of arteries, arterioles (small arteries), veins, venules (small veins), and capillaries. (Principal systemic arteries and veins are illustrated in Figures 13.1 and 13.2.) The capillaries are the tiniest of blood vessels that allow substances such as nutrients (e.g., proteins) and gases (e.g., oxygen), as well as the waste products of metabolism (carbon dioxide and urea), to be exchanged between blood and body cells to sustain life. Remember that cells make up tissues, tissues make up organs, and organs make up systems

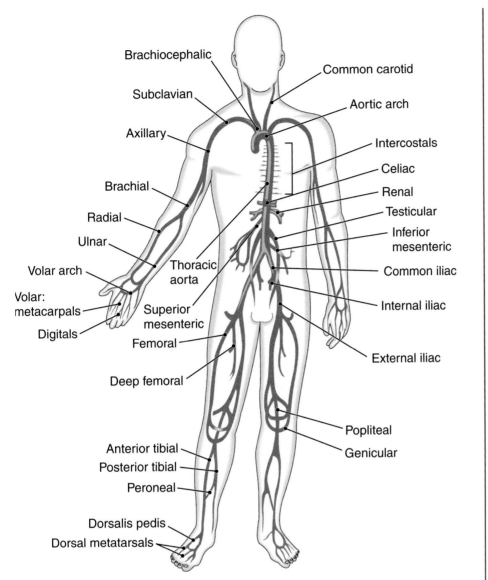

FIGURE 13.1 ■ Principal systemic arteries. (Reprinted with permission from Cohen BJ and Wood DL. Memmler's The Human Body in Health and Disease, 9th Ed. Philadelphia: Lippincott Williams & Wilkins, 2000.)

(e.g., digestive, respiratory) that comprise the total body system. The transport of blood is essential to maintain one's cells and promote overall health.

Some of the more common circulatory system diseases that cause hospital admissions include the following:

▶ coronary artery disease and angina
▶ acute myocardial infarctions (i.e., heart attack)
▶ heart failure
▶ heart arrhythmia and heart blocks
▶ hypertension
▶ atherosclerotic peripheral vascular disease
▶ cerebrovascular accidents (CVA; i.e., stroke)

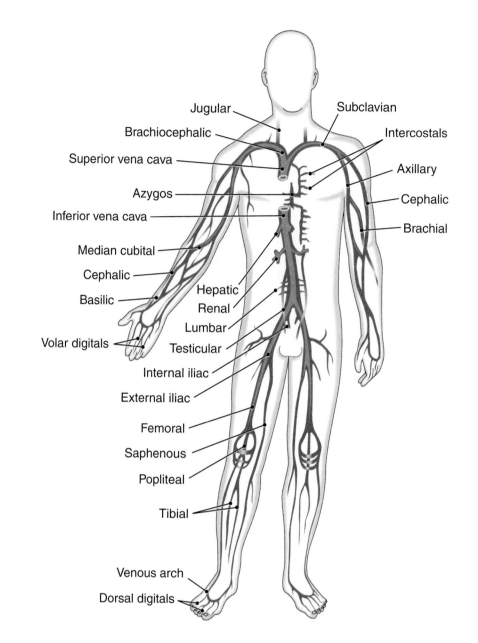

FIGURE 13.2 ■ Principal systemic veins. (Reprinted with permission from Cohen BJ and Wood DL. Memmler's The Human Body in Health and Disease, 9th Ed. Philadelphia: Lippincott Williams & Wilkins, 2000.)

Some of the more common blood and blood-forming organ diseases presented in this chapter include the following:

▶ anemias
▶ pancytopenia
▶ coagulopathies

Circulatory cancers invading blood (leukemia), lymphoid tissue (lymphoma), and bone marrow (myeloma) will be discussed in Chapter 14 of this textbook, "Coding for Neoplasms."

Diseases of the Circulatory System

The circulatory system is subdivided into a network that includes the cardiovascular, cerebrovascular, and peripheral vascular systems. The cardiovascular system (Figure 13.3) includes blood vessels that take blood to and from the heart and support internal organs (viscera), the cerebrovascular system takes blood to and from the brain, and the peripheral vascular system takes blood to and from the extremities. Blood carries oxygen, which is needed by all the cells of the body. Blockages in the cardiovascular, cerebrovascular, or peripheral vascular systems can cause tissue death. The most common cause of blockages of blood vessels is atherosclerosis (arteries become narrowed and clogged with fatty deposits).

Cardiovascular Disease

A cardiovascular disease is any disease of the blood vessels of the heart or a disorder that affects the flow of blood through the heart.

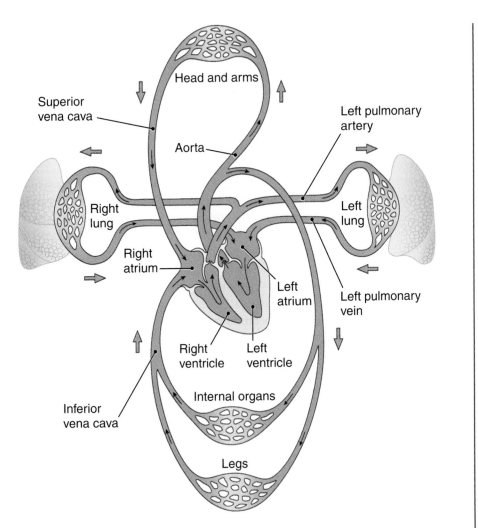

FIGURE 13.3 ■ The cardiovascular system. (Reprinted with permission from Cohen BJ and Wood DL. Memmler's The Human Body in Health and Disease, 9th Ed. Philadelphia: Lippincott Williams & Wilkins, 2000.)

ISCHEMIC HEART DISEASE

Ischemia occurs when there is a decreased blood supply to an area of the body (i.e., a holding back of blood). When blood is held back from cells, cell or tissue death (necrosis) occurs. Ischemic cardiovascular disease is particularly harmful because heart tissue that dies is not regenerative (i.e., it cannot repair itself or be restored). During an acute myocardial infarction (heart attack), necrosis of heart tissue occurs, and depending on the extent of myocardial damage, the infarcted tissue could heal as a scar or the patient could die. Morbidity (diseased condition) and mortality (death) resulting from heart disease are leading causes for hospital inpatient admissions in the United States.

For precise coding, it is helpful to recognize that ischemic heart disease can be organized into three general categories:

- ▶ chronic ischemic heart disease (e.g., coronary artery disease; coronary atherosclerosis)
- ▶ other acute and subacute forms of ischemic heart disease (e.g., unstable angina)
- ▶ acute ischemic heart disease (e.g., acute myocardial infarction)

Each general category can contain more specific cardiac conditions, and the prognosis (i.e., outcome or chance for survival) and treatment for the patient depend on the severity of the disease.

Chronic Ischemic Heart Disease   Chronic ischemic heart disease (category 414) can progress to more dangerous acute manifestations of the disease, such as an acute myocardial infarction (i.e., heart attack). Types of chronic ischemic heart disease that are commonly documented include coronary artery disease and arteriosclerotic or atherosclerotic heart disease.

Coronary artery disease is a nonspecific term that indicates any disorder of the arteries that supply oxygenated blood to the heart. Coronary artery disease is usually the result of narrowing and blocking of the coronary arteries by atherosclerosis. Arteriosclerosis involves hardening of the arteries, and atherosclerosis involves hardening of the arteries with fatty plaque.

Located under the chronic ischemic heart disease category 414 is subcategory 414.0X for coronary atherosclerosis (Figure 13.4). Coronary atherosclerosis provides a fifth-digit subclassification that describes whether atherosclerotic disease is affecting an unspecified coronary vessel (414.00), is affecting a native (one's own) coronary vessel (414.01), is the result of recurring atherosclerotic disease in a previously bypassed coronary vessel (414.02 to 414.05), is in a native coronary artery of a transplanted heart (414.06), or is in a bypassed coronary vessel of a transplanted heart (414.07).

Coronary artery bypass grafting is an operation in which veins (removed from one part of the body) or noncoronary arteries are used to bypass blocked areas of the coronary arteries. Essentially, the purpose of coronary artery bypass grafting is to return oxygenated blood flow to the heart. When arteriosclerotic or atherosclerotic heart disease occurs in a previously bypassed coronary vessel, do not assign a code for complications of surgical and medical care (996 to 999)—it is considered a recurrence of coronary atherosclerotic disease, and you should use codes 414.02 to 414.05.

If no history of a coronary artery bypass graft is documented in the patient's medical record, assign code 414.01, coronary artery disease affecting native vessels. However, with a documented history of a coronary artery

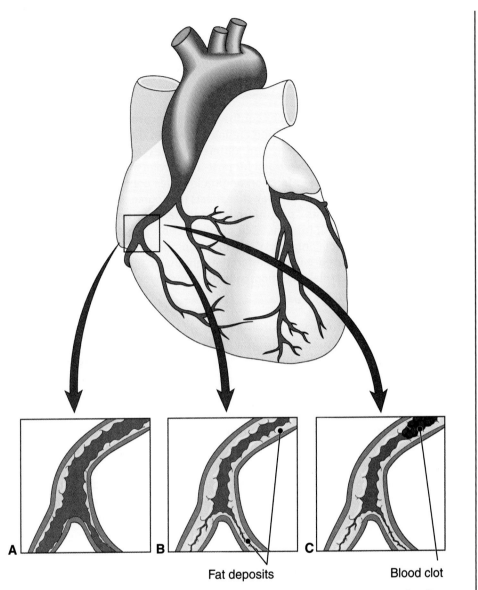

Fat deposits

Blood clot

FIGURE 13.4 ■ Coronary atherosclerosis. **A.** Fat deposits narrow an artery, leading to ischemia. **B.** Blockage (occlusion) of a coronary artery. **C.** Formation of a blood clot (thrombus), leading to myocardial infarction. (Reprinted with permission from Cohen BJ and Wood DL. Memmler's The Human Body in Health and Disease, 9th Ed. Philadelphia: Lippincott Williams & Wilkins, 2000.)

bypass graft, unless a diagnostic or operative procedure (e.g., heart catheterization) is performed during the current episode of care, you cannot determine whether a stated diagnosis of coronary artery disease involves a native vessel or the previously bypassed coronary vessel; therefore, assign code 414.00 (i.e., atherosclerotic heart disease of an unspecified type of vessel).

Other Acute and Subacute Forms of Ischemic Heart Disease and Angina   ICD-9-CM category 411 provides codes for other acute and subacute forms of ischemic heart disease, such as post-myocardial infarction syndrome, also known as Dressler's syndrome (code 411.0). A syndrome is a group of symptoms that together point to a particular disease. After a recent hospital admission for an acute myocardial infarction, a patient returning for care with symptoms that

may include fever, pericarditis (inflammation of the membrane that surrounds the heart), increased white blood cell count, pleuritic pain (chest pain
that occurs with breathing), and pneumonia could indicate a diagnosis of
post-myocardial infarction syndrome (i.e., Dressler's syndrome).

Coders sometimes confuse "post-myocardial infarction syndrome"
with "postinfarc-tion angina"; however, this does not represent the
same condition, and different codes are assigned. Unlike the
symptoms described for post-myocardial infarction syndrome (code
411.0), postinfarction angina involves continuing chest pain after
myocardial infarction that affects the course of care. When a physician
documents "postinfarction angina," assign code 413.9 (angina
pectoris); for "unstable postinfarction angina," assign code 411.1
(unstable angina). When documentation indicates that a patient was
admitted with preinfarction angina that progressed to an acute
myocardial infarction, code the acute myocardial infarction only.

Intermediate coronary syndrome (code 411.1) is more often documented
by physicians as "unstable angina," "crescendo angina," "preinfarction
angina," "new-onset (initial) angina," or "angina at rest." It is characterized
by severe chest pain from an acute anginal episode that does not respond to
conventional medical therapy (e.g., oral medications such as sublingual nitroglycerin) and is not relieved by patient rest or relaxation.

Acute coronary occlusion (thrombus) without myocardial infarction
(code 411.81) or acute coronary insufficiency or acute subendocardial
ischemia (code 411.89) may demonstrate initial findings suggesting that a
possible acute myocardial infarction occurred. Increased creatine phosphoki-
nase-myocardial band or troponin I and T laboratory values reveal enzymes or
muscle proteins that indicate infarcted (i.e., dead) heart muscle tissue. Also,
an abnormal electrocardiogram (abbreviated ECG or EKG), which is used to
record the electricity in the heart, can reveal cardiac damage. However, after
study, the initial abnormal values or readings classified to other acute and
subacute forms of ischemic heart disease do not demonstrate the permanent
damage to the heart that would result from an acute myocardial infarction.

Angina pectoris (code 413.9) is chest pain often associated with underlying coronary artery disease. Unlike unstable angina, conventional treatments
such as the administration of nitroglycerin and patient rest relieve angina
pectoris. Nitroglycerin is a vasodilator, a substance that opens or widens coronary vessels to bring more blood to the heart to relieve the chest pain associated with angina. Nitroglycerin is given as a sublingual tablet (under the
tongue), as a paste on the chest, or as an intravenous infusion. List coronary
artery disease as the principal diagnosis when it is documented as the underlying cause for angina.

Coding Clinic 1997, second quarter, describes more information
regarding coronary artery disease with angina.

Stable angina is a comorbid condition that is treated with medications. It is
often sequenced as an additional (secondary) diagnosis code. Remember, a

comorbid condition is a preexisting condition that was not the reason for admission, but its presence affects the patient's course of care. Therefore, as defined in Uniform Hospital Discharge Data Set (UHDDS) rules, it is reportable.

Acute Ischemic Heart Disease   An acute myocardial infarction (i.e., a heart attack) is an acute ischemic cardiac event that is usually the result of progressive coronary artery disease such as coronary atherosclerosis (hardening of the arteries with fatty plaque), arteriosclerosis (hardening of the arteries), or coronary artery thrombosis (clot formation). These conditions cause coronary artery occlusive disease (ischemia) that can result in an acute myocardial infarction (i.e., an area of infarcted [dead] myocardial tissue).

Code an acute myocardial infarction to category 410. The fourth digit indicates the area of the heart affected by the infarction. For example, 410.41 describes an infarction of the inferior wall (lower portion of the heart wall), and 410.51 describes an infarction of a lateral wall (side of the heart). If the physician documents an acute "non-Q-wave myocardial infarction," you should code it to a subendocardial myocardial infarction (code 410.7X; i.e., an infarction that does not involve the full thickness of the heart wall—just beneath the endocardium, the innermost layer of heart tissue). The fifth-digit subclassification indicates whether this is the initial episode of patient care (fifth digit: 1) for the acute myocardial infarction or a subsequent admission (fifth digit: 2), meaning that the patient had been previously discharged but is now being readmitted within a period of less than 8 weeks from the initial infarction. For example, code 410.41 indicates the initial admission for acute inferior wall myocardial infarction, whereas 410.42 indicates that the patient had been discharged but is now being readmitted less than 8 weeks from the initial myocardial infarction.

Code the acute myocardial infarction as the principal diagnosis in cases in which it is documented that "preinfarction angina" or an "evolving acute myocardial infarction" progresses to the acute infarction. However, if the evolving infarction is prevented (i.e., through early intervention with thrombolytic drugs such as streptokinase or tissue plasminogen activator), code the underlying condition, such as coronary artery disease with preinfarction angina (unstable), as an additional code. Thrombolytic drugs use enzymes that help to dissolve clots.

If a patient experiences an extension of an infarct in which more than one area is affected, assign codes for the separate sites affected unless the Disease Tabular provides a combination code (single code) that describes both sites.

Acute inferolateral wall myocardial infarction: 410.21 (combination code)

Acute anterior and inferior wall myocardial infarction: 410.11 + 410.41 (two codes required)

EXAMPLE

Physicians will sometimes document **acute coronary syndrome** (ACS) that may need further clarification to determine whether this should be coded as an acute myocardial infarction (AMI) or to unstable angina. Patients with acute coronary syndrome can be classified into three categories that include: 1) unstable angina (411.1); 2) Non-ST segment elevation myocardial infarction (410.7x); or 3) ST-segment elevation myocardial infarction (all other codes within AMI category 410). Therefore, if a physician has documented the diagnosis of acute coronary syndrome, review the patient's cardiac enzymes/ Troponin level to determine if it is abnormal. If cardiac enzymes/Troponin are elevated, a query to the physician is needed to determine if the "ACS" was consistent with an acute myocardial infarction or that of unstable angina. If myocardial infarction was ruled-in, then the physician will need to add documentation indicating that the "acute coronary syndrome" was consistent with an acute myocardial infarction.

An old myocardial infarction or a history of myocardial infarction is coded to 412 and is used as an additional code to describe a significant coronary history. It would never be appropriate to use code 412 as a principal diagnosis.

Hypotension (i.e., low blood pressure) associated with an acute myocardial infarction is particularly complicated and can cause instability in an acute myocardial infarction patient. However, some acute myocardial infarction patients are hypertensive (i.e., high blood pressure) on admission and are given drugs to control their hypertension; this can result in iatrogenic hypotension. The term iatrogenic means that the condition results from the treatment of physicians or caregivers. If the hypotension was secondary to drugs given to the patient, assign code 458.29 (iatrogenic hypotension). However, if the patient experiences hypotension that is related to the acute myocardial infarction but not to the medications given, then assign code 458.8.

Procedures for Ischemic Heart Disease

Heart Catheterization. A left and/or right heart catheterization (codes 37.21 to 37.23) is a diagnostic cardiac procedure. During this procedure, a catheter is placed into a patient's vein, artery, or both and is guided into coronary vessels to evaluate whether they are supplying enough oxygenated blood to the heart. Additional cardiac measurements to evaluate blood flow and pressures are performed to determine whether there is evidence for ischemic heart disease or other heart dysfunction. The physician usually places the catheter in the superficial femoral vein to perform a right heart catheterization and into the superficial femoral artery to perform a left heart catheterization.

If the physician has documented only "heart cath" in the procedure note, carefully review the notes for the procedural approach to clarify the coding of left and/or right heart catheterization. The right heart will be accessed through a vein and the left heart through an artery; therefore, determining the procedural approach can help you to identify whether a left and/or right heart catheterization was performed.

Left heart catheterizations or left and right catheterizations are routinely performed in adults, in whom a disorder of the left side of the heart (i.e., left ventricle) is a more common concern. You should also be aware that a coronary angiography with contrast (88.5X), which provides a distinct picture of the coronary vessels, routinely accompanies a heart catheterization procedure and requires additional codes.

Be careful if a doctor documents only "right heart catheterization" in an adult. Physicians will often use the terms **right heart catheterization** and **Swan-Ganz catheterization** interchangeably. Although this is not technically incorrect, the main purpose of performing a Swan-Ganz catheterization (89.64) is to monitor the hemodynamic status of a critically ill patient. In contrast, the main purpose of a right heart catheterization is diagnostic—to evaluate structural defects or dysfunction of the heart. Right heart catheterization is often performed on children suspected of having congenital heart disease, such as atrial or ventricular septal defects, in which shunting of blood occurs between the right and left chambers of the heart. The coding of right heart catheterization can affect diagnosis-related group (MS-DRG) reimbursement to the provider, and this makes it an area of special concern.

Percutaneous Transluminal Coronary Angioplasty or Atherectomy. Starting Oct. 1, 2005, new codes were provided to classify PTCAs and related procedures. A percutaneous transluminal coronary angioplasty or atherectomy (PTCA code 00.66) is a therapeutic procedure performed to treat arteriosclerotic or atherosclerotic heart disease. In this procedure, a catheter with a balloon is maneuvered to a stenosed (narrowed) or thrombosed (clotted) area of a coronary vessel and inflated to open up the affected area and return blood flow (Figure 13.5). In a percutaneous coronary atherectomy, atherosclerotic (fatty) plaque is removed from the inner lining of the vessel by using a device resembling a corkscrew at the tip of the catheter. Sometimes PTCA also involves the placement of a stent device (slotted tube) in the affected area to keep the artery patent (open). Stent placement requires an additional code, 36.06. To perform a PTCA, the coronary vessel must be suitable for this less invasive surgery (i.e., the vessel is accessible and nontortuous; PTCA is less invasive than coronary artery bypass grafting). Note that a more current terminology for percutaneous transluminal coronary angioplasty (PTCA) is **percutaneous coronary intervention** (PCI). Many physicians are now using these terms or abbreviations interchangeably.

A new procedure that accompanies PTCAs is drug-eluting coronary stent placement. Drug-eluting stents contain an active drug that is released after placement. The drug is applied on the surface of the stent and is released over time to reduce the chance of a recurring stenosis of the artery. Drug-eluting stents are not the same as drug-coated or -covered stents, which do not release drugs but are coated with a substance such as heparin to prevent platelets (clotting cells) from forming on the stent. A drug-coated or drug-covered coronary stent is coded to 36.06, whereas a drug-eluting stent is coded to 36.07. The insertion of drug-eluting coronary stents versus other stent placements can change the MS-DRG assignment and, therefore, the reimbursement to the hospital. When there is doubt, you should always verify the precise type of stent that was inserted, either through a physician query or intensive review of the record for manufacturer's information.

As of October 1, 2005, additional code(s) are assigned to indicate 1) the total number of vessels that underwent angioplasty/athrectomy (00.40–00.43) and 2) the total number of stents placed during the procedure

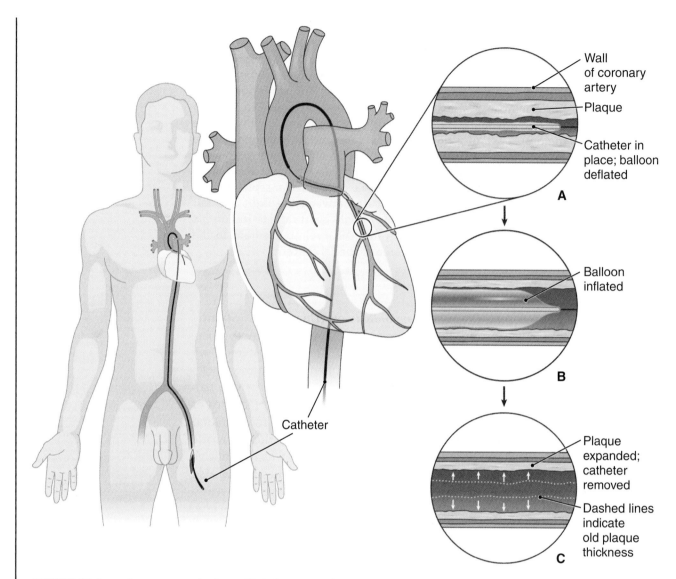

FIGURE 13.5 ■ Coronary angioplasty (PTCA). **A.** A guide catheter is threaded into the coronary artery. **B.** A balloon catheter is inserted through the occlusion. **C.** The balloon is inflated and deflated until plaque is flattened and the vessel is opened. (Reprinted with permission from Cohen BJ. Medical Terminology: An Illustrated Guide, 4th Ed. Baltimore: Lippincott Williams & Wilkins, 2004.)

(00.45–00.48). Remember, the number of vessels undergoing PCI does NOT have to equal the number of stents placed (e.g.- PCI of one vessel with one non-drug eluting stent and one drug eluting stent = 00.66 + 36.06 + 36.07 + 00.40 + 00.46; PTCA of two vessels with one drug-eluting stent = 00.66 + 36.07 + 00.41 + 00.45). As of October 1, 2006 coding changes, an additional code (00.44) was provided to indicate if a procedure was done on a bifurcated vessel (i.e., "branched" such as a femoral bifurcation). This is because a procedure on bifurcated vessels requires more time and resources when compared to procedures on straight vessels. This code can be assigned only once per operative episode regardless of the number of bifurcations present, and it solely describes the presence of a vessel bifurcation, not a specific bifurcation stent.

EXAMPLE

A patient with atherosclerotic coronary artery disease with unstable angina has a single-vessel PCI with drug-eluting stent placement performed: 414.01, 411.1; 00.66, 36.07, 00.40, 00.45

A patient with atherosclerotic coronary artery disease with unstable angina has a three-vessel PCI with stent placement and thrombolytic infusion performed: 414.01, 411.1; 00.66, 36.06, 00.42, 00.45, 99.10

Coders sometimes confuse a PTCA with a percutaneous transluminal angioplasty (PTA) procedure. The latter is a similar procedure that is performed on peripheral vessels (of the extremities) rather than coronary vessels.

Intra-aortic Balloon Pump. An intra-aortic balloon pump insertion (code 37.61) is an invasive cardiovascular procedure in which a specialized catheter with a balloon attached is inserted into the thoracic aorta. Inflations of the balloon are timed to increase coronary perfusion (blood circulation). An intra-aortic balloon pump is an emergent temporary measure used to maintain perfusion of the heart and systemic circulation in an unstable patient with an occluded (blocked) coronary vessel (i.e., evolving infarction) or a dissected coronary vessel that can result as a post-PTCA tear complication, until coronary artery bypass or other open-heart procedures can be performed. Intra-aortic balloon pump (code 37.61) can be located in the Procedure Index under the main term "implantation; pulsation balloon."

Coronary Artery Bypass Graft. Main right and left coronary arteries leave the aorta (the largest artery in the body) and lead to the surface of the heart, where they branch out to provide oxygenated blood (coming from the lungs) to the heart. Atherosclerotic heart disease can progress to coronary artery occlusion and subsequent myocardial infarction. A coronary artery bypass graft is an invasive open-heart procedure to bypass blocked coronary vessels, restore the flow of blood to the heart, and prevent future myocardial damage (Figure 13.6). Coronary artery bypass graft codes include the following:

▶ aortocoronary bypass (vessel bypass from the aorta to the heart) is performed to bypass the occluded coronary vessel, typically by using a harvested saphenous donor vein (from the thigh; codes 36.10 to 36.14)

▶ internal mammary artery (single or double) or other artery bypass is used as a conduit that does not use the aorta but instead uses a noncoronary artery that is rerouted past the occluded coronary vessel to perfuse the heart (36.15 to 36.17)

There are several vascular branches off the main right and left coronary arteries. Some branches (coronary blood vessels) that are often bypassed include the left anterior descending, left circumflex, posterior descending, obtuse marginal, and diagonal arteries. You can locate coronary artery bypass graft codes in the Procedure Index under the main terms "bypass, aortocoronary" and "bypass, internal-mammary-coronary artery."

Extracorporeal circulation, also called **cardiopulmonary bypass** (code 39.61), is assigned as an additional code to the bypass. Extracorporeal circulation

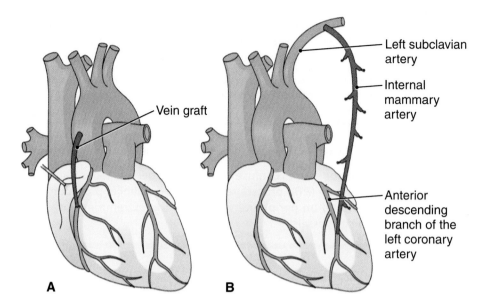

FIGURE 13.6 ■ Coronary artery bypass graft (CABG). **A.** A segment of the saphenous vein carries blood from the aorta to a part of the right coronary artery that is distal to an occlusion. **B.** The mammary artery is used to bypass an obstruction in the left anterior descending coronary artery. (Reprinted with permission from Cohen BJ. Medical Terminology: An Illustrated Guide, 4th Ed. Baltimore: Lippincott Williams & Wilkins, 2004.)

enables the patient's blood to keep circulating while the cardiovascular surgeon operates on the heart. Procedures considered an integral part of the coronary artery bypass graft, such as temporary pacemaker placement, cardioplegia (temporarily stopping the heart to operate), and hypothermia (cooling the body to reduce metabolic demands), are usually not assigned as separate codes.

EXAMPLE

A patient is admitted with unstable angina secondary to severe multivessel atherosclerotic occlusive coronary artery disease. Surgery performed included aortocoronary bypass to the left anterior descending artery, left circumflex artery, and posterior descending artery with a harvested saphenous vein graft and one internal mammary artery, with cardiopulmonary bypass, temporary pacemaker insertion, cardioplegia, and hypothermia: 414.01, 411.1; 36.13, 36.15, 39.61

HEART FAILURE

Heart failure occurs when the heart pumps an inadequate amount of blood to support the needs of the body. In left-sided heart failure (code 428.1), blood pools (i.e., backs up) in the lungs and causes pulmonary edema (fluid in the lungs). Left-sided heart failure can progress to right- and left-sided heart failure, called congestive heart failure (CHF; also referred to as **biventricular heart failure** because both the right and left heart ventricles fail). Because CHF (code 428.0) is one of the most common diagnoses among elderly people in the United States, you should be aware of its symptoms.

Congestive Heart Failure   On physical examination, physicians will document hearing **rales** (i.e., a wet "crackling" sound) on auscultation (listening with a stethoscope) from the pulmonary edema associated with CHF. CHF also causes venous congestion from the back-pressure of the heart with subsequent jugular venous distention (the jugular veins on the neck enlarge and engorge with blood), pitting edema in the lower extremities, and shortness of breath. Also, lungs fill with fluid when CHF patients lie flat; therefore, the patient must prop up with pillows to breathe more easily. The physician often documents this as two-/three-pillow orthopnea.

A lack of clarity in physicians' documentation can sometimes result in a coding error in which the code for **noncardiac** acute pulmonary edema (518.4) or pulmonary edema not otherwise specified (514) is incorrectly assigned when the condition of pulmonary edema associated with heart failure should have been reported (category 428). Coders should note that pulmonary edema, whether documented as acute or not, needs clarification and is a condition often caused by the inability of the heart to pump the blood that the body needs, thus causing CHF. The documentation of "pulmonary edema" or "acute pulmonary edema" by the physician without further specificity is a red flag for coders because physicians often intend this to mean CHF. According to the ICD-9-CM Disease Index, acute pulmonary edema with heart disease or failure is coded to the heart failure code (428.X) only. No additional code is assigned for the pulmonary edema.

You should always review the physician's progress notes, chest radiographs, and any consultant notes to clarify the coding of pulmonary edema. Also, be sure to adequately review the Disease Index to avoid mistakenly coding left heart failure (code 428.1) when the patient has CHF (code 428.0). Within the *Alphabetic Index to Diseases*, locate the main term "edema; pulmonary," which refers you to "edema; lung acute, with mention of heart disease or failure," which assigns the left heart failure code (428.1). A further review of the indented subterms in the *Alphabetic Index to Diseases* and properly reviewing the code in the *Tabular List of Diseases* will show that CHF is coded to 428.0.

TIP Coding Clinic 1988, third quarter, describes more information about acute pulmonary edema with heart disease or failure.

Compensated CHF is a comorbid condition treated with medications. As defined in UHDDS rules, compensated CHF is sequenced as an additional (secondary) code because it affects the care of the patient. A common medication used to control CHF is furosemide (Lasix), a diuretic (which causes urination) that reduces volume overload (fluid retention) and edema, making it easier for the heart to pump blood. Another medication used is digitalis (digoxin; Lanoxin), a cardiotonic, which is a drug that causes the heart to contract more forcefully.

Decompensated CHF means that the patient has an acute exacerbated (severe) CHF episode that may be coded as a principal or a secondary diagnosis, depending on the circumstances of admission.

Below are additional heart failure subcategory codes:

▶ 428.2X describes systolic heart failure (failure of the left ventricle to contract forcefully)

▶ 428.3X describes diastolic heart failure (failure of the left ventricle to relax and fill adequately with blood)

▶ 428.4X describes combined systolic and diastolic heart failure

The fifth-digit subclassification with the subcategory codes 428.2 to 428.4 describes whether the heart failure is unspecified, acute, chronic, or combined acute and chronic.

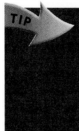

TIP

With the onset of MS-DRGs, it is important that the physician documents the specific type of heart failure, as this detail may effect the payment to the hospital. Nonspecified congestive heart failure (CHF code 428.0) is not classified as a C/C or MCC; whereas, more acute forms of heart failure (e.g., acute diastolic heart failure code 428.31) are classified as MCCs with chronic forms of heart failure (e.g., chronic diastolic heart failure code 428.32) classified as C/Cs. This can significantly change the reimbursement to the hospital, and a physician query may be necessary for precise code assignment.

Heart failure can result from chronic uncontrolled hypertension or high blood pressure. If prolonged and untreated, hypertension can cause the left ventricle of the heart to apply more force during contraction. Because the heart is a muscle, the left ventricle enlarges (i.e., left ventricular hypertrophy) in response to the increased ventricular force necessary to pump blood. Over time, the left ventricle becomes bulky and inflexible and can no longer contract forcefully; this results in heart failure. This condition results in hypertensive cardiovascular disease (code 402.9X). Code 402.9X includes a fifth digit that describes whether it is with (402.91) or without (402.90) heart failure. You must use an additional code with code 402.91 to specify the type of heart failure.

Do not automatically assume a relationship between heart disease and hypertension. A causal relationship between the two must be documented by the physician with terms such as "due to," "secondary to," or "hypertensive cardiovascular disease" for you to code hypertensive heart disease category 402.9X. (Hypertension is covered in depth later in this chapter.)

ARRHYTHMIAS AND HEART BLOCKS

The heart is a muscle often referred to as a double pump. During pulmonary circulation (pump 1), the heart pumps oxygen-poor blood from the right side of the heart to the lungs, where it picks up oxygen and enters the left side of the heart. During systemic circulation (pump 2), the heart pumps oxygen-rich blood from the left side of the heart through the aorta to all parts of the body. Electrical stimulation causes a mechanical contraction of the heart muscle, which consists of four chambers: two upper atria and two lower ventricles. The normal electrical pacemaker of the heart is the sinoatrial node, located near the right upper atrium of the heart. The sinoatrial node initiates an electrical impulse to start the heart (atria) contracting to pump or circulate blood. In a normal heart, the atrioventricular node delays the impulses transmitted from the sinoatrial node to allow the ventricles time to respond (contract). From the atrioventricular node, the impulse passes through the bundle of His/Purkinje network (nerve conduction fibers that cause the heart ventricles to contract). The intrinsic (naturally occurring) electrical impulses from the sinoatrial node measure 60 to 100 per minute. The intrinsic electrical impulses from the atrioventricular nodal area measure 40 to 60 per minute, and the ventricular impulses through the bundle of His/Purkinje network measure 20 to 40 per minute.

The conduction of the heart is evaluated in an electrocardiogram. The P wave represents atrial depolarization (active electrical state to contract atria), the large QRS wave represents ventricular depolarization (active electrical state to contract ventricles), and the T wave represents ventricular repolarization (electrical and ventricular resting state; Figure 13.7).

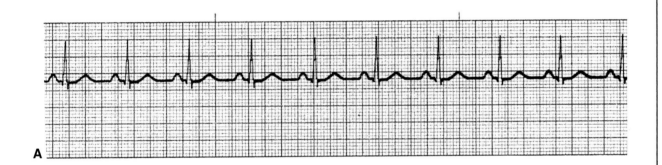

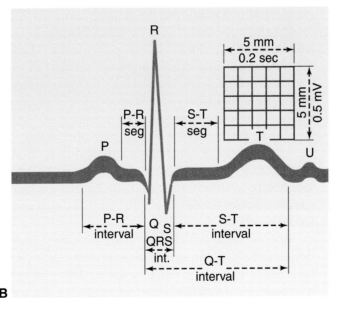

FIGURE 13.7 ■ **A.** An ECG tracing showing normal sinus rhythm. **B.** Commonly measured components of an ECG tracing. (Reprinted with permission from Smeltzer SC, Bare BG. Brunner & Suddarth's Textbook of Medical-Surgical Nursing, 9th Ed. Philadelphia: Lippincott Williams & Wilkins, 2000.)

The sinoatrial node paces the heart because it transmits the fastest intrinsic rate of 60 to 100 impulses per minute. Sinus rhythm is a normal heart rhythm in which the sinus node is initiating the electrical impulse. In the condition known as **sinus bradycardia**, the sinoatrial node initiates the impulse, but the heart rate is slower than 60 bpm. Sinus bradycardia can be a normal response during sleep and is common among conditioned athletes. **Sinus tachycardia** is a condition in which the sinoatrial node initiates the impulse at more than 100 impulses per minute. A fast heart rate can be normal during running or other vigorous activity. It can also result from stimulation of the fight-or-flight response as a reaction to stress or from drinking caffeine.

Arrhythmias In contrast to normal sinus rhythms, arrhythmias are abnormal heart rhythms in which local irritated heart tissue in the atrial or ventricular region of the heart sends out impulses faster that the sinoatrial node, thereby taking over as the pacer for the heart. For example, in atrial fibrillation, the atrial area of the heart may initiate more than 350 impulses per minute. If atrial fibrillation is uncontrolled, drugs and/or electrical cardioversion (defibrillation) are needed to return the patient's heart to a normal sinus rhythm.

People with chronic atrial fibrillation may be prescribed long-term anticoagulant therapy (e.g., warfarin [Coumadin], a blood thinner) to help prevent emboli (traveling clots). Chronic atrial fibrillation is a comorbid condition that is reported because it must be treated with medications. As defined within UHDDS rules, it is sequenced as an additional code because its presence affects the care of the patient.

Ventricular arrhythmia (e.g., ventricular fibrillation, ventricular flutter, or ventricular tachycardia) means that rapid electrical impulses are being initiated from the ventricular area of the heart. Sustained ventricular arrhythmias are referred to as **malignant arrhythmias** because they can be life-threatening. Ventricular fibrillation results in electrical chaos in the heart, producing impulses so rapid that they cannot be measured by taking a pulse. No systemic circulation is possible, so the patient has only 3 to 4 minutes before anoxic encephalopathy occurs (i.e., death of brain cells caused by the lack of oxygen from circulating blood), followed by death. Those who survive instances of ventricular fibrillation are sometimes referred to as **sudden-death survivors**.

Electrophysiologic study (code 37.26) is a diagnostic test often performed to diagnose ventricular fibrillation. Electrophysiologic study is a heart conduction test to evaluate the patient's potential for expressing malignant ventricular arrhythmias (e.g., ventricular fibrillation).

In a malignant ventricular arrhythmia such as ventricular fibrillation, an automatic external defibrillator (AED) can be applied to the chest that provides electric shocks to restart the heart in a sinus rhythm. These electrical countershocks (joules) are referred to as **external electrical cardioversion** (code 99.62).

Because time is a critical factor with ventricular arrhythmias, an internal device called an automatic implantable cardioverter/defibrillator (AICD) can be implanted in the chest to sense and reverse ventricular arrhythmias in at-risk patients. An AICD is mechanically similar to a permanent cardiac pacemaker in that it includes a pulse generator and leads. However, unlike a cardiac pacemaker, which overrides an arrhythmia or heart block, the AICD senses and responds to malignant ventricular arrhythmia only when this is needed. The initial insertion of a total cardioverter/defibrillator system (generator and leads) is coded to 37.94. If the pulse generator or leads are inserted during separate episodes in a staged procedure, then the placement of the leads is coded to 37.95, and the placement of the pulse generator is coded to 37.96. You can locate these codes in the Procedure Index under the main term "implantation, cardioverter/defibrillator."

If a patient is admitted for an adjustment or scheduled replacement of a worn-out AICD pulse generator, assign code V53.32 as the principal diagnosis. V53.32 can be located in the Disease Index under the main term "admission for, adjustment, cardiac device, defibrillator, automatic implantable." The procedure code for the implantation or replacement of a total AICD (code 37.94) can be located in the Procedure Index under the main term "replacement, cardioverter/defibrillator (total system)." Also, listed as subterms are the replacement of leads only (37.97) or of the pulse generator only (37.98). Complications of AICD (i.e., mechanical, infection, or other) will be covered in Chapter 18 of this text: "Complications of Surgical and Medical Care."

You should be aware that there is a difference between an admission for a "firing" and "misfiring" of an AICD. The normal functioning of an AICD causes the device to fire if the patient develops a ventricular arrhythmia. Because of the seriousness of the arrhythmia, patients are admitted to the hospital for evaluation, in which case the arrhythmia code would be sequenced as the principal diagnosis, with V45.02 (cardiac device in situ, defibrillator, automatic implantable) listed as an additional code. An admission for the misfiring of an AICD is coded to a mechanical complication of an AICD (code 996.04).

Heart Block and Tachy-Brady Syndrome   There are many different types of heart block, and some are more severe than others. For example, in a first-, second-, or third-degree atrioventricular heart block, the normal conduction of impulses from the sinoatrial node through the atrioventricular node is either delayed or blocked at the atrioventricular node. A third-degree atrioventricular heart block (code 426.0) is the most severe in that the electrical impulses from the sinoatrial node are completely blocked through the atrioventricular node. Subsequently, the heart functions at the inherent (natural or native) ventricular rate of 20 to 40 impulses per minute, which can cause faintness (syncope) because of the low heart rate and cardiac output. Third-degree atrioventricular block, also called complete heart block, requires the insertion of a permanent cardiac pacemaker to override an inherent (native) pacer dysfunction.

Sinoatrial node dysfunction (also called *tachy-brady syndrome* or *sick sinus syndrome*; code 427.81) is an arrhythmia that requires insertion of a permanent cardiac pacemaker. Medication can be given to speed up the heart in bradycardia or to slow the heart in tachycardia. However, no known medication can adequately respond to a syndrome in which the patient's heart invariably alternates between a slow and fast heart rate. A cardiac pacemaker device is needed to override an intrinsic pacer dysfunction.

CARDIAC PACEMAKERS

External temporary cardiac pacemaker placement (pacer placed outside the body; code 37.78) accompanies electric countershock of the heart to convert an abnormal heart rhythm (e.g., atrial fibrillation) to a normal sinus rhythm. Atrial cardioversion and other electric countershock procedures of the heart are coded to 99.61 and 99.62, respectively. A temporary intraoperative cardiac pacemaker insertion (code 39.64) is considered integral to invasive open-heart surgery and is usually not coded.

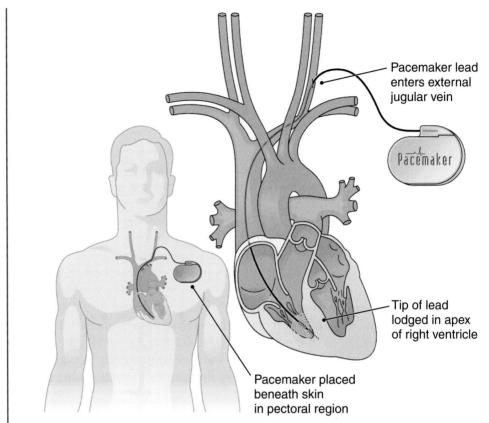

FIGURE 13.8 ◼ Placement of a pacemaker. (Reprinted with permission from Cohen BJ. Medical Terminology: An Illustrated Guide, 4th Ed. Baltimore: Lippincott Williams & Wilkins, 2004.)

Internal permanent cardiac pacemaker placement requires two codes: a code for subcutaneous insertion of the pulse generator (37.80 to 37.83) and a code for inserting the cardiac pacemaker leads (i.e., electrode codes 37.70 to 37.74). The pulse generator is implanted subcutaneously in the chest wall, and the pacemaker leads can be placed on the surface of the heart (epicardial) or within the heart (intra-atrial and/or intraventricular; Figure 13.8). If a pacemaker is specified as a single-chamber device, it requires one lead; a dual-chamber device requires two leads (e.g., atrioventricular lead placement).

Insertion of a cardiac pacemaker can be located in the Procedure Index under the main term "insertion, pacemaker, cardiac," and the insertion of leads can be located under the main term "insertion, electrodes, heart." A common coding error occurs when incompatible codes are assigned for the pulse generator and lead insertion (e.g., incorrectly assigning a code for a single lead insertion with a dual-chamber device, which requires two leads) or when the pulse generator is inserted without the associated lead insertion. This will adversely affect the DRG payment assignment.

EXAMPLE	*A patient is admitted with sick sinus syndrome and has an insertion of a rate-responsive single-chamber cardiac pacemaker device with atrial lead placement: 427.81; 37.82 + 37.73*
	A patient is admitted with a syncopal episode secondary to a complete heart block and has an insertion of a dual-chamber cardiac pacemaker with atrioventricular lead placement: 426.0; 37.83 + 37.72

A cardiac pacemaker battery usually lasts approximately 5 years, and at the end of that time a patient may be admitted for "pacemaker end of life," which means that the pulse generator that includes the battery must be replaced. For admission for pacemaker end of life, assign code V53.31 as the principal diagnosis. You can locate V53.31 in the Disease Index under the main term "admission for; adjustment, pacemaker, cardiac." You can locate the procedure code for the replacement of the pacemaker device (37.85 to 37.87) in the Procedure Index under the main term "replacement; pacemaker, cardiac device." Complications of a cardiac pacemaker (i.e., mechanical, infection, or other) will be covered in Chapter 18 of this text: "Complications of Surgical and Medical Care."

HYPERTENSION

Hypertension is also known as high blood pressure. Blood pressure describes the physical force that circulating blood exerts on arterial walls. Blood pressure is expressed as a fraction (e.g., 120/60 mm Hg), where the top number represents systolic pressure (when the heart ventricles are contracting and pushing blood) and the bottom number represents diastolic pressure (when the heart ventricles are relaxing and filling with blood). Hypertension is characterized by a systolic pressure of more than 140 or diastolic pressure of more than 90. However, a diagnosis of hypertension is not made with a single reading, but from a series of readings of 140/90 mm Hg or more over time.

Hypertension is a prevalent condition that will be encountered frequently by the beginning coder. Hypertension greatly increases an individual's chance of having a stroke and heart disease. According to the American Heart Association, approximately half of the people who have a first heart attack and two thirds who have a first stroke have high blood pressure; moreover, one quarter of the adult population has high blood pressure[1]. The National Center for Health Statistics estimates that in 2001, the number of hypertension-related deaths was approximately 19,250; this represented 8.7 deaths per 100,000 population[2]. Available data indicate that hypertension is a serious and expanding health problem; it is the coder's responsibility to accurately code hypertension-related conditions to make it possible to retrieve patient data for research studies that advance care for the disease.

The Hypertension Table in the Disease Index of the ICD-9-CM gives you quick access to many conditions that are associated with hypertension. The table classifies hypertension into benign, malignant, and unspecified. Doctors rarely describe benign hypertension, and you should not assume that unspecified hypertension is benign. Hypertension without further specificity is coded to unspecified (401.9). Malignant hypertension, also called **accelerated hypertension**, is a serious medical condition that can result in the bursting of an artery, such as in a hemorrhagic stroke (CVA) with infarction. Symptoms often associated with a possible diagnosis of malignant (accelerated) hypertension include papilledema (swelling of the optic disc associated with increased intracranial pressure) and a history of spontaneous epistaxis (nosebleeds associated with capillary hemorrhages).

Be sure to code physician documentation of "uncontrolled hypertension" to hypertension unspecified (code 401.9). Do not assume or code uncontrolled hypertension to accelerated (malignant) hypertension without further documentation from the physician. Also code hypertensive crisis to hypertension, unspecified, unless the physician has documented it as malignant or accelerated.

Primary Versus Secondary Hypertension ICD-9-CM classifies hypertension by type (primary and secondary). Primary hypertension, also called **essential** or **idiopathic**, is the most common type of hypertension, and the cause is unknown. Hypertension is sometimes referred to as the "silent killer" because it can go unnoticed and untreated for years, resulting in damage to organs such as the heart and kidneys (hypertensive heart and renal disease). As described previously, it is best for coders to recognize that primary hypertension can cause disease. For example, over time, untreated hypertension can cause left ventricular hypertrophy (enlargement) in the heart. This is because of the increasing force the left ventricle must exert to push blood against the peripheral resistance caused by the high blood pressure. Against resistance, the left ventricle will gradually enlarge, become muscle bound, and lose contractility. In time, this can lead to CHF, in which the heart can no longer provide adequate blood to support the body's needs.

Whereas primary hypertension can cause disease (e.g., left ventricular hypertrophy), other disease states can also cause secondary hypertension (category 405). As a classic example of secondary hypertension, if one has renal artery stenosis, there would be a decreased blood flow to the kidneys, and the kidneys would respond with an increase in their release of renin. Renin is a hormone that causes arterioles to constrict to increase blood pressure (e.g., hypertension, secondary to renal artery stenosis: 440.1 + 405.91).

To establish hypertensive heart disease, the physician must document causation (e.g., heart disease attributable to hypertension: category 402). However, ICD-9-CM assumes a relationship between a diagnosis of hypertension and renal disease, and causation does not have to be stated (e.g., hypertension and renal failure: 403.90). Any time a patient has both a condition classifiable to category code 402 (e.g., heart disease attributable to hypertension) and a condition classifiable to category code 403 (e.g., hypertension and renal disease), assign a code from category 404 (hypertensive heart and renal disease). The fifth digit describes the presence of heart failure, renal failure, or both. If heart failure is present, an additional code must be added that denotes the specific type of heart failure.

EXAMPLE *Hypertensive cardiovascular disease with CHF and chronic renal failure: 404.91 + 428.0 + 585.9*

CHF, CKD, Stage V and hypertension : 428.0 + 403.91 + 585.5

You should be aware that an increased blood pressure reading (code 796.2) without a diagnosis of hypertension does not indicate a diagnosis of hypertension. Never code an increased blood pressure reading as a principal diagnosis, and code it as an additional diagnosis only if the physician has documented its significance for follow-up and continued monitoring.

HEART VALVE DISORDERS

There are four valves in the heart (tricuspid, pulmonary, mitral, and aortic), all of which prevent the backflow of blood. Conditions (nonrheumatic) affecting these valves—including stenosis, regurgitation, insufficiency, prolapse, and incompetence—are contained within category 424. However, category 396 uses a combination code to describe multiple involvement (disorders) of mitral and aortic valves, whether specified as attributable to rheumatic heart disease or not.

ICD-9-CM assumes that mitral valve stenosis (394.0) and tricuspid valve disorders (397.0) are rheumatic if unspecified. Because there is much confusion over these diagnoses, the best course is not to assume that valvular disorders are rheumatic unless documented by the physician. No longer as prevalent in the United States, rheumatic heart disease (heart disease caused by rheumatic fever that follows a group A β-hemolytic streptococcus infection) usually occurs in childhood after a streptococcal infection and can affect the heart valves, in particular causing mitral valve stenosis with associated CHF. Today, rheumatic fever or its effects are more frequently seen in persons living in third-world countries, immigrants to the United States, and those in the United States older than 50 years (i.e., before antibiotic treatment). However, if a physician specifies mitral valve stenosis, rheumatic, with CHF, assign codes 398.91 and 394.0.

Coding Clinic 2000, second quarter, describes more information about the coding of valvular disorders with no mention of rheumatic heart disease.

Heart Valve Replacements and Valvuloplasty   Heart valve disorders such as stenosis may be treated with a minimally invasive procedure such as percutaneous balloon valvuloplasty (code 35.96), which uses a catheter with an inflatable balloon to repair the valve. Also, invasive open procedures (open-heart valvuloplasty; code 35.1X, 35.2X) can be performed with or without valve replacement to repair the valve. Heart valve replacements can be performed with prosthetic (synthetic) grafts or tissue grafts from porcine or bovine valves. If these invasive open procedures are performed, the procedure code for extracorporeal circulation (code 39.61) should be assigned as an additional code.

If a patient is status post heart valve replacement, report this as an additional diagnosis code when the replaced heart valve has certain implications for the patient's care. For example, use the V43.3 code for status post prosthetic heart valve replacement and an additional code (V58.61) to describe the use of long-term anticoagulant (blood thinner) therapy. A patient with a prosthetic heart valve is at risk for emboli and must receive long-term anticoagulant prophylaxis, which must be considered in his or her overall care. Use code V42.2 for a patient who has had a tissue graft (porcine or bovine) valve replacement.

Mitral valve prolapse (code 424.1) is often coded as an additional diagnosis. Mitral valve prolapse most often occurs in thin young women and is a condition in which the mitral valve prolapses (sags) backward during systole (left ventricular contraction). A physician can hear a mid-systolic click when listening (auscultation). Mitral valve prolapse is most often not a serious medical problem; however, it can affect care and may be reportable. For example, prophylactic antibiotics are often given before surgical procedures (especially dental procedures and teeth cleaning), because during surgery bacteria can enter and circulate in the blood and the valve can become infected, causing acute or subacute bacterial endocarditis.

CARDIAC ARREST

Cardiac arrest (code 427.5) is rarely sequenced as a principal diagnosis because it describes cardiac arrest of an unknown cause. If the underlying cause for the cardiac arrest has been determined, that cause should be sequenced first (e.g., acute myocardial infarction). A diagnosis of cardiac arrest should not be listed as an additional (secondary) diagnosis unless there was an attempt at patient resuscitation. Cardiac arrest should never be added as the cause of patient death in the hospital. For example, if a patient is admitted with cardiac arrest secondary to ventricular tachycardia, sequence the ventricular tachycardia as the principal diagnosis and the cardiac arrest as a secondary diagnosis. If a patient dies during hospitalization and does not undergo resuscitation ("do not resuscitate" or a "no code") and if the physician does not document cardiac arrest in the record, do not code the cardiac arrest as a secondary diagnosis.

CARDIOMYOPATHY

Cardiomyopathy (category code 425) is a progressive degenerative disease of the heart muscle. Often the etiology for the disease is unknown (idiopathic), but cardiomyopathy can sometimes occur secondary to the long-term effects of alcoholism or after a viral illness. The ICD-9-CM provides codes for the many different types of cardiomyopathies (subterms located under the main term "cardiomyopathy"), including the following:

- idiopathic or primary cardiomyopathy: 425.4
- alcoholic cardiomyopathy: 425.5
- ischemic cardiomyopathy: 414.8
- secondary or toxic cardiomyopathy: 425.9
- obstructive hypertrophic cardiomyopathy: 425.1
- cardiomyopathy due to progressive muscular dystrophy: 359.1 + 425.8
- cardiomyopathy due to sarcoidosis: 135 + 425.8
- congestive cardiomyopathy secondary to hypertension with CHF: 402.91 + 425.8 + 428.0

Unless the admission for cardiomyopathy occurs for a newly diagnosed disease or for heart transplantation, do not sequence it as the principal diagnosis. Many of the symptoms that routinely accompany cardiomyopathy, such as CHF and ventricular tachycardia, are the reason for the admission and receive the focus of care. Therefore, they are sequenced as the principal diagnosis, with cardiomyopathy sequenced as an additional code. Because cardiomyopathy results in a low cardiac ejection fraction (i.e., low cardiac output), the care is commonly directed at the symptoms that are the reason for the patient admission and the principal diagnosis. Progressive cardiomyopathy results in a dying heart that can necessitate a heart transplantation.

TIP The diagnosis of ischemic cardiomyopathy (code 414.8) can present a problem for coders because the disease is not classified as a true cardiomyopathy in ICD-9-CM. Although the documentation may be specific and the illness severe, the ICD-9-CM classification does not provide a precise code for this disease. Instead, it classifies ischemic cardiomyopathy under the code for chronic myocardial ischemia not elsewhere classified (414.8). Although caused by the long-term effects of chronic ischemic heart disease, ischemic cardiomyopathy can produce severe low cardiac output (e.g., ejection fraction of 10% to 20%) that is not well described by the chronic myocardial ischemia (414.8) code alone. The classification code of 414.8 is nonspecific and is not recognized by Centers for Medicare and Medicaid Services as a comorbid condition code. With the 414.8 code, the MS–DRG Prospective Payment System inadequately identifies the precise data necessary to measure the medical resources necessary to treat acutely ill patients. Therefore, with a diagnosis of ischemic cardiomyopathy, it is important to review the entire medical record (especially progress notes, nurses' notes, telemetry results, and consultants' notes) for symptoms that capture the severity of the disease and to report these as additional codes. For example, assign additional codes for left heart failure, ventricular arrhythmia, or other conditions that may apply. Be sure to review telemetry tracings, as these patients often manifest premature ventricular contractions (PVCs). A 3-beat run (or more) of PVCs, may indicate the beginnings of ventricular tachycardia (V-tach), which would be a C/C under MS-DRG reimbursement. Query the physician for clarification, and have the physician add supporting documentation to the medical record, if necessary.

Cerebrovascular Disease

A cerebrovascular disease is any disease of the cerebrovascular blood vessels or a disorder that affects the flow of blood through the brain.

CEREBROVASCULAR ACCIDENTS

In a CVA, there is a decreased supply of blood to the brain (acute cerebral ischemia) that can result in an area of infarction (i.e., necrotic cerebral tissue). Because CVA or stroke is a general nonspecific term, you should find out whether the CVA has occurred because of thrombosis, embolism, occlusion (category 433 or 434), or hemorrhage (category 430 to 432). Prior to October 1, 2004, CVA, not otherwise specified (NOS) was coded to 436 (acute but ill-defined cerebrovascular disease).

Many physicians simply document that a patient has experienced a "stroke" or "CVA," when in fact the more precise diagnosis is cerebral "infarction." However, with the October 2004 coding updates, CVA/stroke is now considered an assumed ischemic infarction (Figure 13.9) and is coded to 434.91. You should be aware that some patients may have repeated CVAs (i.e., multiple CVA history). ICD-9-CM provides a mechanism to differentiate between late effects (residual conditions) of old CVAs versus deficits (residual conditions) associated with a current CVA (current episode of care). Deficits that are not associated with the current CVA, but with a previous one, should be coded as late effects by using the CVA combination category code 438 (e.g., hemiplegia with the current CVA would be coded to 342.90; hemiplegia from

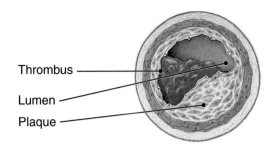

FIGURE 13.9 ■ Ischemic cerebrovascular accident (CVA). (Reprinted with permission from Anatomical Chart Co.)

a previous CVA would be coded to late effects, code 438.20). Remember, codes are intended to tell the story of a patient. Describing residual conditions associated with a current CVA versus an old CVA helps to express the patient's true clinical picture.

EXAMPLE	*Acute embolic CVA with infarction; hemiplegia present at discharge; previous CVA with residual facial droop: 434.11 + 342.90 + 438.83*

CVA deficits present at discharge are coded, whereas deficits that resolve before discharge are not. After inpatient discharge (i.e., discharge from the initial acute care episode), all deficits are expressed as late effects (category 438).

TRANSIENT ISCHEMIC ATTACKS

A transient ischemic attack (TIA; code 435.9) results in a sudden loss of neurologic function that resembles a stroke (right- or left-sided weakness, facial droop, slurred or incoherent speech, memory loss, and confusion). However, in a TIA, the symptoms usually resolve within 24 hours. TIAs often occur before a CVA.

If a patient experiences a TIA and undergoes further testing, such as a carotid ultrasound, that reveals the underlying cause of the unspecified TIA, query the physician to determine whether the more precise diagnosis may be assigned. For example, if the physician documents that the TIA (435.9) was secondary to right carotid stenosis (433.10), assign the more precise code of 433.10 rather than the code for TIA, unspecified. For a patient with a history of TIAs in which a carotid ultrasound, angiography, or testing reveals atherosclerotic carotid stenosis with cerebrovascular ischemia, a carotid endarterectomy (code 38.12) is often performed as a therapeutic procedure.

Peripheral Vascular Diseases

A peripheral vascular disease is any disease of the peripheral blood vessels or a disorder that affects the flow of blood through the extremities.

ATHEROSCLEROSIS OF EXTREMITIES

Atherosclerosis of the extremities (category 440.2X) results in ischemic peripheral vascular disease and can manifest progressively worse symptoms, such as claudication (pain when walking), rest pain (pain in legs when resting), ulcer (open sore on legs), or gangrene (necrosis of tissue). Each fifth-digit code in the category includes the conditions described in the lower fifth-digit codes. Therefore, one would never use more than one code from the 440.2X classification when coding a patient's medical record. For example, code 440.24 would include any of the associated conditions of claudication, rest pain, or ulceration, as described in the lower fifth-digit codes (440.23, 440.22, and 440.21). The fifth-digit codes are classified as follows:

- ▶ atherosclerosis of the extremities, unspecified: 440.20
- ▶ atherosclerosis of the extremities with intermittent claudication: 440.21
- ▶ atherosclerosis of the extremities with rest pain (includes any condition classifiable to 440.21): 440.22
- ▶ atherosclerosis of the extremities with ulceration (includes any condition classifiable to 440.22; however, use an additional code from category 707 to describe the precise location of the ulcer): 440.23
- ▶ atherosclerosis of the extremities with gangrene (includes any condition classifiable to 440.21, 440.22, and 440.23): 440.24

A procedure for treating atherosclerotic peripheral vascular disease is PTA (code 39.50). In this procedure, a catheter with a balloon is maneuvered to a stenosed (narrowed) or thrombosed (clotted) area of a peripheral vessel and inflated to open up the affected area and return blood flow. Sometimes this procedure also involves the placement of a stent device to keep the artery patent (open). The placement of stents requires an additional code (39.90), or if the stent is a drug-eluting stent, the assigned code is 00.55 (insertion of drug-eluting stent in a noncoronary artery). If a thrombolytic agent (drug used to dissolve clots) is used during the PTA, add code 99.10. As of October 2005, additional code(s) are assigned to indicate 1) the total number of vessels that underwent angioplasty/athrectomy (00.40–00.43) and 2) the total number of stents placed during the procedure (00.45–00.48).

A patient was admitted with atherosclerotic femoral artery occlusion with rest pain and underwent PTA of the femoral artery: 440.22; 39.50, 00.40

A patient was admitted with atherosclerotic femoral artery occlusion with rest pain and leg ulceration and underwent PTA with stent placement: 440.23, 707.10; 39.50, 39.90, 00.40, 00.45

EXAMPLE

Another therapeutic procedure is peripheral vascular bypass. This open invasive procedure is coded to 39.29. Also, watch for excisional (surgical) debridements (code 86.22) or hyperbaric oxygenation therapies (code 93.59) for lower extremity ulcers or gangrene.

THROMBOSIS AND THROMBOPHLEBITIS

Thrombosis is a condition in which a clot has formed within a blood vessel. Thrombophlebitis is a clot with inflammation. Thrombosis with thrombophlebitis in veins of the extremities (arms and legs) is coded only to the thrombophlebitis, because this code includes the thrombosis. Although thrombosis and thrombophlebitis are medically treated in the same manner, the codes for thrombosis and thrombophlebitis of the extremities are separated into different MS-DRG prospective payment rates, and thrombosis is given the higher weight. Therefore, coding thrombosis to receive a higher reimbursement under MS-DRGs when thrombophlebitis has been documented would be construed as upcoding, which is an unethical and illegal practice.

Physicians will sometimes use the terms **thrombosis** and **thrombophlebitis** interchangeably. If the term **thrombophlebitis** is documented in the medical record, assign the code for **thrombophlebitis** even if all other documentation is only for thrombosis.

A deep venous thrombosis is a clot that occurs in the veins of the legs. With a deep venous thrombosis, anticoagulant therapy is administered to reduce the risk of a thrombus (clot) dislodging and becoming an embolus that may travel through the veins to the right side of the heart, resulting in a pulmonary (artery) embolism. Sometimes an inferior vena cava umbrella device (Greenfield catheter; code 38.7) is surgically inserted to prevent (filter) the emboli from entering the right heart. The inferior vena cava and superior vena cava are the largest veins in the body; they bring deoxygenated venous blood back to the right side of the heart in order for blood to travel to the lungs to be reoxygenated. The inferior vena cava brings deoxygenated blood from the lower part of the body (e.g., legs) to the heart, and the superior vena cava brings deoxygenated blood from the upper part of the body (e.g., head).

Aneurysms

An aneurysm is an abnormal localized widening of an artery that can occur anywhere in the body (e.g., heart, brain, or extremities). It usually results from a weakness in an area of a vessel that will widen (i.e., balloon out) over time and can burst. However, the aorta is often affected because it is the largest artery in an area that sustains high arterial pressure from the left ventricle during systole. In a dissecting aneurysm, blood lodges in the layers of a vessel (Figure 13.10). In a ruptured aneurysm, the vessel bursts. One of the most emergent inpatient admissions, with a high mortality rate, is an admission for ruptured abdominal aortic aneurysm (ruptured AAA). Patients with a ruptured AAA are hemodynamically unstable (loss of systemic blood circulation), require multiple transfusions, and require resection of the aneurysm and placement of a synthetic graft. Often, because of the high demand for blood and the sensitivity of the brain and kidneys, anoxic encephalopathy or renal failure can occur.

EXAMPLE

Ruptured AAA: 441.3

Acute blood loss anemia: 285.1

Anoxic encephalopathy: 348.1

Renal failure; multiorgan failure: 586

Repair AAA with graft replacement: 38.44

Whole-blood transfusion: 99.03

Codes for aneurysmal repairs are located under the main procedural terms "aneurysmectomy" or "repair, aneurysm." Aneurysm repairs include excision of the aneurysm with anastomosis (reconnection of healthy vessel) or graft replacement of the affected area by clipping or suture.

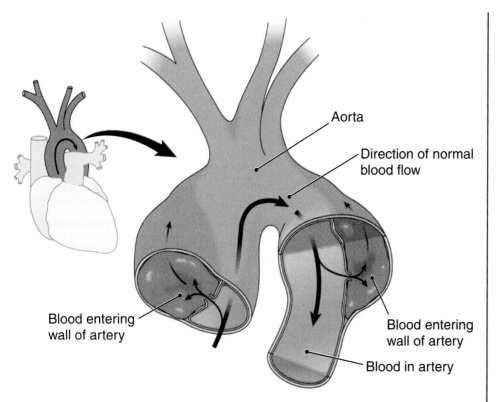

FIGURE 13.10 ■ Dissecting aortic aneurysm. (Reprinted with permission from Cohen BJ. Medical Terminology: An Illustrated Guide, 4th Ed. Baltimore: Lippincott Williams & Wilkins, 2004.)

Miscellaneous Vascular Access Procedures

Many conditions may necessitate venous access to administer drugs quickly into the bloodstream or to remove harmful substances. Venous catheterization, not elsewhere classified (e.g., Hickman catheter), is coded to 38.93 (or to 38.95 if placed for short-term hemodialysis). If a condition such as end-stage renal disease requires more long-term vascular access, a vascular access device is sometimes inserted (code 86.07). Insertion of a totally implantable infusion pump is coded to 86.06. This device contains a reservoir and is surgically placed subcutaneously for long-term systemic administration of drugs. Infusion pumps are typically used for the long-term administration of chemotherapy in cancer patients or for pain control. You can locate these procedures in the Procedure Index under the main term "insertion, catheter, vein," under "insertion, infusion pump," and under "insertion, vascular access device, totally implantable."

 ## Blood and Blood-Forming Organ Diseases

Blood and blood-forming organ diseases are any conditions that adversely affect the function or production of the blood to support the living tissues within the body.

Anemias

Anemia is any condition in which the number of healthy red blood cells in circulating blood is less than normal. Hemoglobin is a protein in red blood cells that carries oxygen. There are many different types of anemia (iron deficiency, aplastic, hemolytic, acute and chronic blood loss, pernicious, sickle cell, hypochromic, microcytic, spherocytic, anemia of chronic disease, and so on). A careful review of all subterms under the main term "anemia" in the Disease Index will help you to assign the correct anemia code.

A literal interpretation of the words that express the type of anemia often helps you to gain a better understanding of the pathology of the disease for coding. A normal red blood cell has a round, disklike shape. Abnormal morphology (shape) of the red blood cell often affects its ability to carry oxygen effectively. For example, in sickle cell anemia, the morphology (shape) of the red blood cell resembles a sickle. Therefore, it is a fragile red blood cell that cannot effectively carry hemoglobin with oxygen. Blood is viscous (sticky) and clumps together, causing tissue infarcts and sickle cell crisis from vaso-occlusion. In macrocytic anemia, the red blood cells are too large; in microcytic anemia, the red blood cells are too small; and in spherocytic anemia, the red blood cells are spherical. In hypochromic anemia (*hypo-*: "decreased"; *chromo-*: "color"), cells lack color. The oxygen in hemoglobin gives blood its bright red color, and someone with hypochromic anemia lacks oxygen in their red blood cells.

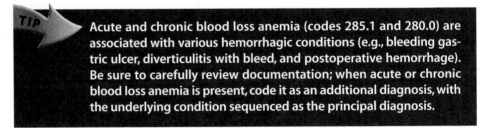

TIP Acute and chronic blood loss anemia (codes 285.1 and 280.0) are associated with various hemorrhagic conditions (e.g., bleeding gastric ulcer, diverticulitis with bleed, and postoperative hemorrhage). Be sure to carefully review documentation; when acute or chronic blood loss anemia is present, code it as an additional diagnosis, with the underlying condition sequenced as the principal diagnosis.

If the sole purpose of the admission is to treat the anemia (e.g., admit for transfusion), anemia is then listed as the principal diagnosis. This occurs more often on an outpatient basis.

ICD-9-CM includes a category for anemia in chronic illnesses (285.2X). This includes the following codes:

▶ anemia in chronic kidney disease: 285.21
▶ anemia in neoplastic disease: 285.22
▶ anemia in other chronic illness: 285.29

The kidneys release a hormone called erythropoietin that helps in the production of red blood cells. Diseased kidneys in end-stage renal disease decrease the normal production of erythropoietin, causing a secondary anemia. In cancers and because of the expected side effects of chemotherapy or radiotherapy, cancer patients can have anemia secondary to neoplastic disease. Many new drugs are available that treat this condition (e.g., epoetin alfa [Epogen; Procrit]). Other diseases, such as chronic alcoholism, can also cause secondary anemia.

Pancytopenia

Immature blood cells begin as stem cells that originate in red bone marrow and start to produce red blood cells, white blood cells, and platelets (clotting cells). These blood cells are the three formed elements of the blood that join with plasma (the liquid portion of the blood). Pancytopenia is a type of aplastic anemia. The term **aplastic** means "no formation," and in aplastic anemia, there is a loss of the formation of stem cells in the bone marrow that results in a failure to properly produce red blood cells, white blood cells, and platelets. *Pan/o-* is a word part that means "all," and pancytopenia occurs when there is a failure to produce all three formed elements of the blood. Therefore, if the patient has leukocytopenia (deficient white blood cells), erythrocytopenia (deficient red blood cells), and thrombocytopenia (deficient platelets), then the patient has pancytopenia. If a physician documents neutropenia (the most predominant type of white blood cell), anemia (deficient red blood cells), and thrombocytopenia (deficient platelets), then the coder should assign the code for pancytopenia only (code 284.1). Treatment for pancytopenia usually includes blood transfusions. However, in some cases, a bone marrow transplantation may be attempted to repopulate the bone marrow with normal blood stem cells.

The *exclusion note* in the Tabular List of Diseases for code 284.1 (pancytopenia) indicates that pancytopenia due to drugs (e.g., chemotherapy) is coded to 284.8. This change in code assignment (284.1 vs. 284.8) may effect your MS-DRG and reimbursement to the hospital. A thorough review of the medical record for precise assignment is essential.

Coagulopathies

A coagulopathy is any condition in which one has a prolonged clotting time and a resulting hemorrhagic disorder. Coagulation (clotting) is a complicated process that involves the timed release of clotting factors I to V and VII to XIII to form a fibrin (protein that forms a clot) clot. Hemophilia (code 286.0) is a specific type of coagulopathy caused by the absence of clotting factor VIII, which is genetically missing in some people; autoimmune thrombocytopenic purpura (code 287.31) is a hemorrhagic disorder attributable to an abnormally decreased platelet count; and disseminated intravascular coagulation syndrome is a severe coagulopathy characterized by fibrinolysis (destruction of fibrin).

A patient who is receiving continuous anticoagulant therapy (blood-thinning drugs) does not necessarily have a coagulation disorder. If a hemorrhage develops that is related to the adverse effect of an anticoagulant medication such as warfarin, code the hemorrhagic condition first, followed by E934.2 (adverse effect of anticoagulant) and V58.61 (long-term use of anticoagulants) as additional codes. Do not assume that the adverse effect is drug related unless it is documented as such by the physician.

Also, use caution when assigning code 286.5, hemorrhagic disorder due to circulating anticoagulants. This is a rare autoimmune disorder in which one acquires antibodies against one's own normal clotting mechanism; it is rarely attributable to the use of anticoagulant drugs.

EXAMPLE	*Patient admitted for diverticular hemorrhage due to the adverse effects of warfarin. Patient on long-term warfarin therapy for chronic atrial fibrillation: 562.12 + E934.2 + 427.31 + V58.61.*
	Patient admitted with diverticular hemorrhage. The patient has pre-existing chronic atrial fibrillation and is on long-term warfarin therapy: 562.12 + 427.31 + V58.61.

SUMMARY

This chapter has addressed diseases of the circulatory system, blood, and blood-forming organs. Among the cardiovascular diseases covered were ischemic heart disease, heart failure, arrhythmias and heart blocks, hypertension, valvular disorders, cardiac arrest, and cardiomyopathy.

The cerebrovascular diseases covered were CVAs and TIAs. The peripheral vascular diseases covered were atherosclerosis of the extremities, thrombosis, and thrombophlebitis. Aneurysms were also addressed in this chapter. The diseases of the blood and blood-forming organs covered were anemias, pancytopenia, and coagulopathies.

This chapter has described the pathology of the common circulatory system, blood, and blood-forming organ disorders. It has also recognized the typical manifestations, complications, and treatments in terms of their implications for coding. Chapter 14 addresses the subjects of neoplasms and oncology.

REFERENCES

1. American Heart Association. Heart Disease and Stroke Statistics—2004 Update. Available at: http://www.americanheart.org/downloadable/heart/1079736729696HDSStats2004 UpdateREV3-19-04.pdf. Accessed: July 30, 2004.
2. National Ambulatory Medical Care Survey, 2001 Summary. National Center for Health Statistics. July 22, 2004. Available at: http://www.cdc.gov/nchs/fastats/hyprtens.htm.

TESTING YOUR COMPREHENSION

1. What comprises the circulatory system?

   _____

2. Name two of the more common blood and blood-forming organ diseases as presented in this chapter.

   _____

3. Why can ischemic cardiovascular disease be so harmful?

   _____

4. Angina pectoris is often associated with what disease?

   _____

5. Severe chest pain that does not respond to conventional medical therapy and is not relieved by rest and relaxation is referred to as what?

   _____

6. An acute ischemic cardiac event that results from progressive coronary artery disease is referred to as what?

   _____

7. If an evolving infarction is prevented through the use of prescription pharmaceuticals, how is this fact coded?

   _____

8. Identify a diagnostic cardiac procedure.

   _____

9. What is the purpose of coronary angiography?

   _____

10. What is the purpose of an intra-aortic balloon pump?

    _____

11. Identify the procedures associated with coronary artery bypass grafting.

    _____

12. Are the procedures identified in item 11 usually coded separately?

    _____

13. Is an additional code assigned for pulmonary edema?

    _____

14. Digitalis is referred to as a cardiotonic drug. Why?

    _____

15. When the left ventricle can no longer contract forcefully, what does this condition cause?

    _____

16. What does electrical stimulation do to the heart muscle?

    _____

17. If atrial fibrillation is uncontrolled, what is needed to return the patient to a normal sinus rhythm?

18. What code is assigned if a patient is admitted for an adjustment or scheduled replacement of a worn-out AICD pulse generator?

19. Why is a third-degree atrioventricular heart block considered the most severe?

20. Two common coding errors occur when pacemaker insertion is addressed. What are they?

21. What are the threshold limits of high blood pressure in terms of the systolic and diastolic pressures?

22. What symptoms are often associated with malignant hypertension?

23. Why is uncontrolled hypertension referred to as the "silent killer"?

24. Identify the four valves in the heart that prevent the backflow of blood.

25. Identify a less invasive treatment for valvular stenosis.

26. What is cardiomyopathy?

27. The onset of cardiomyopathy can occur secondary to the long-term effects of what chronic disease?

28. What can cause a CVA?

29. What is an aneurysm?

30. What is the effect of an abnormal shape of a red blood cell?

31. What hormone released by the kidneys assists in the production of red blood cells?

32. If the physician documents anemia, neutropenia, and thrombocytopenia, what should you code?

CODING PRACTICE I   Chapter Review Exercises

Directions

By using your ICD-9-CM codebook, code the following diagnoses and procedures:

	DIAGNOSIS/PROCEDURES	CODE
1	Sick sinus syndrome. Insertion of a permanent dual-chamber cardiac pacemaker with atrioventricular leads.	
2	Unstable angina secondary to coronary artery disease. Right and left heart catheterization with ventriculogram and coronary angiography. Coronary artery bypass graft _4 with saphenous vein harvesting; aortocoronary bypass to left anterior descending artery and posterior descending artery; double internal mammary bypass.	
3	Acute left-sided embolic cerebrovascular accident with infarction. Right hemiparesis on discharge. Previous CVA with residual aphasia.	
4	Transient ischemic attack secondary to carotid artery stenosis on right. Carotid endarterectomy, right.	
5	Ischemic cardiomyopathy. Congestive heart failure. Ventricular tachycardia.	
6	Atherosclerotic heart disease with new-onset angina. Percutaneous transluminal coronary angioplasty (PTCA) of right coronary artery with placement of stent.	
7	Atherosclerotic peripheral vascular disease, left leg, with claudication and ulcer. Percutaneous transluminal angioplasty of femoral artery, left leg.	
8	Spontaneous epistaxis secondary to uncontrolled hypertension. Anterior and posterior nasal packing.	
9	Acute coronary syndrome with acute anterolateral myocardial infarction. Status post coronary artery bypass graft for coronary artery disease. Essential hypertension. Peripheral vascular disease. Hypertensive cardiovascular disease. Left ventricular hypertrophy. Congestive heart failure. Chronic end-stage renal failure, on hemodialysis.	
10	Cardiac arrest secondary to ventricular fibrillation. Non-insulin-dependent diabetes mellitus. Emphysema/chronic obstructive pulmonary disease by history. Coronary artery disease. Hypothyroidism, on levothyroxine (Synthroid). AICD placement. Electrophysiologic study.	

	DIAGNOSIS/PROCEDURES	CODE
11	Gastrointestinal bleeding secondary to adverse effects of warfarin. Status post prosthetic heart valve replacement, on long-term anticoagulant therapy.	
12	Dissecting thoracoabdominal aneurysm. Resection of thoracoabdominal aneurysm, with graft replacement.	
13	End-stage renal disease. Hypertensive heart disease. Anemia secondary to #1.	
14	Acute pulmonary edema with CHF. Essential hypertension. Mitral valve stenosis and aortic insufficiency.	
15	Seizures due to berry aneurysm.	
16	Deep venous thrombosis with thrombophlebitis, left lower extremity. Placement of a Greenfield catheter (vena cava umbrella device).	
17	Hypertension secondary to malignant pheochromocytoma.	
18	Unstable postinfarction angina. Atherosclerotic heart disease. Status post recent acute inferior wall myocardial infarction 2 weeks previously, status post CABG X4.	
19	CVA secondary to cerebral thrombosis with infarct. Aphasia resolved before discharge but continuing ataxic gait.	
20	Femoral-popliteal occlusive disease, right leg. Right femoral-popliteal bypass.	

Medical Record Case Studies

Instructions

1. Carefully review the medical reports provided for each case study.
2. Research any abbreviations and terms that are unfamiliar or unclear.
3. Identify as many diagnoses and procedures as possible.
4. Because only part of the patient's total record is available, determine what additional documentation you might need.
5. If appropriate, identify any questions you might ask the physician to code this case correctly and completely.
6. Complete the appropriate blanks below for each case study.

CHAPTER 13 CASE STUDIES

Case Study 13.1 (Coder/Abstract Summary Form)

Patient: **John Doe**

Patient documentation: **Review Medical Report 13.1**

1. Principal diagnosis:

   _____

2. Secondary or other diagnoses:

   _____

3. Principal procedure:

   _____

4. Other procedures:

   _____

5. Additional documentation needed:

   _____

   _____

   _____

   _____

Case Study 13.1 (Continued)

6. Questions for the physician:

_____

_____

_____

_____

_____

HISTORY AND PHYSICAL

PATIENT:	Doe, John
DOB:	
MED REC:	1234567
PT ADMN:	
PHYSICIAN:	Smith M.D.
ADMN DATE:	

DATE OF ADMISSION: This 83-year-old white male worked busily outside caring for his lawn. Around noontime, he was called in to have lunch. The wife was sitting in the living room when she heard him cry for help. In the meantime, the patient walked toward his wife, who states he could not speak and appeared pale and weak. The wife immediately called the neighbor next door and EMS was also called at the same time. Shortly thereafter when the wife tried to help him balance, the patient collapsed and fell over her. Both of them hit the ground. EMS arrived shortly thereafter, and the patient was found unresponsive and was brought to the hospital. The patient was not intubated and was found to be breathing on his own. There was no witnessed seizure. There was no bladder or bowel incontinence. The patient has no history of hypertension or diabetes.

ALLERGIES: No known allergies.

MEDICATIONS: Allopurinol 300 mg daily, K-Dur 20 mg daily, Lasix 40 mg daily, 5 mg daily, Plendil 5 mg daily.

PERSONAL HISTORY: The patient is married and lives with his wife. He used to work in construction. He is an active person and likes to do work and "tinker" around the house.

PAST MEDICAL HISTORY: Status post coronary stent placement three years ago by Dr. Heart in the right coronary artery. He has been on Plavix ever since. No other surgeries.

REVIEW OF SYSTEMS: Negative.

PHYSICAL EXAMINATION: Temperature 98 degrees Fahrenheit, pulse 86 per minute, respiratory rate 14, blood pressure 129/84.

HEENT: Pupils equal and reacting to light.

NECK: Supple. No JVD or lymphadenopathy.

CARDIAC EXAM: Heart sounds are normal.

LUNGS: Clear.

ABDOMEN: Soft, bowel sounds are heard.

EXTREMITIES: Reveal no clubbing, cyanosis, or edema. The patient is able to move all four extremities. There is a possible left carotid bruit. The patient tries to respond to verbal commands, but is very drowsy.

LABORATORY DATA: Sodium 136, potassium 4, glucose 111, BUN 18, creatinine .9, albumin 3.8, alkaline phosphatase 98, total bilirubin 2, LDH 103, ALT 13, AST 21, Troponin-I level zero. CPK 78. EKG reveals atrial fibrillation, right bundle branch block, probable anteroseptal infarct, old with Q waves. Posterior parietal lobe infarction. No acute bleed.

IMPRESSION:
1. Acute CVA probably secondary to cerebral embolism.
2. Atrial fibrillation.
3. Coronary artery disease status post-coronary stent placement to the right coronary artery 5 years ago
4. Hypertension.

Continued

MEDICAL REPORT 13.1 (CONTINUED)

5. Elevated bilirubin of uncertain etiology.

6. History of gouty arthropathy, on Allopurinol.

7. History of nephrolithiasis, recurrent. Probably uric stones.

PLAN: Admit the patient to the Intensive Care Unit with cardiology consultation, neurology consultation. In view of the atrial fibrillation and the acute CVA, the question is about IV heparin. The situation was discussed with the patient's wife and daughter who are present at the bedside. Will hold off on his oral medications at this time until further evaluation is done. Will follow.

_____

Signed:

DD:

DT:

NOTES

Case Study 13.2 (Coder/Abstract Summary Form)

Patient: **Frank Jones**

Patient documentation: **Review Medical Reports 13.2 and 13.3**

1. Principal diagnosis:

_____

2. Secondary or other diagnoses:

_____

3. Principal procedure:

_____

4. Other procedures:

_____

5. Additional documentation needed:

_____

_____

_____

_____

6. Questions for the physician:

_____

_____

_____

_____

MEDICAL REPORT 13.2

DISCHARGE SUMMARY

NAME:	Jones, Frank
NUMBER:	9999999
SEX:	M
AGE:	73
ADMIT:	
DIS:	
DATE OF BIRTH:	
ATTENDING PHYSICIAN:	Smith, M.D.

DISCHARGE DIAGNOSES:

1. Hypertensive crisis with acute pulmonary edema and acute respiratory failure.
2. Acute myocardial infarction ruled out.
3. Type 1 insulin-dependent diabetes mellitus.
4. Anemia.
5. History of duodenal outlet obstruction.
6. Gastroesophageal reflux disease.

MEDICATIONS AT DISCHARGE: Prinivil 30 mg p.o. daily, Eldercaps 1 p.o. daily per tube, Rifampin 600 mg per tube daily, Ferrous Sulfate 220 mg liquid per tube b.i.d., Novolin N 12 units every morning and 9 units every evening, Ritalin 10 mg per tube b.i.d., Reglan 10 mg liquid per tube t.i.d., Wellbutrin 75 mg per tube b.i.d., Klorvess 30 mEq per tube b.i.d., Catapres 0.1 mg per tube t.i.d., Prevacid 30 mg per tube daily, Lasix 40 mg per tube b.i.d., sliding scale insulin—blood sugar less than 200 no insulin, 201–250 2 units of Humulin R, 251–300 4 units, 301–350 8 units, 351–400 10 units, greater than 400 CALL MD.

REASON FOR HOSPITALIZATION: This 73-year-old male was admitted to the hospital by way of the emergency department after he presented from the ABC Nursing Home due to acute onset of severe shortness of breath. The patient was found to have marked elevation of his blood pressure at the time of his evaluation in the emergency department. He had blood pressure of 280/170. He was in acute pulmonary edema at that time and received nitroglycerin drip and Lasix and his blood pressure did come under better control. He is admitted to the hospital at this time for further evaluation and therapy.

PHYSICAL EXAMINATION: Blood pressure 280/170. This is a well-developed elderly male who is in marked respiratory distress at the time of his admission to the hospital.

SKIN: Warm and dry. No rash or lesion.

HEENT: Head normocephalic. No evidence of recent trauma. Eyes—Pupils equal, round, reactive to light and accommodation. Extraocular motions intact. Sclerae nonicteric. Conjunctivae pink. Mouth and throat — Oral mucosa pink without lesions or exudates. Tongue and uvula in midline.

NECK: Supple. No jugular venous distention or HJR. Carotids 2+ and equal without bruits. No thyroid enlargement.

CHEST: Clear.

HEART: Regular rate and normal rhythm without click, murmurs, gallops or rubs.

ABDOMEN: Soft, nontender. No masses, organ enlargement, hernias or bruits. The patient has a feeding jejunostomy tube in the left upper abdomen.

EXTREMITIES: No clubbing, cyanosis and edema. The patient moves all extremities. Femoral pulses 2+ and equal. Dorsalis pedis oriented x 3. Cranial nerves II – XII intact. Motor and sensory intact without focal weakness or sensory disturbance.

MEDICAL REPORT 13.2 (CONTINUED)

HOSPITAL COURSE: The patient was hospitalized and evaluated for severe hypertension and acute pulmonary edema. He was started on his nursing home medications during the hospital stay and he received IM Apresoline prn. The patient's blood pressure did come under good control during the hospital stay. Initially, the patient did have some acute respiratory failure with a pH of 7.150, PaCO2 57, PaO2 52.4 with an O2 saturation of 79% on the initial set of blood gases. The patient's blood gases did improve as did his respirations through the rest of the hospital stay. Cardiac isoenzymes were obtained during the hospitalization revealing no evidence of acute myocardial injury.

The patient's initial CBC revealed white blood count 16.1 with a hemoglobin of 11.5, hematocrit 34.3. Repeat CBC revealed hemoglobin of 9.0, hematocrit 26.1. There was no evidence of acute blood loss during the hospitalization. The patient will have a repeat CBC done at the time of discharge from the hospital but the results are pending at this moment. The patient still had some evidence of some systolic hypertension during the latter part of his hospital stay but his Zestril will be increased at the time of discharge from the hospital. The patient will be followed at the nursing home at this time.

Signature affixed via participation in alternative signature program.

D:

T:

CC:

NOTES

MEDICAL REPORT 13.3

HISTORY AND PHYSICAL

NAME:	Jones, Frank
NUMBER:	9999999
SEX:	M
AGE:	73
ADMIT:	
DIS:	
DATE OF BIRTH:	
ATTENDING PHYSICIAN:	Smith, M.D.

CHIEF COMPLAINT: Shortness of breath.

HISTORY OF PRESENT ILLNESS: This 73-year-old male was admitted to the hospital by way of the emergency department after he presented from the Nursing Home because of acute onset of severe shortness of breath. The patient was found to have marked elevation of his blood pressure also at the time of his evaluation in the emergency department. He had a blood pressure of 208/107 with a pulse rate of 130. The patient stated that he has been receiving his medications as needed at the nursing home. The patient does have some chest discomfort. He has had paroxysmal nocturnal dyspnea and orthopnea associated with this shortness of breath.

In the emergency department, the patient received nitroglycerin drip and his blood pressure was brought under control. He is admitted to the hospital at this time for further evaluation and therapy.

PAST MEDICAL HISTORY: Insulin-dependent diabetes mellitus, benign prostatic hypertrophy, arthritis, essential hypertension, iron deficiency anemia, history of gastrointestinal bleeding, depression, status post-feeding jejunostomy because of gastric outlet obstruction secondary to which has now resolved. Status post-resection of duodenum due to gastrointestinal bleeding.

ALLERGIES: The patient has no known drug allergies.

HABITS: The patient is a nonsmoker, nondrinker. There is no drug abuse history.

REVIEW OF SYSTEMS: Noncontributory.

HOME MEDICATIONS:

1. Prinivil 20 mg q.d.
2. Prevacid 30 mg q.d.
3. Atacand 1 q.d.
4. Rifamide 600 mg b.i.d.
5. Lasix 40 mg q.d.
6. Iron sulfate 325 mg per tube b.i.d.
7. Novolin N 12 units q.a.m. and 8 units q.p.m.
8. Ritalin 10 mg p.o. b.i.d.
9. Reglan 10 mg p.o. t.i.d.
10. Wellbutrin 75 mg p.o. b.i.d.
11. Potassium chloride 30 mEq p.o. b.i.d.
12. Clonidine 0.1 mg p.o. t.i.d.
13. Darvocet N-100 1 p.o. q.6.h. p.r.n. pain.

MEDICAL REPORT 13.3 (CONTINUED)

PHYSICAL EXAMINATION

GENERAL: The patient is a well-developed, elderly male in marked respiratory distress at the time he was admitted to the hospital.

VITAL SIGNS: Temperature 97.8, pulse 130, respirations 33, blood pressure 280/170.

SKIN: Warm and dry with no rash or lesion.

HEAD: Normocephalic. No evidence of recent trauma.

EYES: Pupils equal, round, regular, react to light and accommodation. Extraocular muscles intact. Sclerae nonicteric, conjunctivae pink.

MOUTH/THROAT: Oral mucosa pink without lesions or exudates. Tongue and uvula are in the midline.

NECK: Supple, no jugular venous distention or hepatojugular reflex. Carotids are 2+ without bruits. No thyroid enlargement.

CHEST: Rales heard in the lower lung fields bilaterally.

HEART: Regular rate, normal rhythm without clicks, murmurs, gallops or rubs.

ABDOMEN: Soft, nontender, no abdominal masses, rebound, rigidity, organ enlargement, hernias or bruits. The patient had multiple surgical scars present, one longitudinal and some cross transverse abdominal scars also. The patient has a feeding jejunostomy in the left upper abdomen.

EXTREMITIES: No clubbing, cyanosis or edema. The patient moves all extremities. Femoral pulses are 2+ and equal, dorsalis pedis pulses are 2+ and equal.

NEUROLOGICAL: The patient is awake, alert, oriented times three. Cranial nerves II–XII are intact. Motor and sensory are intact without focal weakness or sensory disturbance.

ASSESSMENT
1. Hypertensive crisis with congestive heart failure and acute pulmonary edema.
2. Essential hypertension.
3. Insulin-dependent diabetes mellitus.
4. Gastroesophageal reflux disease.
5. Feeding jejunostomy secondary to history of duodenal outlet obstruction, which has now resolved.

PLAN: Admit to the hospital, IM Apresoline p.r.n., nitroglycerin p.r.n., adjust antihypertensive medications, Lasix. Rule out acute myocardial infarction.

Signature affixed via participation in signature program.

D:
T:

CC:

Case Study 13.3 (Coder/Abstract Summary Form)

Patient: **Bill Peters**

Patient documentation: **Review Medical Reports 13.4 and 13.5**

1. Principal diagnosis:

   _____

2. Secondary or other diagnoses:

   _____

3. Principal procedure:

   _____

4. Other procedures:

   _____

5. Additional documentation needed:

   _____

   _____

   _____

   _____

6. Questions for the physician:

   _____

   _____

   _____

   _____

   _____

HISTORY AND PHYSICAL

PATIENT: Peters, Bill

ROOM:

PATIENT#:

MED REC#:

ADMITTED:

DISCHARGED:

TRAN:

DICT:

CHIEF COMPLAINT: Shortness of breath and leg swelling.

HISTORY OF PRESENT ILLNESS: This 82-year-old male with a prior history of chronic atrial fibrillation, ischemic cardiomy-opathy with multivessel coronary disease (see below) and chronic obstructive lung disease with chronic bronchitis came to the clinic today for pacemaker interrogation. Over the past 2 weeks or so he has had worsening lower extremity swelling, shortness of breath, but at rest and with exertion and has had his diuretic medications adjusted. He also had a home oxygen supply provided for him as of Friday because of shortness of breath. After being seen by his doctor, his oxy-genation was somewhere between 88 and 92% saturated.

Today, he is markedly conversationally dyspneic and unable to complete a sentence without panting. He also has marked leg swelling with 3 + pitting, ankle and pretibial edema bilaterally. His weight remarkably is actually down and on exami-nation pulse oximetry and saturation is 93% on room air. His lung exam revealed decreased breath sounds in both lung fields and no third heart sound was heard on heart exam.

After reviewing the case with Dr. Smith, a decision was made to admit the patient for bedrest, intravenous diuretics and check baseline labs.

ALLERGIES: He has no known drug allergies.

CURRENT MEDICATIONS:
1. Coumadin 2.5 mg daily.
2. Coreg 25 mg twice a day.
3. Lasix 20 mg daily.
4. Celexa 20 mg daily.
5. Glipizide 5 mg in the morning and 2.5 mg in the evening.
6. Isosorbide mononitrate 30 mg daily.
7. Reminyl 4 mg twice a day.
8. Miacalcin Nasal Spray daily.
9. Zantac 115 mg as needed.
10. Claritin 10 mg daily.
11. Flonase nasal spray twice a day.

PRIOR MEDICAL HISTORY: As stated above with cardiac catheterization demonstrating 95% stenosis in the proximal first diagonal branch from the LAD, 90% stenosis in the first obtuse marginal branch of the left circumflex coronary, and dif-fusely diseased with quite dominant right coronary artery with a 70 and 80% proximal stenosis and 90% distal stenosis. The left ventricle showed global with the inferior wall akinetic and an ejection fraction of 25 to 30%. The LAD was apparently not severely diseased, but a small vessel overall. The patient also has chronic bronchitis, oral agent controlled

Continued

MEDICAL REPORT 13.4 (CONTINUED)

diabetes mellitus, history of peptic ulcer disease in the past with Billroth II gastrectomy in 1995, DVT after this Billroth II gastrectomy, chronic atrial fibrillation and BPH. Medical history is otherwise negative for thyroid disease, rheumatic fever or scarlet fever or colitis.

PRIOR SURGICAL HISTORY: Positive for an appendectomy, a gastrectomy as noted above, cardiac catheterization, dual-chamber pacemaker placement a couple of years ago and TURP in 2001. He required short nursing home placement thereafter because of dementia. Other surgeries are denied.

SOCIAL HISTORY: The patient does not smoke cigarettes. Denies alcohol use. His activities of daily living are markedly limited secondary to dyspnea with exertion and especially limited as above. He lives with his wife in a house. He has had no occupational exposures to asbestos or coal dust.

FAMILY HISTORY: Father deceased at 85 from a stroke. A brother died at 50 from an acute myocardial infarction. Mother deceased at 81 after a cholecystectomy with complications thereafter. A sister has rheumatoid arthritis and apparently hemoptysis. Other family history is noncontributory.

REVIEW OF SYSTEMS: As above and he denies lightheadedness, passing out spells, fevers, chills or sweats. He has cough with some left-sided "rattling," but difficulty expectorating sputum. Denies any weight gain. He denies any abdominal swelling, chest pain, pressure, tightness, squeezing or discomfort. He denies any abdominal pain, dysuria, hematuria, frequency, incontinence or hesitancy. He denies any extremity diarrhea, constipation, hematochezia or melena. He has marked lower extremity swelling. He denies calf claudication. He is mildly depressed but denies suicidal ideation. He does have some easy bruising, especially in his arms. He denies any bleeding diathesis. His remaining system review is noncontributory.

PHYSICAL EXAMINATION: On physical exam today in the office the pulse rate was 70 and regular, respirations of 24, blood pressure of 82/64 and he is afebrile. This elderly white male appears rather cachectic and is awake, alert and oriented to time, place and person. Answers questions appropriately with intelligible speech. He is in no acute distress. Skin is warm and dry with good turgor and texture. Multiple ecchymosed areas are noted over the arms. No rashes are noted.

HEENT: The pupils are equal, round and reactive to light. The extraocular muscles are intact. There is no scleral icterus or conjunctival hemorrhage. No xanthelasma are present. The orbits are somewhat sunken. There is a masseter muscle wasting. Mucous membranes are tacky. Dentition is fair. Neck shows no JVD or HJR. The carotids have normal upstroke and amplitude bilaterally without bruits. No thyromegaly is palpated. The lungs have distant breath sounds and a few crackles in both lower fields. The upper fields are without expiratory wheezes.

Expiratory phase is markedly prolonged. The heart is without heave and the PMI is nondisplaced. Heart sounds are distant. The rhythm is regular without murmur or abnormal third heart sound. The abdomen is soft, nontender and nondistended with normoactive bowel sounds and no organomegaly, masses, shifting dullness or bruits. The extremities show 3 + pitting, pedal, ankle and pretibial edema to the knees bilaterally with no calf tenderness noted to palpation. No cervical lymphadenopathy is palpated. The musculoskeletal exam reveals increase in the normal thoracic kyphosis, but no scoliosis and no paravertebral muscular tenderness, ropiness or bogginess to palpation. Neurologic exam is grossly nonfocal.

LABORATORY DATA: Pulse oximetry is 93% on room air. Electrocardiogram demonstrates atrial fibrillation with ventricular pacing and is unchanged from previous office tracings.

IMPRESSION:
1. Congestive heart failure which is acute, mostly right sided, but certainly left sided with hypoxia noted.
2. Chronic obstructive pulmonary disease with chronic bronchitis.
3. Chronic atrial fibrillation.
4. Dementia, which is also chronic for him.
5. Coronary artery disease as noted above.
6. A recent nontraumatic compression fracture of the lumbar spine with pain secondary to this.
7. Hypotension with diuretics and Coreg his only medications that might lower his blood pressure. Isosorbide mononitrate can do this occasionally.

MEDICAL REPORT 13.4 (CONTINUED)

PLAN:

1. Will admit to telemetry.
2. Bedrest will be attempted, except for bathroom privileges.
3. Supplemental oxygen will be administered.
4. Intravenous Lasix will be given.
5. Will check chest x-ray and baseline laboratories.
6. Will decrease Coreg dose with low blood pressure.
7. Will consult Doctor. The case was discussed with him at length.

_____

M.D. Signature

DD:

TD:

NOTES

MEDICAL REPORT 13.5

POST PROCEDURE NOTES

DATE	
	Pre-op diagnosis: left pe
	Post-op diagnosis: left pe
	Procedure: thoracentesis 1000 cm yellow fluid
	Physician: Dr. Smith
	Post-procedure comments:
	Cardiology
	Tolerated thoracentesis
	Feeling better
	BP 131/68 176 T97.2
	TVP = 5-10
	Chest: clear to P + A
	Con: reg; S1 + S2 nl, no S3 or @4, no m
	Ext:
	Na 143 K3.5 BUN 25
	Cxr – no pneumothorax
	Overall, doing reasonably well
	Med
	1. CHF – improving
	2. Pleural effusion
	3. Dementia

Case Study 13.4 (Coder/Abstract Summary Form)

Patient: **David Brooks**

Patient documentation: **Review Medical Reports 13.6 and 13.7**

1. Principal diagnosis:

   _____

2. Secondary or other diagnoses:

   _____

3. Principal procedure:

   _____

4. Other procedures:

   _____

5. Additional documentation needed:

   _____

   _____

   _____

   _____

6. Questions for the physician:

   _____

   _____

   _____

   _____

   _____

MEDICAL REPORT 13.6

HISTORY AND PHYSICAL

PATIENT: Brooks, David

MR#:

RM:

ATT.PHYS: Smith, M.D.

DATE:

HISTORY OF THE PRESENT ILLNESS: The patient is a 71-year-old male known to me with a previous history of percutaneous transluminal coronary angioplasty and stent times two approximately two years ago. Previous coronary artery bypass grafting 12 years ago, now presents with chest pain.

He has been doing well for quite some time. Apparently had substernal chest pain like his angina and his nitroglycerin did not relieve it. The patient went to the emergency room and was given nitroglycerin with some relief. However, had runs of ventricular tachycardia requiring lidocaine and is now transferred for further medical care.

He has had no recent paroxysmal nocturnal dyspnea, dyspnea on exertion, orthopnea, leg edema, or palpitations noted. Decreased exercise tolerance. He is a security guard and walks most of the time and continues to work every day.

REVIEW OF SYSTEMS: No hematochezia. No hematemesis. No chills. No fever. No nocturia, dysuria and no constipation.

ALLERGIES: NO KNOWN DRUG ALLERGIES.

MEDICATIONS:
1. Accupril.
2. Lipitor.

PHYSICAL EXAMINATION

GENERAL: He is a 71-year-old, well-developed, well-nourished white male in no apparent distress.

VITAL SIGNS: Stable.

HEENT: Eyes pupils equal, round and reactive to light and accommodation. Mouth moist. Nose patent. Gross hearing intact.

NECK: Supple, no adenopathy, no jugular venous distention, no bruits.

CARDIOVASCULAR: Regular rate and rhythm and distant S4.

LUNGS: Clear without rales or rhonchi.

ABDOMEN: Protuberant, soft, nontender, normoactive bowel sounds. No masses.

EXTREMITIES: Two plus pulses, full range of motion. No clubbing, cyanosis or edema.

NEURO: Nonfocal.

RECTAL: Not indicated.

ASSESSMENT: Pre-infarct angina with ventricular tachycardia.

MEDICAL REPORT 13.6 (CONTINUED)

PLAN:

1. Lidocaine, nitroglycerin, heparin.
2. Set up for left heart catheterization in a.m.

He understands the risks, benefits and agrees.

Further recommendations to follow.

D:

T:

CC:

NOTES

MEDICAL REPORT 13.7

CARDIAC CATHETERIZATION REPORT

PATIENT: Brooks, David

MR#:

RM:

ATT.PHYS: Smith, M.D.

DATE:

PROCEDURE PERFORMED: Left heart catheterization, percutaneous coronary intervention with stent placement.

PROCEDURE PERFORMED BY: John Smith M.D.

DESCRIPTION OF PROCEDURE: Following informed, witnessed consent, the patient was taken to the Medical Center cardiac catheterization laboratory where the right groin was prepped and draped in sterile fashion. Local anesthesia was given with 1% lidocaine.

A thin-wall needle was inserted into the right femoral artery and subsequently a 6-French sheath inserted into the right femoral artery. Heparin was given to maintain an ACT of approximately 200 to 230 initially. A pigtail catheter was introduced into the right femoral and advanced to the ascending aorta and across the aortic valve into the left ventricle. Left ventricular end-diastolic pressures were recorded. A left ventriculography was performed in the RAO projection. A left ventricular aortic root pullback was obtained. The pigtail catheter was removed and a 6-French 4 left and 4 right coronary catheters were inserted and demonstrated coronary angiography in multiple projections of both the left and right systems. In addition, coronary angiography was performed with the right coronary catheter of the saphenous vein graft and also demonstrated an occluded graft. The catheter was then removed. The pictures were reviewed. Dr. Heart came in and actually looked at the films with me in detail for consideration of possible revascularization options. We elected, subsequent to our discussion, to proceed with percutaneous transluminal coronary angioplasty and stent placement attempt at the saphenous vein graft to the left anterior descending where there was a 99% stenotic area at the anastomosis site of the saphenous vein graft to the left anterior descending.

A 6-French sheath was inserted into the right femoral vein. Heparin at 1000 units was given additionally and then we discontinued the heparin. A hockey-stick guide was then inserted over a wire and advanced to the ascending aorta anastomosis and to the saphenous vein graft. A BMW wire was then inserted and was able to cross the stenosis and anastomotic area into the left anterior descending. Subsequently, a 2.5 cutting balloon was inserted and advanced to the stenotic site. Balloon inflations were initially performed at nominal pressures and then to 10 atmospheres. Repeat angiography demonstrated clearly a significant improvement, but there was still a residual area of stenosis in the proximal vein graft portion of the lesion. We then inserted a 3.0 multilink stent across this area and dilated that further. Because the proximal area of the artery was still somewhat narrowed, we removed the stent and placed a 4.0, 8-mm stent and went in and dilated this to nominal pressures. The proximal area of the vein graft and in the proximal area of the stent to a higher pressure of 14 to 15 mm of pressure. Repeat angiography demonstrated normal flow throughout the vessel and no critical areas of stenosis, residual stenosis of 0%.

The balloon was removed. The wires were removed and repeat angiography demonstrated again normal flow with no evidence of dissection. The sheaths were secure in place and the stent balloon and wire were removed as well as the guiding catheter. The patient was returned to the recovery room in stable condition with stable vital signs.

HEMODYNAMICS: Systemic arterial pressure was initially 138/70 and ranged between that and 142/70 throughout the entire procedure. The left ventricular end-diastolic pressure was measured at 29. No gradient was noted on pullback across the aortic valve.

ANGIOGRAPHY: Fluoroscopy of the left ventricle demonstrates previous areas of stent and bypass surgery and surgical clips, and some calcification noted in the proximal left anterior descending and proximal right coronary artery as well as well as in the aortic root.

LEFT VENTRICULOGRAPHY: Left ventriculography was performed in the RAO projection that demonstrates a normal-size left ventricle with significant hypokinesis noted in the inferior base, less hypokinesis noted in the mid inferior wall, and an

MEDICAL REPORT 13.7 (CONTINUED)

apical dyskinetic area that was small and limited to the apex with a normally appearing anterior anterolateral wall. The overall ejection fraction appeared to be in the 35–40% range. Trace mitral regurgitation was present. The aortic root appeared to be of normal size. The aortic valve appeared to open normally and the mitral valve appeared to move normally as well.

CORONARY ANGIOGRAPHY: Right and left coronary angiography demonstrates a right-dominant system. The left main coronary artery is of normal size and gave rise to a left anterior descending and circumflex system as well as a ramus/proximal diagonal vessel. The left anterior descending was critically narrowed at the junction of the distal portion and bifurcation to 90%. The distal left anterior descending vessel was quite diseased throughout its course and you could see reflux into a stenotic anastomotic site of the saphenous vein graft to the left anterior descending. The diagonal vessel appeared to be quite small with mild, diffuse disease and luminal irregularities, but no critical areas of stenosis. The proximal left anterior descending had an 80–90% area of stenosis, but with flow seen through the left anterior descending and reflux into the saphenous vein graft. The distal left anterior descending was a fair size and was otherwise free of stenotic disease, continuing to the apex. The circumflex vessel was a very small, diminutive system that did not contribute significantly to the coronary circulation and was not suitable for any interventional purpose. It did appear subtotaled with an obtuse marginal branch seen collaterally filling more distally and this probably represents a significantly larger vessel than appreciated today of the circumflex systems. The right coronary artery was a vessel that has had interventions in the past with stents seen through the proximal as well as the mid and distal sections. The right coronary artery had abnormal flow throughout its course. There was a 30% to 40% stenosis proximally with some calcium seen in the ostium of the circumflex. It continued with stent seen in the proximal to mid portion and the distal with stent being placed into the posterior descending artery. This stent was again becoming restenosed and there is a very tight, 75–90% stenosis seen in the distal right coronary artery just prior to the bifurcation of the posterior descending and posterolateral branches. Good flow was seen through both of these branches. The posterior descending artery vessel appears to have some disease, but appears to have normal flow through it as well. The saphenous vein graft to a previous vessel is occluded with a subtotal occlusion area of the circumflex system. Saphenous vein graft to the left anterior descending vessel had very sluggish flow, TIMI-1 to 2 flow, and demonstrated again a good distal left anterior descending vessel. The obstruction in the saphenous vein graft was at the anastomosis to the left anterior descending.

Following stent placement with the 3.0 balloon and the cutting balloon, and a subsequent larger balloon in the proximal portion of the diseased area and into the vein graft, there appeared to be a residual stenosis that was quite minimal in the vein graft and normal, negative stenosis seen throughout the area of the anastomosis. Normal flow was seen throughout the vessel.

CONCLUSIONS:

1. Mild to moderate left ventricular systolic dysfunction (left ventricular ejection fraction = 35–40%) with moderate, severe left ventricular diastolic (left ventricular end-diastolic pressure = 20 mm Hg) dysfunction.

2. Critical multivessel coronary arterial disease with a subtotaled area of the circumflex, critical disease seen at the left anterior descending graft and anastomotic site, and severe disease seen in the distal right coronary artery.

3. Successful percutaneous transluminal coronary intervention with cutting balloon therapy as well as stent placement in the saphenous vein graft and anastomosis site to the left anterior descending and into the left anterior descending itself.

_____

M.D. signature

D:

T:

CC:

Case Study 13.5 (Coder/Abstract Summary Form)

Patient: **Peter Smith**

Patient documentation: **Review Medical Report 13.8**

1. Principal diagnosis:

   _____

2. Secondary or other diagnoses:

   _____

3. Principal procedure:

   _____

4. Other procedures:

   _____

5. Additional documentation needed:

   _____

   _____

   _____

   _____

6. Questions for the physician:

   _____

   _____

   _____

   _____

   _____

   _____

MEDICAL REPORT 13.8

OPERATIVE REPORT

PATIENT: Smith, Peter

ROOM #:

MR#:

PT #:

ADMIT DATE:

PROCEDURE DATE:

PREOPERATIVE DIAGNOSIS: Multivessel coronary artery disease with diminished ejection fraction.

POSTOPERATIVE DIAGNOSIS: Multivessel coronary artery disease with diminished ejection fraction.

PROCEDURE:
1. Coronary artery bypass grafting × 5 with pedicle left internal mammary artery to left anterior descending, reverse saphenous vein graft from aorta to obtuse marginal artery #1, sequential reverse saphenous vein graft from aorta to obtuse marginal #2 and 3, reverse saphenous vein graft from aorta to the posterior descending artery.
2. Transmyocardial laser revascularization, 19 channels in the posterior and apical walls where vessels were nonbypassable.

SURGEON:

ASSISTANT:

ANESTHESIA:

REFERRING PHYSICIAN:

PRIMARY PHYSICIAN:

CROSS-CLAMP TIME: 70 minutes.

BYPASS TIME: 125 minutes. He came off on low dose epinephrine and nitroglycerin in normal sinus rhythm.

INDICATIONS: He is a pleasant 65-year-old gentleman who was admitted to the hospital with unstable angina. He ruled in for myocardial infarction and underwent cardiac catheterization. Left cardiac catheterization with coronary angiography demonstrated multivessel coronary artery disease with diminished ejection fraction. He was referred to me for elective revascularization.

DESCRIPTION OF PROCEDURE: The patient was taken to the operating room and placed in the comfortable supine position on the OR table, and after general endotracheal anesthesia was induced and invasive monitoring was placed, he was prepped and draped in normal sterile fashion.

Transesophageal echocardiogram demonstrated diminished ejection fraction with mild to moderate MR.

The saphenous vein was harvested from his left lower extremity. Standard technique with proximal and distal control was utilized in harvesting the vein. The vein was a poor quality vein but was usable for bypass. His entire left leg saphenous vein was harvested. The wounds were then closed in multiple layers and the vein was prepared on the back table.

The midline sternotomy incision was made. It was taken down sharply. The sternum was divided in the midline. The left pleural space was entered. The internal mammary artery was skeletonized from the subclavian vein to the costal margin. Heparin was administered. It was clipped distally and transected. There was adequate pulsatile flow. It was prepared with topical papaverine and set aside.

The pericardium was then opened in the midline. Pericardial well was fashioned. The aorta was cannulized from the pulmonary artery. The aorta was cannulated with an 8-mm angled cannula. A two-stage venous cannula was placed via the right arterial appendage. Antegrade cardioplegia needle was placed.

Continued

MEDICAL REPORT 13.8 (CONTINUED)

After ACTs were greater than 450, we commenced cardiopulmonary bypass and cooled to 32 degrees. The LAD was heavily diseased vessel, 2 mm in diameter. The PDA was a bifurcated vessel, heavily diseased. The larger of the 2 bifurcated segments, which ran along the great cardiac vein, was 1.1 mm in diameter. The obtuse marginal artery # 1 was an intramyocardial vessel 1.8 mm in diameter. The OM 2 was heavily diseased 1.5-mm vessel. The OM 3 was a 1.0-mm vessel, barely bypassable. His terminal circumflex divided into the 3 small branches that were amenable to bypassing. There was some marbleized muscle indicating recent infarction in the posterior lateral wall. The aorta was cross-clamped. One liter of cold blood cardioplegia was administered in root and the heart arrested in diastole. The PDA artery was opened longitudinally. A standard end-to-side reverse saphenous vein to PDA artery anastomosis was then performed using running 7-0 Prolene suture. Next, the OM3 artery was opened longitudinally. A standard end-to-side reverse saphenous vein to OM3 artery anastomosis was then performed using running 7-0 Prolene suture. A second dose of cardioplegia was administered, and the OM 2 artery was opened longitudinally. A standard side-to-side OM2 artery to saphenous vein anastomosis was then performed using a running 7-0 Prolene suture.

I then trimmed the vein to the appropriate length and sewed the end of the saphenous vein to the OM 1 artery anastomosis using running 7-0 Prolene suture. A third dose of cardioplegia was administered and the mid LAD was opened longitudinally. A standard end-to-side IMA to LAD artery anastomosis was then performed using a running 7-0 Prolene suture. The cross-clamp was removed. The patient was rewarmed.

Three proximal anastomoses were taken off the ascending aorta using a 4-mm punch and 5-0 and 6-0 Prolene sutures. The partial aortic occlusion clamp was removed, de-airing the ascending aorta and then the anastomoses were securely tied. The patient was rewarmed. We had excellent Doppler signal within all our grafts and then turned my attention to the TMR of the posterior wall.

The heart was filled. The heart was elevated and I laid 19 channels with a laser. Nineteen channels involving a portion of the posterolateral wall, posterior wall, and the posterior apex received all the 19 channels. The heart was then returned back through the pericardial space. Atrial and ventricular pacing wires were placed. We were able to wean off cardiopulmonary bypass using low dose epinephrine and nitroglycerin to maintain normal sinus rhythm. Postoperative TEE showed improvement in LV function. Protamine was administered and we decannulated the patient after meticulous hemostasis was obtained. We turned our attention to closure.

The chest was drained with a right, left, and mediastinal chest tube. The sternum was rewired using #5 gauge sternal wire. The fascia was closed with #1 Vicryl sutures. The subcutaneous tissue was closed with 2-0 sutures, and the skin was closed with a running Monocryl stitch. The patient tolerated the procedure well and was taken in stable condition to the cardiac intensive care unit with all sponge and needle counts correct.

_____

M.D. signature

D:

T:

CC:

Coding for Neoplasms

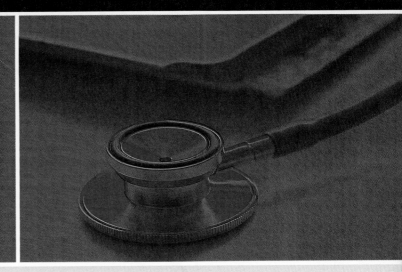

Chapter Outline

Classifying Neoplasm Behaviors
Morphology Codes
Grading and Staging of Cancer
Locating Neoplasm Codes
Coding Solid-Tumor Malignancies
Coding Hematopoietic and Lymphatic Malignancies
Identifying the Principal Diagnosis
Testing Your Comprehension
Coding Practice I: Chapter Review Exercises
Coding Practice II: Medical Record Case Studies

Chapter Objectives

▶ Describe the pathology of common neoplasms.
▶ Recognize the typical manifestations, complications, and treatments of common neoplasms in terms of their implications for coding.
▶ Correctly code common neoplasms and related procedures by using the ICD-9-CM and medical records.

*Coding for neoplasms is included in code section 140 to 239 of chapter 2 in the Disease Tabular of the ICD-9-CM. A **neoplasm**, also called a **tumor**, is an abnormal growth of tissue that arises from healthy tissue. It is important for coders to understand that not all tumors are cancerous. However, no tumor, regardless of its behavior, has a useful function. A neoplasm is abnormal tissue that grows by cellular proliferation more rapidly than normal tissue and continues to grow after the stimuli that initiated the new growth cease. Neoplasms show a partial or complete lack of structural organization and functional coordination with the normal tissue, and they usually form a distinct mass of tissue that may be either benign (benign tumor) or malignant (cancer).[1] To assist in your understanding, the Word Parts Box on page 430 reviews word parts and meanings of medical terms related to neoplasms.*

Word Parts and Meanings of Medical Terms Related to Neoplasms

Word Part	Meaning	Example	Definition of Example
carcin/o-	cancer	carcinoma	Malignant neoplasm involving epithelial tissue that lines skin and internal organs
-oma	tumor; mass	osteoma; lipoma; myoma	Benign (noncancerous) neoplasm of bone; benign neoplasm of fat; benign neoplasm of muscle
aden/o-	gland	adenoma; adenocarcinoma	Benign (noncancerous) neoplasm of glandular epithelial tissue; malignant neoplasm of glandular epithelial tissue
-blast	immature	lymphoblast	An immature lymphocyte (type of white blood cell that produces antibodies)
-plasm	growth	neoplasm	New growth
onc/o-	tumor	oncology	The study of tumors
-therapy	treatment	radiotherapy	Treatment of disease with radiation
meta-	change; beyond	metastasis	Going beyond the original site of cancer
ana-	backward	anaplasia	Reverting (backward) to a more primitive cell form; loss of cell differentiation (structure)
sarc/o-	connective tissue	osteosarcoma; myosarcoma	Malignant neoplasm of bone (a connective tissue); malignant neoplasm of muscle
chem/o-	drugs	chemotherapy	Treatment of disease with drugs

Classifying Neoplasm Behaviors

The neoplasm chapter of the ICD-9-CM is divided into categories that describe **behaviors** for neoplasms:

140–195	Primary malignancies
196–198	Secondary malignancies
199	Malignant neoplasms of unspecified site
200–208	Leukemia, lymphoma, and myeloma
209	Carcinoid tumors (malignant and benign)
210–229	Benign neoplasm
230–234	Carcinoma in situ
235–238	Neoplasms of uncertain behavior
239	Neoplasms of unspecified nature

Malignant Neoplasms

Malignant (cancerous) neoplasms or tumors can be fatal if untreated. Cancer cells occur as a mutation of DNA. DNA provides the blueprint for the production of new body cells (i.e., cell division called **mitosis**) and controls cell growth by producing proteins. Normal body cells wear out and die in a process called **apoptosis** (i.e., programmed cell death) and are replaced through the normal functions of DNA. However, cancer cells are not affected by apoptosis, are nonfunctional and harmful, and are characterized by rapid uncontrolled cell division and tumor growth.

Under a microscope, cancer cells lack structure and appear disorganized (undifferentiated or dedifferentiated) when compared with normal tissue cells that have structure and appear organized (differentiated). Causes of cancer include a hereditary (i.e., genetic) predisposition to the disease; environmental exposure to carcinogens such as tobacco, toxic chemicals, insecticides, and fertilizers; and radiation, including sunlight. Also, certain oncogenic viruses such as HIV can cause cancer (i.e., genetic material is found in some viruses that can cause cancer).

Primary and Secondary (Metastatic) Cancer

Primary malignant tumor cells can originate in one or more locations and can infiltrate deeper tissues within the same organ or **metastasize** (i.e., invade, extend, or spread) to secondary organ sites by traveling through the blood and lymph systems. Whereas the primary site indicates the tissue (i.e., organ) where the cancer originated, the **secondary** (metastatic) sites indicate separate organs to which the primary cancer has spread.

Physicians may sometimes use the term **invasion** to mean metastasis; however, invasion of deeper tissue within the same organ is not considered metastasis. In metastasis, the cancer spreads from the primary site (i.e., organ of origin) to separate (secondary) organ sites. For example, a primary breast cancer invading axillary lymph nodes represents metastasis and is coded to 174.9 + 196.3, whereas kidney cancer of the cortex (outer portion of kidney) invading the medulla (inner portion of the kidney) represents a primary kidney cancer only and is correctly coded to 189.1—not to 189.1 + 198.0. A patient cannot have a primary and secondary cancer of the same organ.

Carcinoma In Situ

Carcinoma in situ describes cancer that is superficial (localized on the surface of the organ) and has not yet invaded deeper tissues.

Benign Neoplasms

Benign neoplasms are noncancerous. In contrast to cancerous tumors, benign neoplasms are characterized by slow growth and do not invade or spread to surrounding tissues (i.e., they are noninvasive). Under a microscope, benign tumor cells appear well differentiated. This means that the tumor cell structure is organized and closely resembles that of normal surrounding tissue cells. Benign tumors do not have the capacity to metastasize (i.e., break away from the original tumor and spread to distant or secondary organ sites or structures). Although benign neoplasms are usually not life-threatening, they can crowd surrounding organs and tissues and sometimes transform into a cancerous condition. A benign neoplasm can usually be surgically removed or destroyed without recurrence.

Neoplasms of Uncertain Behavior

Uncertain behavior means that the tumor cells, under microscopic examination by the pathologist, appear atypical (abnormal) but are noncancerous (i.e., precancerous) at present.

Unspecified Neoplasms

The codes for **unspecified** neoplasms or tumors (i.e., meaning "of unknown behavior") are rarely used for inpatient coding. However, they may be used if the diagnostic workup is incomplete (e.g., the patient leaves the hospital against medical advice or is transferred to another facility before a workup can be completed).

Morphology Codes

At national, state, and local levels, agencies are collecting data to improve the quality of care for cancer patients. Both federal and state funding for state cancer registries require certain providers (e.g., hospitals and ambulatory care facilities) to report newly diagnosed cancer cases (called *analytical cases*) to the state. Also, some health-care facilities offer cancer programs accredited through the American College of Surgeons (ACOS). These facilities strive to adhere to high quality standards for providing care to cancer patients that require more rigorous reporting of patient cancer data, including the use of morphology codes (M codes).

M codes are used in cancer registries and are not required for inpatient reporting for third-party payment. M codes describe the structure (shape) of the cancer cell to identify and classify the tissue cells (histologic type) where the cancer first originated. Each tissue type is made up of similar cells, so by identifying the cell type, pathologists can determine the tissue of origin.

M codes are easy to recognize because they each begin with the capital letter "M" followed by four digits, a forward slash, and a fifth digit. The "M" identifies it as an M code, the next four digits describe the histologic (tissue) type, and the fifth digit represents the behavior of the tumor (primary, secondary, carcinoma in situ, benign, uncertain behavior, or unspecified), which correlates with the columns in the Neoplasm Table in the *Alphabetic Index to Diseases* (volume 2). The ICD-9-CM includes M codes after the main term for a particular cancer type (see excerpt below) in the Disease Index and also at the end of the coding book in the Morphology of Neoplasms appendix. Medical coders working in hospital-based cancer registries need to be proficient in the use of M codes.

Adenocarcinoma (M8140/3)—*see* also
  Neoplasm, by site, malignant

> *Note—The following list of adjectival modifiers is not exhaustive. A description of adenocarcinoma that does not appear in this list should be coded in the same manner as carcinoma with that description. Thus, "mixed acidophil-basophil adenocarcinoma," should be coded in the same manner as "mixed acidophil-basophil carcinoma," which appears in the list under "Carcinoma."*
>
> *Except where otherwise indicated, the morphological varieties of adenocarcinoma in the list should be coded by site as for "Neoplasm, malignant."*

  with
      apocrine metaplasia (M8573/3)
      cartilaginous (and osseous) metaplasia (M8571/3)
      osseous (and cartilaginous) metaplasia (M8571/3)
      spindle cell metaplasia (M8572/3)
      squamous metaplasia (M8570/3)
  acidophil (M8280/3)
      specified site—*see* Neoplasm, by site, malignant
      unspecified site (194.3)
  acinar (M8550/3)

Grading and Staging of Cancer

In coding for oncology, the concepts of grading, staging, protocol, and prognosis are important for coders to understand. Knowledge of these concepts enables you to have more insight into common neoplasms and their treatments (both diagnostic and therapeutic). This insight also allows you to be more aware of what to look for while reviewing the patient's medical record to assign the most accurate codes. For example, diagnosis of carcinoma in situ (noninvasive) of the breast is typically recognized as being treated with a lumpectomy or other localized treatment. However, breast carcinoma metastatic to the axillary lymph nodes often requires more radical treatment, such as a modified mastectomy followed by radiation, chemotherapy, or both.

Grading refers to the maturity (degree of differentiation) of the neoplasm when it is viewed under a microscope. The higher the grade (**dedifferentiation**, or lack of differentiation), the more aggressive the tumor; this, in turn, relates to a poor prognosis (or chance for survival) for the patient. Neoplasms are usually graded on a scale from 1 to 4:

▶ grade 1—the tumor is well differentiated (i.e., cells still have structure and closely resemble normal surrounding tissue cells)
▶ grade 2—the tumor is moderately differentiated (i.e., tissue cells lack structure, are dedifferentiated, or have anaplasia)

    ▶ grade 3—the tumor is poorly differentiated
    ▶ grade 4—the tumor is very poorly differentiated (cells are very undifferentiated [unstructured])

Staging refers to the amount of spread of the cancer (i.e., whether the primary cancer has metastasized to lymph nodes or other distant organ sites). The Tumor, Node, Metastasis (TNM) and the Surveillance, Epidemiology, and End Results (SEER) systems are well-known staging systems that measure the spread of cancer. In the TNM system, developed by the American Joint Committee on Cancer, the T describes the size of the tumor, the N describes whether there is regional lymph node involvement, and the M describes whether there are distant metastases. Cancer registrars collect and report important data for hospital and state cancer registries by using the *International Classification of Disease for Oncology*, published by the World Health Organization, which provides codes for the site, morphology, grade, and behavior of the neoplasm. Cancer registrars also use the Surveillance, Epidemiology, and End Results or the TNM cancer staging system (or both) to report cancer spread. Registries use these data to study and improve the care of cancer patients.

Grading and staging of a cancerous tumor are taken into account when determining the *protocol*, which is a written plan indicating the best course of treatment for the patient, and the *prognosis*, which is the statistically known short- and long-term success rate for cure and life expectancy for the patient.

Locating Neoplasm Codes

In the field of oncology, which involves the study of tumors, it is critically important to determine the primary cancer site to treat the cancer effectively at its originating source. Diagnostic procedures strive to identify where the cancer first began because the originating source can continue to "seed" secondary (metastatic) cancer sites. Although not all cancers metastasize, early detection is crucial to prevent further spread of the cancer and to improve the patient's chances for survival. However, symptoms associated with the secondary (metastatic) sites and not with the primary cancer site often cause the initial admission of a patient to the hospital for care (e.g., abdominal pain with liver metastasis from a primary breast carcinoma). Further evaluation of the metastatic site (e.g., via biopsy and pathologic tissue examination) pinpoints the primary disease site. As a coder, you must be able to correctly distinguish primary from secondary sites.

There are some important keys to precise coding for cancerous neoplasms. The documentation of the cancer cell's morphology (form and structure) by the pathologist or attending physician is an important clue to correctly identifying the neoplasm as a primary or a secondary cancer site. For example, in the phrase "oat cell carcinoma of brain," **oat cell** denotes the morphologic type of cancer. By looking up the main term "carcinoma" and the subterm "oat cell, unspecified" in the Disease Index, you will see that oat cell carcinoma originates from the lung. Because oat cells come from the lung and are not normally found in the brain, the lung is the primary originating source of the cancer in this case, and the brain is a secondary metastatic site (coded 162.9 + 198.3). Morphologic types are easily recognized as modifiers (adjectives) added to the main terms "cancer," "carcinoma," or "adenocarcinoma" in the Disease Index (e.g., "renal cell carcinoma to the liver" means kidney cancer that has metastasized to the liver).

Often, however the physician does not document the cancer's morphologic type, and you must locate neoplasm codes by using the Neoplasm Table provided in the *Alphabetic Index to Diseases* (volume 2). The Neoplasm Table (an excerpt of which is printed below) provides quick access to the location (anatomic site) and behavior of various tumors. Rows within the Neoplasm Table identify the anatomic site of the tumor, such as lung or abdomen. Columns identify the tumor's behavior (primary malignancy, secondary malignancy, carcinoma in situ, benign, uncertain, or unspecified).

Neoplasm, Neoplastic— *Continued*	Malignant			Benign	Uncertain Behavior	Unspecified
	Primary	Secondary	Ca in Situ			
lung	162.9	197.0	231.2	212.3	235.7	239.1
azygos lobe	162.3	197.0	231.2	212.3	235.7	239.1
carina	162.2	197.0	231.2	212.3	235.7	239.1
contiguous sites with bronchus or trachea	162.8	—	—	—	—	—
hilus	162.2	197.0	231.2	212.3	235.7	239.1
lingula	162.3	197.0	231.2	212.3	235.7	239.1
lobe NEC	162.9	197.0	231.2	212.3	235.7	239.1
lower lobe	162.5	197.0	231.2	212.3	235.7	239.1
main bronchus	162.2	197.0	231.2	212.3	235.7	239.1
middle lobe	162.4	197.0	231.2	212.3	235.7	239.1
upper lobe	162.3	197.0	231.2	212.3	235.7	239.1

Ca, carcinoma; NEC, not elsewhere classified.

Coding Solid-Tumor Malignancies

All cancers located in the Neoplasm Table represent solid tumors, and only solid malignant tumors can metastasize (i.e., travel to secondary organ sites). In contrast, hematopoietic and lymphatic malignancies (described in the next section) represent circulatory tumors that are not located in the Neoplasm Table. Also, hematopoietic and lymphatic malignancies do not metastasize as do solid tumors.

Primary Versus Secondary (Metastatic) Malignancies

Sometimes physicians' documentation of metastatic cancer is so vague that it can be difficult to determine whether the cancer sites are primary or secondary. Coders sometimes become frustrated with physicians when they do not clearly document the primary and secondary sites of cancer. However, sometimes the maturity (grade) of the cancer cells is so high (very disorganized or very poorly differentiated cells) that it is difficult for the pathologist to identify the tissue of cancer origin. Not all cancers metastasize, but if the physician documents metastatic cancer, you must assign two (or more) codes that correctly identify both the primary and metastatic sites.

If the previous primary or secondary site has been completely eradicated, it can be described through an additional "history of" code (e.g., bone metastases with a history of prostate cancer, status post radical prostatectomy: 198.5 + V10.46). When either the primary or the secondary site cannot be identified, assign code 199.1 for unspecified primary or secondary site. You can locate code 199.1 within the Neoplasm Table under "Neoplasm, unknown site or unspecified."

EXAMPLE	*Metastatic cancer from the lung: 162.9 + 199.1*
	Metastatic cancer to the lung: 197.0 + 199.1

To correctly code metastatic cancers, pay close attention to the connecting words **to**, **from**, and **of** in the physician's diagnostic statement. The connecting words **to** and **from** reveal where the cancer is coming *from* (primary originating source) and where it traveled *to* (secondary metastatic site). On the other hand, **of** is vague when documented in the context of metastatic cancer, and further clarification from the physician is required. For example, if a physician documents "metastatic cancer of the lung" or "metastatic lung cancer," it is unclear whether the physician intended to identify the lung as a primary or secondary site.

EXAMPLE	*"Metastasis to the lung" indicates a secondary (metastatic) spread to the lung with an unknown primary cancer site: 197.0 (lung secondary) + 199.1 (unknown primary site)*
	"Metastasis from the lung" indicates a primary lung cancer site with an unknown secondary (metastatic) site: 162.9 (lung primary) + 199.1 (unknown secondary site)
	"Metastatic colon cancer to the liver": 153.9 (colon primary) + 197.7 (liver secondary)
	"Metastatic bone cancer from the prostate": 185 (prostate primary) + 198.5 (bone secondary)

TIP *Coding Clinic* offers expert advice regarding what to do when vague documentation is provided for metastatic cancer. For example, *Coding Clinic* describes that certain organ sites—including the liver, bone, brain, peritoneum, lymph nodes, and pleura—are most often recognized as metastatic sites.

In the event that there is vague documentation of metastatic cancer and it is not possible to query the physician, then these sites would be coded as secondary sites. However, if the physician documents an organ site such as the lung, which is not on the list of common secondary sites, without further clarification, you would code that as the primary site. *Coding Clinic* guidelines also state that if multiple sites (two or more) are qualified in the documentation as metastatic, then the sites should be reported as secondary cancer sites with an unknown primary site.

EXAMPLE

Metastatic bone cancer or metastatic cancer of bone: 198.5 + 199.1 (unknown primary cancer site; bone is secondary cancer site)

Metastatic lung cancer or metastatic cancer of the lung: 162.9 + 199.1 (lung is primary cancer site; unknown secondary cancer site)

Metastatic cancer of lung and brain: 197.0 + 198.3 + 199.1 (unknown primary cancer site; multiple secondary cancer sites)

 Coding Clinic 1985, May-June, describes more information regarding neoplasms (140 to 239).

Keep in mind that there is no acceptable margin for error in reporting codes for patients with cancer. Because of the seriousness of the condition and the possible adverse social, work-related, and personal consequences that can result from misinterpreted and misreported cancer data, querying the physician for clarification is always of primary importance. Also remember that accurately coding data for each cancer patient contributes to the overall success of cancer registries that strive to study cancers and cancer treatments to improve the quality of care for all cancer patients.

Contiguous Sites

Contiguous sites are overlapping cancer sites in the same organ. Some organs are divided into sections; for example, the large intestine includes the ascending colon, transverse colon, descending colon, sigmoid, and rectum. When more than one section of the same organ is affected by cancer, it is referred to as **contiguous** or **overlapping** sites. ICD-9-CM classifies this situation through the use of a fourth digit, 8, indicating overlapping or contiguous sites within the same organ. For example, it would be incorrect to code adenocarcinoma of the descending and sigmoid colon to 153.2 and 153.3. Instead, code it to 153.8, meaning malignant neoplasm of contiguous or overlapping sites of the colon for which the point of origin cannot be determined.

Carcinoid Tumors

New codes were introduced to describe carcinoid tumors in 2009. Carcinoid tumors are derived from tissue that is capable of differentiating into benign or malignant neoplasms (e.g., benign carcinoid tumor of the appendix = code 209.51; malignant carcinoid tumor of the appendix = 209.11).

 # Coding Hematopoietic and Lymphatic Malignancies

Hematopoietic and lymphatic cancers, including leukemia (cancer of blood), myeloma (cancer of bone marrow), and lymphoma (cancer of lymph nodes and lymph tissues), are found in the *Alphabetic Index to Diseases* (volume 2) under the main term for the disease and are not located within the Neoplasm Table. This is an important distinction for precise coding. By their nature, hematopoietic and lymphatic cancers are systemic: that is, they circulate but do not metastasize as do solid tumors. Therefore, one should not code a primary circulatory cancer as metastasizing to a solid site. For example, cervical Hodgkin's lymphoma invading the inguinal lymph nodes would be coded to 201.98 (Hodgkin's lymphoma involving lymph nodes of multiple sites) and would not be coded to 201.91 + 196.5 (i.e., one cannot have lymphoma of cervical lymph nodes metastasizing to inguinal lymph nodes).

Cancers of the Blood and Bone Marrow

Leukemia is a cancer of the blood characterized by an increase in the number of malignant white blood cells (leukocytes) in the bone marrow (where blood cells originate) and the bloodstream. The type of white blood cell (leukocyte) affected identifies the type of leukemia.

There are five different mature types of leukocytes: three types of granulocytes and two types of agranulocytes. The three granulocytes (leukocytes that contain granules in their cytoplasm [an area between the nucleus and membrane of a cell] that can be identified with a particular stain) are as follows:

- ▶ neutrophils—a type of leukocyte that fights infection and disease
- ▶ eosinophils—a type of leukocyte that increases in allergic reactions
- ▶ basophils—a type of leukocyte that increases in allergic and inflammatory reactions

The two agranulocytes (leukocytes that do not contain granules in the cytoplasm) are as follows:

- ▶ lymphocytes—a type of leukocyte that produces antibodies to fight infections and disease
- ▶ monocytes—a type of phagocytic leukocyte that surrounds and destroys antigens and their debris (i.e., foreign cells such as bacteria)

Acute forms of leukemia are characterized by an increase of immature white blood cells (**leukoblasts**) in the bloodstream. Chronic forms of the disease involve an increase of mature white blood cells. Symptoms of the disease include fever, fatigue and weakness, enlarged lymph nodes (lymphadenopathy), enlarged spleen (splenomegaly), and enlarged liver (hepatomegaly). Acute forms of the disease result in a rapid onset of symptoms and are more aggressive than chronic forms. Leukemia is often characterized by remissions (no symptoms of the disease) and relapses when the cancerous white blood cells and disease symptoms recur.

EXAMPLE	
	Acute lymphocytic leukemia: 204.00
	Acute lymphocytic leukemia, in remission: 204.01
	Acute lymphoid leukemia, in relapse: 204.02

Four common types of leukemia include the following:

- ▶ Acute lymphocytic leukemia—large numbers of lymphoblasts (immature lymphocytes) are found in the bloodstream. Acute lymphocytic leukemia is a rapidly progressive disease that most often affects children and teenagers.
- ▶ Acute myeloid leukemia (AML)—large numbers of myeloblasts (immature granulocytic neutrophils) are found in the bloodstream.

- Chronic lymphocytic leukemia—increased numbers of mature lymphocytes are found. Chronic lymphocytic leukemia is a slow but progressive disease that most often affects elderly people.
- Chronic myeloid leukemia—increased numbers of mature and immature granulocytic leukocytes are found. Chronic myeloid leukemia is a slow but progressive disease.

Leukemias are most often treated with chemotherapy (drug therapy). Sometimes acute forms of the disease are treated with high-dose chemotherapy to destroy all the leukemic cells, and this is followed by a bone marrow transplantation from a closely matched donor. This procedure is performed to repopulate the bone marrow with normally forming white blood cells.

Multiple myeloma is a cancer caused by malignant plasma cells that are mainly located in the bone marrow. All blood cells originate in the bone marrow from stem cells, and some develop into white blood cells called **lymphocytes**. There are two types of lymphocytes: B-cell lymphocytes and T-cell lymphocytes. Plasma cells develop from B-cell lymphocytes to produce antibodies called **immunoglobulins** that are produced to protect us from different types of foreign organisms. Therefore, plasma cells play an important part in our immune system by fighting infection and disease. In multiple myeloma, malignant plasma cells rapidly divide and grow out of control. They circulate in the bloodstream, accumulate in the bone marrow, and interfere with the normal blood-forming functions of the bone marrow. Symptoms of the disease include recurrent infections, leukopenia (reduction in white blood cells), hypercalcemia (increased calcium in the blood), pain, loss of appetite, fatigue, weakness, mental confusion, anemia, and hyperviscosity syndrome (thickened and sticky blood), and the plasma cells can form bone lesions that result in a weakening of bones. There is no cure for multiple myeloma; however, chemotherapy, radiation therapy, and pain management (with drugs) can help to control and alleviate the symptoms of the disease.

Cancers of the Lymphatic System

Cancers of the lymphatic system include **lymphomas**. Separate from the blood system but closely linked to it, the lymphatic system is a sort of second circulatory system. Like blood, lymph fluid contains lymphocytes and monocytes (white blood cells) that are important in fighting infections; however, lymph does not contain red blood cells or platelets. Lymph fluid filters out of blood vessels throughout the body into surrounding body tissues, where it is called **interstitial fluid**. Interstitial fluid then enters lymph capillaries to become lymph, which flows through lymph vessels and lymph nodes toward large ducts in the chest to eventually return to the bloodstream through veins. There are lymph node concentrations within the body that include the mediastinal (upper chest), inguinal (groin), cervical (neck), and axillary (armpit) areas. An important function of the lymph system is that it serves as a part of our immune system. Lymphocytes and monocytes produced in lymphoid tissues such as lymph nodes and the spleen produce **antibodies**, which circulate throughout the body to attack and destroy harmful foreign organisms such as bacteria and viruses (including cancer cells). Therefore, progressive malignancies involving the lymph nodes and lymph tissue can inhibit the body's ability to fight infection and disease.

Non-Hodgkin's lymphoma (resulting from abnormal lymphocytes with uncontrolled growth) and Hodgkin's disease (resulting from abnormal B-cell lymphocytes called **Reed–Sternberg cells**) comprise most cancers of the lymphatic system. Symptoms of these diseases can include swelling of lymph nodes (lymphadenopathy) caused by the overabundance of lymphocytes that crowd the nodes, enlarged spleen (splenomegaly), fever and chills, fatigue, weight loss, and loss of appetite. Treatment for these lymphomas commonly includes chemotherapy, which is sometimes given in combination with radiation therapy.

EXAMPLE	*Hodgkin's lymphoma invading the lymph nodes of the neck: 201.91*
	Non-Hodgkin's lymphoma with lymphadenopathy of axillary and inguinal lymph nodes: 202.88

Identifying the Principal Diagnosis

Identifying the principal diagnosis for a cancer patient depends on the patient's principal reason for admission.

Treatment of the Primary and Secondary Cancer

The following guidelines will help you to determine whether you should sequence the primary cancer or secondary cancer as the principal diagnosis:

▶ if the principal reason for admission and the main treatment are directed at the primary cancer site, sequence the primary cancer as the principal diagnosis

▶ if the principal reason for admission and the main treatment are directed at the secondary (metastatic) cancer site, sequence the secondary cancer as the principal diagnosis even though the primary cancer may still be present

▶ if the principal reason for admission and the main treatment are directed at both the primary and secondary cancer sites equally, then sequence the primary cancer first

If the admission is for the sole purpose of chemotherapy or radiation therapy (external beam), then assign code V58.11 (admission or encounter for chemotherapy) or V58.0 (admission or encounter for radiation therapy) as the principal diagnosis, and list a current code for the cancer as an additional code. Continue to list the active cancer code until all therapies are discontinued and the cancer is completely eradicated.

A common error is to assign a secondary diagnosis code for "personal history" of cancer when a person is status post surgery and is admitted for adjunct chemotherapy, radiation therapy, or both as a continuation of cancer treatment (e.g., V58.11 [admission for chemotherapy] + V10.3 [personal history of breast cancer]). In this circumstance, it is incorrectly assumed that the cancer was completely eradicated with the initial surgery. Cancer cells can still be circulating after surgery, and treatment with chemotherapy or radiation therapy represents a continuation of a protocol (written treatment plan) for an active cancer condition, so the history code should not be assigned. In this example, the correct code assignment is V58.11 (admission for chemotherapy) + 174.9 (breast cancer).

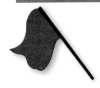 Reporting a "history of" cancer code would indicate that the cancer was completely eradicated and should be sequenced as an additional code only if it bears some significance to the current episode of patient care (e.g., a patient is admitted with gastrointestinal bleeding with a history of colectomy for colon cancer 10 years prior; add code V10.05 for personal history of colon cancer).

An admission for brachytherapy should not be assigned to the admission for radiation therapy code (V58.0). Brachytherapy (92.27) is a procedure in which radioactive substances or "seeds" (small tubes filled with radioactive material such as cesium) are implanted into body tissues (interstitial placement) or a body cavity (intracavitary placement) and result in a localized kill of tumor cells while minimizing radiation damage to healthy surrounding tissues. Sequence the cancer code as the principal diagnosis for a documented admission for a brachytherapy procedure. Often, intracavitary brachytherapy (radioactive substance placed within a body cavity) is used for the treatment of cervix uteri cancer, and interstitial brachytherapy (radioactive substance placed within tissue) can be administered for prostate cancer. Surface application of brachytherapy can be used for skin cancers. The "includes" notes, located under the brachytherapy procedure code (92.27) in the Procedure Tabular, state the need to also code for an incision site when applicable.

A patient with known cervical cancer is admitted for brachytherapy. The patient was taken to surgery, and a cesium implant was inserted into the cervix: 180.0 + 92.27

EXAMPLE

Treatment for Side Effects or Complications Only

Side-effects are expected adverse effects (e.g., symptoms or conditions) that commonly result from the toxic effects of some therapeutic drugs (e.g., nausea and vomiting with dehydration, and anemia or neutropenia that can follow chemotherapy administration; or, drowsiness resulting from the use of antihistamines). If the principal cause of patient admission is for treatment of a sign or symptom associated with a known cancer or a side effect of chemotherapy, sequence the sign or symptom as the principal diagnosis, with the cancer codes listed as additional codes. Recently, a new code was provided (338.3) that can be assigned for neoplasm related pain. This code is assigned for both acute and chronic pain associated with a primary or secondary cancer or tumor. This code may be assigned as the principal diagnosis or as a secondary diagnosis depending on the circumstances of the admission. Per ICD-9-CM Official Guidelines for Coding and Reporting that are effective November 15, 2006, this code is assigned as the principal diagnosis when the stated primary reason for admission/encounter is for pain control/management secondary to a neoplasm. In this circumstance, the underlying neoplasm should then be added as secondary diagnosis. However, when the reason for admission/encounter is for management of the neoplasm, and pain associated with the neoplasm is also documented but not the reason for the admission/encounter; code 338.3 is assigned as a secondary diagnosis (see Official Guidelines for Coding and Reporting Effective November 15, 2006 at http://www.cdc.gov/nchs/datawh/ftpserv/ftpicd9/icdguide06.pdf).

EXAMPLE	*Admission for transfusion for anemia related to chemotherapy for breast cancer. Principal diagnosis: 285.22 (anemia in neoplastic disease) + 174.9 (primary breast cancer) + E933.1 (adverse effect of the therapeutic use of a chemotherapy drug).*
	Admission for IV fluids for dehydration secondary to nausea and vomiting associated with chemotherapy for colon cancer. Principal diagnosis: 276.51 (dehydration) + 787.01 (nausea and vomiting) + 153.9 (colon cancer) + E933.1 (adverse effect of the therapeutic use of a chemotherapy drug).
	Admission for whole-blood transfusion or drug therapy (e.g., filgrastim) for neutropenia (deficient white blood cells) associated with breast cancer and chemotherapy. Principal diagnosis: 288.03 (neutropenia) + 174.9 (breast cancer) + E933.1 (adverse effect of the therapeutic use of a chemotherapy drug).
	A patient with known metastatic lung carcinoma to the ribs and vertebrae was admitted secondary to intractable back pain. The patient's pain was believed to be secondary to metastasis to the bones: 338.3 (neoplasm related to pain) + 198.5 (metastasis to bone) + 162.9 (lung cancer).

When multiple symptoms are associated with the cancer such that no single symptom can be identified as the main or overriding reason for the admission, then the cancer code can be sequenced as the principal diagnosis with the symptoms listed as additional codes.

EXAMPLE	*A patient with known lung carcinoma was admitted secondary to severe weakness, shortness of breath, and weight loss: 162.9 + 780.79 + 786.05 + 783.21*

Follow-Up Treatment

After completion of treatment for a malignancy, it is common to have routine admissions or encounters for follow-up to ensure that there is no recurrence of cancer. When the follow-up results indicate completely negative findings, assign code V67.X for "follow-up examination" as the principal diagnosis with the "personal history of" code for the malignancy. When there has been a combination of therapies (surgery followed by chemotherapy followed by radiation therapy), use the follow-up code for the most recent modality of treatment.

As a general rule, you should always code something before nothing, so assign code V67.X only when there is no recurrence of cancer or evidence of other disease processes (i.e., negative findings). If there is a recurrence of cancer or another disease is present, sequence that condition as the principal diagnosis, and do not use the V67.X code.

EXAMPLE	*A patient with a history of colon resection followed by chemotherapy for colon cancer is admitted for a follow-up colonoscopy to rule out recurrence of the cancer or other pathology. The colonoscopy findings are negative.*
	Principal diagnosis: Follow-up examination after chemotherapy, V67.2
	Additional code: Personal history of colon cancer, V10.05

If the colonoscopy findings in the previous example had indicated a recurrence of cancer or other pathology such as colon polyps or if diverticulosis had been found, then you would not use the code V67.X but would sequence the current condition as the principal diagnosis.

> *A patient with a history of colon cancer is admitted for a follow-up colonoscopy to rule out recurrence of the cancer or other pathology. Colonoscopy reveals extensive diverticulosis and a single benign colon polyp that was removed.*
>
> **EXAMPLE**
>
> **Principal diagnosis:** Diverticulosis, 562.10
> **Additional codes:** Colon polyp, 211.3
> Personal history of colon cancer, V10.05

Cancer Protocols

The four main cancer protocols (treatments) are surgery, chemotherapy, radiation therapy, and immune therapy. These are often offered in combination.

SURGERY

Many cancers are cured by surgical excision (e.g., removal of the lesion or partial removal of the organ) or destruction by means of electrocauterization (burning), fulguration (electrocautery, laser, or other method of destruction), or cryosurgery (freezing tissue). Many of the surgical procedures associated with cancer can be located under general terms in the Procedure Index such as "excision," "resection," or "removal." Also, surgical procedures can be located under specific procedural terms, such as "nephrectomy" or "colectomy"; as eponyms (procedures named after people); or under the main term "operation."

CHEMOTHERAPY

Chemotherapy (code 99.25) uses drugs (e.g., cisplatin, doxorubicin, paclitaxel, or tamoxifen) to destroy cancer cells. Chemotherapy interferes with DNA synthesis of cancer cells through different mechanisms of action. Some cancer drugs have toxic side effects such as hair loss, nausea and vomiting, and myelosuppression (i.e., the bone marrow becomes deficient in producing new blood cells, and patients become anemic [reduction in red blood cells] or neutropenic [reduction in white blood cells]).

One class of chemotherapy drugs attacks rapidly dividing cancer cells. Because hair and gastrointestinal tract cells also divide rapidly, side effects such as hair loss, nausea, and vomiting can result. Certain forms of breast cancer contain estrogen receptors (cancer cells use estrogen for growth), and drugs such as tamoxifen are used to block estrogen and inhibit tumor growth. V-codes are now available to use as additional codes to report a person's estrogen receptor status (V86.0 = ER+; V86.1= ER−), but you must first code the malignant neoplasm of the breast (174.0–174.9, 175.0–175.9). Flutamide is used to block testosterone to depress tumor growth in metastatic prostate cancer. It is important to understand that side effects occur routinely and are not considered adverse effects of drugs. The coding for adverse effects is covered in Chapter 17 of this textbook.

RADIATION THERAPY

Radiation therapy (external beam code 92.2X) focuses ionizing radiation to kill tumor cells while trying to limit damage to normal surrounding tissues (e.g., by using ports and shields). Fractionalization is a way of applying small doses of radiation over time: this results in a cumulative destruction of cancer cells and limited damage to surrounding healthy tissues. A radiation oncologist writes a prescription in rads or grays (100 rads = 1 gray) of radiant energy to destroy tumors.

Adverse effects (unexpected abnormal reactions) that can occur from radiation depend on the part of the body that is irradiated. Adverse effects that occur as an abnormal reaction to therapy should not be confused with side effects (symptoms and conditions; expected adverse effects) that routinely occur from therapy. Radiation fibrosis of the lung (508.1 + E879.2) can result from radiotherapy to the chest. Radiation colitis (558.1 + E879.2) can occur from radiotherapy to the pelvic area. To code an adverse effect of radiation therapy, sequence the adverse condition first, followed by an E code located under "Reaction, abnormal, radiation procedure therapy" from the Index to External Causes.

A common coding error occurs when coders use the code 990 ("effects of radiation, unspecified") when, in fact, the adverse effects are specified, and the definitive diagnosis should be coded with the additional E879.2 code.

Chemotherapy and radiation therapy may be used as individual treatments or may be used in conjunction (combination) with each other or with surgery to ensure that all circulating (systemic) cancer cells are destroyed.

IMMUNOTHERAPY

Immunotherapy uses drugs (e.g., interferon or interleukin) to heighten one's own immune response to kill cancer cells (code 92.28).

Starting October 1, 2005, a new code has been provided to report an admission for antineoplastic immunotherapy – V58.12.

SUMMARY

This chapter has focused on coding for neoplastic conditions. Common clinical procedures related to neoplasms and oncology have been presented as part of the discussion. The application of this knowledge to coding from medical reports and clinical records is emphasized. Also receiving considerable attention is applying this knowledge to identify and correctly assign the principal and, where appropriate, the secondary diagnosis and procedure codes for the respective conditions.

REFERENCES

1. Stedman's Medical Dictionary, 27th Ed. Baltimore: Williams & Wilkins, 2000.

TESTING YOUR COMPREHENSION

1. Define the term **neoplasm**.

   _____

2. True or false? No tumor, regardless of its behavior (malignant or nonmalignant), has a useful function.

   _____

3. What are two common characteristics of benign tumors?

   _____

4. What are the common negative consequences of a benign tumor?

   _____

5. What purpose does a diagnostic test serve in treating a cancerous condition?

   _____

6. What is the nature of all cancers located in the Neoplasm Table?

   _____

7. When more than one section of the same organ is affected by cancer, how is it identified?

   _____

8. What is the meaning of the term **metastases to the lung**?

   _____

9. What is the intended purpose of brachytherapy?

   _____

10. If a cancerous condition displays multiple symptoms, and no single symptom is identified as the precipitating factor for the admission, how is the cancer code sequenced?

    _____

11. What are some of the potential side effects of cancer drugs?

    _____

12. What is the principal determining factor regarding the adverse effects of radiation treatments?

    _____

13. When talking about **grading** of cancer, what does that mean?

    _____

14. When talking about the **staging** of a cancerous condition, what does that mean?

    _____

15. What are the four grade classifications?

    _____

CODING PRACTICE I   Chapter Review Exercises

Directions

By using your ICD-9-CM codebook, code the following diagnoses and procedures:

	DIAGNOSIS/PROCEDURES	CODE
1	Urinary retention secondary to prostate cancer. Transurethral resection of the prostate.	
2	Left upper quadrant breast cancer with axillary lymph node metastases. Modified radical mastectomy with axillary lymph node excision (regional).	
3	Admission for blood transfusion secondary to anemia secondary to colon cancer. Packed red blood cell transfusion.	
4	Small cell carcinoma of the right upper lobe of the lung. Hemoptysis secondary to the small cell carcinoma. Bronchoscopy with transbronchial lung biopsy.	
5	Admission for dehydration with persistent nausea and vomiting secondary to chemotherapy for pancreatic cancer. Intravenous fluid rehydration.	
6	Admission for chemotherapy. Adenocarcinoma of the lung with liver metastases. Chemotherapy.	
7	Hematuria attributable to bladder cancer. Cystoscopy with transurethral bladder lesion cauterization.	
8	Weakness and dizziness secondary to brain metastases. History of breast cancer. Status post radical mastectomy.	
9	Jaundice and biliary obstruction attributable to primary liver cancer.	
10	Carcinoma in situ of lower outer quadrant of the breast. Right breast lumpectomy.	
11	Seizures secondary to metastatic lung cancer to the brain.	

	DIAGNOSIS/PROCEDURES	CODE
12	Bowel obstruction secondary to ascending colon cancer. Right hemicolectomy.	
13	Intractable back pain secondary to acute pathologic fracture of L3 and L4 secondary to bone metastases with a primary tumor of unknown origin.	
14	Renal cell carcinoma. Nephrectomy on left. Ultrasound-guided percutaneous kidney biopsy on left.	
15	Acute lymphocytic leukemia, in relapse. Bone marrow biopsy.	
16	Non-Hodgkin's lymphoma.	
17	Metastatic ovarian cancer with invasion of pelvic lymph nodes and liver. Intramural leiomyoma of uterus. Total abdominal hysterectomy, bilateral salpingo-oophorectomy, pelvic lymph node excision, and open liver biopsy.	
18	Dysphagia secondary to lower esophageal cancer. Malnutrition. Esophagogastroduodenoscopy with esophageal biopsy. Percutaneous endoscopic gastrostomy.	
19	Admit for follow-up. History of colon cancer with no evidence of recurrence this admission. Villous polyp of colon. Colonoscopy with polypectomy.	
20	Abdominal pain with tumor of pancreas noted on computed tomography—patient transferred for further workup.	

CODING PRACTICE II — Medical Record Case Studies

Instructions

1. Carefully review the medical reports provided for each case study.
2. Research any abbreviations and terms that are unfamiliar or unclear.
3. Identify as many diagnoses and procedures as possible.
4. Because only part of the patient's total record is available, determine what additional documentation you might need.
5. If appropriate, identify any questions you might ask the physician to code this case correctly and completely.
6. Complete the appropriate blanks below for each case study.

CHAPTER 14 CASE STUDIES

Case Study 14.1 (Coder/Abstract Summary Form)

Patient: **Jane Doe**

Patient documentation: **Review Medical Reports 14.1, 14.2, and 14.3**

1. Principal diagnosis:

   _____

2. Secondary or other diagnoses:

   _____

3. Principal procedure:

   _____

4. Other procedures:

   _____

5. Additional documentation needed:

   _____

   _____

   _____

   _____

Case Study 14.1 (Continued)

6. Questions for the physician:

_____

_____

_____

_____

_____

_____

MEDICAL REPORT 14.1

DISCHARGE SUMMARY

PATIENT: Jane Doe

MEDICAL RECORD #:   999999

ATTN PHYSICIAN: Smith, M.D.

ADMITTING DIAGNOSIS:

1. Malignant pleural effusion.

2. History of COPD.

3. History of chronic atrial fibrillation.

DISCHARGE DIAGNOSES

1. Malignant pleural effusion.

2. History of COPD.

3. History of atrial fibrillation persistent.

PROCEDURES: The patient underwent chest tube and Port-A-Cath insertion.

HOSPITAL COURSE: This is a 72-year-old white female with a history of a malignant pleural effusion. She had pleurocentesis ×3 done with a re-accumulation of the fluid. She did have two effusions positive for malignant cells. We went ahead and proceeded with a consultation with Dr. Resection the general surgeon. He proceeded with chest tube insertion once we corrected her INR from the use of Coumadin. She tolerated it well. Dr. Tumor, the oncologist, saw her in consultation and is arranging for outpatient chemotherapy once the patient is discharged from the hospital. We still have no tissue diagnosis, but certain that it must be a lung cancer that spread to the pleural lining. We have attempted a pleural biopsy here, but we do not have the correct tools according to Dr. X-ray the radiologist and we will do that on an outpatient basis.

Routine blood work on the patient has been really unremarkable. We have just recently started her back on Coumadin after Port-A-Cath placement and after the chest tube had been removed. We did stop her blood pressure medicine during this hospitalization secondary to a low blood pressure. We have changed her over to digoxin 0.125 mg once a day for rate control of her atrial fibrillation. That has been well controlled with the use of that medication.

It was then decided on this afternoon that the patient could be discharged to home.

DISPOSITION UPON DISCHARGE: The patient was alert, oriented, afebrile and in no apparent distress at the present time. She will go home on a regular diet and activity will be tolerated. We will continue with digoxin 0.125 mg once a day. We will hold off on her Verelan PM and her Tenoretic that she had been on before in the past. I will restart her Coumadin, although we probably need to stop it prior to her pleural biopsy. We will restart it once that is done. She will follow up in the office in one week. We will also consult Dr. Tumor for outpatient chemotherapy, which he will arrange for the patient. Will give her Lortab 5, a half to a whole pill every 4 hours as needed and digoxin 0.125 mg. She will follow up in my office in 1 week.

_____

Smith, M.D.

HISTORY AND PHYSICAL

PATIENT:	Jane Doe
MEDICAL RECORD #:	999999
ATTN PHYSICIAN:	Smith, M.D.

SUBJECTIVE:

CC:
F/U SOB

HPI: Ms. Doe is here for a follow-up. Patient is still having problems with SOB. At times she said it hurts when she breathes. She has a history significant for COPD and atrial fibrillation. A thoracentesis was done this past Tuesday at ABC Medical Center. The patient has had thoracentesis X3 done, and 1 has come up positive for malignant cells. She had a bronchoscopy done this week that was unremarkable. Currently, she is short of breath.

ROS:

CONSTITUTIONAL: Negative for chills, fatigue, fever, and weight change.

E/N/T: Negative for hearing problems, E/N/T pain, congestion, rhinorrhea, epistaxis, hoarseness, and dental problems.

CARDIOVASCULAR: Negative for chest pain.

RESPIRATORY: Positive for dyspnea (with mild exertion). Negative for recent cough, chronic cough, or frequent wheezing.

GASTROINTESTINAL: Negative for abdominal pain, diarrhea, nausea, and vomiting.

GENITOURINARY: Negative for dysuria.

MUSCULOSKELETAL: Negative for arthralgias and myalgias.

INTEGUMENTARY/BREAST: Negative for rash.

HEMATOLOGIC/LYMPHATIC: Negative for lymphadenopathy.

PSYCHIATRIC: Negative for anxiety, depression, and sleep disturbances.

Past Medical History/ Family History/ Social History:

Past Medical History: Hypertension, A-fib, COPD

Surgical History:

Dilation and Curettage: Ectopic pregnancy; Tonsillectomy/Adenoidectomy.

Family History:
Father: Died at age 56 Coronary Artery Disease
Mother: Died at age 88 Cancer (unspecified type)
Brother(s): 4 brothers total; 1 alcoholic deceased
Sister(s): 3 sisters total; 1 Cancer deceased

Social History:

Occupation: Retired (Prior occupation: waitress, retail sales)

Marital Status: Widowed

Children: 3 children (1 deceased)

Continued

MEDICAL REPORT 14.2 (CONTINUED)

Tobacco/Alcohol/Supplements:

Tobacco: She used to smoke up to 1 pack per day. 50 packs/year history. Quit 6 weeks ago.

Alcohol: Drinks alcohol on a social basis.

OBJECTIVE:

Vitals:

Current: T: 97.8 F; BP: 131/175; P: 76; RR: 20

Exams:

PHYSICAL EXAM

GENERAL: well developed and nourished; appropriately groomed; in no apparent distress;

EYES: lids and lacrimal system are normal in appearance; extraocular movements intact; conjunctiva and cornea are normal; PERRLA;

E/N/T: normal EACs, TMs, nasal/oral mucosa, teeth, gingival, and oropharynx;

NECK: supple, full ROM; no thyromegaly; no carotid bruits;

RESPIRATORY: increase A-P diameter resulting in "barrel chest"; normal respiratory rate and pattern with no decreased breath sounds in the right mid-lung field and RLL; diffuse inspiratory wheezes; chest is dull to percussion over the right mid-lung field and RLL;

CARDIOVASCULAR: normal rate; rhythm is irregularly irregular;

GASTROINTESTINAL: nontender, nondistended; no hepatosplenomegaly or masses; no bruits;

LYMPHATIC: no enlargement of cervical or facial nodes;

BREAST/INTEGUMENT: BREASTS: breast exam is normal without masses, skin changes, or nipple discharge; SKIN: no significant rashes or lesion; no suspicious moles;

MUSCULOSKELETAL: Normal range of motion, strength, and tone;

NEUROLOGIC: mental status: alert and oriented x3; cranial nerves II–XII grossly intact;

PSYCHIATRIC: appropriate affect and demeanor; normal speech pattern; grossly normal memory.

ASSESSMENT:

Pleural effusion
Atrial fibrillation
COPD
HTN

PLAN:

Pleural Effusion: Pt will be admitted for chest tube placement. Will also check CT or of Abd/pelvis to r/o other source for her malignant cells.

MEDICAL REPORT 14.3

CONSULTATION

PATIENT: Jane Doe

MEDICAL RECORD #: 999999

ATTN PHYSICIAN: Smith, M.D.

CHIEF COMPLAINT: Large, pleural effusion on the right.

HISTORY OF THE PRESENT ILLNESS: The patient is a 72-year-old, white female with complaints of shortness of breath, with a long smoking history, COPD, atrial fib. She had a thoracentesis done which revealed a malignant pleural effusion. CT scan done immediately after draining the chest revealed no primary in the chest. She is back here because of increased shortness of breath and need for oxygen therapy and drainage of the chest. Dr. Smith asked me to place a chest tube and do chemical pleurodesis afterwards.

PAST MEDICAL HISTORY: Positive for hypertension, as well as COPD and malignant pleural effusion.

PAST SURGICAL HISTORY: Positive for D&C, removal of right ovary and tube secondary to ectopic pregnancy and T&A.

FAMILY HISTORY: Father died at age 56 of coronary artery disease. Mother age 88, with an unknown cancer. She had 4 brothers and 3 sisters. One brother died of alcohol-related disorder and 1 sister died of a malignancy.

SOCIAL HISTORY: The patient is retired, previously worked as a waitress and in retail sales. She is a widow, has 3 children, 1 that passed away. She smoked up to 1 pack of cigarettes a day, 50 packs/year, quit about 6 weeks ago; I think when this effusion was first diagnosed. She is a social alcohol drinker.

REVIEW OF SYSTEMS: Currently, she denies any dizzy spells, fainting spells, or black out spells. She denies any recent changes in vision or hearing. Denies anginal-type chest pain. She does complain of being short of breath and she states this has been progressively more over the past few days, at least since having the chest drained the past time. No change in bowel movement. No change in urinary system. Denies any long bone pain, deformity, and tender joints. Denies any palpable masses in the breast, any skin changes in the breasts. She states Dr. Smith has checked her and he did not find anything wrong with her breast either. No prior history of breast cancer. No family history of breast cancer that she is aware of. Denies any lymphadenopathy. She has easy bleeding due to Coumadin. She denies any suicidal tendency, depression, or paranoia.

PHYSICAL EXAMINATION

GENERAL: An elderly, white female, sitting quietly on the bed, reading the newspaper, when I came into the room. She is well-kept. She does not appear to be in any severe distress currently.

VITAL SIGNS: Since arrival, she has been afebrile. Pulse has been between 88 and 66. Respiratory rate is currently around 20, and the highest recorded was 28. Blood pressure is good at 102/62, last check.

HEENT: Normocephalic and atraumatic. Pupils are equal, round and reactive. Sclerae anicteric. Lids are normal. Irises are normal. Nose, normal to palpitation.

NECK: Supple. I do not detect any thyromegaly or mass. Carotids are 2+ without bruits.

CHEST: Decreased breath sounds on the right. Chest is dull on the right. I do not hear any wheezing on the left.

HEART: Regular rate and rhythm.

ABDOMEN: Soft, nontender. No mass. No organomegaly. Bowel sounds are normal. There is a lower midline incision from surgery for tubal pregnancy.

LYMPHATICS: I do not detect any adenopathy in the neck, axilla, epitrochlear zones, or groin.

Continued

MEDICAL REPORT 14.3 (CONTINUED)

NEUROLOGICAL: She moves all 4 extremities on command. Cranial nerves II through XII appear to be intact. Reflexes are normal in the knees and elbows.

PSYCHIATRIC: Affect and insight are appropriate. She jokes, she smiles, and she carries on an appropriate conversation. She is alert, awake, oriented to time, place, and person.

BREASTS: No palpable masses, skin changes, nipple change, or axillary nodules on either side.

SKIN: She has some sub K, one fairly prominent in the right lower quadrant of the abdomen. No malignant-appearing skin lesions. No open wound, rash, or subcutaneous nodules noted.

IMPRESSION:

1. MALIGNANT PLEURAL EFFUSION ON THE RIGHT, RE-ACCUMULATING.
2. HISTORY OF ATRIAL FIBRILLATION.
3. CHRONIC OBSTRUCTIVE PULMONARY DISEASE.
4. HYPERTENSION.
5. STATUS POST SURGERY FOR RIGHT TUBAL PREGNANCY WITH A RIGHT SALPINGO-OOPHORECTOMY.
6. STATUS POST TONSILLECTOMY AND ADENOIDECTOMY.
7. PATIENT IS ANTI-COAGULATED ON COUMADIN FOR HER ATRIAL FIBRILLATION.

PLAN: Once she is appropriate on her PT, INR, then we will place the chest tube. Once the chest is adequately drained, then we will perform a chemical pleurodesis. I have discussed this plan with the patient.

_____

Dr. Tumor, M.D.

NOTES

Case Study 14.2 (Coder/Abstract Summary Form)

Patient: **John Doe**

Patient documentation: **Review Medical Records 14.4, 14.5, and 14.6**

1. Principal diagnosis:

   _____

2. Secondary or other diagnoses:

   _____

3. Principal procedure:

   _____

4. Other procedures:

   _____

5. Additional documentation needed:

   _____

   _____

   _____

6. Questions for the physician:

   _____

   _____

   _____

   _____

MEDICAL REPORT 14.4

HISTORY AND PHYSICAL

NAME: DOE, JOHN

ACCT #:

MR#:

AGE/SEX:

DOB:

LOCATION:

PHYSICIAN: SMITH, MD

ROOM/BED:

REASON FOR ADMISSION: Small Bowel Obstruction/Ileus/Dehydration

OTHER DIAGNOSIS:

1. Apple core splenic flexure/proximal descending colon carcinoma.
2. Gastroesophageal reflux disease.
3. Elevated CEA.

ALLERGIES: Denies.

OUT-PATIENT MEDICATIONS: Zantac and Prevpac.

HPI: This 53-year-old male known to me from a previous colonoscopy that I performed that revealed a near total obstructing mass in the left proximal descending colon. Follow-up barium enema showing likewise, with biopsy results demonstrating apple core splenic flexure/proximal descending colon invasive moderately differentiated adenocarcinoma. The patient had an elevated CEA at 97. He also had an EGD done on that day, which showed Barrett's esophagus and duodenitis and positive for H-pylori. The patient was started on outpatient Prevpac. The patient over the last day, day and one-half has had some nausea and vomiting, epigastric pain, and had some bloating but is passing gas. I was contacted, as the patient's primary care physician is not available. The patient underwent abdominal x-rays today and laboratory data showing a mild leukocytosis and hemo concentration, and small bowel obstruction/ileus. The patient is thirsty and feels parched.

SOCIAL HISTORY: Denies cigarettes. Social alcohol.

FAMILY HISTORY: No family history of colon cancer.

PHYSICAL EXAMINATION

GENERAL APPEARANCE: Well-nourished male lying on the stretcher in my office in no apparent distress. Looks pale/weak.

HEENT: Dry mucous membranes.

NECK: Supple.

HEART: Rate 100. Sinus tach.

LUNGS: Clear without wheezes or rubs.

ABDOMEN: Soft. Nontender. No masses. No guarding or rebound. No hepatosplenomegaly. Active bowel sounds. No rushes or tinkles heard. No peritoneal signs. The patient states he is passing gas.

PSYCHOLOGICAL: Pleasant affect. Interactive. Intact insight and memory.

MEDICAL REPORT 14.4 (CONTINUED)

SKIN: Warm and dry.

ASSESSMENT: A 53-year-old male with dehydration, nausea and vomiting, and x-ray findings consistent with ileus/small bowel obstruction.

Patient with known apple core, left colon, moderately invasive adenocarcinoma without total obstruction.

PLAN:

1. The patient will be admitted.

2. Rehydrate.

3. Nasogastric tube.

4. Intravenous fluids.

5. The patient had an outpatient computed tomography scan scheduled for tomorrow for evaluation of his abdominal viscera given his elevated CEA at 97.

6. Will continue conservative management with n.p.o. status, IV fluid, nasogastric tube, and repeat laboratories in the a.m. If the patient improves, will perform the computed tomography scan as previously scheduled.

7. Patient aware.

SMITH, MD

NOTES

MEDICAL REPORT 14.5

OPERATIVE REPORT

NAME: DOE, JOHN

ACCT #:

MR#:

AGE/SEX:

DOB:

LOCATION:

PHYSICIAN: SMITH, MD

ROOM/BED:

DATE OF PROCEDURE:

PREOPERATIVE DIAGNOSIS: OBSTRUCTING LEFT COLON CANCER

POSTOPERATIVE DIAGNOSIS: OBSTRUCTING LEFT COLON CANCER; MEDIAL LEFT LIVER LOBE MASS APPROXIMATELY 2-2.5 CM; RETROGASTRIC TRANSVERSE COLON.

PROCEDURE: PARTIAL COLECTOMY; WEDGE RESECTION OF MEDIAL LEFT LOBE OF THE LIVER FOR MASS; PANCREATIC SUTURE REPAIR (PANCREATORRHAPHY); END COLOSTOMY.

SURGEON: SMITH, MD

ASSISTANT: DOE, MD

ANESTHESIA: General Endotracheal Intubation and Local – 0.5% Marcaine with 1/200,000 Epinephrine – 20 CC

IV FLUID: Five Liters of Crystalloid

EBL: 2200 CC (Packed Red Blood Cells 4 Units, FFP 2 Units)

URINE OUTPUT: 500 CC

NG TUBE OUTPUT: 900 CC

FINDINGS: SPLENIC FLEXURE OBSTRUCTING ADENOCARCINOMA WITH SEROSAL METASTASES EXTENDING ONTO THE TRANSVERSE COLON.

PROXIMAL COLONIC – TRANSVERSE COLONIC DILATATION. TRANSVERSE COLON IS RETROGASTRIC IN POSITION WITH A DESMOPLASTIC REACTION OCCURRING BETWEEN THE SPLENIC FLEXURE/PROXIMAL LEFT COLON. ADENOCARCINOMA MASS AND THE TAIL OF THE PANCREAS AND ALSO IN THE LEFT LATERAL ABDOMINAL GUTTER.

MEDIAL LEFT LOBE OF THE LIVER WITH A 2-2.5 CM MASS ANTERIORLY IN THE BODY/SUBSTANCE OF THIS LOBE REGION.

SPECIMEN: TRANSVERSE COLON THROUGH SIGMOID RECTAL JUNCTION COLON; WEDGE RESECTION LEFT LIVER LOBE MASS MEDIALLY.

CULTURES: PERITONEAL FLUID FOR C&S AND GRAM STAIN.

COMPLICATIONS: DISTAL ANTEROINFERIOR ASPECT OF THE PANCREATIC WAS A PARENCHYMAL TEAR REQUIRING SUTURE REPAIR – PANCREATORRHAPHY; ACUTE BLOOD LOSS RESULTING IN ANEMIA.

CONDITION: STABLE/FAIR

OP NOTE IN DETAIL: The patient having been properly identified and plans reconfirmed is brought into the main Operating Room and underwent general endotracheal intubation and was prepped and draped in the usual supine sterile fashion with Foley catheter and central lines placed preoperatively. A midline incision was made from the lower epigastric region through to the suprapubic area with the scalpel through the subcutaneous tissues dissecting down further with

MEDICAL REPORT 14.5 (CONTINUED)

the scalpel through to the fascia and the abdomen was entered. Hemostasis achieved using electrocautery where necessary. A retractor was placed in the abdomen and having been entered showed some cloudy orange peritoneal fluid that was swabbed and sent for a culture and sensitivity and gram stain. The small bowel loops are dilated and with the retractor, the small bowel contents are milked back to the stomach where the NG tube aspirates the contents and is packed away. Having run the bowel, it showed no small bowel obstruction mechanically. The large bowel is moderate to largely dilated and this occurs at approximately the splenic flexure/early proximal descending colon because of the known apple core adenocarcinoma obstructing colon cancer.

The transverse colon, however, is found to be anatomically in retrogastric position and intimate with the pancreas. The left lateral white line of Toldt was mobilized and the sigmoid mesentery was taken down between Kelly clamps and Vicryl ties and a distal sigmoid resection was performed using the GIA stapler. The mesentery of the sigmoid colon is taken down between Kelly clamps and Vicryl ties taking the left colic through to the inferior mesenteric artery and a high ligation is performed using silk and Vicryl ties and stick ligature ties and hemoclips. The mass is with serosal seeding which travels onto the distal transverse colon. The stomach was held anteriorly so that I could have access to the transverse colon and the transverse colon separated from the stomach between Kelly clamps and Vicryl ties. The posterior-inferior aspect of the tumor/splenic flexure area is with a desmoplastic-like reaction through to the distal tail of the pancreas and this was able to be mobilized between Kelly clamps, Vicryl ties and finger dissection. There was a small tear in the distal pancreas at the anteroinferior border and a 3-0 silk suture was placed – mattress for hemostasis control and parenchymal control.

The transverse colon was not invading into the tail of the pancreas at its distal aspect where the serosal seeding and the splenic flexure mass is noted. The transverse colon was mobilized through to the hepatic flexure and the hepatic flexure of the colon is transected using the GIA stapler. The mesentery of the transverse colon from the hepatic flexure through to the splenic flexure was taken down using Kelly clamps and Vicryl ties, stick ligature ties, and hemoclips where necessary. Anatomical resection was done. The specimen was removed and marked with a single long stitch for the sigmoid and a double long stitch for the tumor site.

Inspection of the stomach is unremarkable. Inspection of the liver showed a mass to be present on the anterior aspect of the medial half of the left lobe of the liver at least 5–6 cm from its anterior edge. This mass felt to be approximately 2–3 cm and ovoid and irregular below the surface. Inspection of the rest of the left lobe of the liver and the right lobe of liver are unremarkable. No peritoneal seeding or studding was noted. It was decided to resect this specimen and wide local wedge resection was performed using a electrocautery. Hemostasis was achieved using liver chromic catgut sutures. Hemostasis in effect. Palpation of the gallbladder was unremarkable, no stones felt. The hepatic flexure, having been transected and mobile, was mobilized through to the ascending colon and was easily brought up to the anterior abdominal wall for planned end colostomy. Inspection of the pancreatic tear repair is unremarkable and a drain is placed here and exited out the left lateral aspect of the upper quadrant and secured with nylon suture. This drain is at the tail of the pancreas.

The abdomen was irrigated out and aspirated until clear. Inspection of all quadrants were unremarkable. Hemostasis in effect. The sigmoid and rectal junction GIA staple line is unremarkable and is left of Hartmann's pouch. The omental contents are drawn down over the abdominal visceral contents and the retractor was removed. The right upper quadrant is excised of a plug of skin down to the fascia and a fascial incision was made cruciate form and accommodated with 2–3 fingers for the planned end colostomy for the hepatic flexure/ascending colon end. The Babcock clamps are placed on this right colon and brought up through the planned end colostomy site and then the fascia of the midline abdominal laparotomy incision is closed with 0 loop Biosyn cephalad to caudad and caudad to cephalad. Subcutaneous tissues are irrigated out and locally infiltrated with a total of 20 cc of 0.5% Marcaine with 1/200,000 Epinephrine. Skin edges reapproximated with the stapler. Dry sterile dressings are applied and covered. The end colostomy on the right upper quadrant is matured by removing the GIA staple line and using chromic catgut interrupted sutures and interrupted four-point silk sutures. The end colostomy is pink and viable and easily accommodates my two fingers and there is no blood intraluminally.

Patient tolerated the procedure well and remains intubated and taken to the Intensive Care Unit for postoperative recovery. Of note, the patient received around 4 units intraoperatively of packed red blood cells and two units of fresh frozen plasma. The patient had 500 cc urine output over this 5–6 hour operation and 900 cc out his NG tube.

Smith, MD

MEDICAL REPORT 14.6

PATHOLOGY REPORT

NAME: DOE, JOHN

ACCT #:

MR#:

AGE/SEX:

DOB:

LOCATION:

PHYSICIAN: SMITH, MD

ROOM/BED:

SPECIMEN: **STATUS:**

RECEIVED: **REQ#:**

CLINICAL HISTORY: Bowel obstruction, colon mass

PRE-OPERATIVE DIAGNOSIS: Bowel obstruction, colon mass

POST-OPERATIVE DIAGNOSIS: Bowel obstruction, colon mass

SPECIMEN LABELED:
- **A.** Colon—long single stitch to sigmoid, double long stitch to tumor
- **B.** Liver mass—middle left lobe

GROSS DESCRIPTION:

A. Received in fixative, the specimen consisted of a segment of colon that measured 50 in length and varied from 3.5 cm to 7 cm in diameter. Both ends of the specimen were stapled and a single black ligature was attached to the end toward the sigmoid. A double black ligature was attached to the area of a tumor. Externally, the specimen presented a dark tan to dark brown color, was somewhat tortuous and covered with tags of dark yellow fatty tissues. Numerous metal staples were scattered over the specimen in various areas. On opening, the colonic segment contained some liquid brown fecal material, particularly the two-thirds closest to the end labeled "to sigmoid". Approximately 13 cm from the opposite end was an obstructing encircling tumor mass measuring 4.5 cm in greatest diameter along the longitudinal axis of the colon. This completely encircled the bowel and presented an ulcerated reddish-tan appearance and appeared grossly to infiltrate the thickness of the colonic wall and extended out into the pericolic fatty tissues. The mucosa elsewhere proximal and distal to this, presented a dark tan color with normal appearing folds. Sections from the tumor proper and some of the immediate surrounding pericolic fatty tissue with obvious vari-sized lymph nodes ranging up to 0.6 cm in greatest diameter in cassettes A1 through A11. Sections from the colon at the end which was not tagged by a ligature in cassette A12. Section from the end of the colon tagged with ligature designated "to sigmoid" in cassette A13. Random section from along the colonic segment in cassette A14. In the pericolic fatty tissues, there were several nodes ranging up to 7 to 8 mm in greatest diameter, these submitted in cassettes A15 through A17.

B. Received in fixative, the specimen consisted of a thick wedge of dark tan-dark brown hepatic tissue, which measured 4.3 × 3.8 × up to 2.2 cm. Some areas of this appeared frankly necrotic and extremely friable and in the center of the wedge was a pale tan-white irregular nodule measuring 2 cm in greatest diameter. Representative sections. Three cassettes.

MICROSCOPIC DIAGNOSIS:

A. COLON: Moderately differentiated deeply invasive ulcerated adenocarcinoma or colon with extensive deep complete penetration of the muscularis propria and extending through serosa into pericolic fatty tissues and immediate adjacent small lymph nodes. Lymphovascular invasion present. Pericolic fatty tissue search yielded four vari-sized lymph nodes, two of which contained necrotic metastatic adenocarcinoma. Sections from both extremities of the colonic

MEDICAL REPORT 14.6 (CONTINUED)

segment present normal colotissue (negative for malignancy). Random sections along the colonic segment presented normal colonic tissue (negative for malignancy).

B. **LIVER MASS:** Wedge of hepatic tissue with large metastatic nodule of moderately differentiated colonic adenocarcinoma. Massive central necrosis of metastatic nodule was present.

COMMENT: The tower represents a Duke's stage D-2 with distant metastasis (HEPATIC).

Dr. Smith, M.D.

NOTES

Case Study 14.3 (Coder/Abstract Summary Form)

Patient: **Frank Johnson**

Patient documentation: **Review Medical Report 14.7**

1. Principal diagnosis:

   _____

2. Secondary or other diagnoses:

   _____

3. Principal procedure:

   _____

4. Other procedures:

   _____

5. Additional documentation needed:

   _____

   _____

   _____

   _____

6. Questions for the physician:

   _____

   _____

   _____

   _____

   _____

MEDICAL REPORT 14.7

ADMISSION HISTORY AND PHYSICAL

PATIENT: Johnson, Frank

DOB:

MED REC: 111111

SEX/RACE:

PT ADMN:

LOCATION:

PHYSICIAN: Smith, MD

ADMITTED:

REASON FOR ADMISSION: Patient with history of IGM multiple myeloma admitted for elective chemotherapy with Adriamycin, Vincristine, and dexamethasone.

HISTORY OF PRESENT ILLNESS: The patient is a 53-year-old gentleman who was evaluated this past April where he was admitted for back pain. The patient was found to have a plasma cytoma as well as the patient was noted to have multiple myeloma based on the serum protein electrophoresis which showed a IGM level with M-spike of 2.9. The patient subsequently had a bone marrow biopsy and aspiration proving it to be a increase in the plasma cells. The patient was initially started with radiation to the back area for his lumbar mass there. Radiation was done times 20 treatments that have shrunk the tumor and the patient is clinically having no pain whatsoever. Today, he was admitted for electively starting his chemotherapy with Adriamycin, Vincristine, as well as dexamethasone. Patient currently has no complaints whatsoever.

REVIEW OF SYSTEMS: Denies any headaches, no vision problems such as blurry or double vision. He has no problems swallowing. Has no problem with hearing and has no sinus symptoms. Chest: No shortness of breath or any chest pain. No alternating constipation or diarrhea. No problem passing urine or stool. Has no blood seen in his stool or urine. No focal weakness in any part of the body. No tingling or numbness. Has no back pain whatsoever. No joint pains as well as no feeling of hot or cold. The rest of the systems are negative.

PAST MEDICAL HISTORY: Significant for:
1. Hypertension.

PAST SURGICAL HISTORY: Significant for:
1. Left arm tendon repair.
2. Left leg injury in remote past.

ALLERGIES: No known drug allergy.

MEDICATION:
1. Nifedipine 200 mg p.o. q. day.
2. Lorcet p.r.n.
3. Coumadin 1 mg p.o. q. day.

SOCIAL HISTORY: He used to be a handyman but currently disabled. He used to smoke half a pack per day, denies any smoking at this time. He is not taking any alcohol. He is living with his family.

FAMILY HISTORY: Not significant for any myeloma or lymphoma.

PHYSICAL EXAMINATION: On examination at this time, his vitals include a temperature of 98, pulse 84, respiratory rate of 14, blood pressure 140/80.

HEENT: Atraumatic, normocephalic. Pupils equal, round, and reactive to light. Extraocular muscles are intact. No icterus seen. Mouth is clear. No thrush. No petechia.

Continued

MEDICAL REPORT 14.7 (CONTINUED)

NECK: Supple. No JVD.

CHEST: Bilaterally clear to auscultation. There is a medi-port intact on the left anterior chest wall.

CVS: S1 and S2 are normal. No murmur appreciated.

ABDOMEN: Benign. No hepatosplenomegaly. Bowel sounds positive.

EXTREMITIES: No edema.

LYMPH NODES: No generalized lymphadenopathy.

LAB DATA: The lab work obtained here shows normal BMP with a BUN of 8, creatinine 1.0, calcium 9.3. CBC showed WBC 4.6, hemoglobin 12.0, hematocrit 31.6, platelet 340.

ASSESSMENT/PLAN:

1. Multiple myeloma. Patient will be started on Vincristine, Adriamycin continuous infusion. Will be given dexamethasone as p.o. Will continue watching him for any adverse effect. Patient will be given Zofran for vomiting prevention.

2. Anemia secondary to multiple myeloma. Patient will continue to be watched as he is asymptomatic at this time.

Smith, MD

NOTES

Case Study 14.4 (Coder/Abstract Summary Form)

Patient: **Jones, Steven**

Patient documentation: **Review Medical Reports 14.8, 14.9, and 14.10**

1. Principal diagnosis:

   _____

2. Secondary or other diagnoses:

   _____

3. Principal procedure:

   _____

4. Other procedures:

   _____

5. Additional documentation needed:

   _____

   _____

   _____

   _____

6. Questions for the physician:

   _____

   _____

   _____

   _____

MEDICAL REPORT 14.8

HISTORY AND PHYSICAL

PATIENT: Jones, Steven

DOB:

MED REC: 999999

SEX/RACE: M

PT ADMN:

LOCATION:

ATTENDING PHYSICIAN: SMITH, MD

HISTORY OF PRESENT ILLNESS: This is a 70-year-old male I saw about a year ago. The patient had cancer of the bladder with muscle invasion. Chemotherapy performed by Dr. Med. I checked him one year ago and he was o.k. but I checked him a month ago and found that he had a recurrent cancer. The only problem that bothers me is the cancer coming back right in through the diverticulum on the right side. I am kind of worried about that might split out and that is going to be a disaster. We decided to perform a radical cystectomy.

PAST MEDICAL HISTORY: The patient had a double bypass about ten years ago and also had a stent placement in the heart about a month ago.

ALLERGIES: The patient has allergies to seafood and iodine.

SOCIAL HISTORY: The patient quit smoking about ten years ago and smoked almost half pack a day.

REVIEW OF SYSTEMS: The review of systems is significant for colon cancer in the father.

PHYSICAL EXAMINATION: Generally, is alert. HEENT is within normal limits. The neck was supple. The lungs were clear to auscultation and percussion. The heart was normal sinus rhythm, no murmur. The abdomen was soft, no palpable mass or organomegaly. Extremities were symmetrical, good pulses. External genitalia is normal. The prostate was very small—less than 20 grams size and soft.

IMPRESSION: Cancer of the bladder recurrent and muscular invasion.

PLAN: Radical cystectomy with ileal conduit. He knows all the complications including bleeding and also adjacent organ damage and possible blood clot. He decided to have the operation done.

_____

Smith, M.D.

MEDICAL REPORT 14.9

REPORT OF CONSULTATION

PATIENT: Jones, Steven

DOB:

MED REC: 999999

SEX/RACE: M

PT ADMN:

LOCATION:

PHYSICIAN:

ADMITTED:

REASON FOR CONSULTATION: This patient underwent cystectomy for malignancy. He is a known case of coronary artery disease status post bypass surgery done about 14 years ago and status post stent procedure. Recently was hospitalized for the elective procedure for cystectomy for the infiltrating malignancy of the bladder. The patient denies any chest pain, shortness of breath, palpitations, dizziness or syncopal episode.

PAST MEDICAL HISTORY: There is no history of hypertension or diabetes mellitus. The patient had a bypass procedure done about 15 years ago and he is known to have peripheral vascular disease for which he had a femoral popliteal procedure done on both sides 15 years ago. The patient recently had a repeat cardiac catheterization because of recurrent symptoms and was found to have critical lesion and had stent procedure done.

FAMILY HISTORY: The family history is not significant for diabetes mellitus, hypertension, cerebrovascular accident, or myocardial infarction. The patient's father had carcinoma of the colon.

SOCIAL HISTORY: The patient quit smoking nearly 15 to 16 years ago and occasionally drinks beer. He used to take one or two cups of coffee and he worked as a cook.

ALLERGIES: The patient has allergies to iodine.

MEDICATIONS: The current medications are listed as noted.

REVIEW OF SYSTEMS: The review of systems is otherwise essentially negative.

PHYSICAL EXAMINATION: The patient is well-developed, moderately-nourished and not in acute distress. He understands, communicates, and is cooperative. The pulse is 90, blood pressure 138/80 and the temperature was normal. The head and neck was supple. Pupils equal, round, and reactive to light and accommodation. Conjunctiva was normal, no jugular venous distension. Carotids are equal and good. There are no bruits appreciated. The chest was symmetrical. The heart was irregular rhythm with occasional irregularity, 2/6 systolic murmur at the apex. The lung air entry is equal and fair. Rhonchi is heard anteriorly and posteriorly. There is no evidence of rales. The abdomen was benign, no areas of rigidity tenderness, no organomegaly, and bowel sounds are normal. Extremity pulses are felt and are fairly equal on both sides, no pitting edema, no varicosities or ulcerations. Musculoskeletal showed a negative. CNS had no localizing signs.

IMPRESSION:

1. Status post cystectomy for malignancy.
2. Coronary artery disease status post bypass procedure 14 years ago and recent stent procedure.
3. Peripheral vascular disease status post bypass procedure.
4. Ex-smoker.

PLAN AND RECOMMENDATIONS: Available labs, electrocardiogram, chest x-ray, and necessary and pertinent orders will be written in the chart.

MEDICAL REPORT 14.10

REPORT OF OPERATION

PATIENT: Jones, Steven

DOB:

MED REC: 999999

SEX/RACE: M

PT ADMN:

LOCATION:

SURGEON:

ADMITTED:

PREOPERATIVE DIAGNOSIS: Cancer of the bladder.

POSTOPERATIVE DIAGNOSIS: Cancer of the bladder.

OPERATION: Radical cystectomy and ileal conduit, cystoscopy, and insertion of the left ureteral stent.

ANESTHESIA: General/epidural.

ANESTHESIOLOGIST:

ESTIMATED BLOOD LOSS: Less than 500 cc.

COMPLICATIONS: None.

DRAINS: None.

PROCEDURE: The patient was first brought to the suite and placed in the dorsal lithotomy position and prepped the genitalia with Betadine and draped in the usual sterile fashion. The # 21 cystoscope was inserted into the bladder. The left sided stent placement was done with the # 7 French universal contour stent.

Then the patient was brought to the operating room. I couldn't do it on the right side because I cannot identify the ureteral orifice. The patient was placed in the supine position and prepped the genitalia, abdomen with Betadine and draped in the usual sterile fashion. The lower midline incision was made, the same incision that was done before and carried through to the subcutaneous tissue and rectus fascia. The rectus fascia was opened and the rectus muscles were split. When I went in the peritoneum there was quite a bit of dilatation because of previous aorta bifemoral operation. We took our time to perform lysis of a significant amount of adhesions. Then we identified both ureters and there were no problems.

We decided to do the cystectomy. I found there were no lymph nodes identified in both iliac and aortic nodes. Between the retroperitoneum and the bladder sac was cut completely. Then both pedicles of the bladder were cut. Some of them used the ligature and some were tied with 3-0 Vicryl sutures. After completion of both pedicles, the ureters were identified and sent out for frozen section to be sure the margins were clear of any tumor and they told me there was no tumor in the ureter whatsoever. The right ureter was o.k. but was dilated maybe triple the size of a normal ureter. The left side was stuck in there because of previous operations. We had to take time before we could free it all the way to the top of the L4-5 area. Then the endopelvic fascia was cut and the puboprostatic ligament was burned with the ligature on both sides and cut. The ureter was completely transected. The ureteral catheter was pulled out. Then the urethra and dorsal vein complex was approximated with 0 chromic and a couple of figure-of-eight sutures. The bleeding was completely stopped. The specimen was obtained and sent out. In the meantime, we created the ileum for the conduit about six inches or less. Then I had the left ureter brought to the right side under the sigmoid colon and then both ureters were spatulated. Then the end of the ureter was approximated with 3-0 chromic and then the ureter end was hooked up to the conduit proximal end and the anastomosis was done with 3-0 chromic mostly interrupted sutures, some of them running sutures. Then I put

MEDICAL REPORT 14.10 (CONTINUED)

in normal saline and there was a couple of leaking spaces that were reinforced with 3-0 chromic sutures. The conduit was delivered to the right lower quadrant stab wound for ileal stoma and also the fascia was cut. The peritoneum was perforated. The conduit was brought outside. It seems it was not quite everted right but it did o.k. but we couldn't do too much because of so much adhesions inside. The conduit was fixed to the peritoneum inside with 0 chromic and then the fascia conduit approximated with 0 Vicryl several interrupted sutures everted and the conduit was approximated with 0 chromic running sutures halfway because we covered the peritoneum in the lower part. Then the rectus fascia was approximated with 0 Maxon running sutures and subcutaneous tissue with 3-0 plain and skin with clips. In the meantime, I put the conduit stent placement in before the anastomosis on each side, which was delivered all the way to the outside, and the conduit stent was held with 3-0 silk on each side.

The patient tolerated the procedure well and was sent to the recovery room in good condition.

Dr. Smith, M.D.

NOTES

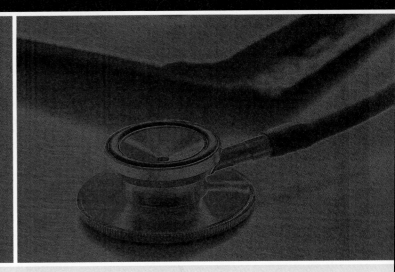

Coding for Complications of Pregnancy, Childbirth, and the Puerperium

Chapter Outline

The Obstetric Record
Distinguishing Time in Pregnancy Coding
Stages of Labor
Locating Pregnancy Codes in the Disease Index
Outcome-of-Delivery Codes
Uncomplicated Pregnancy With Normal Delivery
Complications of Pregnancy and Delivery
Common Labor and Delivery Procedures
Delivery Prior to Admission
Pregnancy Supervision Codes
Pregnancy With Abortive Outcome
Molar and Ectopic Pregnancy
Testing Your Comprehension

Coding Practice I: Chapter Review Exercises
Coding Practice II: Medical Record Case Studies

Chapter Objectives

▶ Describe the pathology of common complications of pregnancy, childbirth, and the puerperium.
▶ Recognize the typical manifestations, complications, and treatments of pregnancy, childbirth, and the puerperium in terms of their implications for coding.
▶ Correctly code common complications of pregnancy, childbirth, the puerperium, and related procedures by using the ICD-9-CM and medical records.

Complications of pregnancy, childbirth, and the puerperium are included in code section 630 to 677 of chapter 11 of the Disease Tabular of the ICD-9-CM. Pregnancy codes are used exclusively during the period that begins after conception and ends 6 weeks after delivery of the newborn.

Word Parts and Meanings of Medical Terms Related to Pregnancy and Childbirth

Word Part	Meaning	Example	Definition of Example
-gravida	Pregnancy	multigravida	Many pregnancies
hyster/o-	Uterus	hysterectomy	Surgical removal of the uterus
mast/o-	Breast	mastectomy;	Surgical removal of the breast; surgical
mamm/o-		mammoplasty	repair of breast
oophor/o-	Ovary	bilateral oophorectomy	Surgical removal of both ovaries
salping/o-	fallopian tubes	bilateral salpingectomy	Surgical removal of both fallopian tubes
perine/o-	perineum (area between the vagina and anus)	perineorrhaphy	Suture of the perineum
episi/o-	vulva (part of the external female genitalia; perineum)	episiotomy	Incision of the vulva (perineum) to enlarge the vaginal opening to aid in the delivery of the baby
-para -parous	to bear (give birth; delivery)	multipara	Woman who has had many births (deliveries)
-rrhea	Discharge	menorrhea	Menstruation
men/o	Menstruation	dysmenorrhea	Painful menstruation
-rrhagia	excessive bleeding	menorrhagia	Excessive bleeding during menstruation
metr/o metri/o	Uterus	endometriosis	An abnormal condition of the inner lining of the uterus

It is important to know that pregnancy codes (630 to 677) from chapter 11 take precedence over codes from other ICD-9-CM chapters because pregnancy, generally speaking, complicates all other conditions. Although codes from other ICD-9-CM chapters can be added to provide more detail, codes from the pregnancy chapter are sequenced first. To assist in your understanding, the Word Parts Box on this page reviews word parts and meanings of medical terms related to pregnancy and childbirth, and Figure 15.1 illustrates the female reproductive system.

The Obstetric Record

Mothers and their newborns always have separate medical records. In this chapter and Chapter 16 of this textbook, you will learn that certain codes and rules are specific to an obstetric record (i.e., the mother's record), whereas other codes and rules are specific to the newborn's record. Coding for the newborn record is covered in Chapter 16 of this textbook.

Mother's and baby's codes should not be interchanged (do not use the mother's codes on a newborn record or vice versa).

The format and content of an obstetric record are unique when compared with other medical records. Becoming familiar with the format will help you to locate conditions when reviewing the record. If an episode of

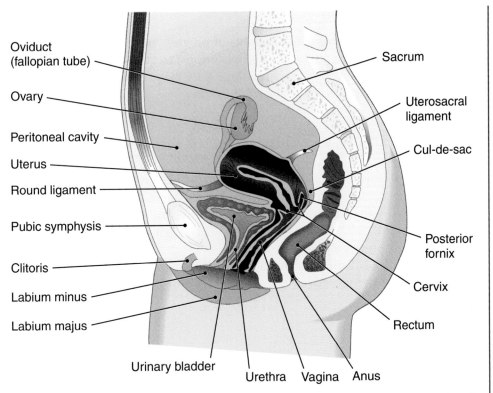

FIGURE 15.1 ■ Female reproductive system, as seen in sagittal section. (Reprinted with permission from Cohen BJ and Wood DL. Memmler's The Human Body in Health and Disease, 9th Ed. Philadelphia: Lippincott Williams & Wilkins, 2000.)

obstetric care results in delivery, the record is composed of three main sections: the prenatal section, the labor and delivery section, and the postpartum section.

Prenatal Section

The prenatal record is usually started in the obstetrician's office and is the equivalent of a History and Physical record; it contains important information on past and present conditions that can affect the management of the pregnancy. The prenatal record is usually sent to the hospital 6 weeks before the estimated date of delivery to ensure that the record is available when the patient presents for delivery.

To understand the prenatal record, it is helpful to understand the terms **gravida** and **para**. Gravida describes the number of pregnancies a woman has had, and para describes the number of deliveries. This obstetric history can affect the management of the current pregnancy. A woman may have more pregnancies than deliveries because of miscarriages or other abortive outcomes (such as a poor reproductive history or prior spontaneous abortions).

Labor and Delivery Section

Information needed for precise coding is also found in the labor and delivery section of the record, which contains documentation of any complications or procedures performed during the labor and delivery episode of care.

Postpartum Section

The postpartum section mainly consists of progress notes that document the patient's course of care, including complications, treatments, and response to treatments after delivery. A final discharge note may replace a discharge summary if the delivery was without complications.

Distinguishing Time in Pregnancy Coding

The length of time associated with a **term** pregnancy is 9 months (a full-term gestational period). Pregnancy is measured in stages called **trimesters**. The first trimester is the first 3-month period, the second trimester is the second 3-month period, and the third trimester is the last 3 months of gestation. Figure 15.2 illustrates a pregnant uterus.

Each trimester indicates important milestones in the evolution of the pregnancy and the growth of the developing fetus. Therefore, the length of

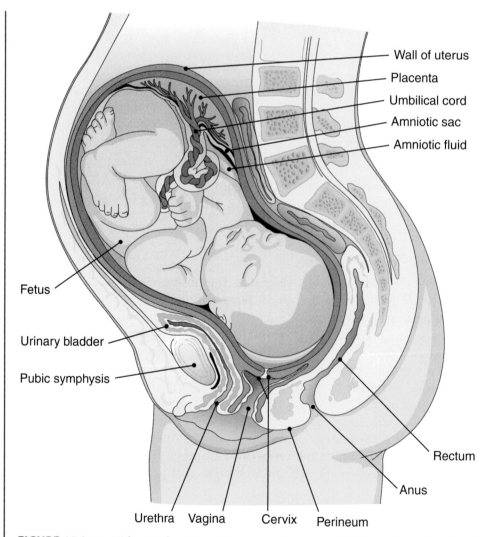

FIGURE 15.2 ■ Midsagittal section of a pregnant uterus with intact fetus. (Reprinted with permission from Cohen BJ and Wood DL. Memmler's The Human Body in Health and Disease, 9th Ed. Philadelphia: Lippincott Williams & Wilkins, 2000.)

TABLE 15.1	Gestation Time		
Gestation Time (weeks before delivery)		**Classification**	**Code**
Less than 37 completed weeks		Preterm	644.21
At least 37 weeks, but less than 40 completed weeks		Term	650 if normal delivery with no complications
40 to 42 completed weeks		Postterm	645.11
More than 42 completed weeks		Prolonged	645.21

gestation is extremely important for precise pregnancy coding. In ICD-9-CM, the time frame for a normal (term) gestation is at least 37 but less than 40 completed weeks. Therefore, if a woman delivers after 22 completed weeks but before 37 completed weeks (e.g., 36 weeks and 6 days), the delivery is considered "preterm." Delivery at 40 completed weeks or more is "postterm." Less than 22 weeks' gestation is considered an abortive outcome rather than a delivery.

During the episode of care in which a woman delivers, physicians often document only the weeks and days of the woman's gestational period in their final diagnosis; you must determine whether the pregnancy is considered term to assign the correct codes. For example, if the physician documented a "36-week pregnancy, delivered," you should be aware that this indicates a preterm pregnancy and affects the coding of the record. Knowing the gestational time required for a term birth helps you to determine how the delivery should be classified and coded (Table 15.1).

The length of gestation affects the coding of the mother's medical record as well as the newborn's. In the development of an infant, a fertilized egg is described as an **embryo** for the first 2 months of gestation and then as a **fetus** after month 2. From birth through the first 28 days of life, the child is described as a **newborn** or **neonate** and thereafter as an **infant** for the first year.

Stages of Labor

Women may experience complications during the different stages of labor. Because the stage of labor affects coding, understanding the three stages of labor will help you to apply the most accurate codes.

Stage 1: from the beginning of uterine contractions to full dilation of the cervical os (opening to the uterus)
Stage 2: from full dilation of the cervical os to delivery of the newborn
Stage 3: from delivery of the placenta (afterbirth) to the end of uterine contractions

Upon completion of the third stage of labor, a 6-week puerperium, or postpartum (i.e., after delivery), period begins.

Labor complication codes are often specific to each of the three stages. For example, primary uterine inertia indicates weakness of uterine contractions in the first stage of labor (661.0X), and secondary uterine inertia indicates weakness of uterine contractions in the second stage of labor (661.1X). Further, nursing documentation in the labor room of the woman's stating, "I'm tired of pushing," should prompt the coder to review the record further for the obstetrician's documentation of a possibly prolonged second stage of labor (662.2X).

TIP Documentation of a prolonged or lengthy labor experience may also indicate the need for a focused review of the record to determine whether it relates to complications of the first, second, or third stage of labor.

Locating Pregnancy Codes in the Disease Index

Many coders have difficulty in coding pregnancy records, perhaps because they code them infrequently and lack practice. Another problem may be that they limit their search of main terms for pregnancy codes in the Disease Index. Some coders get in the habit of looking under the main term "delivery; complicated by" in the Disease Index, yet several other useful main terms are available for locating conditions associated with pregnancy. Aside from the main term "delivery," the main terms of "pregnancy," "labor," "puerperal or postpartum," "prolonged," "premature," "post-term," and the condition itself (e.g., hypertension or diabetes) are excellent sources for finding maternal conditions.

The main term "pregnancy; complicated by, current disease or condition" is an excellent source for finding many conditions that complicate pregnancy. You can also look under the main term for a condition and then review subterms that reference pregnancy.

EXAMPLE

"Pregnancy, complicated by" type 1 insulin-dependent diabetes mellitus, undelivered during current episode of care: 648.03 + 250.01

"Diabetes; complicating pregnancy, childbirth, or puerperium," delivered during the current episode of care: 648.01 + 250.00

Outcome-of-Delivery Codes

If a woman delivers during the current episode of care, then you must always sequence an outcome-of-delivery code (V27.X) as an additional code after the pregnancy codes from chapter 11 of the ICD-9-CM. Outcome-of-delivery codes are used because the pregnancy codes alone cannot express the outcome of delivery. These codes can be located in the Disease Index under the main term "outcome."

EXAMPLE

Single liveborn outcome of delivery: V27.0

Twin, both liveborn outcome of delivery: V27.2

Single stillborn outcome of delivery: V27.1

Never assign an outcome-of-delivery code as the principal diagnosis.

Uncomplicated Pregnancy with Normal Delivery

Code 650, which is located under the main term "delivery; uncomplicated" in the Disease Index, is used as the principal diagnosis when there is a completely normal delivery (i.e., term gestation and spontaneous vaginal delivery, with or without an episiotomy). To qualify as a completely normal delivery, the outcome of delivery must always be a single liveborn infant, indicated by the additional code V27.0, and the presentation of the fetus must always be headfirst (e.g., **vertex**, **cephalic**, or **occipital** presentation are common terms that describe a normal headfirst presentation of the fetus within the cervical opening for delivery) (Figure 15.3).

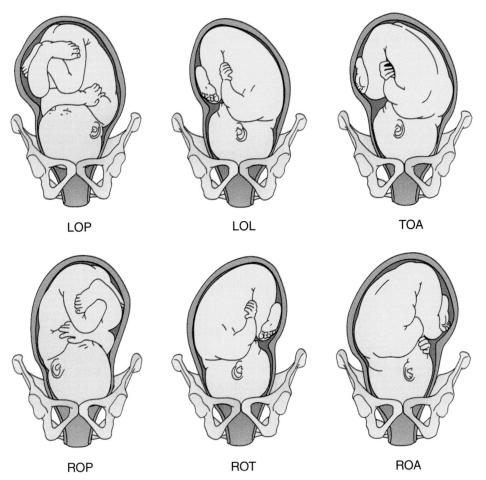

FIGURE 15.3 ■ Fetal position. All are vertex presentations. A = anterior; L = left; O = occiput; P = posterior; R = right; T = transverse. (Reprinted with permission from Pillitteri, A.[2003], Maternal and Child Nursing, 4th Ed., Philadelphia: Lippincott, Williams & Wilkins.)

Any complication during the current episode of care excludes the use of code 650 on the record (e.g., no perineal lacerations or other complications). Also, any antepartum (before delivery) conditions must have been completely resolved before the admission for delivery to use code 650. If applicable, you can assign code V25.2 as an additional diagnosis if the woman elected to have a sterilization procedure performed (e.g., tubal ligation) during the current episode of care. This is not considered a complication of care.

Routine procedures that might accompany code 650 include the following:

▶ Manually assisted vaginal delivery (code 73.59). This encompasses manipulation of the fetus through the birth canal by the physician or midwife.

▶ Routine episiotomy (code 73.6) with no tear (e.g., extension). In this procedure, an obstetrician performs a posterior incision of the perineum to increase the size of the vaginal opening to aid in labor and delivery. A routine episiotomy allows a clean, straight cut and suture repair, as opposed to a ragged perineal tear that may cause extensive damage to tissues.

▶ Artificial rupture of membrane (code 73.0X). In this procedure, the amniotic sac (bag of water) surrounding the fetus is broken to precipitate (begin) labor.

▶ Electrode placement to monitor the fetal heart rate (code 75.32 for internal placement and 75.34 for external placement). Fetal monitors check whether the fetus is in distress (possibly indicated by a sustained fetal heart rate of <90 or >140 bpm).

Any reference to procedures including instrumentation (e.g., forceps or vacuum extraction of the fetus), fetal manipulation or cephalic version (rotating or turning the fetus to proper position), suturing of perineal lacerations, or cesarean delivery disallows the use of code 650.

Complications of Pregnancy and Delivery

In contrast to the three-digit code for uncomplicated pregnancy (650), all pregnancy complication codes require a fifth digit to describe the current episode of care for the condition, as follows:

▶ 0 for an unspecified episode of care (rarely used on an inpatient record)
▶ 1 for a newborn delivered during the current episode of care, with or without mention of an antepartum condition
▶ 2 for a newborn delivered during the current episode of care, with mention of a postpartum complication
▶ 3 for an antepartum condition, undelivered (i.e., the newborn was not delivered during the current episode of care)
▶ 4 for a postpartum condition, undelivered (i.e., the newborn was delivered during a previous admission, and the patient is returning for care)

 TIP   The mandatory use of a fifth digit is usually denoted in the Disease Tabular of the ICD-9-CM codebook by the section symbol (§) next to the pregnancy three-digit category code.

For pregnancy complication codes, some fifth digits are like oil and water—they cannot be used together to describe the same admission. Only the fifth digits of <u>1</u> and <u>2</u> can be used in combination within the same episode of care. Any other fifth-digit combinations are incompatible. For example, you cannot list a fifth digit of <u>1</u> and <u>3</u> on the same record, because <u>1</u> denotes that the delivery occurred during the current episode of care, whereas <u>3</u> denotes that the delivery did not occur.

Pregnancy coding can be especially difficult when there are multiple complications or conditions and, therefore, multiple codes assigned. Some coders mistakenly assume that when a patient has a condition that requires a fifth digit of <u>2</u> (delivered, with mention of postpartum complication), then all pregnancy codes must be assigned a fifth digit of <u>2</u>. However, even if there is a mention of a postpartum complication, some of the complications may have occurred before delivery and therefore must be assigned the fifth digit of <u>1</u>.

EXAMPLE

Correct:

664.11	*Second-degree perineal laceration, with delivery*
666.12	*Other immediate postpartum hemorrhage, with delivery*
V27.0	*Single liveborn outcome of delivery*

Incorrect:

664.1<u>2</u>	*Invalid fifth digit (a tear during delivery is not a postpartum complication)*
666.12	*Other immediate postpartum hemorrhage, with delivery*
V27.0	*Single liveborn outcome of delivery*

TIP To help avoid incorrect fifth-digit assignment, always check the acceptable fifth digits, which are noted in brackets under the subcategory code in the Disease Tabular.

The *Tabular List of Diseases* indicates that for code 664.1X (second-degree perineal laceration), only <u>0</u>, <u>1</u>, and <u>4</u> are valid fifth digits. For code 666.1X (other immediate postpartum hemorrhage), only <u>0</u>, <u>2</u>, and <u>4</u> are valid fifth digits. Therefore, if a woman delivers during the current episode of care and the above-noted conditions occurred, 664.11 and 666.12 are the only acceptable choices (see excerpt below).

---

§ 664.1   **Second Degree Perineal Laceration**
[0,1,4]   Perineal laceration, rupture, or tear (following episiotomy) involving:
      pelvic floor
          perineal muscles
          vaginal muscles
| *Excludes* | that involving anal sphincter (664.2) |

§ 666.1   **Other Immediate Postpartum Hemorrhage**
[0,2,4]   Atony of uterus
      Hemorrhage within the first 24 hours following delivery of
        placenta
      Postpartum hemorrhage (atonic) NOS

Unless the delivery is completely normal and uncomplicated, the designation of the principal diagnosis in obstetric records is determined by the main complication of the delivery. If no complication of delivery occurred (e.g., perineal laceration or cesarean delivery for obstructed labor), then the main complication of the pregnancy (e.g., hypertension or diabetes) should be sequenced as the principal diagnosis. When delivery is performed via a cesarean section, the principal diagnosis is the reason for the cesarean section.

The pregnancy complication category codes 647 ("infectious and parasitic condition in the mother classifiable elsewhere, but complicating pregnancy, childbirth, or the puerperium") and 648 ("other current conditions in the mother classifiable elsewhere, but complicating pregnancy, childbirth, or the puerperium") usually require an additional code to further specify the precise condition.

EXAMPLE	*Genitourinary gonorrhea in pregnancy, antepartum condition: 647.13 + 098.0*
	Iron-deficiency anemia in pregnancy, antepartum condition: 648.23 + 280.9

Common Complication Codes

A common pregnancy complication code is used for maternal/fetal Rh factor incompatibility (code 656.11). Rh is a naturally occurring antigen (foreign substance) that is on the surface of red blood cells in some individuals. It is denoted by a plus sign after one's blood type (e.g., O positive, or O$^+$; A positive, or A$^+$). An Rh-negative (Rh-) individual does not have the Rh factor.

Maternal and fetal blood do not mix during pregnancy, but there is an exchange of nutrients and oxygen via the placenta and umbilical cord. However, during birth, fetal and maternal blood can mix. If a pregnant woman is Rh- and the fetus is Rh$^+$, the Rh$^-$ woman subsequently develops Rh$^+$ antibodies that attack the foreign Rh$^+$ antigens. This is a classic antigen/antibody reaction.

Problems can occur if an Rh- woman has a second Rh$^+$ child. During the second pregnancy, Rh$^+$ antibodies in the pregnant woman attack and destroy the red blood cells of the Rh$^+$ baby, causing a condition in the newborn called hemolytic disease of the newborn, or erythroblastosis fetalis. To prevent hemolytic disease of the newborn, the Rh- woman is given an injection of the drug Rh$_o$(D) immune globulin (RhoGAM) (code 99.11) during early pregnancy and again shortly after delivery. Administration of this drug prevents the Rh- woman from producing Rh$^+$ antibodies.

TIP Carefully review the prenatal record to determine a woman's Rh status and review the medication administration record to confirm whether RhoGAM was administered.

Another common complication of pregnancy occurs when a woman has tested positive for group B streptococcus bacteria (via vaginal swab with culture). Although a positive streptococcus B finding may not represent an acute infection, there is a potential for transmission and harm to the infant during delivery. Therefore, code this as an "other current condition affecting pregnancy" (648.9X), with the group B streptococcus carrier status code of V02.51.

Coding Clinic 1998, fourth quarter, describes more information about group B streptococcus carriers in pregnancy.

Table 15.2 highlights common complications of pregnancy and the corresponding codes.

TABLE 15.2   Codes for Complications of Pregnancy

Complication	Example	Code
Abnormal fetal heart rate	Pregnancy at 35 weeks, undelivered, complicated by fetal decelerations	659.73
Anemia	Antepartum iron deficiency in pregnancy	648.23 + 280.9
Cephalopelvic disproportion	Term pregnancy complicated by maternal cephalopelvic disproportion requiring low transverse cesarean section	653.41 + V27.0 + 74.1
Cervical incompetence or disproportion	Admission for placement of Shirodkar cerclage for cervical incompetence	654.53 + 67.59
Diabetes mellitus	Antepartum type 1 insulin-dependent diabetes mellitus, out of control, in pregnancy	648.03 + 250.03
Difficulties in labor	37.5-week term pregnancy with desultory labor, single liveborn delivery with manually assisted vaginal delivery	661.21 + V27.0 + 73.59
Elderly multigravida (second or more pregnancy, aged ≥35 years)	Term pregnancy, elderly multigravida, single liveborn delivery	659.61 + V27.0
Elderly primigravida (first pregnancy, aged ≥35 years)	Term pregnancy, elderly primigravida, single liveborn delivery	659.51 + V27.0
Young maternal age (<16 years)	Term pregnancy, mother age 14, single liveborn delivery	659.81 + V27.0
Fetal conditions	Term pregnancy complicated by oversized infant, single liveborn delivered, episiotomy	653.51 + V27.0 + 73.6
	Term pregnancy delivered, nuchal cord with compression	663.11 + V27.0
	Term pregnancy with delivery of trisomy 21 baby (Down's syndrome)	655.11 + V27.0
Fetal distress	Cesarean section for fetal distress during labor with delivery of liveborn infant	656.31 + V27.0 + 74.1
Fetal malposition (e.g., breech, brow, shoulder, or face presentation)	Term pregnancy, low-transverse cesarean section for breech presentation and obstruction of labor, single liveborn	652.21 + 660.01 + V27.0 + 74.1
Hyperemesis gravidarum (vomiting in pregnancy)	Mild hyperemesis gravidarum at 20 weeks, discharged after treatment of same	643.03
Hypertension	Pregnancy with severe antepartum preeclampsia	642.53

(continued)

TABLE 15.2 (*continued*)

Complication	Example	Code
Infection	Pregnancy complicated by antepartum Escherichia coli urinary tract infection	646.63 + 599.0 + 041.4
	Admission for pelvic cellulitis, postterm pregnancy with delivery 1 week prior	670.04
Insufficient prenatal care	Term pregnancy, delivery of single liveborn infant, small for dates, no prenatal care, smoking during pregnancy	656.51 + 648.41 + 305.1 + V23.7 + V27.0
Intrauterine fetal death	Term pregnancy resulting in stillborn delivery (after completion of 22 weeks' gestation)	656.41 + V27.1
Maternal conditions	Pregnancy complicated by antepartum maternal heart disease with mitral and aortic valvular insufficiency	648.63 + 396.3
Multiple gestation	38.5-week twin delivery, both liveborn; routine episiotomy	651.01 + V27.2 + 73.6
Perineum tears (during delivery)	Term pregnancy, single liveborn, complicated by first-degree perineal tear requiring repair	664.01 + V27.0 + 75.69
	38-week term pregnancy resulting in single liveborn infant; routine episiotomy with second-degree extension	664.11 + V27.0 + 75.69
	38-week term pregnancy resulting in single liveborn infant; second-degree episiotomy	650 + V27.0 + 73.6
Postpartum hemorrhage	Term pregnancy, delivered single liveborn infant, complicated by delayed postpartum hemorrhage with subsequent acute blood-loss anemia	666.22 + 648.22 + 285.1 + V27.0
Preterm and postterm delivery	33 weeks' gestation with manually assisted delivery of 5 lbs. 3 oz. newborn	644.21 + V27.0
Rh-factor incompatibility	Term pregnancy, delivered, Rh incompatibility; vaginal assisted delivery, RhoGAM administration	656.11 + V27.0 + 73.59 + 99.11
Uterine scar from previous cesarean delivery	Term pregnancy, single newborn delivery, previous cesarean section, vaginal birth after cesarean section with manually assisted delivery	654.21 + V27.0 + 73.59

As of October 2006, a new category was created for Chapter 11, Complications of Pregnancy, Childbirth, and the Puerperium. This new category (649) would include codes to specify smoking, obesity, bariatric surgery status, coagulation defects, epilepsy, spotting, and uterine size and date discrepancies that complicate pregnancy.

Examples:

Term pregnancy, single newborn delivery, complicated by maternal tobacco abuse = 649.01 + V27.0

28 week pregnancy admitted with seizures secondary to known epilepsy = 649.43 + 345.90

Term pregnancy, single newborn delivery, complicated by maternal obesity, BMI 33 = 649.11 + 278.00 + V85.33 + V27.0

Pregnancy at 31 weeks, undelivered, complicated by spotting = 649.53

Common Labor and Delivery Procedures

Common labor and delivery procedures include manually assisted vaginal deliveries, episiotomies, laceration repairs, and cesarean deliveries. If a delivery occurs, at least one procedure code will be assigned. However, multiple procedure codes may be assigned, depending on the type of delivery and any complications of labor or delivery that developed.

Manually assisted vaginal delivery (code 73.59) describes a routine assisted spontaneous vaginal delivery. An assisted vaginal delivery can occur with or without complications of pregnancy.

Episiotomy (code 73.6) involves an incision of the perineum and subsequent suture repair (episiorrhaphy) after delivery. If the incision extends or tears during the delivery, it is classified as an obstetric laceration. Code 75.69 (repair of a current obstetric perineal laceration) excludes the repair of a routine episiotomy. Therefore, use code 75.69 only to report the repair of an episiotomy with extension. However, if the physician extends the episiotomy to expedite delivery, it is considered an episiotomy and not a laceration because it was extended by the physician and not by the delivery itself. Code 73.6 excludes an episiotomy in association with a forceps or vacuum delivery (see "forceps or vacuum delivery with episiotomy").

EXAMPLE

Second-degree episiotomy: 73.6

Midline episiotomy with second-degree extension: 75.69

Low forceps delivery with third-degree episiotomy: 72.1

Low forceps delivery with episiotomy with third-degree extension: 72.1 + 75.69

An episiotomy (73.6) is considered a routine part of a manually assisted spontaneous vaginal delivery (73.59). Therefore, code 73.59 is generally not coded in addition to the 73.6 episiotomy code. However, some health-care facilities require both codes.

Repair of current obstetric lacerations can involve tears of the perineum, vagina, vulva, bladder, rectum, or uterus and always has an associated pregnancy complication diagnosis code. These codes can be located in the Procedure Index under the main term "repair," followed by a subterm for the site of the tear and then the further indented subterm for "current obstetrical laceration."

EXAMPLE

Repair current obstetric second-degree perineum laceration: 75.69

Repair current obstetric vaginal laceration: 75.69

Repair current obstetric urethral laceration: 76.61

Cesarean section (category code 74; abbreviated C/S or C-section) is an operation that removes the fetus through an incision into the uterus. In the Procedure Index under the main term "cesarean section" are various types of cesarean sections that denote the operative approach or technique. For example, the classic cesarean section (which usually occurs in an emergency situation) uses a vertical cut through the abdominal wall into the uterus, whereas the low cervical cesarean section uses a low transverse abdominal incision into the uterus. The low cervical approach is performed more often because it is less damaging to abdominal muscles and results in a better appearance. This approach is sometimes referred to as the **bikini cut.**

Cesarean sections must always be medically warranted, and an associated pregnancy complication diagnosis code indicating the medical need for the procedure is required. Common complications indicating the need for a cesarean section include the following:

- ▶ fetal malpresentation (the normal presentation of the fetus must always be headfirst; fetal malpresentations include breech [buttocks], brow, shoulder, face, and transverse lie [sideways] presentations)
- ▶ previous cesarean section delivery (uterine incisional scar from previous cesarean delivery)
- ▶ fetal distress during labor
- ▶ maternal sexually transmitted disease (e.g. herpetic, gonococcal, or syphilitic infection)
- ▶ cephalopelvic disproportion (the fetal head is too large for the maternal pelvic brim)
- ▶ placental disorders (e.g., placenta previa [placenta implanted over cervical os] or abruptio placentae [placenta breaks away from uterine wall])

Never assign diagnosis code 650 with a cesarean section; a normal delivery is completely incompatible with this procedure.

Forceps and vacuum extraction (code category 72) and fetal version procedures (code category 73) are generally performed to assist in the delivery of a malpresented fetus and should be reported with the applicable pregnancy complication diagnosis code. Any use of the pregnancy complication code 669.51 (which describes forceps or vacuum extractor delivery without mention of indication) should be referred to the medical record or patient care review committee for the facility, because medical necessity must be documented by the obstetrician. Code 669.51 reveals a lack of supporting physician documentation to justify forceps or vacuum extractor delivery. Therefore, coders should take steps to report this through the appropriate administrative channels within the hospital so that corrective action can be applied through medical staff committees.

Delivery Prior to Admission

On occasion, a woman gives birth en route to a hospital or prior to admission and is admitted for postpartum care only. In this case, keep in mind that the birth did not occur at the health-care facility, and, therefore, the codes must not report that it did. If the delivery outside of the facility is without complications and the woman is admitted for postpartum observation only, use code V24.0 (located in the Disease Index under "admission (for); postpartum observation, immediately after delivery"). If a woman is admitted with any complications, use the pregnancy complication code with a fifth digit of 4 (denoting a postpartum condition or complication as the reason for the current episode of care). For example, if the admission is for repair of a third-degree perineal laceration after delivering in a taxi en route to a hospital, assign code 664.04 and a procedure code for the repair of the obstetric laceration.

Pregnancy Supervision Codes

As the term implies, pregnancy supervision codes are assigned to report routine prenatal outpatient service visits provided in the obstetrician's office or obstetric clinic. As shown in the excerpt below, pregnancy supervision codes are located in the *Alphabetic Index to Diseases* under the main term "pregnancy; supervision (of) (for)."

Pregnancy
    supervision (of)(for)—*see also* Pregnancy, management affected by
        elderly
            multigravida V23.82
            primigravida V23.81
            high-risk V23.9
            insufficient prenatal care V23.7
            specified problem NEC V23.8
            multiparity V23.3
            normal NEC V22.1
            first V22.0
        poor
            obstetric history V23.49
                preterm labor V23.41
            reproductive history V23.5
        young
            multigravida V23.84
            primigravida V23.83

In some circumstances, you will assign pregnancy supervision codes as additional codes to report relevant historical information for an inpatient stay. For example, insufficient prenatal care (code V23.7) is of special concern and puts the patient at higher risk. Also, the V23.2 code for multiparity is sometimes used as an additional code to help explain a woman's request for elective sterilization during the episode of care. However, if the conditions complicate the pregnancy, pregnancy codes are often available (e.g., young maternal age affecting management of pregnancy, 659.8X; delivery complicated by multiparity, 659.4X).

Coders should be cautioned about the misuse of code V22.2 for incidental pregnancy. To use code V22.2, the physician must document that the pregnancy is incidental and has no bearing on the presenting condition or the treatment rendered. Code V22.2 used as an additional code means that the pregnancy did not complicate the care for the presenting condition. However, even an emergency department encounter for a broken toe, which may seem

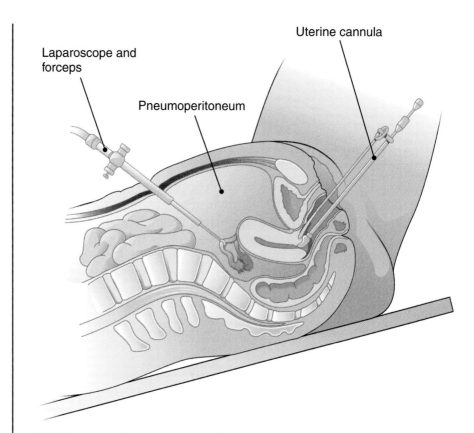

FIGURE 15.4 ■ Laparoscopic sterilization. (Reprinted with permission from Cohen BJ. Medical Terminology: An Illustrated Guide, 4th Ed. Baltimore: Lippincott Williams & Wilkins, 2004.)

irrelevant, could change the course of care because radiographs of the foot could harm the fetus. Alternatively, if a pregnant woman is admitted with abdominal pain, an ultrasound may be performed rather than a computed tomographic scan. In contrast to diagnostic computed tomographic scans or radiographs that emit radiation, ultrasounds use sound waves to produce an image of an organ or tissue and will not harm the fetus.

Admission or Encounter for Sterilization

Code V25.2, indicating an admission or encounter for sterilization, can be used as a principal or secondary diagnosis code (depending on the circumstances) for women as well as men. The procedure for women is often a tubal ligation, in which the fallopian tubes are cut and tied off, resulting in sterility (Figure 15.4). Other techniques that include endoscopic procedures that surgically occlude (block) the fallopian tubes are coded to categories 66.2X to 66.3X. For men, vasectomy and ligation (tying off) of the vas deferens (tube that carries sperm) can be performed to render sterility (code category 63.7X).

Code V26.0 is used when the current reason for the encounter is a sterilization-reversal procedure. In the *Alphabetic Index to Diseases*, code V26.0 can be located under the main term "admission (encounter) for; restoration of organ continuity (poststerilization) (tuboplasty) (vasoplasty)." The reversal procedure for women can be located in the *Alphabetic Index to Procedures* under the main term "repair; fallopian tube, by reanastomosis" (code 66.79). For men, it is located in the *Alphabetic Index to Procedures* under the main term "repair; vas deferens, by anastomosis" or is located under the main term for the operation "vasovasostomy" (code 63.82).

Pregnancy With Abortive Outcome

An abortion is the expulsion of a nonviable (cannot exist on its own) embryo or fetus from the uterus at or before 20 weeks of gestation or the expulsion of a fetus weighing less than 500 g. ICD-9-CM classifies terminations of pregnancy less than 22 weeks as abortive outcomes. Located under the main term "abortion" in the *Alphabetic Index to Diseases*, there are different types of abortions that include the following:

▶ **Spontaneous abortion** (category code 634), also called a miscarriage, results in the premature expulsion of the fetus for an unknown cause.
▶ **Legal abortion** (category code 635) can be performed for therapeutic reasons (i.e., when there are health concerns for the pregnant woman or there is suspected damage to the fetus) or for elective reasons in a licensed abortion clinic or other health-care facility.
▶ **Illegal abortion** (category 636) is one performed in an unlicensed facility or by an unlicensed practitioner. This code is used by a health-care facility only to report aftercare for the treatment of complications resulting from an illegal abortion that was performed outside of the facility.
▶ **Unspecified abortion** (category 637) occurs when a surgical procedure on the uterus results in the unplanned removal of the fetus.
▶ **Failed (legal) abortion** (category 638) occurs when a legal abortion fails to result in the expulsion of the products of conception.

The abortions classified in category codes 634 to 638 include a fourth-digit subcategory to describe any complications associated with the abortion (occurring during the current episode of care), as well as a fifth-digit subcategory to describe whether the abortion was incomplete (1) or complete (2). An abortion is considered incomplete when the uterus retains any products of conception. Abortion complication codes usually require an additional code to further describe a precise condition.

Spontaneous abortion, incomplete, with acute endometritis: 634.01 + 615.0

Spontaneous abortion, incomplete, with urinary tract infection due to Escherichia coli: 634.71 + 599.0 + 041.4

EXAMPLE

Hospital inpatient admissions for abortion are often for spontaneous incomplete abortions (code 634.91). An abortion caused by major trauma (e.g., automobile accident) is classified as a spontaneous abortion and requires an E code to explain the external cause of the injury. As in the case of all trauma coding, the most severe injury is listed as the principal diagnosis.

Diagnoses: motor vehicle accident (MVA) with blunt abdominal trauma and ruptured spleen, four broken ribs, 15-week gestation with resulting spontaneous abortion secondary to MVA.

Procedures: exploratory laparotomy, splenectomy, dilation and curettage: 865.04 ; 807.04 ; 634.91; 41.5 ; 69.02 ; E819.9

EXAMPLE

If an unplanned abortion results from an operation on the uterus, the condition causing the admission is sequenced as the principal diagnosis (e.g., hysterectomy for cancer of the cervix uterus); the code for unspecified abortion (637.92) is sequenced as an additional code. If an unintended abortion results as a consequence of major surgery on an organ other than the uterus (e.g., cholecystectomy for gallstones), then the condition causing the surgery would be sequenced as the principal diagnosis, with the code for spontaneous abortion (634.92) given as an additional code.

To accurately code therapeutic abortions (category 635), you must determine whether there is a documented maternal or fetal reason for the abortion. If there is a maternal reason for the therapeutic abortion, sequence the therapeutic abortion code first, followed by a pregnancy complication code with the fifth digit <u>3</u>. Locate the pregnancy complication code in the Disease Index under the main term "pregnancy; complicated (by), current disease or condition (nonobstetric)." If there is a fetal reason for the therapeutic abortion (i.e., suspected damage to the fetus), sequence the therapeutic abortion code first, followed by a pregnancy complication code with the fifth digit <u>3</u>. Locate these codes in the Disease Index under the main term "pregnancy; affected by, abnormality, fetus (suspected)."

EXAMPLE	*Therapeutic abortion related to maternal primary cardiomyopathy: 635.92 + 648.63 + 425.4*
	Therapeutic abortion due to suspected Down's syndrome in fetus: 635.92 + 655.13

Codes for other types of abortion procedures, located under the main term "abortion" in the Procedure Index, include the following: dilation and curettage (code 69.0X), injection of saline (75.0), insertion of laminaria (69.93) or prostaglandin suppository (96.49) into the cervix uteri, and aspiration curettage (69.51). The use of a laminaria or prostaglandin suppository (placed in cervix) produces strong uterine contractions to induce or complete an abortion.

To classify readmissions for complications after a prior discharge for an abortion, use category code 639.

EXAMPLE	*After abortion 1 week previously, patient was readmitted for pelvic peritonitis: 639.0*

Other types of abortions include the following:

- ▶ **Missed abortion** (code 632): fetal death occurs before 22 weeks of gestation, with retention of the dead fetus and products of conception. An expulsion of the dead fetus that results with a spontaneous abortion was missed, and the dead fetus is retained in the uterus. Retention of a dead fetus after 22 weeks is coded to intrauterine fetal death (656.4X) and is not classified to abortion. Intrauterine fetal death (after 22 weeks' gestation) is a complication of pregnancy, and the outcome of delivery should include a code for stillbirth (e.g., V27.1—single stillborn).
- ▶ **Threatened abortion** (code 640.0X): hemorrhage in early pregnancy (before 22 weeks' gestation) that may or may not result in expulsion of the fetus.

Molar and Ectopic Pregnancy

Molar pregnancy (codes 630 and 631) classifies hydatidiform moles (i.e., cystic uterine masses) or other abnormal products of conception (e.g., blighted ovum or fleshy uterine mass). Hysterotomy with removal of a hydatidiform mole is coded to 68.0. The procedure for the removal of other molar pregnancies would be coded by locating the main term "excision, lesion" for the site (e.g., uterus or ovary) and then reviewing the subterms that indicate whether it used an open (invasive with incision) or endoscopic (less invasive, with a scope) procedure (e.g., see "excision, lesion, ovary" [65.29] versus "excision, lesion, ovary, by laparoscope" [65.25]).

Anything that is **ectopic** is outside of its normal location. In an ectopic pregnancy (category code 633), the fertilized egg implants in an area outside of the uterus, such as in the fallopian tube, ovary, or abdominal cavity (Figure 15.5).

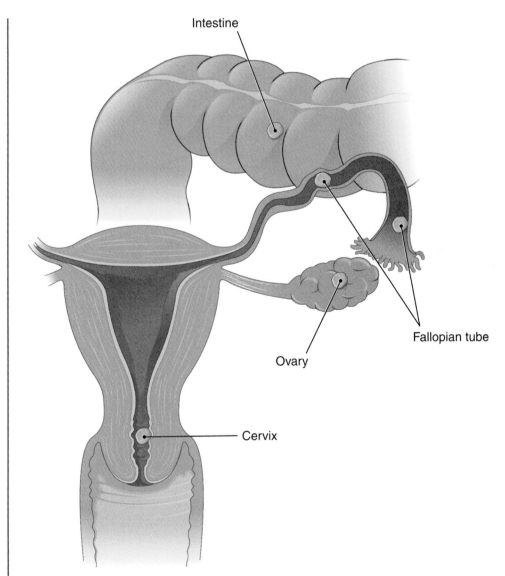

FIGURE 15.5 ■ Sites at which an ectopic pregnancy can occur. (Reprinted with permission from Cohen BJ. Medical Terminology: An Illustrated Guide, 4th Ed. Baltimore: Lippincott Williams & Wilkins, 2004.)

The most common ectopic pregnancy is a tubal pregnancy (code 633.1X). Because the fallopian tube can rupture, surgery with removal of the ectopic pregnancy is indicated (e.g., salpingectomy with removal of tubal pregnancy [code 66.62]). New fifth digits provide specificity in cases in which there is a concurrent intrauterine pregnancy (e.g., tubal pregnancy with [coexisting] intrauterine pregnancy: 633.1<u>1</u>).

For molar or ectopic pregnancy complications, use category code 639 to describe a complication during the current episode of care or a subsequent episode of care (return after discharge).

SUMMARY

This chapter has described the pathology of common complications experienced in pregnancy, childbirth, and the puerperium and has also provided a basis for recognizing the manifestations of these complications and their treatments. Correctly coding the respective complications has also been emphasized.

TESTING YOUR COMPREHENSION

1. What common time period is used for the use of pregnancy codes?

2. Why do pregnancy codes take precedence over other codes?

3. Once a delivery takes place, how is the typical medical record structured?

4. What time period defines a preterm delivery?

5. Identify the three stages of labor.

6. What determines the designation of the principal diagnosis in obstetric records?

7. True or False? An assisted vaginal delivery occurs only when complications are noted in the delivery process.

8. What code is used to report the repair of an episiotomy with extension?

9. What is considered a routine part of a manually assisted spontaneous vaginal delivery?

10. A procedure that removes the fetus through an incision to the uterus is referred to as what type of operation?

11. When forceps, vacuum extraction, and fetal version procedures are used, there must be an accompanying pregnancy complication diagnosis code. If the reason for the use of these procedures is not documented in the medical record, what should be done?

12. What code is used to explain a woman's request for elective sterilization?

13. Termination of pregnancy at less than 22 weeks is referred to as what type of outcome?

14. What are the different types of abortions?

15. Intrauterine fetal death after 22 weeks of pregnancy is referred to as a complication of pregnancy and should be coded according to what category?

_____

16. If something is referred to as ectopic, what does this mean?

_____

17. What is the most common type of ectopic pregnancy?

_____

CODING PRACTICE I   Chapter Review Exercises

Directions

By using your ICD-9-CM codebook, code the following diagnoses and procedures:

	DIAGNOSIS/PROCEDURES	CODE
1	Vaginal birth after previous cesarean section. Live term newborn. Spontaneous vaginal delivery with routine episiotomy.	
2	Premature rupture of membranes. Second-degree perineal laceration. Live term newborn. Medical induction labor. Episiotomy with second-degree extension.	
3	Forty-one weeks' gestation for induction of labor. Fetal decelerations. Term live birth. Medical induction of labor. Internal and external fetal monitoring. Low transverse cesarean section.	
4	Forty weeks' gestation. Vaginal delivery with no complications. Single liveborn. Assisted spontaneous vaginal delivery.	
5	Breech presentation with delivery of single liveborn infant. Low cervical cesarean section.	
6	Fourth-degree laceration. Gestational diabetes. Large infant. Live term newborn. Vaginal delivery with repair of fourth-degree laceration.	
7	Ectopic (tubal) pregnancy. Salpingectomy with removal of tubal pregnancy.	
8	Ten weeks' gestation with admission for intractable nausea and vomiting with dehydration.	
9	Spontaneous incomplete abortion. Dilation and curettage with removal of retained products of conception.	

	DIAGNOSIS/PROCEDURES	CODE
10	Readmit for postpartum mastitis. Delivered 1 week prior.	
11	Pregnancy-induced hypertension—36 weeks' gestation, undelivered.	
12	Severe preeclampsia, 35.5 weeks' gestation. Live-born delivery. Low transverse cesarean section.	
13	Missed abortion. Insertion of prostaglandin suppository.	
14	Twenty-five weeks' gestation. Pyelonephritis, undelivered.	
15	Shoulder dystocia. Rh incompatibility. Delayed postpartum hemorrhage. Blood-loss anemia. Term liveborn delivery. Low forceps delivery with episiotomy. RhoGAM administration. Transfusion of packed red blood cells.	
16	Fetopelvic disproportion with obstruction. Hypothyroidism. Postoperative blood-loss anemia. Term liveborn delivery. Low transverse cesarean section.	
17	Advanced maternal age at 40 years. Failure to progress, second stage. Desire for sterilization. Live newborn at term. Low cervical cesarean section. Bilateral tubal ligation (Pomeroy).	

	DIAGNOSIS/PROCEDURES	CODE
18	Forty-two weeks' gestation. Periurethral laceration. Term liveborn delivery. Artificial rupture of membranes. Assisted spontaneous vaginal delivery with repair of periurethral tear.	
19	Thirty-two weeks' gestation. Intrauterine death. Stillborn delivery. Medical induction of labor. Vaginal delivery.	
20	Premature labor at 35.5 weeks. Twin pregnancy, both liveborn. Fetal distress in twin B. Vaginal delivery, twin A. Classic cesarean section, twin B.	

CODING PRACTICE II   Medical Record Case Studies

Instructions

1. Carefully review the medical reports provided for each case study.
2. Research any abbreviations and terms that are unfamiliar or unclear.
3. Identify as many diagnoses and procedures as possible.
4. Because only part of the patient's total record is available, determine what additional documentation you might need.
5. If appropriate, identify any questions you might ask the physician to code this case correctly and completely.
6. Complete the appropriate blanks below for each case study.

CHAPTER 15 CASE STUDIES

Case Study 15.1 (Coder/Abstract Summary Form)

Patient: **Jane Doe**

Patient documentation: **Review Medical Reports 15.1 and 15.2**

1. Principal diagnosis:

   _____

2. Secondary or other diagnoses:

   _____

3. Principal procedure:

   _____

4. Other procedures:

   _____

5. Additional documentation needed:

   _____

   _____

   _____

Case Study 15.1 (Continued)

6. Questions for the physician:

_____

_____

_____

_____

_____

DISCHARGE SUMMARY

PATIENT:	Doe, Jane
DOB:	
MED REC:	999999
SEX/RACE:	F/1
PT ROOM:	
ADM DATE:	6/30
DISCHG DT:	7/03

HISTORY: This is a 25-year-old white female, gravida 2, para 1, with 1 living child, whose EDC is 10/21. The week prior to admission, the patient has been seen in the office and treated for a urinary tract infection. She had two previous early in the pregnancy and had been treated with Keflex. This time, she was placed on Augmentin. The patient came to the emergency room on the early morning 06/27 with headache, nausea and vomiting, and fever. She had lab work done and was treated symptomatically. She called me later in the day complaining of persistence of her symptoms and therefore, she was admitted for further treatment and evaluation. She was placed on the floor in the hospital and during the night placed on IV Claforan, subcutaneous Terbutaline was started while she was transferred to the suites as she was having contractions. She persisted with nausea and vomiting and headache, and these were initially treated symptomatically. She also had pelvic pressure and examination revealed a closed cervix. With persistent headache and nausea and vomiting, consultation was obtained by Dr. Fever, who felt that the patient probably had viral meningitis. Tests were drawn for West Nile and St. Louis encephalitis. Over time, the patient's headache gradually improved as well as her fever that had a downward trend. The vomiting stopped; and her fever subsided. At this time, she had significant weakness and she could barely get up to go to the bathroom. Her laboratory work appeared normal. By 6/31, her weakness had improved but she still had some nausea. She was changed from sq Terbutaline to p.o. on 7/1. Because of increasing contractions p.o. Terbutaline every 6 hrs was subsequently changed to every 3 1/2 hours given 2.5 mg. The patient had symptoms of oral and vaginal yeast infection and was treated symptomatically. She was discharged on the morning of 7/3 feeling much stronger with no more headache, nausea, and vomiting. She still had some occasional contractions but had done much better on 2.5 Terbutaline every 3 1/2 hrs.

DISPOSITION: She will be placed on bed rest at home with follow-up in my office in one week. Discharge activity was discussed with the patient in detail as well as warning symptoms.

DISCHARGE DIAGNOSES:
1. PROBABLE VIRAL MENINGITIS.
2. PREGNANCY, UNDELIVERED AT 24 WEEKS.
3. PREMATURE LABOR, ARRESTED.
4. ORAL & VAGINAL YEAST INFECTION.
5. URINARY TRACT INFECTION, ON AUGMENTIN.

DISCHARGE MEDICATIONS:
1. Terbutaline 2.5 mg. Every 3 hrs.
2. Fioricet for headache, as needed.
3. Oral medication for yeast – Terazol
4. Continue Augmentin

Dr. Smith, M.D.

DD:

DT:

MEDICAL REPORT 15.2

INTERNAL MEDICINE CONSULTATION

PATIENT:	Doe, Jane
DOB:	
MED REC:	999999
SEX/RACE:	F/1
PT ROOM:	
ADM DATE:	6/30
DISCHG DT:	7/03

CC: Headache

HPI: This 25-year-old WF, who is 23 weeks pregnant developed suprapubic pressure, diarrhea and increased urinary frequency on 6/23. The following day, Dr. Smith found that she had a urinary tract infection and treated this with Augmentin. After 2 days of it, the diarrhea resolved. However on 6/26, she had a severe headache that she thought was a migraine. Fioricet helped some, but by that evening, the headache was much worse and vomiting started. After several hours of this, at 03:00, she woke her husband up and they came to the ED. Phenergan and Demerol were given and she was discharged. As her symptoms continued, she returned later that afternoon and was subsequently admitted and given IV antibiotics. Temperatures have continued between 101 and 103.

The patient explains that she has a history of migraine headaches twice a year. Three weeks ago, she took a Zpak for URI. About a month ago, she had some tick exposure. She has not traveled out of the country and had no exposure to someone with a similar illness. She states she feels better today than she has been over the past 2 days.

PMH: Ruptured ovarian cyst leading to the need for 4 units of transfused blood. Several laparoscopic surgeries in the past.

SH: She works as a legal assistant.

ROS: HEENT: painful to focus in extremes of vision. Recurrent mouth ulcers. Dry mouth. CV: indigestion treated with Zantac last week. PULM: mild dyspnea. GI: no BM in several days. GU: mild suprapubic pain continues. MS: lots of "aches and pains" through the illness. NEURO: Generalized weakness.

PR: This WDWN Pregnant WF was in NAD and was ambulatory to BR.

HEENT: PERL, EOMI, Mouth negative.

NECK: Supple, no adenopathy or goiter.

LUNGS: Clear to auscultation and percussion.

HEART: RRR without murmur, rub, or gallop.

BREASTS: Not examined.

ABD: Pregnant with tenderness in the suprapubic area.

EXTRM: Pedal pulses present. No edema or calf tenderness.

NEURO: Grossly normal.

SKIN: No rashes seen.

LAB: On admission, the WBC was elevated. Today 6.5, Hct 26, Plts 185, gluc 98, BUN 2, Creat 0, Protein & albumin were both low. UA now normal.

Continued

MEDICAL REPORT 15.2 (CONTINUED)

IMPRESSION: Fever and headache. Probable viral meningitis. Since she is feeling better today, I would not recommend a LP at this time. Sinus infection has been treated.

PLAN: Although it is doubtful that these would be positive, I would recommend to draw tests to look for West Nile and St. Louis Encephalitis. Will follow along and would recommend to continue the Claforan for now.

_____

Dr. Fever, M.D.

DD:

DT:

NOTES

Case Study 15.2 (Coder/Abstract Summary Form)

Patient: **Linda Jones**

Patient documentation: **Review Medical Reports 15.3 and 15.4**

1. Principal diagnosis:

   _____

2. Secondary or other diagnoses:

   _____

3. Principal procedure:

   _____

4. Other procedures:

   _____

5. Additional documentation needed:

   _____

   _____

   _____

6. Questions for the physician:

   _____

   _____

   _____

   _____

MEDICAL REPORT 15.3

DISCHARGE SUMMARY

PATIENT: JONES, LINDA

DOB:

MED REC: 999999

SEX/RACE: F/2

PT ACCT:

LOCATION:

ADM DATE:

DISCHG DT:

ADMISSION DIAGNOSIS: ABNORMAL FETAL TRACING-BRADYCARDIA
DELIVERY OF VIABLE INFANT
GROUP B STREP CARRIER

This is a 35-year-old G1 P0 who came into the office for a routine visit and had a sonogram done because she is at about 40 weeks gestation. During the sonogram the patient demonstrated fetal heart rate down to the 60's. She was taken to L&D and it had returned to the 150's. Shortly after being in labor and delivery room, she had another deceleration to the 60's. It was decided to do a primary cesarean section. However, the patient's cervix was only fingertip.

REVIEW OF SYSTEMS: As listed.

PAST MEDICAL HISTORY: Varicose veins.

PAST SURGICAL HISTORY: T&A.

REVIEW OF SYSTEMS: Unremarkable.

FAMILY HISTORY: Hypertension.

SOCIAL HISTORY: No habits.

ALLERGIES: Keflex.

PHYSICAL EXAMINATION

Vital Signs – blood pressure 146/74, pulse 87, respirations 20.

HEENT – normal.

Heart – regular rate and rhythm.

Abdomen – gravid uterus.

Breasts – deferred.

Lungs – normal.

Cervix – fingertip and long.

HOSPITAL COURSE: The patient did well postop. Postop day #1, she was without complaints. Positive flatus.

Vital Signs – afebrile, vital signs stable.

CV – regular rate and rhythm.

Chest – clear.

Abdomen – soft, positive bowel sounds, incision clean, dry and intact.

Hemoglobin – 12.4, A+ blood type.

MEDICAL REPORT 15.3 (CONTINUED)

Postop day #2 – the patients states she has good pain control, positive flatus, no bowel movement, afebrile.

Vital Signs stable.

CV – regular rate and rhythm.

Chest – clear.

Abdomen – soft, positive bowel sounds, firm fundus.

Extremities – no clubbing, cyanosis, or edema.

She is to be discharged to home on Tylox 1-2 po q. 4 to 6 hours prn pain, Anaprox one po q. 12 hours prn #30 three refills. Follow-up in my office scheduled in three weeks.

Dr. Smith, M.D.

DD:

DT:

NOTES

MEDICAL REPORT 15.4

OPERATIVE REPORT

PATIENT: JONES, LINDA

DOB:

MED REC: 999999

SEX/RACE: F/2

PT ACCT:

LOCATION:

ADM DATE:

DISCHG DT:

DATE OF SURGERY:

SURGEON: DR. C. SECTION

ASSISTANT:

ANESTHESIOLOGIST:

ANESTHESIA:

ESTIMATED BLOOD LOSS: 1000 CCS.

COUNT: CORRECT TIMES 2

COMPLICATIONS: NONE

PREOPERATIVE DIAGNOSIS: 35-YEAR-OLD G1 AT 39 AND 6/7THS WEEKS. REPORTED TO THE OFFICE FOR ROUTINE VISIT AND HAD A SONOGRAM DONE TO CHECK FLUID. DURING THE SONOGRAM, FETAL HEART TONES WERE IN THE 60'S AND THE PATIENT WAS SENT TO LABOR AND DELIVERY. HEART TONES INCREASED TO THE 150'S BUT LATER HAD ANOTHER SPONTANEOUS DECELERATION. SHE WAS BROUGHT BACK FOR ABNORMAL TRACING FOR DELIVERY.

POSTOPERATIVE DIAGNOSIS: SAME AS ABOVE.

OPERATION: LOW-CERVICAL CESAREAN SECTION

Findings at surgery: Viable female infant Apgars 7 and 8, Apgars 9 and 9.

OPERATIVE PROCEDURE: The patient was taken to the operating room and after adequate anesthesia was prepped and draped in the usual sterile fashion. A Pfannenstiel incision was made and carried down to the fascia. The fascia was nicked and extended laterally. The fascia was separated from the rectus muscles. The rectus muscles were separated. The peritoneum was entered and extended superiorly and inferiorly. The bladder flap was formed. The lower uterine incision was made and extended laterally, and the infant's head was delivered. Shoulders and body without complications. The nasopharynx was suctioned. The cord was clamped and cut. The infant was passed to the awaiting neonatology staff. Cord blood was obtained, and the placenta was removed manually and sent to pathology. The uterus was curetted with a moist lap. The uterus was closed in a single layer fashion using #1 Chromic on a CT. The figure-of-eight stitches were used to obtain hemostasis. The pericolic and the gutters in the cul-de-sac were cleaned with a moist lap, and the uterus was allowed to fall back into the pelvic cavity. The fascia was closed with #1 Vicryl and the subcu was irrigated and the skin was closed with staples. The patient tolerated the procedure well and was sent to the recovery room in stable condition.

_____

DR. C. SECTION, M.D.

DD:

DT:

Case Study 15.3 (Coder/Abstract Summary Form)

Patient: **Karen Hopkins**

Patient documentation: **Review Medical Reports 15.5, 15.6, 15.7, and 15.8**

1. Principal diagnosis:

_____

2. Secondary or other diagnoses:

_____

3. Principal procedure:

_____

4. Other procedures:

_____

5. Additional documentation needed:

_____

_____

_____

6. Questions for the physician:

_____

_____

_____

_____

_____

MEDICAL REPORT 15.5

OBSTETRIC DISCHARGE SUMMARY

PATIENT: HOPKINS, KAREN

MR#:   999999

AGE: 24

SEX: F

DOB:

ROOM LOC:

                SMITH, MD.

1. Reasons for Admission

Labor and Delivery

( )   Vaginal delivery

( )   Cesarean section

( )   Undelivered

Prenatal Observation and Evaluation

( )   Amniocentesis   __/__/__

( )   Cerclage   __/__/__

( )   Diabetes screen __/__/__

( )   OCT   __/__/__

( )   Toxemia mgmt.   __/__/__

( )   Ultrasound   __/__/__

( )   _____   __/__/__

Abortion

( )   Dilatation & curettage

( )   Suction curettage

Blood loss _____ cc.

2. Complications and Procedures

Prenatal summary risk assessment

( )   No risk factors noted

( )   At risk: Pre-term labor

       _____

( )   High risk: _____

       _____

Intrapartum *(see L&D Summary for details)*

Postpartum Complications

( )   None

( )   Spinal headache

( )   P.P. eclampsia

( )   Hemorrhage

( )   Phlebitis

( )   Pelvic infection

( )   Urinary infection

( )   Pulmonary infection

( )   Wound infection

Procedures

( )   Transfusion _____

( )   P.P. tubal ligation

( )   Curettage

( )   Antibiotics

( )   Rho (D) Ig

( )   Rubella Ig

( )   _____

3. Newborn Data

( ) Male   ( ) Female

( ) Circ   ( ) No circ

Disposition of well NB

( ) Home with mother

Other status of NB

( ) Remains in nursery

( ) Remains in NICU

( ) Deceased

Complications

( ) Preterm ( ) RDS

( ) Jaundice ( ) Sepsis

( ) Other:

MEDICAL REPORT 15.5 (CONTINUED)

(or)

( ) Placed for adoption

at:

( ) Transferred

to:

_____

_____

_____

4. Discharge Plans

Medications:

( ) None

( ) OR:_____

Special Instructions:

( ) None

( ) OR:_____

Discharge to:

( ) Home

( ) OR:_____

Family Planning

( ) None

( ) OR:_____

Follow up in: 6 weeks

at: office.

Discharge date: ___/___/___.

at ____:____ AM/PM.

Hct / Hgb /   Date

36.9 /12.1 /   ___/___/___

5. Diagnoses:

IUP 36.3 weeks.

SROM.

Pre-term labor.

Desire for permanent sterilization.

Spontaneous assisted delivery.

Median episiotomy.

Postpartum tubal.

_____

Dr. Smith, M.D. / Date

NOTES

MEDICAL REPORT 15.6

PRENATAL HEALTH HISTORY SUMMARY

PATIENT: HOPKINS, KAREN
MR#: 999999
AGE: 24
SEX: F
DOB:
ROOM LOC:

SMITH, MD.

Age: 24   Race: white   Religion: _____   Marital status: married

Years married: 7   Education: 4   Occupation: Clerk

Home address: _____ Home tel. _____ Work tel. _____
Nearest relative: _____
Relative's employer: _____ Work tel.: _____
Referring physician: _____ Attending physician: _____

Pt	Fam	Medical History	Pre-existing Risk Guide
		01. Congenital anomalies	36. ( ) age <15 or >35
		02. Genetic diseases	37. ( ) less than 8th grade education
		03. Multiple births	38. ( ) cardiac disease
		04. Diabetes mellitus	39. ( ) tuberculosis active
		05. Malignancies	40. ( ) chronic pulmonary disease
	✓	06. Hypertension (mother)	41. ( ) thrombophlebitis
		07. Heart disease	42. ( ) endocrinopathy
		08. Rheumatic fever	43. ( ) epilepsy (on medication)
		09. Pulmonary disease	44. ( ) infertility (treated)
		10. GI problems	45. ( ) 2 abortions (spontan/induced)
		11. Renal disease	46. ( ) greater than 7 deliveries
		12. Other urinary tract problems	47. ( ) previous preterm or SGA infant
		13. Genitourinary anomalies	48. ( ) infant => 4000 grams
		14. Abnormal uterine bleeding	49. ( ) isoimmunization (ABO)
		15. Infertility	50. ( ) hemorr. during previous preg.
		16. Venereal disease	51. ( ) previous preeclampsia
		17. Phlebitis, varicosities	52. ( ) surgically scarred uterus
		18. Nervous/mental disorder	53. ( ) other
		19. Convulsive disorder	54. ( ) age =>40 years
		20. Metabolic/endocrine disorder	55. ( ) diabetes mellitus
		21. Anemia/hemoglobinopathy	56. ( ) hypertension
		22. Blood dyscrasias	57. ( ) cardiac disease class 3 or 4

MEDICAL REPORT 15.6 (CONTINUED)

Pt	Fam	Medical History		Pre-existing Risk Guide	
		23.	Drug addiction	58. ( )	chronic renal disease
		24.	Smoking/alcohol	59. ( )	congen. chromosomal anomalies
		25.	Infectious diseases	60. ( )	hemoglobinopathies
✓		26.	Operations/accidents (T&A)	61. ( )	isoimmunization (Rh)
		27.	Blood transfusions	62. ( )	drug addiction/alcoholism
		28.	Other hospitalizations	63. ( )	habitual abortions
		29.	No known disease	64. ( )	incompetent cervix
		Sensitivities		65. ( )	prior fetal or neonatal death
		30.	( ) None known (NKA)	66. ( )	prior neurolog. damaged infant
		31. ( )	Antibiotics	67. ( )	other:
		32. ( )	Analgesics	Initial risk assessment	
		33. ( )	Sedatives	68. ( )	no risk factors noted
		34. ( )	Anesthesia	69. ( )	at risk
		35. ( )	Other	70. ( )	at high risk

Menstrual History:

Onset: 13 age

Cycle: 28–30 days

Length: 4–5 days

Amount: Average

LMP: __/__/__

Pregnancy History:

Grav: 6

Term: 2

Pret: 1

Abort: 2

Live: 3

EDC: __/__/__

No	Month/year	Sex	Wt. at birth	Wks. gest.	Hrs. in labor	Type of delivery	Details of delivery
1	4/96			8 1/2			miscarriage
2	6/97	M	6lbs 8oz	40	38	vaginal	
3	4/00	F	6lbs 9oz	40	10	vaginal	
4	10/01	M	6lbs 5oz	37	4	vaginal	
5	9/02			9 1/2			miscarriage
6							
7							
8							

Signature

MEDICAL REPORT 15.7

XYZ WOMENS' HOSPITAL NUR **LIVE**

PATIENT ASSESSMENT

LABOR & DELIVERY SUMMARY

PATIENT: HOPKINS, Karen

AGE/SEX: 24/F

ACCOUNT #:

LOCATION: OB

UNIT #:

ROOM/BED:

ADMIT DATE:

STATUS: ADM IN

ATTENDING: Smith, MD

LABOR & DELIVERY SUMMARY

LABOR SUMMARY:

Gravida 6   Para 3   Term 2   Preterm 1   Abort 2   Living 3

Blood Type O Pos   Presentation: Vertex

Position   Complications? N

Comment:

Induction of Labor? N   AROM Induction? N   Oxytocic Induction? N

Augmentation of Labor? Y   AROM Augmentation? N   Oxytocic Augmentation? Y

Monitor During Labor? Y   EFM? Y   External UC Monitor? Y   Internal FM? N

Internal UC Monitor? N   Ambu bag & suction available at time of delivery? Y

Medications During Labor: STADOL 1 MG IV

Time of Last Narcotic 2205

DELIVERY DATA

METHOD OF DELIVERY:

Vertex? Y   Vertex Type: Spontaneous Comment:

Forcep Type: N

Breech? N Breech Type:

Comment:

Cesarean? N Cesarean Type:

Placenta Delivery Type: Spontaneous

Blood Loss: <500 ml

Configuration: Normal

Placenta Weighed? N   Placenta GMS: Nuchal Cord × 0   True Knot? N

Umbilical Vessels × 3? Y   Umbilical Vessels × 2? N   Cord Blood to Lab? Y

Episiotomy Type: Median   Suture Type: Chromic

MEDICAL REPORT 15.7 (CONTINUED)

Laceration Type: None   Laceration Location:

Comment:

Surgical Procedures: Tubal ligation

Comment:

Delivery Anesthesia: Local   Delivery Room Meds: Pitocin

Comment:

CHRONOLOGY

EDC:

Admit to Hospital:

Membranes Ruptured:

Date Contractions Began:

Complete Cervical Dilation:

Delivery of Infant:

Delivery of Placenta:

INFANT DATA

APGAR SCORES:

Heart Rate – 1min 2

Respirations – 1min 2

Muscle Tone – 1min 2

Reflex Irritation – 1min 2

Skin Color – 1min 1

Apgar One Minute: 9   Heart Rate – 5min 2

Respirations – 5min 2

Muscle Tone – 5min 2

Reflex Irritation – 5min 2

Skin Color – 5min 2

Apgar One Minute: 10

Comment:

Initial Newborn Exam No Observed Abnormalities

Comment:

BASIC DATA

ID Bracelet No.

Gender: Female   Birth Order: 1 of 1

Weight: 6lbs. 11oz.   Length: 20.0   Vitamin K? Y   Dose: 0.5 CC

Erythromycin Opth Oint OU? Y

Continued

MEDICAL REPORT 15.7 (CONTINUED)

Meds by:

Output   Comment:

Living at Transfer to Crib#: 2   Deceased:

Date: __ / __ / __ Time: __/__ AM/PM

Comment: INFANT TO UNIT. INITIAL NEWBORN CARE INITIATED BY R.N. PATIENT MLE REPAIRED BY DR. SMITH WITH 2.0 CHROMIC, 2 PACKS USED. PATIENT GIVEN PERI CARE AFTER PLACENTA, AMERICAINE OINT APPLIED AND DERMOPLAST SPRAY APPLIED TO MLE AND COOL PAD PLACED. PERINEUM VERY SWOLLEN WITH HEMORRHOIDS NOTED. PATIENT SITTING UP IN BED. FUNDUS FIRM SMALL TO MOD LOCHIA NOTED. PATIENT DENIES ANY OTHER C/OS. STADOL 1 ESC TO EXIT.

OCCURRENCE DATE __ / __ / __

ATTENDING NURSE NAME: _____ R.N.

_____

SMITH, MD

NOTES

_____

MEDICAL REPORT 15.8

OPERATIVE REPORT

DATE OF OPERATION: __ / __ / __

SURGEON: SMITH, MD

PREOPERATIVE DIAGNOSIS: STERILIZATION

POSTOPERATIVE DIAGNOSIS: POSTPARTUM STERILIZATION

OPERATION: INFRA UMBILICAL MINI LAPAROTOMY WITH BILATERAL TUBAL LIGATION

OPERATIVE PROCEDURE: This patient was placed on the table under spinal anesthesia, prepped and draped in the usual manner. A small incision under the umbilicus, incision deepened down into the skin and subcutaneous tissue down to the peritoneum, which was entered. The left tube was brought out, excising a section of the midportion of the tube. The ends were then doubly ligated and cauterized. The same procedure was then done on the right side, excising a segment of the right tube. The tubes were returned to the abdominal cavity with closure in layers, approximating the peritoneum with 0 Dexon, the fascia with #1 Dexon and the skin was closed with 4-0 subcuticular Vicryl sutures and a dry dressing was applied. All tissue removed was sent to Pathology for examination.

The patient tolerated the procedure well and was sent to the Recovery Room in satisfactory condition.

_____

SMITH, MD

DD:

DT:

Patient: HOPKINS, Karen   Age/Sex: 24/F

Account #   XYZ Women's Hospital

Admit Date:

Status : ADM IN

Attending: Smith, MD

NOTES

Case Study 15.4 (Coder/Abstract Summary Form)

Patient: **Tracy Dale**

Patient documentation: **Review Medical Reports 15.9, 15.10, and 15.11**

1. Principal diagnosis:

   _____

2. Secondary or other diagnoses:

   _____

3. Principal procedure:

   _____

4. Other procedures:

   _____

5. Additional documentation needed:

   _____

   _____

   _____

   _____

6. Questions for the physician:

   _____

   _____

   _____

   _____

   _____

MEDICAL REPORT 15.9

OBSTETRIC DISCHARGE SUMMARY

NAME:	DALE, TRACY
MR#:	999999
AGE:	25
SEX:	F
DOB:	
ROOM LOC:	
	SMITH, MD.

3. Reasons for Admission

Labor and Delivery
( ) Vaginal delivery
( ) Cesarean section
( ) Undelivered

Prenatal Observation and Evaluation
( ) Amniocentesis   __ / __ / __
( ) Cerclage   __ / __ / __
( ) Diabetes screen __ / __ / __
( ) OCT   __ / __ / __
( ) Toxemia mgmt.   __ / __ / __
( ) Ultrasound   __ / __ / __
( )   __ / __ / __

Abortion
( ) Dilatation & curettage
( ) Suction curettage
Blood loss _____ cc.

4. Complications and Procedures

Prenatal summary risk assessment
( )   No risk factors noted
( )   At risk: Previous C-section
          Depression; Tobacco use
( )   High risk:

Intrapartum *(see L&D Summary for details)*
Postpartum Complications
( )   None
( )   Spinal headache
( )   P.P. eclampsia
( )   Hemorrhage
( )   Phlebitis
( )   Pelvic infection
( )   Urinary infection
( )   Pulmonary infection
( )   Wound infection
Procedures
( )   Transfusion _____
( )   P.P. tubal ligation
( )   Curettage
( )   Antibiotics
( )   Rho (D) Ig
( )   Rubella Ig
( )

Continued

Medical Report 15.9 (Continued)

Newborn Data

( ) Male ( ) Female

( ) Circ ( ) No circ

Disposition of well NB

( ) Home with mother

(or)

( ) Placed for adoption

at:

Other status of NB

( ) Remains in nursery

( ) Remains in NICU

( ) Deceased

( ) Transferred

to:

Complications

( ) Preterm ( ) RDS

( ) Jaundice ( ) Sepsis

( ) Other:

( ) **Discharge Plans**

Medications:

( ) None

( ) OR: Vit

Special Instructions:

( ) None

( ) OR: _____

Discharge to:

( ) Home

( ) OR: _____

Family Planning

( ) None

( ) OR: _____

Follow up in: 6 weeks

at: office.

Discharge date: ___/___/___.

at ____:____ AM/PM.

Hct / Hgb /   Date

31.9 /11.0 /   ___/___/___

5. Diagnoses:

IUP at term.

Previous C-section.

Cord prolapse.

Desire for permanent sterilization.

Low cervical: transverse C-section.

Postpartum tubal ligation.

_____

Dr. Smith, M.D. / Date

NOTES

MEDICAL REPORT 15.10

PRENATAL HEALTH HISTORY SUMMARY

NAME: DALE, TRACY

MR#: 999999

AGE: 25

SEX: F

DOB:

ROOM LOC:

SMITH, MD.

Age: 24   Race: cauc   Religion: Catholic   Marital status: married

Years married: 2   Education: 4   Occupation: _____

Home address: _____ Home tel. _____ Work tel. _____

Nearest relative: _____

Relative's employer: _____ Work tel.: _____

Referring physician: _____ Attending physician: _____

Pt	Fam	Medical History	Pre-existing Risk Guide
		01. Congenital anomalies	36. ( ) age <15 or >35
		02. Genetic diseases	37. ( ) less than 8th grade education
	✓	03. Multiple births (mother)	38. ( ) cardiac disease
		04. Diabetes mellitus	39. ( ) tuberculosis active
		05. Malignancies	40. ( ) chronic pulmonary disease
	✓	06. Hypertension (mother)	41. ( ) thrombophlebitis
	✓	07. Heart disease (mother-MI)	42. ( ) endocrinopathy
		08. Rheumatic fever	43. ( ) epilepsy (on medication)
		09. Pulmonary disease	44. ( ) infertility (treated)
		10. GI problems	45. ( ) 2 abortions (spontan/induced)
		11. Renal disease	46. ( ) greater than 7 deliveries
✓		12. Other urinary tract problems	47. ( ) previous preterm or SGA infant
		13. Genitourinary anomalies	48. ( ) infant => 4000 grams
		14. Abnormal uterine bleeding	49. ( ) isoimmunization (ABO)
		15. Infertility	50. ( ) hemorr. during previous preg.
		16. Venereal disease	51. ( ) previous preeclampsia
	✓	17. Phlebitis, varicosities (grandmo)	52. ( ) surgically scarred uterus
✓		18. Nervous/mental disorder (depress)	53. ( ) other
		19. Convulsive disorder	54. ( ) age =>40 years
		20. Metabolic/endocrine disorder	55. ( ) diabetes mellitus
✓		21. Anemia/hemoglobinopathy	56. ( ) hypertension
		22. Blood dyscrasias	57. ( ) cardiac disease class 3 or 4

Continued

MEDICAL REPORT 15.10 (CONTINUED)

Pt	Fam	Medical History	Pre-existing Risk Guide
		23. Drug addiction	58. ( ) chronic renal disease
✓		24. Smoking/alcohol (10cig/day)	59. ( ) congen. chromosomal anomalies
	✓	25. Infectious diseases	60. ( ) hemoglobinopathies
✓		26. Operations/accidents (D&C)	61. ( ) isoimmunization (Rh)
		27. Blood transfusions	62. ( ) drug addiction/alcoholism
		28. Other hospitalizations	63. ( ) habitual abortions
		29. No known disease	64. ( ) incompetent cervix
		Sensitivities	65. ( ) prior fetal or neonatal death
		30. ( ) None known (NKA)	66. ( ) prior neurolog. damaged infant
		31. ( ) Antibiotics	67. ( ) other:
		32. ( ) Analgesics	Initial risk assessment
		33. ( ) Sedatives	68. ( ) no risk factors noted
		34. ( ) Anesthesia	69. ( ) at risk
		35. ( ) Other	70. ( ) at high risk

Menstrual History:

Onset: 13 age

Cycle: 28 days

Length: 5-7 days

Amount: Heavy

LMP: __/__/__

Pregnancy History:

Grav: 6

Term: 3

Pret: 0

Abort: 2

Live: 3

EDC: __/__/__

No.	Month/ year	Sex	Wt. at birth	Wks. gest.	Hrs. in labor	Type of delivery	Details of delivery
1	3/01	F	7lbs 3oz	39		c-section	breech
2	4/00	F	7lbs 9oz	40	12	vaginal	
3	11/97	F	9lbs 2oz	40	24	vaginal	
4							
5							
6							
7							
8							

Signature

MEDICAL REPORT 15.11

XYZ WOMENS' HOSPITAL NUR **LIVE**

PATIENT ASSESSMENT
LABOR & DELIVERY SUMMARY

PATIENT: DALE, Tracy

AGE/SEX: 25/F

ACCOUNT #

LOCATION: OB

UNIT #:

ROOM/BED:

ADMIT DATE:

STATUS: ADM IN

ATTENDING: Smith, MD

LABOR & DELIVERY SUMMARY

LABOR SUMMARY:

Gravida 6   Para 3   Term 3   Preterm 0   Abort 2   Living 3

Blood Type A Pos   Presentation: Vertex

Position   Complications? N

Comment:

Induction of Labor? N   AROM Induction? N   Oxytocic Induction? N

Augmentation of Labor?   AROM Augmentation? Y   Oxytocic Augmentation? N

Monitor During Labor? Y   EFM? Y   External UC Monitor? Y   Internal FM? N

Internal UC Monitor? N   Ambu bag & suction available at time of delivery? Y

Medications During Labor: NONE

Time of Last Narcotic

DELIVERY DATA

METHOD OF DELIVERY:

Vertex?   Vertex Type: Spontaneous   Comment:

Forcep Type: N

Breech? N Breech Type:

Comment:

Cesarean? Y   Cesarean Type: Low Cervical: transverse

Placenta Delivery Type:

Blood Loss: <500 ml   Comment: PROLAPSE CORD

Configuration: Normal

Placenta Weighed?   Placenta GMS: Nuchal Cord ✕   True Knot?

Umbilical Vessels ✕ 3? Y   Umbilical Vessels ✕ 2?   Cord Blood to Lab? Y

Episiotomy Type: Suture Type:

Continued

MEDICAL REPORT 15.11 (CONTINUED)

Laceration Type: Laceration Location:

Comment:

Surgical Procedures: Tubal ligation (Pomeroy)

Comment:

Delivery Anesthesia: General   Delivery Room Meds: Pitocin

Comment:

CHRONOLOGY

EDC:

Admit to Hospital:

Membranes Ruptured:

Date Contractions Began:

Complete Cervical Dilation:

Delivery of Infant:

Delivery of Placenta:

INFANT DATA

APGAR SCORES:

Heart Rate – 1min 2

Respirations – 1min 2

Muscle Tone – 1min 2

Reflex Irritation – 1min 2

Skin Color – 1min 0

Apgar One Minute: 8   Heart Rate – 5min 2

Respirations – 5min 2

Muscle Tone – 5min 2

Reflex Irritation – 5min 2

Skin Color – 5min 1

Apgar One Minute: 9

Resuscitation   Minutes to Sustained respirations 0

Infant Medications:

Comment:

Initial Newborn Exam

Comment:

MEDICAL REPORT 15.11 (CONTINUED)

BASIC DATA

ID Bracelet No.

Gender: Male   Birth Order: 1 of 1

Weight: 8lbs. 5oz.   Length: 20.0   Vitamin K? Y   Dose: 1MG

Erythromycin Opth Oint OU? Y

Meds by:

Output   Comment:

Living at transfer to Crib#: 5   Deceased:

Date: __ / __ / __   Time: __ / __ AM/PM

Comment:

ESC TO EXIT.

OCCURRENCE DATE __ / __ / __

ATTENDING NURSE NAME: _____ R.N.

_____

Dr. SMITH, M.D.

NOTES

_____

Coding for Conditions in the Perinatal Period and Congenital Anomalies

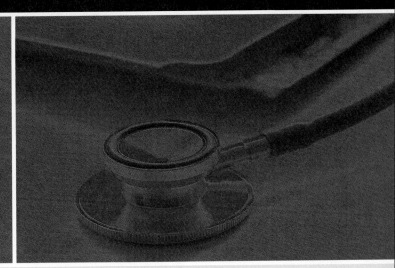

Chapter Outline

Congenital Codes and Patient Age

Neonate Medical Record Format and Apgar Score

Admission-for-Birth Codes

Common Perinatal Conditions and Congenital Anomalies

Birth Before Admission

Neonate Supervision Code

Routine Neonatal Procedures

Testing Your Comprehension

Coding Practice I: Chapter Review Exercises

Coding Practice II: Medical Record Case Studies

Chapter Objectives

▶ Describe the pathology of common perinatal conditions and congenital anomalies.

▶ Recognize the typical manifestations, complications, and treatments of perinatal conditions and congenital anomalies in terms of their implications for coding.

▶ Correctly code common complications of perinatal conditions and congenital anomalies and related procedures by using the ICD-9-CM and medical records.

Codes for conditions in the perinatal period and congenital anomalies are included in chapter 15, code section 760 to 779, and chapter 14, code section 740 to 759, respectively, of the Disease Tabular of the ICD-9-CM. To assist in your understanding, the Word Parts Box on page 524 reviews word parts and meanings of medical terms related to the perinatal period and congenital anomalies.

Word Parts and Meanings of Medical Terms Related to the Perinatal Period and Congenital Anomalies

Word Part	Meaning	Example	Definition of Example
neo-	new	neonate	Newly born (literally meaning *new birth*)
nat/i	birth	neonatal	Pertaining to a newborn
Peri-	surrounding; around	perinatal	Surrounding or around the time of birth
-lytic	destroy	hemolytic	To destroy blood cells
-lysis			
-pnea	breathing	apnea	No breathing
cyan/o-	blue	cyanosis	-Bluish discoloration of the skin associated with diminished oxygenation of blood
jaund/o-	yellow	jaundice	Yellow discoloration of the skin
Con-	together, with	conception	-To bring together; the beginning of pregnancy
genit/o	beginning, producing, or forming	congenital	Pertaining to the beginning or formation; occurring at birth
-al	pertaining to	fetal	Pertaining to the fetus
-cele	hernia	meningocele	Hernia (abnormal bulging or protrusion) of meninges
mening/o-	meninges (membranes that cover the spinal cord and brain)	meningitis	Inflammation of the meninges
myel/o-	spinal cord or bone marrow	myelomeningocele	Hernia of the spinal cord and meninges

"Peri-" means **surrounding**, and "nat/i-" means **birth** (Table 16.1). Therefore, the perinatal period means **surrounding the time of birth**. ICD-9-CM defines the perinatal period as beginning before birth and lasting through the first 28 days of the infant's life. This is an important time frame, because the coding for some conditions can change at day 29 (e.g., newborn sepsis up through day 28, 771.81; sepsis after 28 days, 038.9).

During the perinatal period, codes are assigned to report the following:

▶ initial admission for birth
▶ perinatal conditions
▶ congenital and perinatal deformities

A congenital anomaly is a deformity that an infant is born with. Congenital deformities can result from genetic factors (i.e., inherited through the chromosomes of the mother or father) or from factors related to complications of the pregnancy or delivery (e.g., malposition of the fetus or birth trauma).

Congenital Codes and Patient Age

Congenital codes are routinely used on the newborn's medical record. However, congenital conditions can sometimes affect care throughout the patient's lifetime (e.g., Down's syndrome, code 758.0). Therefore, depending on the circumstances, congenital codes can sometimes be reported for adults. However, you should always exercise caution when assigning these codes to an adult record.

Every time you assign a code from category 740 to 759, double-check to determine whether the condition is truly congenital (i.e., a condition the infant is born with) versus acquired (i.e., a condition developed later as an adult), because this affects the code assignment. Congenital codes (coming from category 740 to 759) can be easily recognized when final-checking codes before billing. In contrast to congenital codes, acquired codes are found in the applicable system chapter relating to the disorder (e.g., digestive or respiratory).

EXAMPLE

Congenital gastrointestinal arteriovenous malformation: 747.61

Acquired arteriovenous malformation: 569.84

Diverticulosis, esophagus (congenital): 750.4

Diverticulosis, esophagus, acquired: 530.6

Newborn Medical Record Format and Apgar Score

The format and content of a newborn record are unique. You should become familiar with the format to help locate newborn conditions when reviewing the record. If an episode of care results in birth, the record is basically composed of three main sections that include newborn identifying information, newborn delivery and assessment, and newborn progress notes (sometimes including special newborn admission and discharge forms).

Newborn Identifying Information

Newborn identification information forms contained within the medical record include the following:

▸ name and sex of baby
▸ date and time of birth
▸ newborn admission (medical record) number
▸ footprints or fingerprints
▸ neonate identification band information for baby and mother
▸ attending obstetrician's name

Newborn Delivery and Assessment

The newborn delivery section of the newborn's record is sometimes a copy (part form) of the mother's labor and delivery record. This section contains a history of the delivery and an assessment of the newborn's physical status (i.e., physical examination) that documents any abnormal conditions or complications of the mother's labor and delivery that may have affected the newborn.

The **Apgar score**, documented in the newborn's delivery record, is an assessment of the newborn's physical status taken at 1 and 5 minutes after birth (Table 16.1). Apgar assigns a score for the newborn's heart rate, respiration,

TABLE 16.1 Apgar Scoring Chart			
Category*	**0**	**1**	**2**
Heart rate (Pulse)	Absent	Slow (less than 100 beats/min)	More than 100 beats/min
Respiratory effort (Respirations)	Absent	Slow, irregular	Good, crying
Muscle tone (Activity)	Flaccid	Some flexion of extremities	Active motion
Reflex irritability (Grimace)	No response	Weak cry or grimace	Vigorous cry
Color (Appearance)	Blue, pale	Body pink, extremities blue	Completely pink

* Each category is rated as 0, 1, or 2. The rating for each category is then totaled to a maximum score of 10. Normal newborns score between 7 and 10. Newborns who score between 4 and 6 require special assistance; those who score below 4 are in need of immediate life-saving support.

color, muscle tone, and response to stimulus. The highest score that can be received in any category is a 2, and the maximum score is 10.

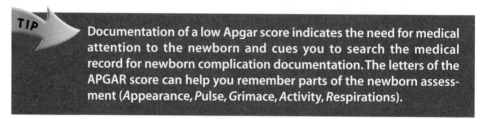

TIP Documentation of a low Apgar score indicates the need for medical attention to the newborn and cues you to search the medical record for newborn complication documentation. The letters of the APGAR score can help you remember parts of the newborn assessment (*Appearance, Pulse, Grimace, Activity, Respirations*).

Remember that newborns will always have separate medical records from the mother and that you should never assign pregnancy codes (assigned to the mother) to the newborn's record.

Newborn Progress Notes

Newborn progress notes contained within the medical record include nurses' observations in the nursery; these are documented as often as the newborn's condition warrants. Newborn progress notes usually include the newborn's color (e.g., pink, jaundiced, or cyanotic [bluish in color]) and vital signs, including temperature, respiratory rate, and heart rate. Also, newborn weight, irritability or shakiness, arousability or consciousness, intake and output of fluids, frequency of urination and meconium stool (passing first stool), adequacy of suckling (feeding), and appearance of the umbilical stump are recorded. Any medications or treatments given would also be recorded.

Admission-for-Birth Codes

The principal reason for the newborn's admission is birth. Codes in category V30 to V39 describe the type of birth (e.g., single liveborn) and are used only during the episode of care in which the infant is born. These codes are always assigned as the principal diagnosis and can be located under the main term "newborn" in the *Alphabetic Index to Diseases*. Admission-for-birth category codes (V30 to V39) include a fourth-digit subcategory code of <u>0</u> or <u>1</u> that describes whether the infant was born in the hospital. A fifth-digit subclassification of <u>0</u> or <u>1</u> describes whether the infant was born with or without a cesarean section and can be used only when a fourth digit of <u>0</u> was assigned, indicating that the birth occurred in the hospital.

Admission-for-birth codes include the following:

▶ single liveborn, born in the hospital, delivered without mention of cesarean section: V30.00
▶ single liveborn admission, born in the hospital, delivered with mention of cesarean section: V30.01
▶ twin, mate liveborn, born in the hospital, delivered without mention of cesarean section: V31.00
▶ twin, mate stillborn, delivered with mention of cesarean section: V32.01
▶ single liveborn, born before admission to the hospital: V30.1
▶ other multiple, mates all liveborn, delivered without mention of cesarean section: V34.00
▶ other multiple, mates liveborn and stillborn, delivered with mention of cesarean section: V36.01

Common Perinatal Conditions and Congenital Anomalies

For an admission resulting in birth, assign any perinatal conditions (disorders) and any congenital or perinatal deformities (anomalies) of the newborn as additional codes after the applicable category V30 to V39 principal diagnosis code. Many perinatal conditions or disorders are usually transient and resolve with or without treatment in the first 28 days after birth (i.e., the perinatal period), such as transient neonatal jaundice (yellow coloration of the newborn's skin caused by excessive bile in the blood) that resolves with phototherapy or transient neonatal sepsis that resolves with antibiotic therapy. In contrast, some congenital deformities or anomalies result from inherited chromosomal (genetic) disorders (e.g., Down's syndrome) or maternal conditions that can affect the individual throughout his or her lifetime (e.g., mental retardation associated with maternal cocaine abuse during pregnancy: 319 + 760.75). Other congenital or perinatal deformities or anomalies can result from malposition of the fetus (e.g., bilateral congenital hip dislocations caused by breech malposition of the fetus) or can be related to birth trauma or injuries (e.g., fractured clavicle) that resolve with treatment.

EXAMPLE

Neonatal hypoglycemia: 775.6

Abnormal fetal heart rate: 763.83

Neonatal sepsis: 771.81

Physiologic jaundice: 774.6

Congenital hydrocephalus: 742.3

Down's syndrome: 758.0

Cleft lip and palate: 749.20

Marfan's syndrome: 759.82

Congenital hip dislocation (due to fetal malposition): 754.30

Fractured clavicle (due to birth trauma): 767.2

Hypoxic-ischemic encephalopathy (HIE): 768.7

Assign codes for any conditions that affect the infant's current episode of care (for birth) or that will affect the newborn's future care as additional diagnoses even if they are not treated during the current stay. If the newborn is transferred to another facility for treatment of the condition, the condition is sequenced as the principal diagnosis for the facility that received the patient in transfer, because that is what occasioned the admission.

EXAMPLE	

Hospital A

Principal Diagnosis: Term newborn boy, V30.00

Secondary Diagnosis: Atrial septal defect, 745.5

Transferred to Hospital B for atrial septal defect repair

Hospital B

Principal Diagnosis: Atrial septal defect, 745.5

Procedure: Atrial septal defect repair, 35.71

Gestation Time and Birth Weight

Although the newborn's and mother's medical records are separate and follow different coding guidelines, you should check the coding of both records to ensure that they are consistent in regard to gestation time (e.g., the newborn's record is reported as preterm and the mother's record is reported as preterm pregnancy, delivered).

Live births before term gestation (less than 37 completed weeks) with a birth weight of 1,000 to 2,499 g are considered preterm (code 765.1X). Extreme immaturity (code 765.0X) indicates a birth weight of less than 1,000 g. Extreme immaturity and preterm codes include a fifth-digit subclassification to report the birth weight. Preterm births also require an additional code to specify the weeks of gestation (*765.2X). Live births after term gestation (42 or more completed weeks; code 766.2) are considered **postterm**.

EXAMPLE	

*Single liveborn by vaginal delivery, 35 weeks' gestation, delivered, 2,100 g: V30.00 + 765.18 + *765.28*

TIP

Make sure the fifth-digit assignment describing the newborn's weight is consistent with the Disease Tabular notes under the assigned code. For example, code 765.09 describes an extremely immature newborn with a birth weight of 2,500 g or more, which is inconsistent with the Disease Tabular notes for code 765.0X, which describe an extremely immature newborn as weighing less than 1,000 g.

Regardless of the length of gestation, "light for dates" or "small for dates" (category code 764) indicates that the newborn was affected by slow fetal growth, with or without fetal malnutrition. The fifth-digit subclassification used with 764 indicates the newborn's birth weight.

Term birth, single liveborn at 38 weeks, vaginal delivery, light for dates at 1,700 g: V30.00 + 764.06	**EXAMPLE**

Regardless of the length of gestation, "heavy for dates" or "large for dates" (766.1) indicates that the newborn is overly large (i.e., oversized). "Exceptionally large baby" (code 766.0) represents a birth weight of 4,500 g or more ($\geq$10 lbs.).

Term birth, single liveborn at 38 weeks, delivered by low transverse cesarean section, exceptionally large baby at 10 lbs. 7 oz.: V30.01 + 766.0	**EXAMPLE**

TIP 28.35 g = 1 oz.; therefore, a baby who weighs 10 lbs. 7 oz. weighs 4,734.45 g. The birth weight may be recorded in the medical record in either pounds/ounces or grams, depending on each facility's preferences. However, ICD-9-CM classifies a baby's weight in grams only. If a facility records the newborn's weight only in pounds/ounces, it will be necessary to convert the weight to grams for accurate coding.

Neonatal Jaundice

Bilirubin is a substance that is normally produced as red blood cells degrade and are broken down in the body. When functioning properly, the liver removes excess bilirubin from the blood by attaching it to bile (from the liver), with which it travels through bile ducts to the intestines and is excreted with feces. However, excessive bilirubin in the blood (i.e., hyperbilirubinemia) causes jaundice (also called **icterus**). A common symptom of jaundice is a yellowing of the skin and whites of the eyes. Perinatal jaundice can result from many conditions, including the following:

- ▶ hemolytic diseases that destroy red blood cells (773.X), such as hemolytic disease of the newborn (hemolytic disease of the newborn not otherwise specified: 773.2)
- ▶ congenital blockage of the bile duct (751.61)
- ▶ jaundice associated with prematurity (774.2), resulting from a physiologically immature liver that cannot remove excess bile (which contains bilirubin) from the body
- ▶ transient physiologic jaundice (774.6)

Newborns affected by preterm or physiologic jaundice are often treated with phototherapy (code 99.83). Phototherapy (treatment with concentrated light) aids in the breakdown and release of bilirubin in the body.

Do not code jaundice if it is not treated and therefore does not affect the episode of care.

Perinatal Sepsis

Neonatal sepsis (code 771.81), located under the main term "septicemia; newborn" in the *Alphabetic Index to Diseases*, classifies a persistent bacterial infection in the newborn's blood. Assign an additional code to identify the offending organism if it is known (e.g., *Escherichia coli*, code 041.4). Use code 771.81 throughout the perinatal period (28 days). After 28 days, the infant is no longer considered a newborn or in the perinatal period, and sepsis is then coded to category 038. If neonatal sepsis is suspected but documented as ruled out, assign code V29.0.

The V29.X category (observation for suspected conditions that are ruled out) is important because it explains the use of health-care resources not routinely associated with a normal newborn admission. For example, if the newborn's mother is currently being treated for an infection, the newborn is at risk for infection and therefore may have a workup and may be given antibiotics for suspected sepsis. If the suspected condition is ruled out, then the V29.X codes will help classify and report the legitimate reason for an extended hospital stay and the additional medical resources used. Depending on the circumstances of the admission, category V29.X can be used as a principal or secondary diagnosis.

Fetal Distress

Code 768.(2-4), located under the main term "distress; fetal" in the *Alphabetic Index to Diseases*, describes fetal metabolic acidemia (increase in acidity of the blood) as a life-threatening condition in the fetus. The fourth digit indicates whether the condition was noted before labor (768.2) or during labor (768.3) or was unspecified regarding the time of labor (768.4).

Maternal Conditions Affecting the Fetus or Newborn

Code categories 760 through 763 and 775 classify maternal complications of pregnancy that affect the fetus or newborn. These include conditions such as the following:

▶ maternal hypertension affecting the fetus or newborn: 760.0
▶ fetus or newborn affected by noxious substances transferred via the placenta or breast milk, located under the main term "noxious" in the Disease Index (e.g., neonatal drug screen positive for cocaine: 760.75); neonatal drug screen positive for anticonvulsants: 760.77
▶ drug withdrawal syndrome in newborn: 779.5
▶ maternal diabetes affecting fetus or newborn with hypoglycemia: 775.0
▶ maternal diabetes with manifest disease in the infant: 775.1
▶ fetal alcohol syndrome: 760.71

Rh Incompatibility

Code 773.0 classifies Rh incompatibility affecting the fetus or newborn. Called **hemolytic disease of the newborn or erythroblastosis fetalis due to Rh**, this condition destroys red blood cells in the newborn because of a blood group incompatibility between the fetus and mother. A Coombs test is a laboratory test that can detect Rh^+ antibodies in the infant to confirm the diagnosis of hemolytic disease of the newborn. (Also see the explanation of Rh incompatibility in Chapter 15 of this textbook.)

Respiratory Distress Syndrome

Respiratory distress syndrome, or hyaline membrane disease (code 769), is a respiratory disorder in the preterm infant caused by immature lungs that collapse. The lungs are hyaline (shiny) in appearance and lack surfactant, a substance that is normally produced by the lungs. Newborns who have this condition are usually treated with oxygen administration and a drug replacement of surfactant, which reduces the viscosity (stickiness) in the lungs and allows them to expand more easily. The newborn must be intubated (insertion of an endotracheal tube) and may be placed on a mechanical ventilator to assist in breathing. The surfactant is inhaled through the breathing tube.

A premature infant was born via cesarean section with respiratory distress syndrome. The infant was 32 weeks' gestation, and birth weight was 1,669 g. The infant was intubated, placed on mechanical ventilation for >96 hours, and received surfactant: V30.01 + 769 + 765.16 + 765.26; 96.04 + 96.72

EXAMPLE

Fetal and Newborn Aspiration

Meconium is the baby's first stool. If the fetus excretes the first stool before or at the time of birth, the newborn can aspirate (inhale) meconium-stained amniotic and vaginal fluids with his or her first breath. Meconium aspiration syndrome (code 770.12) describes symptoms such as dyspnea (difficult breathing), tachypnea (rapid breathing), and apneic spells (cessation of breathing) that can last for a short time or be persistent. Treatments for meconium aspiration syndrome include suction of the oropharyngeal airway, administration of oxygen, and antibiotics. These are classified as miscellaneous therapeutic procedures that are not routinely coded for inpatient admissions.

Starting October 1, 2005, nine new codes were added for the subcategory 770.1X that includes meconium aspiration and other fetal and newborn aspiration, which allows for more precise coding of these conditions. Also, codes for meconium staining (779.84) and aspiration of postnatal stomach contents with or without respiratory complications were added to subcategory 770.8X (Other respiratory problems after birth). These codes include:

770.10 Fetal and newborn aspiration, unspecified
770.11 Meconium aspiration without respiratory symptoms
770.12 Meconium aspiration with respiratory symptoms
770.13 Aspiration of clear amniotic fluid without respiratory symptoms
770.14 Aspiration of clear amniotic fluid with respiratory symptoms
770.15 Aspiration of blood without respiratory symptoms
770.16 Aspiration of blood with respiratory symptoms
770.17 Other fetal and newborn aspiration without respiratory symptoms
770.18 Other fetal and newborn aspiration with respiratory symptoms
770.85 Aspiration of postnatal stomach contents without respiratory symptoms
770.86 Aspiration of postnatal stomach contents with respiratory symptoms
779.84 Meconium staining

Meconium documented as "meconium in liquor" or "meconium staining" on the neonatal delivery record should not be confused with or coded to meconium aspiration syndrome. Meconium aspiration syndrome is a serious condition, as noted by the symptoms listed previously.

Transitory Tachypnea of Newborn

Transitory tachypnea of newborn (770.6), abbreviated TTNB or TTN, results in rapid breathing in the newborn that lasts for a short time. Transitory tachypnea of newborn occurs because of a slow reabsorption of fluid in the newborn's lungs. Treatment may consist of the administration of oxygen and continuous positive airway pressure (code 93.90), which delivers oxygen under pressure to aid in the reabsorption and clearing of the lung fluid.

Neonatal Apnea

Neonatal apnea (770.8X) refers to periods of cessation of breathing (apnea) in a newborn infant that may be the result of insufficient nerve impulses to the respiratory system or of airway obstruction or may be of an unknown etiology.

Neonatal Cyanosis

Neonatal cyanosis (770.83) is an abnormal condition of poor oxygenation of the blood that causes a bluish skin discoloration (cyanosis) and may be attributable to conditions such as congenital heart or lung disease (e.g., septal defects of the heart or tetralogy of Fallot (Figure 16.1)).

Patent Ductus Arteriosus

The lungs are not used for respiration while the fetus is in utero. During intrauterine growth, oxygenated blood passes through an open duct between the pulmonary artery and aorta (ductus arteriosus), bypassing the lungs of the fetus. Starting with the newborn's first breath, the ductus arteriosus must begin to close as the newborn uses the lungs for oxygenation of blood.

Patent ductus arteriosus (code 747.0) is a condition in which the duct remains open (patent) after birth (Figure 16.2); this leads to deoxygenation of the blood and increased pulmonary artery pressure, which can cause heart failure. Indomethacin is a common drug used to treat patent ductus arteriosus. However, if the medication fails to close the duct, thoracoscopic surgery through a small incision in the newborn's chest can be performed to ligate (tie off) the patent ductus arteriosus (see the main term "repair" or "closure," patent ductus arteriosus, code 38.85, in the *Alphabetic Index to Procedures*).

Congenital Atrial and Ventricular Septal Defects

Septa are chamber walls of the heart that separate the right side of the heart (with deoxygenated venous blood) from the left side of the heart (with oxygenated arterial blood). In congenital septal defects, a small septal hole exists between the upper atrial and/or lower ventricular chambers of the heart (atrial septal defects, code 745.5, and ventricular septal defects, code 745.4).

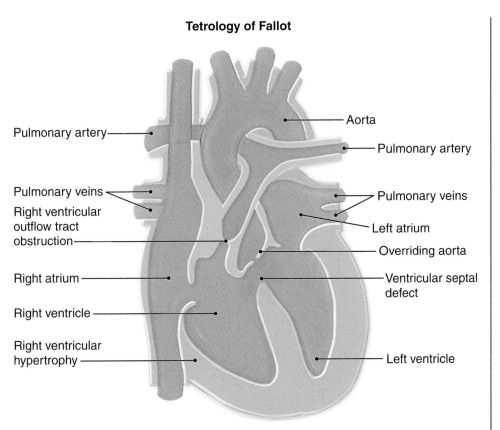

Tetrology of Fallot

Pulmonary artery

Pulmonary veins

Right ventricular
outflow tract
obstruction

Right atrium

Right ventricle

Right ventricular
hypertrophy

Aorta

Pulmonary artery

Pulmonary veins

Left atrium

Overriding aorta

Ventricular septal
defect

Left ventricle

FIGURE 16.1 ■ Congenital heart defects. Tetralogy of Fallot. (Reprinted with permission from Anatomical Chart Co.)

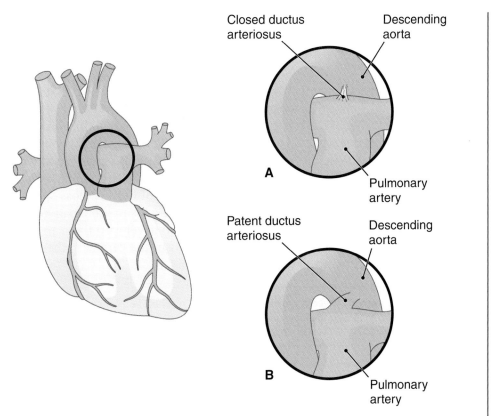

Closed ductus
arteriosus

Descending
aorta

A

Pulmonary
artery

Patent ductus
arteriosus

Descending
aorta

B

Pulmonary
artery

FIGURE 16.2 ■ Patent ductus arteriosus. A. Normal. B. The ductus arteriosus fails to close. (Reprinted with permission from Cohen BJ. Medical Terminology: An Illustrated Guide, 4th Ed. Baltimore: Lippincott Williams & Wilkins, 2004.)

Atrial septal defect

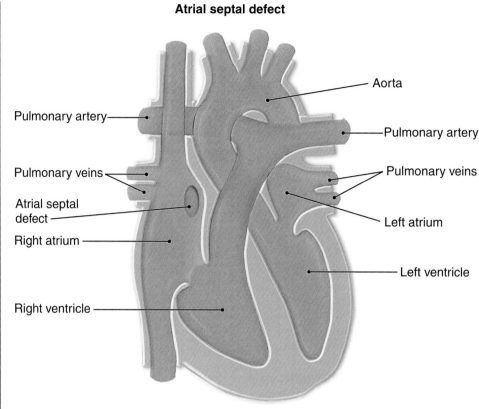

FIGURE 16.3 ■ Congenital heart defects. Atrial septal defect. (Reprinted with permission from Anatomical Chart Co.)

Atrial or ventricular septal defects (abnormal holes between the atrial or ventricular septal walls of the heart) cause a shunting (shift) of blood between the right and left side of the heart and result in an abnormal mixing of deoxygenated blood with oxygenated blood (Figure 16.3). Whether from pulmonary volume overload or from the abnormal mixing of venus blood with arterial blood that results in heart failure, shunting in either direction can cause serious harm to the newborn. Sometimes septal defects close spontaneously after birth, whereas others require surgical closure or repair with a patch graft. New less invasive procedures have been developed that can close the defects by advancing catheters through vessels in the cardiac catheterization laboratory to correct the defect.

EXAMPLE	*An infant was born at 38 weeks' gestation via cesarean section. The infant was noted to have a ventricular septal defect and underwent ventricular septal defect repair with prosthesis: V30.01 + 745.4 + 765.29; 35.53*

Congenital Pyloric Stenosis

Congenital pyloric stenosis (750.5) is a condition marked by a narrowing of the pyloric sphincter (outlet from the stomach to the duodenum) (Figure 16.4). A symptom associated with this in a newborn is projectile vomiting during feeding. This condition usually requires surgical correction.

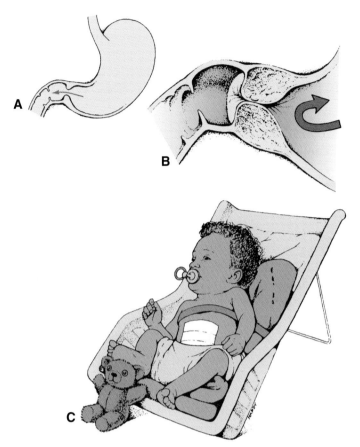

FIGURE 16.4 ■ Pyloric stenosis. (A) Normal passage through pyloric sphincter; (B) Stoppage of flow due to stenotic sphincter; (C) Postoperative treatment: child propped upright, slightly on right side, aids in gastric emptying. (Reprinted with permission from Nettina, Sandra M., MSN, RN, CS, ANP, The Lippincott Manual of Nursing Practice, 7th ed. Lippincott, Williams & Wilkins, 2001.)

Feeding Problems in the Newborn

Feeding problems in the newborn (code 779.3) is a condition sometimes documented by the physician as "poor" or "weak" suckle. Trying different nipples or formulas or changing from breast-feeding to bottle-feeding can effectively treat this condition. Sometimes during the perinatal period or in childhood, an infant or child presents for a failure to thrive (code 783.41), indicating an insufficient weight gain for his or her age. A swallow evaluation study may be indicated.

An infant was born at 39 weeks' gestation by vaginal delivery. The infant was described as a "poor feeder" in progress notes. The infant was changed from breast-feeding to bottle-feeding, with good results: V30.00 + 779.3

EXAMPLE

Congenital Hydrocephalus

Congenital hydrocephalus (742.3) results when cerebrospinal fluid does not properly drain from the ventricles of the brain. The bones of the neonatal skull are not fused, to allow for growth of the head. Therefore, with congenital hydrocephalus ("water on the brain"), the newborn's head can become abnormally large as cerebrospinal fluid accumulates. Treatment usually involves the placement of a ventriculoperitoneal shunt, a tube inserted in the ventricles of the brain that drains excess cerebrospinal fluid into the peritoneal cavity. To locate the main term for the placement of a ventriculoperitoneal shunt, see the main term "shunt; ventricular to abdominal cavity," code 02.34, in the *Alphabetic Index to Procedures* (see excerpt below).

SHUNT—*SEE ALSO* ANASTOMOSIS *AND* BYPASS, VASCULAR
 Ventricular (cerebral) (with valve) 02.2
 to
 abdominal cavity or organ 02.34

Hemangioma

Hemangioma (288.0X) is a dense, abnormal mass of small blood vessels (capillaries). Hemangiomas can appear on the skin or internal organs but are particularly upsetting to parents when they appear on the newborn's face. Over time, superficial hemangiomas usually disappear without treatment. However, large hemangiomas may require surgical intervention to excise, debulk, or destroy the small vessel mass.

Congenital Spina Bifida

Congenital spina bifida (category 741) is a herniation, or abnormal bulging, of the meninges (membranes surrounding the spinal cord and brain) that occurs in the spine (Figure 16.5). Spina bifida can involve a herniation of meninges, known as a **meningocele**, or a herniation of the meninges and spinal cord, known as a **meningomyelocele**. These conditions are often associated with hydrocephalus (741.0X) and lower body paralysis (i.e., paraplegia). Surgery is commonly used to remove the herniated tissue. Spina bifida occulta (756.17) is a minor form of the disorder usually noted only by a dimple in the skin covering the spine.

EXAMPLE	*Spina bifida, lumbar region, with hydrocephalus: 741.03*
	Spina bifida, thoracic region, without hydrocephalus: 741.92

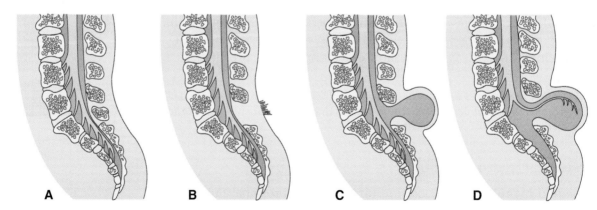

FIGURE 16.5 ■ Spinal defects. **A.** Normal spinal cord. **B.** Spina bifida occulta. **C.** Meningocele. **D.** Myelomeningocele. (Reprinted with permission from Pillitteri A. Maternal and Child Health Nursing: Care of the Childbearing and Childrearing Family, 4th Ed. Philadelphia: Lippincott Williams & Wilkins, 2003.)

Birth Before Admission

Sometimes a live birth occurs en route to the hospital, and the newborn infant is admitted for observation only. In such cases, the codes must not report that a live birth occurred in the institution. The neonatal codes (category V30 to V39) include a fourth digit <u>1</u> that indicates that the infant was "born before admission to the hospital." When the fourth digit <u>1</u> is used, no fifth digit is required because there is no need to specify whether the newborn was delivered by cesarean section. If the newborn has any perinatal conditions or congenital or perinatal deformities, assign these as additional diagnoses.

Newborn Supervision Code

Newborn supervision code V20.2 is used to explain a follow-up visit for well baby and general child care. It is often assigned to report a routine outpatient service visit to the pediatrician's office or child clinic and is not used for inpatient services. The newborn supervision code can be located in the *Alphabetic Index to Diseases* under the main term "admission for; examination, well baby and child care." If a complicating condition is present (e.g., upper respiratory infection), code the condition only, and do not assign code V20.2.

Routine Neonatal Procedures

Newborns are routinely vaccinated for hepatitis B during an admission for birth. Sequence V05.3 as an additional diagnostic code to explain the need for a prophylactic vaccination. Assign code 99.55 as a procedure code to report the vaccine administration. Both codes can be located under the main term "vaccination" in the Disease and Procedure Indexes.

A term infant was born by vaginal delivery; hepatitis B vaccination was given before discharge: V30.00 + V05.3; 99.55	EXAMPLE

For a male infant, review the medical record for the performance of a routine circumcision (code 64.0). A circumcision removes the foreskin (the fold of skin covering the tip of the penis). As of October 1, 2005, new codes have been provided to explain the reasons why a patient did not receive a routine vaccination (subcategory V64.0X) (eg – vaccination not given due to religious reasons V64.07; vaccination not given due to parent refused V64.05).

SUMMARY

This chapter has described the pathology of common perinatal conditions and congenital anomalies. The common manifestations, complications, and treatments of perinatal conditions and congenital anomalies also have been identified in terms of their implications for coding.

TESTING YOUR COMPREHENSION

1. Define the perinatal period of an infant's life.

2. How are congenital deformities contracted?

3. What comprises the Apgar score?

4. Provide five examples of congenital anomalies.

5. What determines an extreme immaturity code of 765.0X?

6. What does too much bilirubin in the blood cause?

7. What laboratory test can be performed to determine an Rh blood group incompatibility between the fetus and the mother?

8. What is the term used to describe the baby's first stool?

9. What is the abnormal condition of poor oxygenation of the blood that causes a bluish skin discoloration?

10. What is the result of an atrial or ventricular septal defect?

11. What symptom manifests as congenital pyloric stenosis?

12. When cerebrospinal fluid does not properly drain from the ventricles of the brain, what condition can result?

13. Identify the condition that results from a dense abnormal mass of small blood vessels.

14. A herniation of the meninges or meninges and spinal cord results in what condition?

15. What prophylactic vaccination is routinely administered at birth?

CODING PRACTICE I Chapter Review Exercises

Directions

By using your ICD-9-CM codebook, code the following diagnoses and procedures:

	DIAGNOSIS/PROCEDURES	CODE
1	Term appropriate for gestational age newborn. Cesarean section for breech presentation. Bilateral congenital hip dislocations.	
2	Thirty-four-week preterm newborn, delivered by cesarean section, 1,800 g. Hyperbilirubinemia of prematurity. Respiratory distress syndrome. Endotracheal intubation with ventilator for 5 days. Umbilical vein catheterization. Phototherapy.	
3	Term appropriate for gestational age male newborn, vaginal delivery. Hepatitis B immunization. Circumcision. Hepatitis B vaccine.	
4	Term newborn, vaginal delivery. Large for gestational age. Infant of diabetic mother.	
5	Unilateral cleft lip and palate. Repair cleft lip and palate.	
6	Twin A via vaginal delivery. Premature infant at 36 weeks, 2,250 g. Observation for sepsis, ruled out. Twin B via cesarean section. Premature infant at 36 weeks, 2,000 g. Fetal distress noted during labor. Transient tachypnea of newborn. Observation for sepsis, ruled out.	
7	Term newborn, vaginal delivery. Fractured clavicle. Large for gestational age infant.	

	DIAGNOSIS/PROCEDURES	CODE
8	Term newborn, vaginal delivery. Heart murmur, possible patent ductus arteriosus. Transferred for workup.	
9	Term newborn by cesarean section. Fetal decelerations noted in labor. Cord tight around neck.	
10	Postterm newborn, vaginal delivery. Down's syndrome (trisomy 21). Ventricular septal defect.	
11	Term male newborn, vaginal delivery. Congenital hydrocele. Hypospadias.	
12	Term newborn by cesarean section. Respiratory distress, type II. Neonatal sepsis. ABO incompatibility. Umbilical vein catheterization. Intravenous antibiotics. Exchange transfusion.	
13	Premature infant at 35 weeks, vaginal delivery, 2,312 g. Maternal cocaine use during pregnancy, with positive fetal drug screen. Transitory tachypnea of newborn. Jittery baby, suspected drug withdrawal syndrome.	
14	Observation for term newborn, born in taxi en route to hospital. Healthy female infant.	
15	Term newborn, vaginal delivery. Small for gestational age, 1,850 g. Fetal alcohol syndrome. Poor suckle—feeding problems.	
16	Premature infant transferred from XYZ hospital for failure to thrive, 2,346 g.	
17	Spina bifida with hydrocephalus. Insertion of ventriculoperitoneal shunt.	

	DIAGNOSIS/PROCEDURES	CODE
18	Term newborn, vaginal delivery. Hemangioma of face. Removal of hemangioma, left cheek.	
19	Twenty-year-old patient with Marfan's syndrome. Mitral stenosis. Mitral valve prosthetic replacement.	
20	Cerebral palsy.	

CODING PRACTICE II | Medical Record Case Studies

Instructions

1. Carefully review the medical reports provided for each case study.
2. Research any abbreviations and terms that are unfamiliar or unclear.
3. Identify as many diagnoses and procedures as possible.
4. Because only part of the patient's total record is available, determine what additional documentation you might need.
5. If appropriate, identify any questions you might ask the physician to code this case correctly and completely.
6. Complete the appropriate blanks below for each case study.

CHAPTER 16 CASE STUDIES

Case Study 16.1 (Coder/Abstract Summary Form)

Patient: **Doe, Baby Girl**

Patient documentation: **Review Medical Reports 16.1 and 16.2**

1. Principal diagnosis:

   _____

2. Secondary or other diagnoses:

   _____

3. Principal procedure:

   _____

4. Other procedures:

   _____

5. Additional documentation needed:

   _____

   _____

   _____

   _____

Case Study 16.1 (Continued)

6. Questions for the physician:

_____

_____

_____

_____

_____

NEWBORN DISCHARGE SUMMARY

PATIENT: DOE, BABY GIRL

MED REC NO: 999999

ACCT NO: V01234567890

PHYSICAL EXAMINATION:

Date of exam: 5/31   Time of exam: Baby's age at exam:

Temperature: Respiration rate: 40   Pulse rate: 150

(Code: X = No abnormalities   O = Abnormalities present)

1.	X	Reflexes	6.	X	Thorax	11.	X	Genitals
2.	O	Skin	7.	X	Lungs	12.	X	Anus
3.	X	Head/Neck	8.	X	Heart	13.	X	Trunk/Spine
4.	X	Eyes	9.	X	Abdomen	14.	X	Extremities/Joints
5.	X	ENT	10.	X	Umbilicus	15.	X	Tone/Appearance

Description of Abnormal Findings: Please describe your findings objectively. Reserve your impressions or diagnoses for the Discharge section below. Please begin your findings with reference number preceding the circled category.

Jaundice to Umbilicus

_____

_____

_____

BASIC DATA

Blood Type: B+   Energix B Vaccine

Coombs: Positive

Sex: Female   Hearing Screen (PASS)

Race: Caucasian

Date of Birth:

Time of Birth:

Place of Birth: In Hospital

Newborn Discharged on:

Follow-up visit scheduled for: Dr. Newborne

DISCHARGE STATUS: Use this section to summarize the baby's present condition. Describe briefly existing and received neonatal problems. If the baby is deceased, explain the reasons for death.

Problem 1 – Coombs positive
Developed: At Birth
Status: ABO incompatibility

Problem 2 – Jaundice
Developed: In nursery
Status: Stable

MEDICAL REPORT 16.1 (CONTINUED)

Problem 3 – Premature 4 weeks
Developed:
Status:

Course of Treatment & Impressions: Please refer to problem 1, 2, 3, or 4 in your summary. Note also your final impressions of the baby at discharge.

Phototherapy

Hep B vaccine

_____

Date / Physician's Signature

NOTES

MEDICAL REPORT 16.2

PATIENT ASSESSMENT

NEWBORN ASSESSMENT

PATIENT: Doe, Baby Girl

AGE/SEX:

ACCOUNT#: V01234567890

UNIT#:

LOCATION: NURSERY

ROOM/BED:

ADMIT DATE: 5/31

STATUS:

ATTENDING: Newborne, MD

NEWBORN ASSESSMENT

Delivery of Infant: 05/31   Time: 2209   Gender: Female

Estimated Weeks Gestation: 36   Weight: 5 lb 11.2 oz   Length: 20.0

Head Circumference: 34   Chest Circumference: 30   Abdomen Circumference: 29

NB Physician: Newborne, MD   Pediatrician Notified: Newborne, MD

Pediatrician Notified By: Smith, RN   Time: 0620

Living@ Transfer to Crib#: ID Bracelet No. 3456

Apgar One Minute: 9   Apgar Five Minutes: 10   Apgar Ten Minutes:

Delivery Type: Spontaneous Vaginal Del   Spontaneous Respirations? Y

Oxygen? Y   Type: Free Flow   Resuscitation? N   Meconium Stained? N

Newborn Resuscitation

Umbilical Vessels x 3? Y   Cord Blood to Lab? Y   Nuchal Cord x

Routine Meds Given? Y   Dextrose Stix:

Systems:

T: 98.6   Source: Rectal   P: 140 R: 48   POX

Alert? Y   Muscle Tone: Flexed   Heart Rate: Regular

Lungs Clear? Clear

Bowel Sounds: Present

Breastfeeding? Y

Bottle Feeding?   Formula Type:

WIC? Y

Additional VS:

Comments:

ALERT AND ACTIVE WITH LUSTY CRY RESPIRATIONS 40-50S NO RETRACTIONS, GRUNTING OR NASAL FLARING NOTED. 2245-WRAPPED IN WARM BLANKETS TO MOM FOR BONDING. 0015-TO BREAST NURSED 5 MINS.

Occurred Date:

5/31

Monogram:

Case Study 16.2 (Coder/Abstract Summary Form)

Patient: **Doe, Baby Boy**

Patient documentation: **Review Medical Reports 16.3, 16.4, and 16.5**

1. Principal diagnosis:

_____

2. Secondary or other diagnoses:

_____

3. Principal procedure:

_____

4. Other procedures:

_____

5. Additional documentation needed:

_____

_____

_____

6. Questions for the physician:

_____

_____

_____

_____

MEDICAL REPORT 16.3

NEWBORN DISCHARGE SUMMARY

PATIENT: DOE, BABY BOY
MED REC NO: 999999
ACCT NO: V01234567890

PHYSICAL EXAMINATION

Date of exam: 5/31   Time of exam: Baby's age at exam:

Temperature: Respiration rate: Pulse rate:

(Code: X = No abnormalities   O = Abnormalities present)

1.	X	Reflexes	6.	X	Thorax	11. X	Genitals
2.	X	Skin	7.	X	Lungs	12. X	Anus
3.	X	Head/Neck	8.	X	Heart	13. X	Trunk/Spine
4.	X	Eyes	9.	X	Abdomen	14. O	Extremities/Joints
5.	X	ENT	10.	X	Umbilicus	15. X	Tone/Appearance

Description of Abnormal Findings: Please describe your findings objectively. Reserve your impressions or diagnoses for the Discharge section below. Please begin your findings with reference number preceding the circled category.

14-R Club Foot

BASIC DATA
Blood Type: Energix B Vaccine
Coombs:
Sex: Male   Hearing Screen (PASS)
Race: Caucasian
Date of Birth:
Time of Birth:
Place of Birth: In Hospital

Newborn Discharged on:
Follow-up visit scheduled for: Dr. Newborne

DISCHARGE STATUS: Use this section to summarize the baby's present condition. Describe briefly existing and received neonatal problems. If the baby is deceased, explain the reasons for death.

Problem 1 – Club Foot
Developed: At Birth
Status: Stable

MEDICAL REPORT 16.3 (CONTINUED)

Course of Treatment & Impressions: Please refer to problem 1, 2, 3, or 4 in your summary. Note also your final impressions of the baby at discharge.

Hep B vaccine

_____

Date / Physician's Signature:

NOTES

MEDICAL REPORT 16.4

PATIENT ASSESSMENT

NEWBORN ASSESSMENT

PATIENT: Doe, Baby Boy

AGE/SEX:

ACCOUNT#:   V01234567890

UNIT#:

LOCATION: NURSERY

ROOM/BED:

ADMIT DATE:

STATUS:

ATTENDING: Newborne, MD

NEWBORN ASSESSMENT

Delivery of Infant: 05/31   Time: 0915   Gender: Male

Estimated Weeks Gestation: 39   Weight: 8 lb 9.2 oz   Length: 20.05

Head Circumference: 35   Chest Circumference: 35   Abdomen Circumference: 33

NB Physician: Newborne, MD   Pediatrician Notified: Newborne, MD

Pediatrician Notified By: Smith, RN   Time: 0930

Living @ Transfer to Crib #:   ID Bracelet No. 7890

Apgar One Minute: 9   Apgar Five Minutes: 9   Apgar Ten Minutes:

Delivery Type: Repeat CS   Spontaneous Respirations? Y

Oxygen? Y   Type: Free Flow   Resuscitation? N   Meconium Stained? N

Newborn Resuscitation

Umbilical Vessels x 3? Y   Cord Blood to Lab? Y   Nuchal Cord x

Routine Meds Given? Y   Dextrose Stix:

Systems:

T: 98.4   Source: Rectal   P: 162   R: 46   POX

Alert? Y   Muscle Tone: Flexed   Heart Rate: Regular

Lungs Clear? Clear

Bowel Sounds: Present

Breastfeeding? N

Bottle Feeding? Y   Formula Type: Simc FE

WIC? Y

Additional VS:

Comments:

PARENTS AWARE OF THE RIGHT CLUB FOOT.

Occurred Date:

5/31

Monogram:

MEDICAL REPORT 16.5

OPERATIVE REPORT

PATIENT: DOE, BABY BOY

MED REC NO: 999999

ACCT NO: V01234567890

DATE OF PROCEDURE: 05/31

PREOPERATIVE DIAGNOSIS: CIRCUMCISION

POSTOPERATIVE DIAGNOSIS: CIRCUMCISION

SURGEON: NEWBORNE, MD

ANESTHESIA: .5 CC 1% XYLOCAINE

PROCEDURE: The baby was placed in the supine position with legs strapped down. The genital area was prepped with iodine and the drapes were placed properly.

After that, .5 cc of 1% Xylocaine was injected subcutaneously at the 3 and 9 o'clock positions respectively at the base of the penis. A few minutes were given for the anesthesia to take effect.

Following that, two small clamps were placed on the prepuce at 3 and 9 o'clock and with another one, the skin overlying the glans—for approximately 1 cm—was clamped with a straight Heaney clamp for hemostasis. After it was clamped, the line of pressure was cut with a small scissors. The glans was retracted and separated from the foreskin. After that a Plastibell was placed over the glans and the foreskin was tied over the Plastibell. The excess skin was removed and hemostasis was completed. The glans fell freely under the plastic bell.

We then used Betadine and returned the patient to the Nursery uneventfully.

_____

Date / Signature of Surgeon

NOTES

Case Study 16.3 (Coder/Abstract Summary Form)

Patient: **Jones, Adam**

Patient documentation: **Review Medical Reports 16.6 and 16.7**

1. Principal diagnosis:

   _____

2. Secondary or other diagnoses:

   _____

3. Principal procedure:

   _____

4. Other procedures:

   _____

5. Additional documentation needed:

   _____

   _____

   _____

   _____

6. Questions for the physician:

   _____

   _____

   _____

   _____

   _____

MEDICAL REPORT 16.6

NEWBORN DIVISION

DISCHARGE SUMMARY

INFANT'S NAME: Jones, Adam

PARENT'S NAME: Jane Jones

ADDRESS:

ATTENDING: Dr. Newborne

PREGNANCY:

38 and 2/7 wks. Gestation   26 yr. old   Gravida 3   Para 2
Complications:

DELIVERY:

Vaginal

Under 12 hours

APGAR: 1min 10   5min 10

Complications:

COURSE:

Date of Birth   Birth weight 6-15   Birth length 19.5

Male Term

Discharge: Weight 6/9   Head circ. 36cm   Red reflex

Circumcision   Hepatitis Vaccine

Mat. HbsAG

MBT O+

BBT O+

Coombs neg

HCT 52.8

Genetic Screen

DISCHARGE DIAGNOSES:

Term

Hearing Screen passed

NEWBORN INSTRUCTION:

Feeding: Breast

_____

Date / Physician Signature

MEDICAL REPORT 16.7

OPERATIVE REPORT

INFANT'S NAME: Jones, Adam

PARENT'S NAME: Jane Jones

ADDRESS:

ATTENDING: Dr. Newborne

Name of Procedure: Circumcision
Date:
Anesthesia: 1% Lidocaine
Pre-operative Diagnosis: Phimosis of newborn
Post-operative Diagnosis: Same
Tissue Removed: Foreskin
Sponge Count: None

DESCRIPTION OF PROCEDURE: Under sterile conditions, the patient was prepared and draped and the circumcision was performed in a usual manner, using the Plastibell technique. Hemostasis was insured, and the patient returned to the nursery in satisfactory condition. There were no deviations from the description and there were no complications.

_____

Date / Signature of Surgeon

NOTES

Case Study 16.4 (Coder/Abstract Summary Form)

Patient: **Miller, Thomas**

Patient documentation: **Review Medical Reports 16.8 and 16.9**

1. Principal diagnosis:

   _____

2. Secondary or other diagnoses:

   _____

3. Principal procedure:

   _____

4. Other procedures:

   _____

5. Additional documentation needed:

   _____

   _____

   _____

   _____

6. Questions for the physician:

   _____

   _____

   _____

   _____

   _____

MEDICAL REPORT 16.8

ADMISSION/REGISTRATION RECORD

PATIENT: MILLER, Thomas

MED REC NO: 999999

ACCT NO: V01234567890

ADMIT DATE/TIME: 06/28 9:26

ROOM NO.

DATE OF BIRTH: 06/28

GUAR:

RESPONSIBLE PARTY & ADDRESS: Miller, John and Jane

EMERGENCY CONTACT NAME:

INSURANCE: In-Care/Blue-Care

MISC:

DR. ATTENDING/ADMITTING: Newborne, MD

ADMISSION DIAGNOSIS/SIGNS & SYMPTOMS: Newborn

PRINCIPAL DIAGNOSIS: (The condition established after study to be chiefly responsible for occasioning the admission of the patient to the Hospital for care)

Term Birth Living Infant

Complications: N/A

Comorbidities: N/A

Procedures:
CBC
ABO
RH
Direct Coombs
on cord blood

DISCHARGE DATE/TIME: 06/30

_____

Date / Physician's Signature:

MEDICAL REPORT 16.9

PHYSICIAN RECORD OF NEWBORN INFANT

PATIENT: Miller, Thomas
MED REC NO: 999999
ACCT NO: V01234567890

Mother's Name: Jane Miller   Father's Name: John Miller

Delivery Physician: Attending Physician: Birth Date 06/28

Sex: Male   Race: White

Gest. Age by Asses: Term 39   Weight 8-11   Length 20   Head Circum 36

Chest 36   Abd. 36   Apgar 1 min/5min: 8/9

Mother's Age: 23   Grav2 Para1

Prog. Problem:

Mother Blood Type: A+

Membr Rupt. 0926   Presentation Vertex   Anesthesia Spinal   Type Delivery C/S

Resuscitation   O2   Breast/Formula Formula

ADMISSION EXAMINATION

Description of Abnormal Findings

_____

_____

_____

_____

Term Birth Living Infant

DISCHARGE EXAMINATION

Description of Abnormal Findings
Mild Jaundice

_____

_____

_____

_____

Term Birth Living Infant

_____

Date / Physician's Signature:

Coding for Injury and Poisoning

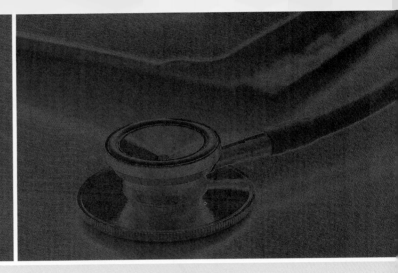

Chapter Outline

Sequencing Codes for Multiple Injuries
Fractures
Dislocations
Sprains and Strains of Joints and Muscles
Open Wounds
Amputations
Intracranial Injuries
Injuries to Internal Organs
Superficial Injuries
Injuries to Blood Vessels, Nerves, and Spinal Cord
Contusions and Crushing Injuries
Foreign Body Entering Orifice
Burns
Early Complications of Trauma
Poisoning by Drugs and Adverse Effects of Drugs

Late Effects of Injuries and Poisonings
Classifying Child and Adult Abuse
Testing Your Comprehension
Coding Practice I: Chapter Review Exercises
Coding Practice II: Medical Record Case Studies

Chapter Objectives

▶ Describe the pathology of common injuries and poisonings.
▶ Recognize the typical manifestations, complications, and treatments of injuries and poisonings in terms of their implications for coding.
▶ Correctly code common complications of injuries and poisonings and related procedures by using the ICD-9-CM and medical records.

Injuries and poisonings are covered in category codes 800 through 995 of chapter 17 of the Disease Tabular of the ICD-9-CM. These codes cover a range of conditions including fractures, injuries to internal organs, open wounds, burns, and poisonings by drugs, chemicals, and other agents. To assist in your understanding, the Word Parts Box on page 560 reviews word parts and meanings of medical terms related to injury and poisoning.

Word Parts and Meanings of Medical Terms Related to Injury and Poisoning

Word Part	Meaning	Example	Definition of Example
re-	back; again	reduction	-To put back again; a reduction procedure can realign broken bones
patho-	Disease	pathologic fracture	-A spontaneous fracture caused by disease of the bone
ortho-	Straight	orthopedist	-A physician who straightens bones (i.e., treats bone diseases and injuries)
dys-	abnormal; bad; painful	dysfunction	Abnormal function
-rrhaphy	to suture	tenorrhaphy	Suture of a tendon
de-	removal of; down	debridement	A procedure to remove nonviable (diseased) tissue
-plasty	surgical repair	myoplasty	Surgical repair of a muscle
tox/o- toxic/o-	Poison	Toxic	Pertaining to poison
per-	Through	percutaneous	Through the skin
mal-	Bad	malunion of a fracture	-Bad union (healing) of a fracture
intra-	within; into	intracranial	Within the head
-thorax	chest; pleural cavity	traumatic pneumothorax	An abnormal entry of air into the chest (pleural space) due to injury

Sequencing Codes for Multiple Injuries

Multiple traumatic injuries can be present at the time of a patient's admission to a hospital. When multiple injuries exist, the code for the most severe injury, as determined by the attending physician, is sequenced as the principal diagnosis. Unless unforeseen complications arise, the most severe injury will usually receive the primary focus of treatment. Other coexisting injuries, preexisting comorbid conditions, or complicating conditions during the hospital stay should be assigned as additional codes.

EXAMPLE

An elderly male was involved in a motor vehicle accident on the highway and received blunt trauma to the chest and abdomen from hitting the steering wheel. The patient was the driver of the car and was not wearing his seat belt. The patient was admitted to the hospital through the emergency department for a ruptured spleen, four broken ribs, whiplash, and multiple contusions. The patient had a known history of emphysema. The patient was immediately taken to surgery for removal of the ruptured spleen.

Principal Diagnosis:	*865.04*	*Ruptured spleen, traumatic (most severe injury)*
Secondary Diagnosis:	*807.04*	*Fractured ribs × 4*
	847.0	*Whiplash (cervical sprain)*
	924.8	*Multiple contusions*
	492.8	*Emphysema*
	E819.0	*Motor vehicle accident of unspecified nature, driver*
Principal procedure:	*41.5*	*Splenectomy (total)*

To perform a final accuracy check of the codes being reported, notice that injury codes coming from chapter 17 of the ICD-9-CM codebook are different from condition codes coming from other ICD-9-CM chapters on diseases. For example, emphysema code 492.8 (a specific type of chronic obstructive lung disease) comes from chapter 8 in the ICD-9-CM codebook (diseases of the respiratory system), whereas traumatic emphysema code 958.7 (abnormal air or gas in subcutaneous tissues attributable to an injury) comes from chapter 17 (injury and poisoning).

Avoid making the error of reporting traumatic injuries as non-traumatic conditions and vice versa.

Using E Codes to Report Causes and Locations of Injuries

E codes are located in the External Causes of Injury and Poisoning Index within the *Alphabetic Index to Diseases* and classify causes of injuries, including burns. Common injury E codes include the following:

E881.0	Fall from ladder
E886.0	Fall in sports (e.g., injured while being tackled in football)
E927	Twisting injury
E905.3	Stung by bee
E816.0	Motor vehicle accident attributable to loss of control, without collision on highway, driver
E890.3	Burned by conflagration (fire) in private dwelling
E960.0	Assault in brawl (e.g., beaten in fight)

E codes can also describe the location where an injury or accident occurred. Located under the main term "Accident; occurring at" in the External Causes of Injury and Poisoning Index, E codes can describe sites that include the following:

E849.7	Hospital
E849.1	Farm
E849.6	Restaurant
E849.4	Skating rink
E849.0	Home
E849.3	Construction site

Never sequence E codes as the principal diagnosis. Sequence them only as additional codes to report the nature (external cause) of an accident or the circumstance most directly responsible for an injury or poisoning (i.e., the proximate cause).

EXAMPLE

After arrival at the emergency department for care, the patient stated that he had been chased by a dog while biking and had fallen. He was then bitten on the right hand and also sustained a bruise to the right knee from the fall. The dog owner reported that the animal was up to date with immunizations, and the patient was treated in the emergency department for a puncture wound to the right hand from the dog bite. The patient's hand wound was cleansed, and he received a tetanus shot before discharge. The knee radiograph demonstrated negative findings.

Principal Diagnosis:	*882.0*	*Puncture wound, right hand*
Secondary Diagnosis:	*924.11*	*Contusion, knee*
	E906.0	*Dog bite as the proximate cause for the most significant injury requiring primary treatment*
	E826.1	*Fall from bicycle*

Depending on the established coding policies and procedures for each facility, Health Information Management departments may sometimes limit the reporting of E codes to aid in coder productivity. However, many state laws require E codes for mandatory reporting to state-funded trauma registries because the information obtained from these coded data is used to help legislators set public policy to prevent and reduce harm to the public from serious accidents (e.g., a reported increase in head injuries attributable to motorcycle accidents may cause state legislators to address the need for helmet laws).

Using E Codes to Report Sentinel Events

State hospital licensure laws mandate the reporting of **sentinel events.** Sentinel events are unexpected circumstances that cause serious injury or death to a patient within the health-care facility. The health-care facility must submit mandatory forms that use E codes to notify state agencies of the circumstances surrounding sentinel events. State agencies use the reported information to investigate the causes for sentinel events, direct agency actions to prevent future sentinel events, and monitor other quality-of-care concerns within health-care facilities.

EXAMPLE

A patient was admitted to the hospital for treatment of pneumonia. On the second hospital day, the patient accidentally fell out of bed. This resulted in a hip fracture, and the patient was taken to the operating room for an open reduction, internal fixation (ORIF), right hip.

Principal Diagnosis:	*486*	*Pneumonia*
Secondary Diagnosis:	*820.8*	*Traumatic hip fracture*
	E884.4	*Fall from bed*
	E849.7	*Occurring in hospital*
Principal Procedure:	*79.35*	*ORIF, right hip*
Other Procedure:	*99.21*	*Intravenous antibiotics*

Using E Codes to Classify Collisions

Another rule for E codes states that collisions between different types of vehicles, persons, or objects must be classified in a hierarchical order (i.e., in order of importance). This order is explained in the italicized notes in the box under the main term "Collision" in the External Causes of Injury and Poisoning Index. In classifying collisions, always select the higher code according to the following order of precedence:

Aircraft

Watercraft

Motor vehicle

Railway

Pedal cycle

Animal-drawn vehicle or animal being ridden

Streetcar or nonmotor vehicle

Other vehicle

Pedestrian or person using pedestrian conveyance

Object

For example, according to this hierarchy, if an automobile collided with a train, it would be classified as a motor vehicle collision, not a railway collision.

Fractures

A fracture is a broken bone. Located in the *Alphabetic Index to Diseases* under the main term "Fracture," indented subterms describe fractures according to anatomic site (e.g., femur, tibia, skull, and vertebra), and further-indented subterms classify whether the fracture was open or closed. **Open fracture** indicates that the fracture penetrated or broke the skin, whereas a **closed fracture** does not break the skin (Figure 17.1). To assign the correct diagnosis code for a traumatic fracture (attributable to an injury), review the medical record documentation to determine whether the fracture was open or closed.

Traumatic fractures should not be confused with pathologic (spontaneous; nontraumatic) fractures that result from weakened bone attributable to disease (e.g., osteoporosis). Pathologic fracture codes (category 733) do not result from an external traumatic injury and are coded from the ICD-9-CM codebook chapter 13 (on diseases of the musculoskeletal system and connective tissue) and would not be coded from the ICD-9-CM codebook chapter 17 (on injury and poisoning).

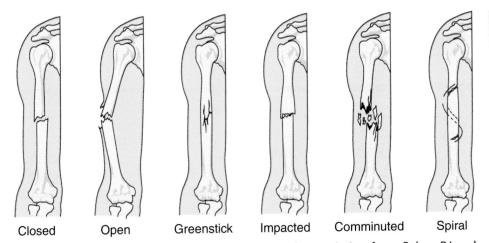

| Closed | Open | Greenstick | Impacted | Comminuted | Spiral |

FIGURE 17.1 ■ Types of fractures. (Reprinted with permission from Cohen BJ and Wood DL. Memmler's The Human Body in Health and Disease, 9th Ed. Philadelphia: Lippincott Williams & Wilkins, 2000.)

Closed tibial fracture:	*823.80*
Open tibial fracture:	*823.90*
Compression fracture of	
the L3 vertebra secondary	
to osteoporosis:	*733.13 + 733.00*

Physicians sometimes use other descriptive terms to indicate open or closed fractures. In the *Alphabetic Index to Diseases*, italicized notes in the box located under the main term "Fracture" and general notes at the beginning of fracture categories 800 to 829 in the *Tabular List of Diseases* describe various terms that indicate the fracture as closed or open.

Terms that describe types of closed fractures include the following:

▶ simple
▶ comminuted
▶ greenstick
▶ impacted
▶ linear
▶ spiral

Terms that describe types of open fractures include the following:

▶ compound
▶ infected
▶ missile
▶ puncture
▶ with foreign body

Without further documentation from the physician, classify an unspecified fracture as closed.

Common Procedures for Treating Fractures

Fracture treatment may be open or closed.

Be aware that a diagnosis of open or closed fracture has no bearing on whether the fracture treatment is open or closed.

TREATMENT FOR DISPLACED FRACTURES

In a displaced fracture, the broken bone is out of anatomic alignment. Therefore, the intent of treatment for a displaced fracture is to bring the bone back into anatomic alignment. This is done through a reduction procedure in which the physician physically manipulates the fractured bone back into its normal position, i.e., reduces the displacement (Figure 17.2). A **closed reduction** is a manipulative procedure that is performed without an incision to bring the bone back into anatomic alignment. An **open reduction** is a manipulative procedure that is preceded by an incision into the fracture site.

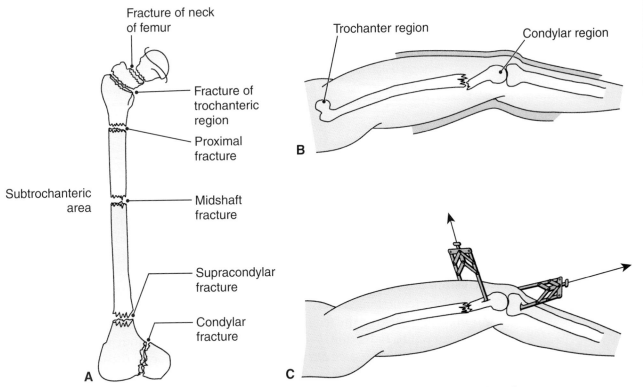

FIGURE 17.2 ■ **A.** Types of femoral fractures. One method of correction for a fracture of the femur in the distal third is two-wire skeletal traction. **B.** Example of deformity on admission to hospital. **C.** Adequate reduction is achieved when additional wire is inserted in the lower femoral fragment, and vertical lift is secured. (Reprinted with permission from Smeltzer SC and Bare BG. Brunner & Suddarth's Textbook of Medical-Surgical Nursing, 10th Ed. Philadelphia: Lippincott Williams & Wilkins, 2004.)

Fracture-reduction codes can be located under the main term "Reduction" in the *Alphabetic Index to Procedures* and then under the subterm for the site of the fracture. In both open and closed fracture reduction procedures, carefully review further-indented subterms that specify the placement of pins, rods, or other hardware (e.g., internal fixation devices) to stabilize the fracture, because this will change the code assignment.

Closed reduction of radial fracture:	79.02	**EXAMPLE**
Closed reduction of radial fracture with internal fixation:	79.12	

Fracture-reduction codes include the initial casting, so an additional code is not required for the cast. In the *Alphabetic Index to Procedures* after the main term "Reduction, fracture," you will note nonessential modifiers in parentheses that include "with casting." Also, the "includes notes" under category code 79 for Reduction of Fracture in the *Tabular List of Procedures* include "application of cast."

Treatment for open fractures can also include an additional code for debridement of the exposed bone; this involves the surgical removal or cutting away of devitalized bone tissue. You can locate these codes under the main term "Debridement; open fracture (compound)" by site in the *Alphabetic Index to Procedures.*

<table>
<tr><td>**EXAMPLE**</td><td>*Principal Diagnosis:*</td><td>*820.31*</td><td>*Compound intertrochanteric fracture of femur*</td></tr>
<tr><td></td><td>*Principal Procedure:*</td><td>*79.35*</td><td>*ORIF, femoral fracture*</td></tr>
<tr><td></td><td>*Other Procedure:*</td><td>*79.65*</td><td>*With debridement*</td></tr>
<tr><td></td><td>*Principal Diagnosis:*</td><td>*813.31*</td><td>*Colles fracture, left wrist*</td></tr>
<tr><td></td><td>*Principal Procedure:*</td><td>*79.02*</td><td>*Closed reduction with casting, fracture, left distal radius*</td></tr>
</table>

TREATMENT FOR NONDISPLACED FRACTURES

Some fractures are nondisplaced (i.e., remain in anatomic alignment). In this case, a reduction procedure would not be necessary. However, when deemed medically necessary by the physician, external or internal fixation without fracture reduction may be performed. External fixation involves casting, splinting, or skeletal traction on the surface of the skin to apply pressure to stabilize the bones. Internal fixation involves the placement of metal pins or rods within bones. You should be aware that pinning (i.e., internal fixation without fracture reduction) is routinely used for nondisplaced fractures of weight-bearing bones, such as the femur. Refer to the main term "Fixation; internal (without fracture reduction)" or "Fixation; external (without manipulation for reduction)" in the *Alphabetic Index to Procedures* to locate these codes.

<table>
<tr><td>**EXAMPLE**</td><td>*Principal Diagnosis:*</td><td>*820.8*</td><td>*Nondisplaced fracture of the femoral neck*</td></tr>
<tr><td></td><td>*Principal Procedure:*</td><td>*78.55*</td><td>*Percutaneous pinning without reduction, femoral neck fracture*</td></tr>
<tr><td></td><td>*Principal Diagnosis:*</td><td>*813.07*</td><td>*Closed radial fracture, proximal end*</td></tr>
<tr><td></td><td>*Principal Procedure:*</td><td>*93.53*</td><td>*Application of cast, without reduction*</td></tr>
<tr><td></td><td>*Principal Diagnosis:*</td><td>*810.00*</td><td>*Closed fracture, right clavicle*</td></tr>
<tr><td></td><td>*Principal Procedure:*</td><td>*93.54*</td><td>*Application of splint for immobilization*</td></tr>
</table>

Dislocations

Dislocation occurs when a bone becomes displaced from its joint capsule; this usually results from trauma. Common sites for dislocations are the shoulder and hip joints. Dislocations that occur without a fracture are coded to category codes 830 to 839. Indented subterms, located under the main term "Dislocation" in the *Alphabetic Index to Diseases*, identify the dislocation site and classify whether the dislocation was open or closed. An open dislocation indicates that the dislocated bone has broken through the skin.

<table>
<tr><td>**EXAMPLE**</td><td>*Closed shoulder dislocation:*</td><td>*831.00*</td></tr>
<tr><td></td><td>*Open shoulder dislocation:*</td><td>*883.10*</td></tr>
</table>

TIP Injuries documented as "fracture-dislocations" by the physician are coded to the fracture code only. This can be noted under the main term "Dislocation" in the *Alphabetic Index to Diseases*, in which there is a cross-reference: "with fracture—see Fracture by site."

Common Procedures for Treating Dislocations

Dislocation treatment usually involves a closed (without incision) or open (with incision) reduction of the dislocation. These codes are located under the main term "Reduction; dislocation" by site within the *Alphabetic Index to Procedures*.

		EXAMPLE
Closed reduction of shoulder dislocation:	*79.71*	
Open reduction of shoulder dislocation:	*79.81*	

Sprains and Strains of Joints and Muscles

Sprains and strains are common injuries of the musculoskeletal system. **Sprains** result in the overstretching or tearing (beyond its normal range of motion) of a joint capsule, ligament, or both. Joint capsules, which include the ankle, knee, shoulder, hip, and vertebrae, allow for the movement of an otherwise rigid skeleton. Ligaments help attach bones to bones. Symptoms of a sprain include joint pain, swelling, instability, and/or immobility of the joint.

		EXAMPLE
844.2	*Current acute anterior cruciate ligament tear, right knee*	
E886.0	*Patient tackled and fell while playing football this morning*	
845.00	*Ankle sprain*	
E927	*Patient twisted ankle while stepping off curb*	

Strains result in the overstretching or tearing of a muscle, tendon, or both. Tendons attach muscles to bones and allow for musculoskeletal movement. Symptoms of a strain include muscle pain, spasms, swelling, and decreased range of motion.

		EXAMPLE
846.9	*Low back strain*	
E927	*Injury from lifting boxes*	
840.4	*Current rotator cuff tear, right shoulder*	
E927	*Injury while playing tennis (i.e., strenuous movements in recreational activities)*	

Open Wounds

Category codes 870 to 894 classify open wounds that result from lacerations, cuts, penetrations, perforations, punctures, avulsions (i.e., torn tissue), or other external breaks of the skin. Located under the main term "Wound" in the *Alphabetic Index to Diseases*, subterms describe wound sites, and further-indented subterms under the site code describe whether the open wound included "tendon involvement" or was "complicated." The italicized notes in the box located under the main term "Wound, open" in the *Alphabetic Index to Diseases* describe "complicated" wounds as those that include delayed healing or treatment, the presence of a foreign body, or primary infection (e.g., cellulitis).

EXAMPLE

Laceration to the palm of the right hand from knife requiring 10 stitches. The patient was carving a Halloween pumpkin when he slipped with the knife.

Principal Diagnosis:	882.0	*Laceration, palm*
Secondary Diagnosis:	E920.3	*Accident caused by cut from knife*
Principal Procedure:	86.59	*Suture, skin of hand*

A patient fell while skateboarding, resulting in an open wound to the elbow with beginning cellulitis (an infection of the skin and subcutaneous tissue). The wound required cleansing and stitches; oral antibiotics were prescribed, and the patient was instructed to return to the emergency department if the site became increasingly warm or developed red streaking.

Principal Diagnosis:	881.11	*Wound open, elbow, complicated*
Secondary Diagnosis:	682.3	*Cellulitis, elbow*
	E885.2	*Fall while skateboarding*
Principal Procedure:	86.59	*Suture, skin of elbow*

Sequencing of codes for open wounds and cellulitis depends on the circumstances of admission. If the primary focus of care was for cellulitis associated with a wound (e.g., cellulitis with admission for intravenous antibiotics with minimal wound care), sequence the cellulitis code first, with the wound (complicated) sequenced as an additional code. However, if the primary focus of care was directed at the wound, sequence the wound (complicated) as the principal diagnosis.

For open wounds associated with open fracture, penetrating wounds of internal organs, contusions, crush injuries, or superficial injuries (e.g., abrasion, friction burn, blister, or scratch), the cross-reference *"see"* after the main term "Wound, open" in the *Alphabetic Index to Diseases* directs you to see the other condition (listed previously), as applicable.

Amputations

Codes for traumatic amputation (loss of a body part because of an injury; code categories 895 to 897) can be located under the main term "Amputation" in the *Alphabetic Index to Diseases* according to the subterms for the anatomic sites. Further-indented subterms specify whether the amputation is "complicated" by delayed healing or treatment, the presence of a foreign body, or an infection.

EXAMPLE

Traumatic amputation, arm, complicated:	*887.3*
Traumatic amputation, right index finger:	*886.0*

Current traumatic amputations are often followed by a revision amputation procedure for the current amputation site or a reattachment procedure. Amputation procedure codes can be located under the main term "Amputation" in the *Alphabetic Index to Procedures*. An amputation specified as a disarticulation means the amputation was through the joint capsule.

EXAMPLE

The patient was admitted for a traumatic nonsalvageable amputation of the foot that was treated with ankle disarticulation.

Principal Diagnosis:	896.0	*Traumatic amputation, right foot*
Principal Procedure:	84.13	*Ankle disarticulation*

Traumatic amputation reattachment procedures are located under the main term "Reattachment" in the *Alphabetic Index to Procedures* and are further classified according to anatomic site.

Principal Diagnosis:	*896.0*	*Traumatic amputation of left foot*	**EXAMPLE**
Principal Procedure:	*84.26*	*Reattachment, foot*	

Intracranial Injuries

Codes for intracranial injuries (internal head injuries) without a related skull fracture are coded to categories 850 to 854 and can be located under the main term "Injury; internal, intracranial" in the *Alphabetic Index to Diseases* or under the main term for the specific condition (e.g., contusion, brain).

When locating intracranial injury codes under the name of the condition (e.g., hemorrhage, brain), be careful to locate the subterm that correctly describes the condition as attributable to an injury or trauma, as opposed to nontraumatic conditions that come from other system chapters. That is, if the injury is traumatic, the code should come from the injury chapter, but if the injury is nontraumatic, then the code should come from the related system chapter (e.g., "Diseases of the Circulatory System").

Hemorrhage; brain; traumatic:	*853.0X from chapter 17 ("Injuries")*	**EXAMPLE**
Hemorrhage; brain; nontraumatic:	*431 from chapter 7 ("Circulatory System")*	

Subterms under the main term "Injury; internal, intracranial" identify the specific intracranial site (such as the brain stem, cerebellum, or cortex), the specific type of intracranial injury (e.g., contusion, hemorrhage, or laceration), and whether there was an open intracranial wound. Fifth digits indicate whether there was a loss of consciousness and can describe the duration of unconsciousness.

Cerebral contusion from being struck in the head with a hardball while playing baseball, no loss of consciousness: 851.81 + E917.0 + E849.4	**EXAMPLE**

Category code 850, cerebral concussion, includes fourth and fifth digits that describe the duration of unconsciousness. A cerebral concussion results in temporary brain deficits (i.e., dysfunction) that usually clear within 24 hours or less. Other intracranial injuries, such as cerebral contusions or lacerations, can result in deficits that last more than 24 hours and may cause permanent neurologic deficits, such as epilepsy.

When coding intracranial injuries associated with a skull fracture (category codes 800 to 804), you must refer to the skull fracture by site. The fifth digit also describes any associated loss of consciousness.

Fracture at the base of the skull with an intracranial laceration from being hit by a thrown bat while playing baseball. Brief loss of consciousness: 801.12 + E917.5	**EXAMPLE**

Injuries to Internal Organs

You can locate codes that classify injuries to internal organs (e.g., liver, lung, heart, colon, or kidney) within the *Alphabetic Index to Diseases* under the main term "Injuries; internal" and then by locating the subterm for the organ site. A fourth digit specifies whether the injury to the internal organ is associated with an open wound.

EXAMPLE

Stab wound to the right upper quadrant of the abdomen with a penetrating wound to the liver. The patient was stabbed with a knife during a barroom brawl: 864.15 + E966 + E849.6

The patient fell from a ladder while painting his house and was impaled by a picket fence; this resulted in a penetrating wound into the left lower quadrant of the abdomen that lacerated his descending colon: 863.50 + E888.0 + E920.8 + E849.0

Superficial Injuries

Conditions such as blisters, friction burns, scratches, and abrasions are considered superficial injuries (category codes 910 to 919). These codes can be located in the *Alphabetic Index to Diseases* under the main term "Injury; superficial," with subterms to indicate the site.

EXAMPLE

Friction burn to the left thigh from skidding into home plate while playing baseball.
    916.0   Friction burn, thigh
    E885.9   Fall from other slipping, tripping, or stumbling

Infected blisters, both feet, from poorly fitting new shoes.
    917.1   Blister, infected, feet
    E928.5   External constriction caused by other object (ill-fitting shoes)

Injuries to Blood Vessels, Nerves, and Spinal Cord

Codes for injuries to the blood vessels, nerves, and spinal cord are located in the *Alphabetic Index to Diseases* under the main term "Injury" by site. Injuries to blood vessels are classified in code categories 900 to 904; injuries to nerves and the spinal cord are classified in code categories 950 to 957. Depending on the circumstances for admission (i.e., the injuries that warranted the admission to the hospital) and the primary focus of care, these codes may be sequenced as the principal diagnosis or secondary diagnosis according to definitions from the Uniform Hospital Discharge Data Set rules covered in Chapter 2 of this textbook.

EXAMPLE

Puncture wound, left lower thigh, from a stray dart, severing the superficial femoral artery. Suture repair, left superficial artery: 904.1 + E920.8 + 39.31

Damage to digital nerve, ring finger, left hand. Finger pinched in automatic car window: 955.6 + E918

Transient paraplegia secondary to damage to nerve root, lumbar, from twisting injury while doing yard work: 952.2 + E927 (Note—For an injury to the spinal cord with a vertebral fracture, the coder is directed to see "Fracture, vertebrae, by site, with spinal cord injury")

Tackle football injury with tingling, numbness, and "dead arm" sensation from the overstretching of the brachial plexus, right shoulder area: 953.4 + E886.0

Contusions and Crushing Injuries

Contusions (bruises) are classified in category codes 920 to 924. Contusions often result from blows (i.e., blunt trauma) to the body. Although there is no break in the skin, a contusion manifests in a typical "black and blue" discoloration that results from damaged and ruptured small blood vessels leaking into surrounding tissues beneath the surface of the skin.

Painful contusion, sacrum, from riding on a mechanical bull: 922.32 + E927

EXAMPLE

For contusions associated with crush injury, joint dislocation, fracture, internal organ injury, intracranial injury, nerve injury, or open wound, the cross-reference "*see*" after the main term "Contusion" in the *Alphabetic Index to Diseases* directs you to see the other condition (listed previously), as applicable.

Crushing injuries (category codes 925 to 929) are attributable to severe trauma and are located under the main term "Crush" in the *Alphabetic Index to Diseases*, followed by the subterm for the body site. Minor crush injuries can occur, for example, from slamming a finger in a car door, hitting one's hand with a hammer, or dropping a heavy object on one's foot. Because there are many nerves in the extremities that allow fine movement, increased sensitivity, and dexterity, crush injuries can result in extreme pain. Severe crush injuries can cause extensive harm to the skin, damage to underlying muscle and soft tissues, avulsion (torn tissue) injuries, and injuries to nerves, bones, and internal organs, with organ rupture and hemorrhage.

For crush injuries associated with fracture, joint dislocation, internal organ injury, intracranial injury, nerve injury, or an open wound, the cross-reference "*see*" after the main term "Crush (injury)" in the *Alphabetic Index to* Diseases directs you to see the other condition (listed previously), as applicable.

The patient was a passenger in a motor vehicle accident involving losing control and striking a tree, resulting in massive crushed chest injury with bilateral hemothorax: 860.2 + E816.1 (this is an example of when you would code the specific condition—hemothorax—and not the crushing injury)

EXAMPLE

Foreign Body Entering Orifice

Foreign bodies are not part of one's natural tissues and may include objects, such as coins, glass or gravel (in an open wound), or food that becomes lodged in orifices (e.g., openings such as the throat) or that penetrate body tissues. In the *Alphabetic Index to Diseases*, subterms located under the main term "Foreign body; entering through orifice (current) (old)" specify the anatomic site. For foreign bodies involving open wounds, you should refer to "Wound, open" by site, complicated.

EXAMPLE		
	934.1	*Aspiration of peanut into the left lower lobe bronchial airway*
	E911	*Aspiration of food causing obstruction of the respiratory tract*
	33.23	*Bronchoscopy*
	98.15	*Removal of foreign body from bronchus without incision*

Burns

Category codes 940 to 949 classify burns. Subterms, located under the main term "Burn," are provided to identify burn sites. Further-indented subterms under the site code classify burns according to the degree of burn (Figure 17.3).

▸ **first-degree** burns result in erythema (redness)
▸ **second-degree** burns result in blistering
▸ **third-degree** burns involve a full-thickness loss of skin and may involve deeper necrosis (death) of tissues and loss of body parts

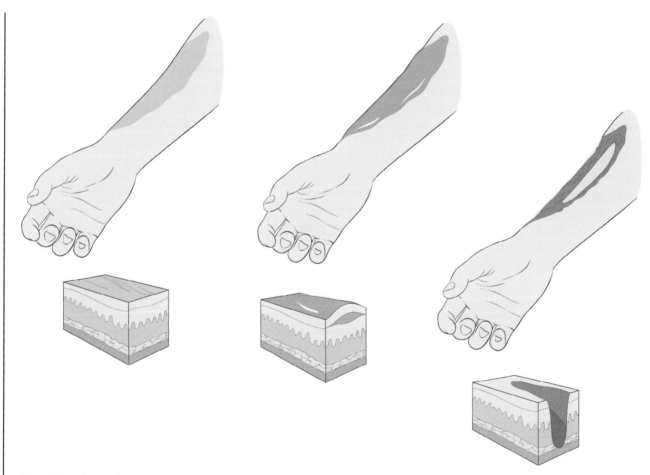

FIGURE 17.3 ■ Three types of burns shown on an arm and in a cross-section of skin. (Left) superficial burn, (center) partial-thickness burn, (right) full-thickness burn. (LifeART image copyright © 2008 Lippincott Williams & Wilkins. All rights reserved.)

Serious or extensive burns can result in secondary infection, dehydration, scarring, and death.

Sequencing Burn Codes

As a general rule, when more than one burn is present, the highest degree of burn is sequenced first. Less severe burns, as well as coexisting injuries, preexisting comorbid conditions, or complications during the hospital stay, should be assigned as additional codes. Code burns of the same anatomic site (and therefore the same three-digit category code) but of different degrees to the highest degree of burn for that site only.

Second- and third-degree burns to the left forearm: 943.31 (code only the third-degree burns)	**EXAMPLE**

Category code 948, under the main term "Burn; extent," provides a fourth digit that describes the body-surface area involved in burns (e.g., arm, leg, or torso). The fifth digit provides added detail about the percentage of the total body surface with third-degree burns. Paramedics and emergency department physicians commonly use a chart called the "rule of nines" to quickly assess the percentage of total body surface burned and the percentage involved with third-degree burns (Figure 17.4). Each arm accounts for 9%; each leg, 18%; head, 9%; front and back torso, 18% each; and genitals, 1%. This chart establishes a total burn score to assess the threat to life and the probability of survival of the patient so that medical personnel can deliver fast and appropriate treatment. Category code 948 is most often used as an additional code to describe the extent of total body surface burned but can sometimes be reported as a single code if the extent of the burns is so widespread that codes identifying each specific part of the body burned cannot be adequately established.

While at home, an elderly patient fell asleep while smoking in bed. The mattress subsequently caught fire, and the patient experienced second- and third-degree burns to the trunk and first- and second-degree burns to the right arm. It was estimated that the burns covered 34% of the patient's total body surface, with 20% third-degree and 10% second-degree burns to his trunk and 4% first- and second-degree burns to his arm.	**EXAMPLE**

Principal Diagnosis:	942.30	*Third-degree burns to trunk*
Secondary Diagnosis:	943.20	*Second-degree burns to arm*
	948.32	*30% to 39% of body surface burned, with 20% thereof with third-degree burn*
	E898.1	*Bed set on fire from cigarette*
	E849.0	*Accident occurring at home*

Remember to add E codes to classify the cause of the burns; these codes can be located in the External Causes of Injury and Poisoning Index in the *Alphabetic Index to Diseases*.

Early Complications of Trauma

Usually sequenced as additional codes during the initial episode of care for the acute injury, category 958 codes classify early complications of trauma (i.e., secondary [subsequent] complications that quickly follow the acute injury).

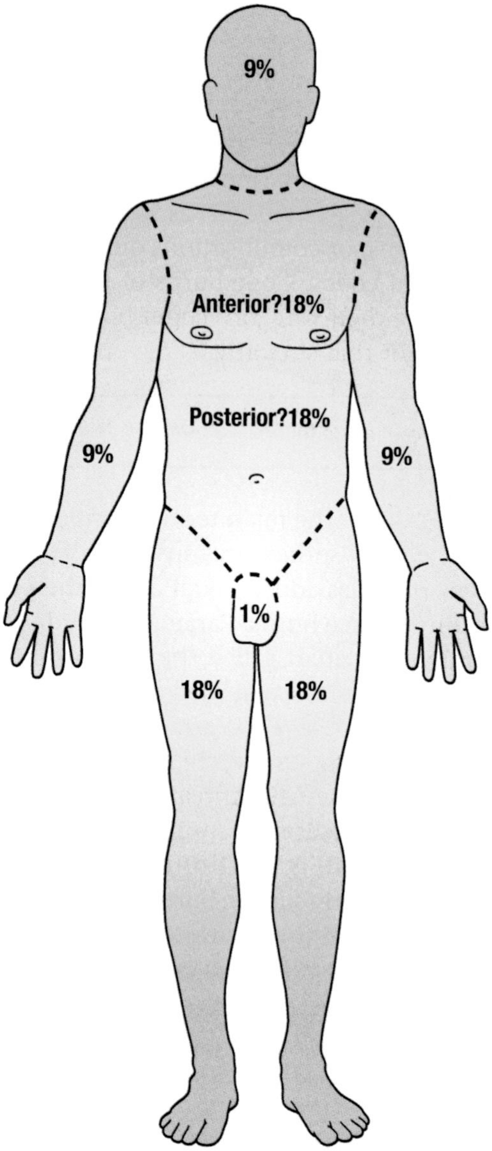

FIGURE 17.4 ■ The rule of nines: Estimated percentage of total body surface area (TBSA) in the adult figured by sectioning the body surface into areas with a numerical value related to nine. (Note: The anterior and posterior head total 9% of TBSA.) In burn victims, the total estimated percentage of TBSA injured is used to calculate the patient's fluid replacement needs. (Reprinted with permission from Smeltzer SC and Bare BG. Brunner & Suddarth's Textbook of Medical-Surgical Nursing, 10th Ed. Philadelphia: Lippincott Williams & Wilkins, 2004.)

You must carefully review the subterms (usually the subterm "traumatic") under the main term for the condition in the *Alphabetic Index to Diseases* to locate the correct code.

EXAMPLE	*Shock, traumatic:*	*958.4*
	Fat embolism:	*958.1*
	Emphysema, traumatic subcutaneous:	*958.7*

Poisoning by Drugs and Adverse Effects of Drugs

The terms **poisoning** and **adverse effects** of drugs, chemicals, or other agents indicate different coding situations.

When coding a poisoning or a reaction to the improper use of a medication (e.g., the patient did not take the medication as prescribed by the physician), chemical, or other agent, sequence the poisoning codes first, followed by a code for the manifestation (e.g., confusion, tachycardia, or hypotension) and then the E code that identifies the drug, agent, or chemical substance and circumstances of the poisoning (e.g., accident, suicide attempt, assault, or undetermined). The poisoning code and E code are located under the specific agent, drug, or other chemical substance in the Table of Drugs and Chemicals in the *Alphabetic Index to Diseases*.

 TIP Common terms that indicate poisoning or the incorrect use of drugs include "drug overdose," "drug intoxication," or administration of the "wrong medication" or "wrong dosage."

When coding an adverse effect (i.e., abnormal reaction) to the proper use of a medication (i.e., the patient *did* take the medication as prescribed by the physician), sequence the adverse effect code or codes first (e.g., dermatitis or bradycardia), followed by an E code from the Table of Drugs and Chemicals that identifies the prescribed drug, agent, or chemical substance that caused the adverse effect (see excerpt below). In the Table of Drugs and Chemicals, the E code is located under the name of the specific agent, drug, or other chemical substance in the column heading for "therapeutic use."

EXTERNAL CAUSE (E-CODE)

Substance	Poisoning	Accident	Therapeutic Use	Suicide Attempt	Assault	Undetermined
Digoxin	972.1	E858.3	E942.1	E950.4	E962.0	E980.4
Dihydrocodeine	965.09	E850.2	E935.2	E950.0	E962.0	E980.0

 TIP Common terms used on medical reports that indicate adverse effects resulting from the correct use of prescribed drugs include "allergic reaction or response," "drug hypersensitivity," "idiosyncratic reaction" as an unexpected effect in an individual, and "drug toxicity" as a cumulative effect.

A young patient is admitted for orthostatic hypotension attributable to ingestion of his mother's hypertension pills, which he believed were over-the-counter vitamins.

EXAMPLE

972.6 *Accidental overdose of antihypertensive medication*
458.0 *Orthostatic hypotension secondary to #1*
E858.3 *Accidental overdose, antihypertensive drug*

A patient was admitted for a diffuse skin rash attributable to ampicillin. Prophylactic ampicillin was prescribed before a dental cleaning procedure because of a known history of mitral valve prolapse.

    693.0   Rash secondary to ampicillin taken prophylactically for dental cleaning
    E930.0   Adverse effect, therapeutic use of penicillin
    424.1   Mitral valve prolapse

A **cumulative effect** occurs when the concentration or the amount of the drug in one's body steadily increases over time and eventually reaches toxic levels. This can occur even when the drug is being taken as prescribed. Cumulative effects of drugs often happen in the elderly because of the slowing of their metabolism, which naturally occurs with age. Lower metabolism can slow the breakdown or release of drugs in the body. Some comorbid conditions also may inhibit the breakdown of drugs in the body (e.g., diseased kidney function may hinder the release of some drugs that are excreted in urine). As an example, digoxin (digitalis; Lanoxin) is often prescribed for chronic congestive heart failure (CHF) and atrial fibrillation in the elderly. If the physician documents "digoxin toxicity" and the patient has taken the drug as prescribed, do not code it as a poisoning. Instead, code the digoxin toxicity as an adverse effect, because this represents toxicity as a cumulative effect.

Elderly people living with chronic diseases are often prescribed many different medications to treat their conditions. Taking many medications can be confusing for most people. However, the elderly are especially vulnerable to errors in the self-administration of their medications and often require assistance with their care. Also, non–English-speaking people living in the United States can be prone to accidental medication errors attributable to language barriers.

    Remember to use the E code that denotes accidental poisoning when a patient is admitted for taking the wrong pills or wrong dosages; do not assume other causes (e.g., suicide attempt, undetermined).

Contrast the examples below.

EXAMPLE

Patient A was admitted for dehydration, nausea and vomiting, diarrhea, and altered mental status secondary to digoxin toxicity (cumulative effect). The patient had a history of compensated CHF controlled with medications (digoxin and furosemide [Lasix]).

    Principal Diagnosis: 276.51   Dehydration
    Secondary Diagnosis: 787.01   Nausea and vomiting
                         787.91   Diarrhea*
                         780.97   Altered mental status*
                         E942.1   Adverse effect (therapeutic use), digoxin*
                         428.0   Compensated CHF (as a comorbid condition)*

Patient B was admitted with dehydration, nausea and vomiting, diarrhea, and altered mental status secondary to digoxin overdose. The patient had mistakenly taken a double dose of his medications. He had forgotten that he had already taken them earlier in the day. The patient had a history of compensated CHF controlled with medication (digoxin and furosemide).

Principal Diagnosis:	*972.1*	*Digoxin poisoning*
	276.51	*Dehydration*
	787.01	*Nausea and vomiting*
	787.91	*Diarrhea*
	780.97	*Altered mental status*
	E858.3	*Accidental poisoning, digoxin (see excerpt below)*
	428.0	*Compensated CHF*

The combination of prescribed drugs with alcoholic beverages can be harmful and is discouraged. Therefore, the reaction to a medication combined with alcohol is coded as a poisoning. Sequence the poisoning code for the drug(s) or alcohol first, followed by a code for the manifestation (e.g., somnolence, stupor, drowsiness, dizziness, or convulsions) and then the E code that identifies the drug(s) and alcohol and circumstances for the poisoning (e.g., accident, suicide attempt, assault, or undetermined).

A patient was prescribed Ambien (zolpidem tartrate) by his family physician for insomnia. The patient's wife reported that over the course of an evening at home, the patient ingested the Ambien with approximately six beers. The patient's wife noticed he had become dizzy and had slurred speech. He was nearly semicomatose, so she rushed him to the emergency department, where he was admitted secondary to a reaction to the Ambien ingested with alcohol.

Principal Diagnosis:	*967.8*	*Ambien (zolpidem tartrate) poisoning*
Secondary Diagnosis:	*980.0*	*Alcohol poisoning*
	780.4	*Dizziness*
	784.5	*Slurred speech*
	780.09	*Semicoma*
	E852.9	*Accidental poisoning, Ambien (other specified sleep pill)*
	E860.0	*Accidental poisoning, alcohol (beverage alcohol)*

Late Effects of Injuries and Poisonings

Late effects describe residual conditions that occur after the acute illness or injury has been treated. There is no time limit for reporting late effects. They are reported as often as the residual conditions warrant continuing medical treatment. As a general rule (i.e., unless the *Alphabetic Index to Diseases* directs otherwise), when reporting late effects, sequence the residual condition first, followed by the late-effects code. The late-effects code describes the past acute illness or injury that caused the residual condition to occur, and can be located under the main term "late effects" in the *Alphabetic Index to Diseases*. When coding for late effects, do not report the codes for the initial acute illness or injury, because these conditions no longer exist. Medical care is now being directed at the residual conditions (sequelae) of past illnesses or injuries. Although not often used by hospitals, a late-effect E code is available in the *Alphabetic Index to External Causes of Injury and Poisoning* that can be sequenced as an additional code to describe the past external circumstances that caused the initial injury to occur (e.g., late effect of an accidental fall: E929.3).

EXAMPLE	

Short limb secondary to fracture of the tibia and fibula on the right that occurred 10 years ago as a child from a head-on motor vehicle accident. The patient is now 20 years old.

736.81	*Short leg, acquired*
905.4	*Late effect of a fracture to the lower extremity*
E929.0	*Late effect of motor vehicle accident*

Malunion of a radial fracture, left arm. Three months before, the patient tripped and fell in a parking garage, fracturing the arm.

733.81	*Malunion of a fracture*
905.2	*Late effect of a fracture to an upper extremity*
E929.3	*Late effect of a fall*

Chronic liver dysfunction resulting from accidental overdose of acetaminophen (Tylenol) 2 years ago.

573.9	*Liver dysfunction*
909.0	*Late effect of poisoning*
E929.2	*Late effect of accidental poisoning*

Chronic renal insufficiency resulting from an adverse reaction to a previously prescribed nonsteroidal antiinflammatory antiarthritic medication taken 5 years ago.

585.9	*Chronic renal insufficiency*
909.5	*Late effect of an adverse effect of a drug*
E935.6	*Adverse effect of nonsteroidal antirheumatics, therapeutic use (under the main term "Late effect," the E Codes Index does not provide E codes to describe adverse effects attributable to the therapeutic use of a drug. Therefore, you must use the Table of Drugs and Chemicals to locate and identify the responsible drug [e.g., nonsteroidal antiinflammatory drug] and circumstance [e.g., therapeutic use])*

Classifying Child and Adult Abuse

Abuse, whether emotional, nutritional (i.e., neglect), physical, sexual, or psychological, is the intentional mistreatment of a person who lacks the physical prowess or the emotional capacity to resist the aggressive behavior of another person or persons. Children, elderly adults, and female spouses are most often the victims of abuse. Every state has legislation that requires the mandatory reporting of child and adult abuse by health-care providers to law-enforcement authorities. According to the Administration for Children and Families, for the calendar year 2002, an estimated 1,800,000 referrals alleging child abuse or neglect were accepted by state and local child protective services agencies for investigation. The referrals included more than 3 million children, and of those, approximately 896,000 children were determined to be victims of child abuse or neglect by child protective services agencies.[1] From the data that are being published regarding both child and adult abuse, it remains a serious problem. It is the coder's responsibility to accurately code conditions involving abuse to make it possible to report and retrieve patient data that advance the prevention of its occurrence.

Because the reporting of child and adult abuse is of primary importance, coders must follow specific coding guidelines for the sequencing of these cases. Sequencing of these codes follows this order:

1. the code for child or adult abuse is the principal diagnosis (located in the Disease Index under the main term "Abuse")
2. codes for injuries

3. the E code for the proximate cause of the injury (i.e., the circumstance that is directly responsible for the injury; located in the Alphabetic Index to External Causes of Injury and Poisoning)

4. the perpetrator E code, which describes who was responsible for the injury (located in the E Codes Index under the main term "Abuse")

A 5-year-old child was battered by her father for wetting the bed and was admitted for a skull fracture with intracerebral hemorrhage and fractured humerus. After 24 hours, the patient remained unconscious and nonarousable and was transferred to XYZ Children's Critical Care Hospital.

EXAMPLE

Principal Diagnosis:	*995.54*	*Abuse, child, physical*
	803.35	*Skull fracture with intracerebral hemorrhage, >24-hour loss of consciousness without return to preexisting conscious level*
	812.20	*Fractured humerus*
	E960.0	*Beatings, not otherwise specified*
	E967.0	*Abuse by father*

SUMMARY

This chapter has addressed the subject of coding for injuries and incidents of poisoning. Included is the following information: the pathology of common injuries and poisonings; the typical manifestations, complications, and treatments of injuries and poisonings in terms of their implications for coding; and the proper method of coding these complications.

REFERENCE

1. U.S. Department of Health and Human Services, Administration for Children & Families Summary Child Maltreatment 2002. Available at: http://www.acf.dhhs.gov/programs/ cb/publications/cm02/summary.htm. Accessed: September 21, 2004.

TESTING YOUR COMPREHENSION

1. When multiple injuries are present, which code is sequenced as the principal diagnosis?

2. What is the purpose of using E codes in terms of serious injuries?

3. What is considered a sentinel event in terms of reporting to a state authority?

4. If an automobile collides with a train, is the collision considered a motor vehicle mishap or a railway collision?

5. Distinguish a traumatic fracture from a pathologic fracture.

6. What is the intent of treatment for a displaced fracture?

7. What is an open reduction?

8. What are considered common sites for dislocations?

9. What is commonly involved in treating a dislocation?

10. What attaches muscles to bones?

11. What determines the sequencing of codes for open wounds or cellulitis?

12. What chapter should be consulted when attempting to locate a traumatic intracranial injury?

13. What chapter should be consulted when attempting to locate a nontraumatic intracranial injury?

14. What code category is used to classify injuries to blood vessels?

15. What code category is used to classify injuries to the nerves and the spinal cord?

16. What is often used by physicians to quickly assess the percentage of total body surface burned and the percentage involved with third-degree burns?

   _____

17. What is the purpose of the rule of nines?

   _____

18. Identify common terms on medical reports that indicate adverse effects resulting from the correct use of prescribed drugs.

   _____

19. How is a reaction to a prescribed medicine taken in conjunction with alcohol coded?

   _____

CODING PRACTICE I   Chapter Review Exercises

Directions

By using your ICD-9-CM codebook, code the following diagnoses and procedures:

	DIAGNOSIS/PROCEDURES	CODE
1	Subcapital hip fracture, right. Patient fell down steps while attending church. Right hip hemiarthroplasty (bipolar endoprosthesis).	
2	Right anterior shoulder dislocation. Patient fell off swing at playground. Reduction, right shoulder dislocation.	
3	Painful right ankle sprain. Twisted ankle while doing yard work at home.	
4	Lumbar strain secondary to lifting hay bales on his uncle's farm.	
5	Subdural hemorrhage, brief loss of consciousness. Patient fell in his bathroom and hit his head against the bathtub. Computed tomographic scan of head.	
6	Traumatic pneumothorax. Fracture of ribs $\times$ 5. Chest wall contusion. Status post auto collision—driver. Chest tube insertion (tube thoracostomy).	
7	Open wound, right forearm, with radial artery laceration. Chainsaw injury. Suture repair, radial artery.	
8	Open wound, right thumb, with laceration of digital nerve. Cut by electric knife while carving Thanksgiving turkey. Suture digital nerve.	
9	C6 vertebral fracture with spinal cord injury. Quadriplegia. Spinal shock. Injured diving into pool. Endotracheal intubation with prolonged mechanical ventilation >96 hours.	

	DIAGNOSIS/PROCEDURES	CODE
10	Status post fall on right hip. Fracture ruled out, hip contusion.	
11	Crush injury to left foot with large toe fracture. Patient dropped barbells on foot at gym.	
12	Fall from horse, with chest wall, left hip, and left orbital contusions. Open fracture, right distal tibia and fibula. Open reduction, internal fixation, tibial and fibular fracture, with casting. Debridement, open fracture site.	
13	Cat bite on right hand, infected.	
14	Traumatic amputation, left forearm. Traumatic shock. Farm accident. Hand caught in wood chipper. Disarticulation amputation of elbow.	
15	Second- and third-degree burns to the chest wall. Second-degree burns to face. Patient threw gasoline on charcoal grill.	
16	Sertraline (Zoloft) overdose secondary to suicide attempt. Depression, respiratory distress, diaphoresis, tremors.	
17	Gastrointestinal hemorrhage attributable to warfarin (Coumadin) toxicity. Coumadin prescribed for chronic atrial fibrillation. Chronic renal insufficiency. Liver dysfunction. Hypertension. Compensated CHF. Chronic obstructive pulmonary disease. Smoker. Long-term coumadinization.	
18	Keloid scar, chin, from previous burn injury. Scar revision, right cheek.	
19	Bimalleolar fracture, right ankle. Fall from bicycle. ORIF, right ankle fracture.	

	DIAGNOSIS/PROCEDURES	CODE
20	First- and second-degree sunburn to face, chest, and legs. Patient forgot her sun lotion and fell asleep at the beach today.	
21	Inhalation burn to lungs from chlorine fumes attributable to accidental chlorine spill while at work cleaning municipal swimming pool.	
22	Nondisplaced femoral neck fracture, right. Slipped on ice while shoveling snow in his driveway. Percutaneous pinning, right hip.	
23	Puncture wound with foreign body (nail), left hand. Patient accidentally shot hand with nail gun while working at construction site. Removal of foreign body (nail) imbedded in soft tissue, left hand.	
24	Gross hematuria secondary to kidney contusion on right. Patient was kicked in the back during a fight.	
25	Acute right knee injury with medial meniscus tear. Patient felt a sharp pain in the knee when kicking a soccer ball during a game yesterday. Arthroscopy with meniscectomy.	
26	First- and second-degree burns to face, neck, arms, and chest. Third-degree burn to tip of nose. Thirty percent total body burn. Burned from hot grease spill while cooking at home.	

CODING PRACTICE II   Medical Record Case Studies

Instructions

1. Carefully review the medical reports provided for each case study.
2. Research any abbreviations and terms that are unfamiliar or unclear.
3. Identify as many diagnoses and procedures as possible.
4. Because only part of the patient's total record is available, determine what additional documentation you might need.
5. If appropriate, identify any questions you might ask the physician to code this case correctly and completely.
6. Complete the appropriate blanks below for each case study.

CHAPTER 17 CASE STUDIES

Case Study 17.1 (Coder/Abstract Summary Form)

Patient: **Jane Doe**

Patient documentation: **Review Medical Reports 17.1, 17.2, and 17.3**

1. Principal diagnosis:

   _____

2. Secondary or other diagnoses:

   _____

3. Principal procedure:

   _____

4. Other procedures:

   _____

5. Additional documentation needed:

   _____

   _____

   _____

   _____

Case Study 17.1 (Continued)

6. Questions for the physician:

_____

_____

_____

_____

_____

MEDICAL REPORT 17.1

DISCHARGE SUMMARY

PATIENT:	DOE, JANE
MED REC NO:	999999
ATTN PHYSICIAN:	SMITH, MD

DISCHARGE DIAGNOSIS:

1. Impacted subcapital fracture, left hip.

2. Displaced surgical neck fracture, left proximal humerus.

3. Marked emphysema.

HOSPITAL COURSE: This 76-year-old lady fell and sustained a fracture of the left shoulder and the left hip, and was admitted to the hospital for care. The patient has a history of quite severe emphysema and is oxygen dependent three liters per minute. Examination revealed pain about the left shoulder and some swelling. Also pain about the left hip. Review of x-rays showed a displaced surgical neck fracture of the left shoulder and left hip is impacted slightly valgus subcapital fracture. It should also be noted that she had a stroke several years ago which has left the left upper extremity useless and she does not use it at all. Also, she is weak on the left side but has been able to walk. With the severe emphysema, it was felt that general anesthesia was too much of a risk so spinal anesthesia was selected and the hip was pinned and the left shoulder was treated with a sling.

On day two under spinal anesthesia, the left hip was pinned percutaneously with three cannulated screws. Postoperatively she did well and was quite stable. Hematocrit was 32.0, hemoglobin 10.9.

On the second postoperative day the patient's dressing was removed from the left hip and there was no active drainage and there was no redness. The compression bandage was removed and left off. The patient is being discharged to skilled nursing facility for rehabilitation with touch-down weightbearing only on the left. She will continue wearing a sling. The patient should have a follow-up x-ray of the left shoulder within two weeks, a follow-up x-ray of the left hip should be obtained within a month. The patient has sutures of the left hip that should be removed in about ten days. The patient will be continued on the same medication that she has been taking at home. Also Extra-Strength Tylenol one to two every four hours p.r.n. for pain.

_____

DR. SMITH, M.D.

NOTES

MEDICAL REPORT 17.2

PREOPERATIVE HISTORY AND PHYSICAL

PATIENT:	DOE, JANE
MED REC NO:	999999
ATTN PHYSICIAN:	SMITH, MD

CHIEF COMPLAINT: Pain left shoulder and left hip.

HISTORY OF PRESENT ILLNESS: This 76-year-old lady tripped and fell in her mobile home today and states that she fell very hard on the left shoulder and the left side of her body. After the fall, she had pain in the left shoulder and left hip. The patient was brought to the Emergency Room of ABC Memorial Hospital for care and was complaining of pain in the left hip and left shoulder, and was admitted for care. The patient has had some difficulties with her health including emphysema and usually is on 3 L of oxygen most all the time.

MEDICAL/SURGICAL HISTORY: Operations: She has had two cesarean sections, carotid endarterectomy right side 1996, tonsillectomy as a child, a femoral-popliteal graft on the left side in 1997. Medical: A stroke about 1999, mainly affecting her left side, mostly her left arm. She has been ambulatory. Diabetes mellitus, hyperlipidemia, depression.

MEDICATIONS: Medications are Zocor 20 mg one daily, Nexium one tablet daily for a hiatal hernia with GERDs. She takes enteric aspirin 325 mg daily, Zoloft 50 mg daily. She takes a nebulizer four times a day, she says is a 150 Duo-Neb 3m/5mg INH 3 ml DE4.

ALLERGIES: SHE IS ALLERGIC TO PENICILLIN.

REVIEW OF BODY SYSTEMS:

HEENT: Bilateral cataracts. Hearing is good.

CHEST: Emphysema. She smoked for more than fifty years, 1-1/2 packs a day. She quit about thirteen years ago.

GI: Good appetite: She states she has a hiatal hernia.

GU: No complaints.

NEUROMUSCULAR: Weak on the left side.

PHYSICAL EXAMINATION:

GENERAL: Physical examination reveals a well-developed, well-nourished lady that appears to be in reasonable health for her age.

VITAL SIGNS: Temperature 98.0, pulse 108, respirations 24, blood pressure 220/70. Weight 107 lbs, 5 foot tall.

HEAD: Examination of her head: Normocephalic. The patient has slight tenderness on the left side of her head.

EYES: Pupils appear equal.

NOSE: Midline.

THROAT: No injection.

NECK: Fairly good motion without pain.

CHEST: No congestion of her lungs.

HEART: Regular rhythm. Did not hear a murmur.

ABDOMEN: Flat, soft, nontender.

MEDICAL REPORT 17.2 (CONTINUED)

EXTREMITIES: Left hand is curled up into sharp flexion and it does not appear that she uses this. There is pain and swelling around the left shoulder, slight tenderness over the left hip.

DIAGNOSTIC DATA: X-rays of the left shoulder show a surgical neck fracture that is transverse and the shaft is displaced medially. X-rays of the left hip show slightly valgus, impacted subcapital fracture.

ADMISSION DIAGNOSIS:

1. Displaced fracture left proximal humeral neck.
2. Impacted surgical neck fracture, left hip.
3. Emphysema, oxygen-dependent.
4. Stroke, left side.

PLAN: I talked with the patient and with her son about the situation. It appears that consideration of stabilizing her humeral fracture with a rod may make her care more simple. There is some risk of putting the rod in. The patient is having pain in her arm.

The left hip plan is to do a percutaneous or a small incision with compression or multiple screw fixation in situ. The patient is slightly at more risk because of her lung situation. Risks, benefits, alternatives discussed. Gives informed consent.

_____

DR. SMITH, M.D.

NOTES

OPERATIVE REPORT

PATIENT: DOE, JANE

MED REC NO: 999999

ATTN PHYSICIAN: SMITH, MD

DATE OF SURGERY:

PREOPERATIVE DIAGNOSIS: Impacted valgus subcapital fracture of the left hip.

POSTOPERATIVE DIAGNOSIS: Impacted valgus subcapital fracture of the left hip.

OPERATION: Left hip pinning, with 6.5 cannulated screws.

DESCRIPTION OF OPERATION: After satisfactory spinal anesthesia, the patient in the supine position on the C-arm table, the left hip and entire left lower extremity was prepared and draped free in the usual manner. The arm was brought into position and the pin was placed in the hip joint area, to find the proper lateral opening to go up through the neck and head. A #11 blade was used to make room for inserting a Steinmann pin. An eighth-inch Steinmann pin was brought to the lateral surface of the femur, which was palpated with the end of the pin, and the center was found. The C-arm was then used to pick the right spot to enter, and then the pin, as handle, was brought up somewhat more superior, so that a more straight-in entrance could be made for starting the pin, and then it was scooted up through the head. A second pin laterally was started slightly superior and run up through the center of the head, and the superior pin also was placed. The patient was brought up into frog-legged position to check the lateral, which was satisfactory. The drilling was then carried out over the pins to start them, and also drilling was carried up along the calcar; 85- and 95-mm screws were used. These went in snugly, and the pinning looked very good. Anterior and posterior films were received.

The wounds were washed and then a single 3-0 Ethilon suture was used to bring each of the 3 stab wounds in the skin together, 4s were applied, with Elastoplast tape. The patient tolerated the procedure well.

_____

DR. SMITH, M.D.

NOTES

Case Study 17.2 (Coder/Abstract Summary Form)

Patient: **Helen Jackson**

Patient documentation: **Review Medical Reports 17.4 and 17.5**

1. Principal diagnosis:

   _____

2. Secondary or other diagnoses:

   _____

3. Principal procedure:

   _____

4. Other procedures:

   _____

5. Additional documentation needed:

   _____

   _____

   _____

   _____

6. Questions for the physician:

   _____

   _____

   _____

   _____

MEDICAL REPORT 17.4

HISTORY AND PHYSICAL

PATIENT: JACKSON, Helen
DOB:
MED REC: 111111
PT ADMN:
ADMN DTE:
LOCATION:
PHYSICIAN: SMITH, MD

CHIEF COMPLAINT: Ms. Jackson is a 71-year-old female patient who lost her balance and fell down a hill onto her left upper extremity.

HISTORY OF PRESENT ILLNESS: The patient presented to the ER where she was evaluated and found to have a comminuted fracture of the right humeral head and proximal humeral shaft.

MEDICAL HISTORY: The patient's medical history is significant for diabetes mellitus and hypertension.

ALLERGIES: The patient has an allergy to penicillin.

CURRENT MEDICATIONS: Glucophage, insulin, Humalog 15 units q.a.m., and Humulin N 42 units q.a.m. and 55 units q.p.m. The patient also takes Zestoretic. Tenormin. Atacand/HCTZ tablets.

PHYSICAL EXAM: The patient is alert and oriented × 3. She has no history of loss of consciousness.

SKIN: Significant for contusion over the left thumb. Swelling at the left thumb at the metacarpal phalangeal joint.

EXTREMITIES: The patient's right upper extremity is contained within a shoulder immobilizer. The patient has intact neurovascular status to the right upper extremity. Sensation is intact. The patient has contusion, ecchymosis, and a positive radial stress test of the left thumb.

HEENT: The patient is normocephalic, atraumatic. Pupils are equally round and reactive to light. Sclera is white. ENT clear. The patient's neck is supple. Trachea is midline.

CHEST: Clear to auscultation and percussion.

CARDIAC: Exam regular rhythm and rate.

ABDOMEN: Round, soft, bowel sounds present.

GENITOURINARY AND RECTAL: Omitted.

DIAGNOSTIC IMPRESSION:
1. Comminuted humeral head and proximal shaft fracture, right upper extremity.
2. Rotator cuff tear.

PLAN: At this time, the patient will be scheduled for prosthetic replacement. The risks and benefits of said procedure were reviewed with the patient. The patient has a severely comminuted fracture. There is no alternative. The patient will require reconstruction of the rotator cuff and metaphysis with a prosthetic device.

_____
DR. SMITH, M.D.

MEDICAL REPORT 17.5

OPERATIVE REPORT

PATIENT: JACKSON, Helen

DOB:

MED REC: 111111

PT ADMN:

ADMN DTE:

LOCATION:

PHYSICIAN: SMITH, MD

Date of Operation:

PREOPERATIVE DIAGNOSIS: Comminuted right humeral head fracture, torn rotator cuff, right shoulder.

POSTOPERATIVE DIAGNOSIS: Comminuted right humeral head fracture, torn rotator cuff, right shoulder.

PROCEDURE PERFORMED:

1. Hemiarthroplasty, right shoulder.
2. Reconstruction of right rotator cuff.

SURGEON:

ANESTHESIA: General.

ANESTHESIOLOGIST:

EBL: 250-300 cc.

COMPLICATIONS: None.

PROCEDURE IN DETAIL: The patient was taken to the OR where she was placed in the supine position and general anesthetic was initiated. After endotracheal tube was established, the patient was brought to the beach chair position and the patient's right upper extremity was prepped and draped in the usual sterile fashion. Using a #10 blade, an anterior saber type incision was made at the level of the junction of the pectoralis and deltoid. Using a combination of sharp and blunt dissection technique, the subcutaneous tissues were incised and explored. The interval between the anterior deltoid and pectoralis was entered and the dissection to the deltopectoral groove was developed. The cephalic vein was identified and retracted out of harms way. Contributories to the brachiocephalic vein were tied, ligated or coagulated as they were encountered. This revealed the fracture site. It is noteworthy that at the level of the supraspinatus and subscapularis there was a vertical split and at the rotator cuff, there was a fragmented portion of the humeral head which was anterior, inferior, and presented the shell of the humeral head and its attachment to the subscapularis and portion of the supraspinatus.

The remainder of the supraspinatus and infraspinatus went posteriorly. There were a large number of bone fragments contained at the fracture site. The fracture site was then debrided extensively of all bone fragments. The patient's remaining humeral head and neck was resected using an oscillating saw and using the prosthetic bursa as a reference for cutting. The patient's femoral canal was then drilled to accept a size 11 component. The bursa accepted a size 11 component.

Continued

Trial components were placed. Great care was taken to maintain adequate height, to avoid compromising the deltoid function postoperatively. Great care was made to maintain proper aversion, so that we would avoid compression, anteversion, and retroversion. The trial component was placed and found to be in excellent position. Stable with abduction, forward flexion. The patient's wound was then irrigated copiously with normal saline. The distal bone fragments were removed. The canal was prepped and dried, and the Bigliani modular humeral stem was then placed and cemented to the humeral shaft. The humeral head was attached. It was a 46 spherical humeral head x 24 mm height. The patient's shoulder was again reduced and found to be stable. The rotator cuff was repaired using interrupted sutures of 2-0 Tycron to repair the defect at the junction of the subscapularis and supraspinatus tendon. Prior to repairing the defect, sutures had been passed through the Bigliani component, fins with holes, for attachment of the rotator cuff to the component. The patient's wound was then irrigated copiously with normal saline lavage. A large bore drain was placed into the substance of the wound. The rotator cuff was observed to be attached well to the component. The interval at the level of the deltopectoral groove was repaired using interrupted sutures of #0 Vicryl. The subcutaneous tissue was approximated with 2-0 Vicryl, and the skin was approximated with staples. Compressive dressing applied to the patient's shoulder. The patient was returned to the Recovery Room in stable, satisfactory condition.

DR. SMITH, M.D.

NOTES

Case Study 17.3 (Coder/Abstract Summary Form)

Patient: **Anna Campbell**

Patient documentation: **Review Medical Reports 17.6 and 17.7**

1. Principal diagnosis:

   _____

   _____

2. Secondary or other diagnoses:

   _____

3. Principal procedure:

   _____

4. Other procedures:

   _____

5. Additional documentation needed:

   _____

   _____

   _____

6. Questions for the physician:

   _____

   _____

   _____

MEDICAL REPORT 17.6

DISCHARGE SUMMARY

PT NAME: CAMPBELL, Anna
MR#:   222222
ADMISSION DATE:
DISCHARGE DATE:
ATTENDING PHYSICIAN: Smith, M.D.
ADMISSION DIAGNOSIS: UNRESPONSIVENESS
DISCHARGE DIAGNOSIS: PHENOBARBITAL OVERDOSE
                         NONCOMPLIANCE
                         ORGANIC BRAIN SYNDROME
                         SEIZURE DISORDER
                         TRANSIENT NEUTROPENIA
                         CHRONIC OBSTRUCTIVE PULMONARY DISEASE
                         ATELECTASIS
                         NICOTINE DEPENDENCE
                         ANEMIA OF CHRONIC DISEASE
                         VENTILATOR DEPENDENCE
                         MILD AORTIC STENOSIS
                         POSSIBLE LEFT LOWER LUNG PNEUMONIA

PROGNOSIS: Probably good.

HPI/HOSPITAL COURSE: This is an 80-year-old woman who presented unresponsive and was supported with mechanical ventilation for three or four days. She gradually became better, was able to breathe, and has slowly awakened. She was found to have a phenobarbital level greater than 100. This had been a problem in the past with noncompliance with her medications. She was observed without any seizure medications on the long term care unit. Likely, she will be started with a low dose seizure treatment, perhaps once a day phenobarbital, but she will be observed to see how she does without any medications at all. She is expected to do well and is continuing to approach her baseline mental status.

LABORATORY DATA: Please refer to above HPI/Hospital Course and patient's chart.

DISCHARGE INSTRUCTIONS: Diet: As tolerated. Activity: As tolerated with seizure precautions. Medications: Tylenol p.r.n. Follow-up is in long term care unit.

_____

Smith, MD

HISTORY AND PHYSICAL

PT NAME: CAMPBELL, Anna

MR#: 222222

ADMISSION DATE:

ATTENDING PHYSICIAN: Smith, M.D.

CHIEF COMPLAINT: UNRESPONSIVENESS

HPI: The patient is an 80-year-old widowed housewife with a history of lifelong seizure disorder. She did not answer telephone calls from her brother from about 4:30 on, and a neighbor went over to check on her and found her unresponsive in a chair. Apparently, she was dressed. There was no note of any incontinence. An ambulance was called and she was intubated in the field. She was said to have nonreactive pinpoint pupils, but this improved with ventilation and she now has midpoint reactive pupils. Basically, she has only reflex movements and was unresponsive for several hours.

Her niece reports that she had been complaining of a fair amount of dizziness lately and was using her walker. About a month ago, her Phenobarbital level was quite high and some adjustments were made in her medication. The Phenobarbital level from about two weeks ago was satisfactory at 37 and 40, but the one today is 107. Her Dilantin level was low a month ago, is not satisfactory at 14. Her brother does not think that the patient is confused and mixing up her pills. Nor does he feel that she is depressed and would have taken an overdose.

MEDICAL HISTORY: She has had seizure disorder since a child. She had hip fracture repaired in 1998. Apparently, at that time, she was having dizziness and falls. Both the Dilantin and phenobarbital levels were somewhat high at 24.88 and 51.6, respectively, at that time.

ALLERGIES: None are recorded.

MEDICATIONS: Phenobarbital 200 mg twice daily, Dilantin 100 mg twice daily, as well as Slow-Mag 3 times daily.

SOCIAL HISTORY: The patient has been widowed for over 20 years. She lives alone. She no longer drives a car, but does walk to the store and does her own cooking. She is still a smoker of about a half pack per day. She is not a drinker at all.

FAMILY HISTORY: Longevity, with her brother aged 88 and living independently. She had a sister who was diabetic and died at age 70. There are several other siblings who have passed on at advanced ages and two died young in accidents.

PHYSICAL EXAMINATION—GENERAL APPEARANCE: The patient is a rather tall, somewhat gaunt, older female on a ventilator.

VITAL SIGN: BP in the ER was 120/67, Temp 95.2.

HEENT: Eyes are closed, when held open they deviate from each other. Pupils are about 3 mm and reactive. Movements did not elicit any extraocular movements. Fundi are obscured by opacity bilaterally. She is edentulous. There is an endotracheal tube in the mouth.

NECK: No cervical adenopathy or thyromegaly. No bruits are heard in the neck. Carotid pulse adequate.

PMI: Adequate. Heart is not palpable—rhythm is regular.

LUNGS: Fairly good air entry with ventilator cycle.

BREAST: Negative.

ABDOMEN: Flat to scaphoid. There is a lower midline incision, which is well healed. There are ventral hernias bilaterally.

EXTREMITIES: Pulses are decreased. The legs appear puffy but are nonpitting. Elicited vague disturbed posturing in the arms. Toes are up-going bilaterally.

LABORATORY STUDIES: Normal sinus rhythm with 1 PCA. Chest x-ray is at a rather poorly positioned rotated film, but is probably clear. Chest CT is said to be normal.

Continued

MEDICAL REPORT 17.7 (CONTINUED)

Phenobarbital level of 170. pH: 14. White count: 3,300. Platelets: 13.7. Hemoglobin: 12.3. MCV: Elevated at 102.5.

IMPRESSION: UNCONSCIOUS OF UNCLEAR ETIOLOGY—POSSIBLE POSTICTAL STATE FROM A BREAKTHROUGH SEIZURE— But with the supratherapeutic levels, that seems unlikely. She may be in a barbiturate coma with a level that high. She may have anoxic encephalopathy secondary to either of the above or possibly to a cardiac arrhythmia.

PLAN: The patient will be maintained on the ventilator overnight and we will attempt to wean her, if the gasses allow. Continue Dilantin IV. Hold phenobarbital. Her living will was discussed with the patient's brother and he agrees that the stipulations with permanent unconsciousness do not apply. Therefore, the patient is a candidate for resuscitation in the event of cardiac arrest.

_____

Smith, MD

NOTES

Case Study 17.4 (Coder/Abstract Summary Form)

Patient: **Trudy Simpson**

Patient documentation: **Review Medical Reports 17.8, 17.9, and 17.10**

1. Principal diagnosis:

   _____

2. Secondary or other diagnoses:

   _____

3. Principal procedure:

   _____

4. Other procedures:

   _____

5. Additional documentation needed:

   _____

   _____

   _____

6. Questions for the physician:

   _____

   _____

   _____

   _____

MEDICAL REPORT 17.8

DISCHARGE SUMMARY

PATIENT: SIMPSON, Trudy

DOB:

MED REC: 333333

PT ADM/NO:

ADMIT DATE:

LOCATION:

PHYSICIAN: SMITH, MD

DATE OF ADMISSION:

DATE OF DISCHARGE:

FINAL DIAGNOSES:

1. Left femoral neck fracture.

2. Paroxysmal atrial fibrillation, converted to sinus rhythm.

3. Electrolyte imbalance. Spasms.

4. Urinary tract infection. Rash secondary to Bactrim.

5. History of previous multiple cerebrovascular accidents with a mild dementia.

6. Hypertensive heart disease without congestive heart failure.

7. Abnormal PT.

REASON FOR ADMISSION: Fall with inability to ambulate and left hip pain. The patient is a 79-year-old woman with a history of previous CVA, hypertensive heart disease, and a mild dementia. She was fine until the day of her admission, when she fell while trying to ambulate with her walker. She subsequently presented to the ER where she was found to have a probable compression fracture of L1. She was subsequently admitted to the medical floor. On the second day of admission she was noted to have marked tenderness on the left hip. Subsequent x-ray of the left hip revealed a femoral neck fracture. Please refer to the admission history and physical. At that time Dr. Ortho did a repair of the left hip fracture. He did an open reduction and internal fixation of the left intertrochanteric hip fracture. She had two units of blood for falling hematocrit/blood loss anemia postoperatively. A second consultation with Dr. Nerve of the neuro service saw the patient for spasms, and he evaluated with studies that included carotid Doppler and EEG and that did not show any significant pathology.

PERTINENT LABORATORY STUDIES: An x-ray of the left hip showed a left intertrochanteric fracture. An MRI of the spine showed multilevel degenerative disk disease with no acute fracture. Echocardiogram showed an abnormal left ventricular function with an EF of 65%.

HOSPITAL COURSE: The patient was placed on Lasix while Coumadin was put on hold. Postoperatively she developed an atrial fibrillation that was controlled with Toprol, Digoxin, and Verapamil. Currently, the patient is in sinus rhythm; she is currently on Toprol and Digoxin. In view of the minimal LV function, the Digoxin will be put on hold. She was on anticoagulation prior to admission for two previous ischemic strokes. In view of the history of atrial fibrillation, the need for Coumadin therapy is apparent. On admission, she had a spasm of the left hand and wrist. Serum calcium was obtained that was normal, however, magnesium and phosphates were severely low. Apparently, as of now, the abnormalities are corrected. The patient developed a urinary tract infection postoperatively with culture demonstrating >100,000 colonies of E-coli. She was started on Bactrim p.o. but developed a diffuse rash so this was changed to Keflex. The patient is stable now, she is afebrile and she will be discharged to rehab facility. For now, she is able to transfer from the bed to the chair with assistance but she is not able to ambulate.

MEDICAL REPORT 17.8 (CONTINUED)

DISCHARGE MEDICATIONS: (1) Lactulose 60 mg p.r.n. q.h.s., (2) Darvocet 1 tablet q.6h p.r.n. pain. (3) Levothroid 0.075 mg q.d. (4) Lipitor 10 mg q.d. (5) Remeron 15 mg q.hs. (6) OsCal 500+D l t.i.d. (7) Coumadin 3 mg q.d. (8) Diovan 160 mg q.d. (9) Magnesium chloride 400-l t.i.d. (10) Neutra-Phos 1 tab q.i.d. (11) Megace 100 mg q.i.d. (12) Toprol 50-mg q.d. (Metoprolol 50 mg. b.i.d. may be substituted for Toprol).

Smith, MD

NOTES

CONSULTATION

PATIENT:	SIMPSON, Trudy
DOB:	
MED REC:	333333
PT ADM/NO:	
ADMIT DATE:	
LOCATION:	
PHYSICIAN:	SMITH, MD

DATE OF CONSULTATION:

REFERRING PHYSICIAN: Smith, MD

CONSULTING PHYSICIAN: Ortho, MD

CHIEF COMPLAINT: Back and left hip pain.

HISTORY: This is a 79-year-old female who apparently fell. She was seen at the ER and admitted to the medical service with a compression fracture. The patient continued to complain of left hip pain. Orthopedics was consulted after x-rays demonstrated a left intertrochanteric hip fracture.

PHYSICAL EXAMINATION: Demonstrates an alert, elderly white female complaining of left hip pain. Her neck and back are nontender. Pelvis is nontender. She has an obvious deformity to the left hip with the leg abducted. Motor sensory intact distally.

X-ray of the left hip demonstrates a comminuted osteopenic left intertrochanteric hip fracture.

PERTINENT LABORATORY: The patient had a history of Coumadin anticoagulation and PT is 19.9 with an INR of 2.7 earlier today.

IMPRESSION: Closed left intertrochanteric hip fracture.

PLAN: Open reduction and internal fixation of the left intertrochanteric hip fracture when PT returns to within normal limits. Will start vitamin K and follow serial PT, PTT.

_____

Smith, MD

MEDICAL REPORT 17.10

OPERATIVE REPORT

PATIENT: SIMPSON, Trudy

DOB:

MED REC: 333333

PT ADM/NO:

ADMIT DATE:

LOCATION:

PHYSICIAN: SMITH, MD

DATE OF PROCEDURE:

SURGEON: Dr. Ortho

PREOPERATIVE DIAGNOSIS: Closed osteopenic left intertrochanteric hip fracture.

POSTOPERATIVE DIAGNOSIS: Closed osteopenic left intertrochanteric hip fracture.

PROCEDURE PERFORMED: Open reduction and internal fixation, left intertrochanteric hip fracture (Osteonics OHS 135-degree four-hole side plate with 80 mm lag screw).

ANESTHESIA: General endotracheal.

ESTIMATED BLOOD LOSS: 75 cc.

DRAINS: One Hemovac.

COMPLICATIONS: None.

INDICATIONS: The patient is a 79-year-old female who fell, sustaining an injury to her left hip. She was admitted to the medical service of the hospital. Orthopedics was consulted for her left hip fracture. The patient was found to have a left intertrochanteric hip fracture. The patient has been on Coumadin anticoagulation prior to her admission. Therefore, she was maintained on bed rest until her prothrombin time returned to normal limits. After reviewing the severity of the injury with the patient, including the risks, benefits, and rehabilitative course of the planned procedure, she presents for open reduction and internal fixation of the left intertrochanteric hip fracture.

Informed consent was obtained.

DESCRIPTION OF PROCEDURE: After satisfactory general endotracheal anesthesia was established by the anesthesiologist, the patient was placed on the fracture table. The right lower extremity was placed in a padded leg holder. The left lower extremity was placed in a padded fracture boot. A preoperative reduction maneuver was performed. Satisfactory reduction of the comminuted fracture was confirmed in both the AP and lateral C-arm planes.

Therefore, the left hip area was prepped and draped in the usual sterile manner. Ancef 1 gm was administered preoperatively intravenously.

A longitudinal incision over the lateral proximal hip was made. Dissection was carried down to the subcutaneous tissues, the fascia lata and vastus lateralis fascia. Bleeding was controlled with electrocautery. Blunt dissection was used to divide the vastus lateralis muscle in line with its fibers. Subperiosteal dissection was used to expose the lateral cortex of the proximal femur.

Under C-arm guidance, a guide pin was placed across the fracture site into the center of the femoral head. Satisfactory guide pin placement was confirmed in both the AP and lateral C-arm planes. The guide pin was then measured, reamed, and an 80-mm lag screw placed, followed by a 135-degree four-hold side plate. The side plate screw holes were drilled, measured, and screws placed in the standard fashion. A compression screw was placed with satisfactory compression noted.

Prior to closure of the surgical site, satisfactory reduction of the fracture and alignment of the hardware construct were confirmed in both the AP and lateral C-arm planes.

Continued

MEDICAL REPORT 17.10 (CONTINUED)

The wound was irrigated with normal saline. A Hemovac drain was placed deep to the fascia. The vastus lateralis fascia was closed with running #1 Vicryl. The fascia lata was closed with running #1 Vicryl. The subcutaneous tissue was closed with running 2-0 Vicryl. The skin was closed with staples. Xeroform and sterile dressing were applied.

The patient tolerated the procedure well and was taken to the recovery room in stable condition.

_____

Ortho, MD

NOTES

Case Study 17.5 (Coder/Abstract Summary Form)

Patient: **John Doe**

Patient documentation: **Review Medical Reports 17.11, 17.12, and 17.13**

1. Principal diagnosis:

   _____

2. Secondary or other diagnoses:

   _____

3. Principal procedure:

   _____

4. Other procedures:

   _____

5. Additional documentation needed:

   _____

   _____

   _____

6. Questions for the physician:

   _____

   _____

   _____

   _____

MEDICAL REPORT 17.11

DISCHARGE SUMMARY

PATIENT: DOE, JOHN

DOB:

MED REC:

PT ADM/NO:

ADMIT DATE:

LOCATION:

PHYSICIAN: SMITH, MD

DATE OF ADMISSION:

DATE OF DISCHARGE:

PRINCIPAL DIAGNOSIS:

1. Metabolic acidosis, secondary to toxin ingestion and beta-blocker overdose.

This 60-year-old patient ingested multiple meds including Lopressor, Seroquel, Dilantin, Protonix, and aspirin and presented to the emergency room essentially comatose, blood pressure of 86 systolic with pulse in the low 40s. He had admitted he had been depressed and was using this as a suicide attempt.

He was admitted to the intensive care unit where he was given dopamine. His hypokalemia was corrected. He was given glucose supplementation for resolution of his ketoacidosis secondary to sopropyl alcohol. His cardiac catheterization reports were reviewed and angioplasty in the past. Fortunately, he had no evidence of myocardial infarction while in the hospital. His T4 was initially slightly high and his T3 thyroxine index was normal.

All electrolyte values returned to normal. His BUN was 2, creatinine 0.7, calcium was 8.5, still slightly low. Other metabolic parameters were normal.

His electrocardiogram shows normal sinus rhythm, with moderate voltage criteria of left ventricular hypertrophy. He can resume his Lopressor, Protonix, Seroquel, and Bextra as before. I have some samples of Aciphex or Prevacid that I can give him to substitute for the Protonix and I believe we have some extra samples that he can use as needed. No tranquilizers, narcotics, or anxiolytics were prescribed.

The patient is to follow up with his psychiatrist. He can resume care with his previous primary care physician for follow-up of his blood pressure.

CONDITION OF DISCHARGE: Stable.

Smith, MD

HISTORY AND PHYSICAL

PATIENT: DOE, JOHN

DOB:

MED REC:

PT ADM/NO:

ADMIT DATE:

LOCATION:

PHYSICIAN: SMITH, MD

DATE OF ADMISSION:

REASON FOR ADMISSION: Suicide attempt.

HISTORY OF PRESENT ILLNESS: This is a 60-year-old white male, on Lopressor and other medications, who developed feelings of uselessness and therefore took a bag of his medications including Lopressor. Thirty minutes after he ingested the pills, he came to the emergency room and received lavage. However, his pressure and pulse proceeded to deteriorate. His pulse dropped to the 40s. His sensorium became drowsy. He entered a semicomatose state. His blood pressure plummeted to less than 90 systolic and he required a dopamine drip as well as atropine. He was admitted to the intensive care unit.

MEDICAL HISTORY: This reveals he has been on Lopressor for control of blood pressure.

FAMILY HISTORY: Family history of heart disease.

SOCIAL HISTORY: He is divorced and lives alone. No children.

REVIEW OF SYSTEMS: Review shows emaciation, pallor, and weakness. Currently he is semicomatose. He is breathing spontaneously and has a gag reflex. The patient has no grimace. He does not appear to have chest pain or dyspnea. No dysuria. He does have apparently a history of genitourinary surgery. No melena. No leg swelling. He is semicomatose.

PHYSICAL EXAMINATION

VITAL SIGNS: On admission his vital signs were initially stable, and then they deteriorated, with blood pressure down to 88/56, pulse down in the 40s range on monitor—approximately 45, respirations 20, temperature afebrile.

SKIN: Pale.

HEENT: Unremarkable. Pupils are equal.

NECK: Supple.

HEART: S1 and S2; slow rate.

LUNGS: Coarse.

CHEST: Barrel chest.

ABDOMEN: No organomegaly.

GU: Grossly intact. Condom catheter in place.

EXTREMITIES: Decreased range of motion.

NEUROLOGICAL: Semicomatose; cannot cooperate with the rest of the examination. Facies appears to be symmetric.

Continued

MEDICAL REPORT 17.12 (CONTINUED)

ASSESSMENT & PLAN: Lopressor overdose with resultant hypotension and bradycardia. Admit to the intensive care unit. Obtain counseling about his depression, suicide attempt, and feelings. Will try to improve his self-esteem. Consult psychiatry for his depression/suicide attempt. Intravenous fluids. Follow closely. He may need intubation if his respiratory tract becomes compromised.

Smith, MD

NOTES

MEDICAL REPORT 17.13

CONSULTATION

PATIENT: DOE, JOHN

DOB:

MED REC:

PT ADM/NO:

ADMIT DATE:

LOCATION:

PHYSICIAN: SMITH, MD

DATE OF CONSULTATION:

ATTENDING PHYSICIAN: SMITH, MD

REQUESTING PHYSICIAN: SMITH, MD

CONSULTING PHYSICIAN: JONES, MD

REASON FOR CONSULTATION: Acute renal failure in a patient who took a multisubstance overdose.

HISTORY OF PRESENT ILLNESS: The patient is a 60-year-old gentleman who is retired who was admitted after he ingested aspirin, Lopressor, Protonix, and Seroquel and apparently also drank a bottle of rubbing alcohol. On admission, he was confused and was found to be acidotic. Nephrology was consulted but was not on call this weekend and will see the patient two days later. During the ensuing two days, his creatinine has gone from 1.1 up to 2.5. He remains non-oliguric. He has stable vital signs at the present time.

The patient presently complains of a severe headache and some abdominal discomfort. He does have an NG tube in place and there is a slight amount of NG suction. He denies any history of renal disease.

LABORATORY DATA: On admission: sodium 144; potassium 3.3; CO 108; CO2 26; BUN 19; creatinine 1.1; normal liver function tests. Lab work from yesterday showed sodium 143; potassium 3.2; CO 112; CO2 23; creatinine 2.5; BUN 21. URINALYSIS: Specific gravity 1.020; pH 6; ketones 15; protein 30 mg/dL. Blood 2-4 red blood cells/high power field, although this was a catheterized urine. SALICYLATE LEVEL: less than 4.0 on admission. pH showed 7.25; pCO2 56; pO2 79.

MEDICAL HISTORY: Hypertension. Significant depression. Mild degenerative joint disease.

REVIEW OF SYSTEMS: No visual disturbances. There has been no fever or chills. He has been feeling quite depressed. He is presently having a headache and abdominal discomfort. No vomiting or gagging. He notes no chest pain.

PHYSICAL EXAMINATION

GENERAL: The patient is a well-developed, thin male who appears unkempt.

VITAL SIGNS: Blood pressure 112/78; pulse 74 and regular; respirations 20.

HEENT: Sclerae anicteric. Conjunctivae pink. Buccal mucosa is moist. There is an NG tube in place.

NECK: Reveals flat neck veins.

CHEST: Symmetric.

LUNGS: Bilateral rhonchi on expiration.

HEART: Regular rate and rhythm, without gallop, rub, or murmur.

ABDOMEN: Soft, nontender. Bowel sounds are active.

Continued

MEDICAL REPORT 17.13 (CONTINUED)

EXTREMITIES: Reveal no edema.

NEUROLOGIC: Grossly intact.

ASSESSMENT:

1. Acute renal failure—perhaps prerenal, but could be related to ingestion of nephrotoxic agent.
2. Multisubstance overdose.
3. Respiratory acidosis associated with bronchospasm and CO_2 retention.

RECOMMENDATIONS:

1. Repeat urinalysis.
2. Repeat basic metabolic profile.
3. Ultrasound of the kidneys.

Thank you for this consultation. Will follow up the patient with you and make further recommendations as necessary.

_____

Jones, MD

NOTES

Coding for Complications of Surgical and Medical Care

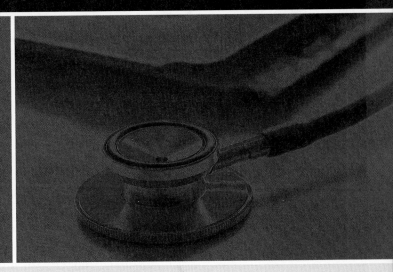

Chapter Outline

Nosocomial Versus Iatrogenic Adverse Effects or Events

Medical Staff Bylaws

Sequencing Complication Codes

Complications of Medical Devices, Implants, and Grafts

Complications of Transplanted Organs

Nonspecific Complication Codes That Describe General Body Systems

Complications Causing Outpatient to Inpatient Admission Within 72 Hours

Other Indicators of Complications of Surgical and Medical Care

Testing Your Comprehension

Coding Practice I: Chapter Review Exercises

Coding Practice II: Medical Record Case Studies

Chapter Objectives

▶ Describe common complications of surgical and medical care.

▶ Recognize the typical manifestations, complications, and treatments of complications of surgical and medical care in terms of their implications for coding.

▶ Correctly code common complications of surgical and medical care and related procedures by using the ICD-9-CM and medical records.

Complications of surgical and medical care, including complications of medical devices, implants, and grafts, are included in code categories 996 to 999 of chapter 17 of the Tabular List of Diseases of ICD-9-CM. Complications of surgery and medical care codes can be generally located under the main term "Complications" in the Alphabetic Index to Diseases or under the main term for the condition followed by the subterm "postoperative." For example, code 998.12 for postoperative hematoma is located under the main term "Complications; surgical, hematoma" and under "Hematoma; postoperative." There is no time limit to the reporting of complication codes, because problems related to surgical or medical care can occur soon after an intervention or several years later.

As always, carefully review the medical record documentation and strive for accuracy. Codes from categories 996 to 999 can help to identify problem areas in patient care that can be improved in the health-care facility, which has a commitment to provide high-quality patient care. Reporting of category 996 to 999 complication codes does not always imply poor-quality care at the facility. However, you should be aware that state agencies, Medicare reviewers (quality improvement organizations; QIOs), insurance companies, managed care organizations, and other third-party payers closely scrutinize these codes as possible indicators of quality-of-care concerns. These codes can delay payment to the provider, and payers may request copies of medical records to review cases to determine whether the quality of patient care was poor. If it was, this situation can result in payments being denied to the provider. It is important that coders do not assume that all conditions after surgical and medical care are complications of that care unless they are expressly documented as such by the attending physician.

EXAMPLE	*Postoperative acute blood loss anemia: 285.1—this condition is routinely associated with hip replacement surgery and is not assumed to be a complication of care*
	Postcholecystectomy syndrome: 576.0—this is a condition in which the original biliary symptoms, such as abdominal pain and jaundice, persist after the removal of the gallbladder, and it is not assumed to be a complication of gallbladder surgery
	Infected colostomy site: 569.61—this, and other complications of the stoma, is not considered a complication of surgery

Nosocomial versus Iatrogenic Adverse Effects or Events

Medical coders are in a good position to screen medical records (i.e., occurrence screening) for documented nosocomial and iatrogenic adverse effects or events. **Nosocomial** and **iatrogenic** are key words that indicate adverse effects or events related to treatment. Nosocomial means that adverse effects were produced by the hospital. For example, a nosocomial infection such as nosocomial pneumonia means that the pneumonia was acquired by the patient in the hospital. Iatrogenic means that the adverse effects were produced by the physician or were directly related to medical treatment. For example, an iatrogenic rash could occur if the physician prescribed the wrong medication.

You should be aware that, although the classification of category codes 996 to 998 may or may not be an indicator of a possible quality-of-patient-care concern, category 999 always indicates sentinel events in patient care that must be investigated through internal mechanisms (e.g., risk manager, safety or infection control officer, or medical staff committees). Sentinel events are unexpected occurrences that result in serious injury to or death of the patient (e.g., the surgeon amputated the wrong leg or a significant drug error by the physician or nurse resulted in patient death). These events are sentinel because they require immediate investigation to determine the causes so that the facility can take corrective actions to prevent them from occurring again.

For example, if an intravenous infiltration results in sloughing (breakdown) of skin, 999.9 is the proper code to assign. If a patient receives an incompatible blood transfusion, code 999.6 is assigned. As category 999 codes, these are examples of a complications directly related to medical treatment, and they are sentinel events that would need internal investigation and corrective action. In contrast, if a patient is readmitted for intravenous antibiotics because of a postoperative sternal wound infection with chest wall cellulitis 1 week after coronary artery bypass grafting, this is coded to 998.59 + 682.2 + V45.81 + 99.29. As a category 998 code, this is an example of a complication that may or may not be an indicator of a possible quality-of-patient-care concern. That is, upon review of the patient's medical record, the medical staff (peer) review committee may find that the infection indicates the need to improve internal operating room (OR) procedures or that the infection resulted from the patient's noncompliance with his discharge wound care instructions. In either case, this diagnosis should be closely reviewed by a medical staff committee to determine whether a nosocomial or iatrogenic event has occurred.

TIP Codes from categories 996 to 999 can be viewed as a unique opportunity to proactively address quality-of-care issues that may occur in the health-care facility.

Medical Staff Bylaws

In every hospital, written medical staff bylaws outline the organization and guiding principles of the medical staff. Covered within the provisions of the bylaws, physician peer review committees often review patient cases that have been coded from the complications of surgical and medical care category of ICD-9-CM and determine whether these cases represent possible coding errors or deviations from recognized patient care standards (i.e., substandard care).

Medical staff committees that review medical records to determine the appropriateness and quality of patient care may include the following:

- Surgical Case Review Committee
- Medical Case Review Committee
- Infection Control Committee
- Medical Records Committee
- Blood Utilization Review Committee
- Pharmacy and Therapeutics Committee
- Utilization Review Committee
- Risk Management Committee
- Quality Assurance Committee
- Patient Care Committee

Both federal and state laws offer protection to health-care facilities currently engaging in quality-assurance or quality-improvement activities. These laws ensure that facilities can act in "good faith" to identify and correct internal problems in patient care without being under a constant threat of lawsuits. If health-care facilities were under constant public scrutiny, they might ignore or cover up problems rather than act in good faith to correct them.

Coders should be knowledgeable of the concepts of corporate liability and the importance of the physician credentialing files in which health-care facilities act as "good corporate citizens" or have a fiduciary (entrusted) responsibility to monitor and ensure the competence of all employees and medical staff. This is to protect the public from harm and to provide an environment conducive to providing quality patient care. Hospitals are "corporately liable" for exercising reasonable care in providing such things as proper medical supplies and equipment, healthy food, and a safe physical environment and in exercising reasonable care in hiring and retaining competent employees and granting medical privileges to qualified physicians. It is the hospital's administrative duty to supervise the actions of the medical staff and ensure that patient care is of acceptable quality. The hospital must maintain a physician's credentialing file, which is a key component in demonstrating and maintaining high-quality patient services. The physician's credentialing file includes evidence of appropriate education, state licensure, insurance (malpractice) coverage, maintenance of continuing education, prior malpractice claims information, Drug Enforcement Agency number, and results of internal quality peer reviews for every physician allowed medical privileges in the facility.

Coders should be aware of these (federal) FY2008 Final Rules that relate to quality and the need for precise coding: These final rules include:

Present-on admission (POA) indicator: Starting October 1, 2007, CMS requires hospitals to report whether or not diagnoses were POA. For FY2008, together with the Centers for Disease Control and Prevention, CMS identified 8 high volume, hospital acquired conditions that could have reasonably been prevented. October 1, 2008, CMS will begin imposing financial penalties for their occurrence (e.g., pressure ulcers code 707.0X; catheter associated urinary tract infections code 996.64; object left in surgery code 998.4; air embolism code 999.1; surgical site infections code 998.59 and mediastinitis after CABG surgery code 519.2; vascular catheter-associated infection code 999.31; blood incompatibility code 999.6; and, falls with injuries). At the time of this textbook's publishing, CMS is proposing to increase the current list of 8 HACs to 17 for FY2009.

Core measures: As part of the Hospital Quality Data for Annual Payment Update (RHQDAPU) program for 2008, CMS requires hospitals to report on 27 different quality of care measures, and the data (results) are available to the public in order for consumers to compare the performance of hospitals. Results data can be accessed on a dedicated web site (www.hospitalcompare.hhs.gov). Examples of measures include results of patient satisfaction surveys, 30–Day Risk Adjusted Heart Attack Mortality, 30–Day Risk Adjusted Heart Failure Mortality, and appropriate initial antibiotic selection for pneumonia. Hospitals can receive up to a two percent (2%) reduction in payment for FY2008 for nonparticipation and poor scores. At the time of this textbook's publishing, CMS is proposing to add 43 more measures to the mandatory quality reporting for FY2009.

Both the POA indicators and Core Measures reporting are part of a national initiative to promote "value-based purchasing" in healthcare (i.e., pay-for-performance [P4P] systems), which incentivize providers to apply evidence based protocols ("best care practices") that promote high quality clinical care and services at reduced cost.

Sequencing Complication Codes

According to Uniform Hospital Discharge Data Set (UHDDS) rules and depending on the circumstances of admission, complications of surgical and medical care codes from categories 996 to 999 can be used as the principal diagnosis or secondary diagnosis. As a review from Chapter 2 of this textbook, remember that the UHDDS establishes definitions for official hospital reporting and defines the principal diagnosis as "the condition, after study, chiefly responsible for occasioning the admission of the patient to the hospital for care." Although a complication is usually sequenced as an secondary diagnosis, if the acute reason for an inpatient admission is a complication, then the complication code is sequenced as the principal diagnosis. This can occur when a patient undergoing an outpatient encounter is admitted to inpatient status secondary to a complication, is readmitted to the same facility for a complication related to a previous admission, or is transferred from another facility because of a complication.

> *A patient underwent outpatient colonoscopy with accidental iatrogenic puncture of the colon. The patient was subsequently admitted to inpatient status because of the accidental puncture.*
>
> *Principal diagnosis:*   *998.2*
>
> *A patient who was discharged 3 days earlier after cholecystectomy presented with abdominal pain and distention. Workup revealed that the patient had an ileus (bowel obstruction), and the patient was readmitted for further care/treatment. On patient discharge, the attending physician documented that the ileus was attributable to the patient's recent surgery.*
>
> *Principal diagnosis:*   *997.4*
> *Secondary diagnosis:*   *560.1*

EXAMPLE

Complications of Medical Devices, Implants, and Grafts

Medical devices, implants, and grafts can include cardiac pacemakers, heart valve replacements, breast prostheses, catheters, shunts, joint prostheses, orthopedic rods and pins, synthetic and tissue grafts, and so on. Codes 996.0X to 996.7X classify complications of medical devices, implants, and grafts. Complications generally fall into three categories:

1. **mechanical complications**—these include breakdown, displacement, leakage, obstruction, perforation, and protrusion of any medical device, implant, and graft (see the main term "Complications; mechanical" and the specified type of device, implant, or graft in the *Alphabetic Index to Diseases*)
2. **infection and inflammatory complications**—these occur as an abnormal reaction to any medical device, implant, or graft (see the main term "Complications; infection and inflammation" and the specified type of device, implant, or graft in the *Alphabetic Index to Diseases*)
3. **other complications**—these include embolism (i.e., traveling clot in a blood vessel), fibrosis (e.g., tissue scarring), hemorrhage, pain, stenosis (e.g., narrowing of blood vessels), thrombus (blood clot), or complica-

tions not otherwise specified (NOS) attributable to any medical device, implant, or graft (see the main term "Complications; due to (presence of) any device, implant, or graft; specified type NEC [not elsewhere classified]" in the *Alphabetic Index to Diseases*)

Coders usually do not have difficulty in determining whether a medical device, implant, or graft resulted in an "Infection and/or inflammatory complication" (subcategory 996.6X), because this type of complication is usually straightforward and well documented by physicians. However, sometimes coders have difficulty determining whether a documented complication of a medical device should be classified as a "Mechanical complication" (subcategories 996.0X to 996.5X) or "Other complication" (subcategory 996.7X). Following the process of elimination can help you to clarify the correct coding for these situations. For example, if the complication listed is not attributed to an infection or inflammation (996.6X) and the specific type of complication documented by the physician is not described in the "includes notes" in the *Tabular List of Diseases* for mechanical complications (996.0X–996.5X) that include "Breakdown, displacement, leakage, obstruction, perforation, or protrusion," then you may use the "Other complication" category (996.7X), which includes "Complication NOS, embolism, fibrosis, hemorrhage, pain, stenosis, and thrombus."

Starting October 1, 2005, new codes (996.40–996.47; 996.49) were added to describe specific causes for the mechanical breakdown of a joint prosthesis (e.g. –996.41 = mechanical loosening of prosthetic joint; 996.42 = dislocation of prosthetic joint; 996.44 = periprosthetic fracture around prosthetic joint).

EXAMPLE

Status post cardiac pacemaker with protrusion:
* *996.01* *Mechanical complication of cardiac pacemaker*
* *V45.01* *Status post cardiac pacemaker*

Pain secondary to retained hardware (pins), status post femoral neck fracture:
* *996.78* *Other complication of internal orthopedic implant*
* *905.3* *Late effects of femoral neck fracture*

Infected total hip replacement on left:
* *996.66* *Infection attributable to internal joint prosthesis*
* *V43.64* *Status post hip replacement*

Complications of Transplanted Organs

Subcategory 996.8X includes complications of transplanted organs, including failure and rejection. In coding these situations, sequence the complication code subcategory 996.8X for the transplanted organ first, and then add a code to specify the precise nature of the complication.

EXAMPLE

Status post kidney transplantation for end-stage renal disease with rejection: 996.81 + 585.6

Bone marrow transplant infection attributable to aspergillosis: 996.85 + 117.3 (a bone marrow transplantation is performed to repopulate normal blood cells in a patient with a disease such as leukemia [cancer of the white blood cells]—after chemotherapy, total body irradiation, or both, a relative or closely matching donor's bone marrow cells are transplanted to the recipient)

Acute graft-versus-host disease, status post bone marrow transplantation for acute myel-ogenous leukemia: 279.51 + 205.00 (graft-versus-host disease occurs as an immune response [i.e., rejection] to donor bone marrow cells in the recipient)

Nonspecific Complication Codes That Describe General Body Systems

As a general rule for coding complications of surgical or medical care (categories 996 to 999), if the specific condition is included in the complication code description itself, then no additional code is required to add detail. However, if the specific condition is not included in the complication code description itself, then an additional code is used to add detail.

The category 997 complication codes are usually nonspecific and often require an additional code to add more specificity or detail to identify the specific complicating condition. For example, category 997 includes nonspecific codes to describe complications affecting general body systems (e.g., postoperative respiratory system complication: 997.39; postoperative digestive system complication: 997.4). In the *Tabular List of Diseases*, the includes notes under category 997 state "use additional code to identify the complication." As an exception to this general rule for category 997, postoperative hypertension (code 997.91) requires the assignment of only one code for the complication of surgery because the specific condition (hypertension) is described in the complication code itself; no additional code is required to add detail. Also, using an additional code for preexisting hypertension (codes 401 to 405) is excluded when reporting the code for postoperative hypertension (see exclusion notes under code 997.91).

Category 998 usually includes codes for complications of procedures not elsewhere classified. These codes are usually more specific than codes from the 997 category and most often do not require an additional code for detail.

			EXAMPLE
Postoperative cardiac arrest:	*997.1*	*Postoperative cardiac complication*	
	427.5	*Cardiac arrest (added for detail)*	
Postoperative pneumonia:	*997.31*	*Ventilator associated pneumonia*	
	482.40	*Staphylococcal pneumonia*	
Postoperative hypertension:	*997.91*		
Postoperative hemorrhage:	*998.11*		

Postoperative wound dehiscence: 998.30

Accidental puncture or laceration during a procedure: 998.2

Postoperative septicemia attributable to Staphylococcus aureus:

998.59	*Postoperative septicemia*
038.11	*Staphylococcus aureus sepsis (added for detail because the specific condition [Staphylococcus aureus] is not included in the complication code)*

Complications Causing Outpatient to Inpatient Admission Within 72 Hours

Outpatient encounters (e.g., ambulatory surgery or medical visit) can result in complications that require inpatient admission to the hospital (i.e., from outpatient to inpatient admission).

 TIP Medicare mandates that all outpatient encounters occurring within 72 hours of inpatient admission to the same hospital be combined with and billed under the inpatient stay only.

When coding outpatient to inpatient encounters, remember to code the reason for the inpatient admission—not the reason for the original outpatient encounter—as the principal diagnosis.

EXAMPLE

Outpatient to inpatient admission for postoperative hemorrhage after colonoscopy with polypectomy. Exploratory laparotomy revealed iatrogenic perforation of the large bowel requiring suture repair.

998.2	*Accidental puncture or laceration during a procedure*
998.11	*Postoperative hemorrhage*
211.3	*Colon polyp*
46.75	*Suture repair, large bowel*
45.42	*Endoscopic polypectomy*

Other Indicators of Complications of Surgical and Medical Care

As a review from previous chapters in this textbook, remember that diagnosis-related groups (now MS-DRGs) are a case-mix system adopted by the federal government and many other third-party payers to reimburse hospitals for inpatient services. As a case-mix system, MS-DRGs describe the type and volume of patients treated by the hospital. As a prospective payment system, MS–DRGs establish a predetermined rate of reimbursement to hospitals in advance of the health-care services provided according to the types of patients treated. This is reported through medical codes that represent patient diagnoses and procedures submitted by the hospital to Medicare or other third-party payers.

In addition to the category codes 996 to 999 presented in this chapter that describe complications of surgical and medical care, you should be aware that a MS-DRG assignment may point to a possible complication or quality-of-care concern. For example, inpatient admissions or outpatient encounters that change to inpatient admissions can generate MS-DRGs, which describe: extensive operating room (OR) procedure unrelated to principal diagnosis; nonextensive OR procedure unrelated to principal diagnosis; and, complications of treatment. These MS-DRGs can be with or without CCs/MCCs, and may indicate a possible problem in patient care.

A patient with a known history of senile dementia was admitted with acute congestive heart failure. During the admission, the patient fell out of bed and sustained a femoral neck fracture. The patient was then taken to surgery and underwent open reduction/internal fixation of the femoral fracture.

Principal Diagnosis:	*428.0*
Secondary Diagnosis:	*290.0 and 820.8*
Procedure:	*79.35*
DRG:	*981 (extensive OR procedure unrelated to the principal diagnosis with MCC)*

A patient underwent outpatient tonsillectomy for chronic tonsillitis on February 1. The patient was discharged home from outpatient surgery in good condition. The following day, the patient developed postoperative bleeding and was subsequently admitted as an inpatient on February 2.

Principal Diagnosis:	*998.11*
Secondary Diagnosis:	*474.00*
Procedure:	*28.2*
DRG:	*989 (nonextensive OR procedure unrelated to the principal diagnosis without CC/MCC)*

A patient with known end-stage renal disease and hypertension was admitted secondary to suppurative peritonitis. The peritonitis was documented as being attributable to the patient's peritoneal catheter. The patient was admitted and placed on intravenous antibiotics.

Principal diagnosis:	*996.68*
Secondary Diagnosis:	*567.29, 403.91, 585.6*
Procedure:	*99.21*
DRG:	*919 (complications of treatment with MCC)*

Because Medicare mandates that all outpatient encounters occurring within 72 hours of inpatient admission to the same hospital be combined with and billed under the inpatient stay, the date of the patient's actual outpatient procedure can be outside the parameters of the patient's actual inpatient admission date. Also, readmissions for treatment within 30 days to the same facility may indicate inadequate treatment during the initial stay. The reporting of complication codes (categories 996 to 999), certain MS-DRGs, and dates of admission and discharge enable the Quality Improvement Organization (QIO)—an independent agency that is contracted by the Centers for Medicare and Medicaid Services—to track potential quality-of-care concerns in the review of Medicare and Medicaid provider services. Generally, the QIO reviews patients' medical records to ensure that the provider adhered to recognized professional standards for the quality of patient care; that medical necessity was established for the inpatient admission; that appropriate health-care resources were used to treat the patient; and that the correct MS-DRG was assigned to ensure proper payment to the provider (i.e., MS-DRG validation to prevent "upcoding").

As a coder, your job is to code precisely. As an employee, your job is to support the mission of the hospital to provide quality patient care. In the performance of competent coding, it is important for you to recognize when medical record documentation, codes, MS-DRGs, and dates of service indicate possible patient-care problems so you can ensure that these cases are referred to appropriate internal channels that support quality improvement. These coder competencies and actions help to prevent the disconnection of hospital communication, which is necessary to promote the mission of providing high-quality patient care.

SUMMARY

This chapter has addressed coding for complications related to surgical and medical care. Nosocomial versus iatrogenic adverse effects or events have been explored. Complications involving medical devices, implants, and grafts were considered, as were complications from transplanted organs. The chapter also addressed complications affecting specific body systems and complications that cause outpatient to inpatient admission within 72 hours. The subject of medical staff bylaws was also reviewed.

TESTING YOUR COMPREHENSION

1. What code category addresses complications of surgical and medical care?

2. What is the time limit for reporting complication codes?

3. With what procedure is postoperative anemia often associated?

4. If postcholecystectomy syndrome occurs after the removal of a patient's gallbladder, is this considered a complication of that surgical procedure?

5. What is an iatrogenic event?

6. Complications of medical devices, implants, and grafts generally fall into three categories. What are they?

7. What is the purpose of bone marrow transplantation?

8. Identify a general rule for coding complications of surgical or medical care if the specific condition is included in the complication code description.

9. What does Medicare require for an outpatient encounter within 72 hours of an inpatient admission to the same hospital?

CODING PRACTICE I — Chapter Review Exercises

Directions

By using your ICD-9-CM codebook, code the following diagnoses and procedures:

	DIAGNOSIS/PROCEDURES	CODE
1	Postoperative atelectasis.	
2	Postoperative ileus.	
3	*Escherichia coli* urinary tract infection secondary to chronic indwelling Foley catheter. Status post cerebrovascular accident with residual right-sided hemiplegia. Neurogenic bladder.	
4	Status post left knee replacement with recurrent dislocation. Closed reduction, knee dislocation.	
5	Phlebitis, left arm, secondary to intravenous infiltration.	
6	Clotted AV hemodialysis graft. Chronic renal failure, end-stage. Hypertension. Declotting of AV graft with revision.	
7	Painful knee prosthesis. Total knee revision.	
8	Infected right above-knee amputation stump. Diabetic peripheral vascular disease. Debridement (revision) of stump.	
9	Coronary artery disease. Unstable angina. Postprocedure groin hematoma. Left heart catheterization. Left ventricular angiogram. Coronary angiography.	

	DIAGNOSIS/PROCEDURES	CODE
10	Small-bowel obstruction secondary to adhesions. Chronic obstructive pulmonary disease. Hypertension. Iatrogenic bowel enterotomy. Lysis of adhesions. Suture of small intestine.	
11	Status post recent appendectomy with postoperative external wound dehiscence.	
12	Arteriosclerosis of left lower extremity with ulcer. Coronary artery disease. Hypertension. Type 1 insulin-dependent diabetes mellitus. Intraoperative myocardial infarction. Acute respiratory distress syndrome. Status post previous coronary artery bypass grafting. Above-knee amputation, left. Endotracheal intubation with mechanical ventilation <96 hours.	
13	Bilateral carotid stenosis. Hypertension. Postoperative cerebrovascular accident. Carotid endarterectomy, left.	
14	Dysfunctional uterine bleeding. Uterine leiomyoma. Chronic blood-loss anemia. Dysmenorrhea. Postop urinary retention. Total abdominal hysterectomy/bilateral salpingo-oophorectomy.	
15	Sepsis secondary to AV graft infection (i.e., line infection). Chronic renal failure secondary to type 2 diabetes mellitus.	
16	Cholecystitis with cholelithiasis. GERDS. Hypothyroidism. Postoperative fever of unknown etiology. Laparoscopic cholecystectomy. Intraoperative cholangiogram.	

	DIAGNOSIS/PROCEDURES	CODE
17	Kidney transplant failure/rejection leading to acute renal failure. End-stage renal disease. Hypertension. Diabetic nephropathy. Venous catheter insertion for dialysis. Hemodialysis.	
18	Outpatient to inpatient admission for urticaria attributable to serum. Chronic blood-loss anemia. Menorrhagia. Uterine fibroids. Packed red blood cell transfusion.	
19	Status post cardiac pacemaker insertion with admission for infected pacer pocket. Debridement of pacer pocket.	
20	Nonhealing surgical wound. Status post open reduction/internal fixation of femur fracture. Intravenous antibiotic.	

CODING PRACTICE II   Medical Record Case Studies

Instructions

1. Carefully review the medical reports provided for each case study.

2. Research any abbreviations and terms that are unfamiliar or unclear.

3. Identify as many diagnoses and procedures as possible.

4. Because only part of the patient's total record is available, determine what additional documentation you might need.

5. If appropriate, identify any questions you might ask the physician to code this case correctly and completely.

6. Complete the appropriate blanks below for each case study.

CHAPTER 18 CASE STUDIES

Case Study 18.1 (Coder/Abstract Summary Form)

Patient: **John Doe**

Patient documentation: **Review Medical Reports 18.1 and 18.2**

1. Principal diagnosis:

   _____

2. Secondary or other diagnoses:

   _____

3. Principal procedure:

   _____

4. Other procedures:

   _____

5. Additional documentation needed:

   _____

   _____

   _____

   _____

Case Study 18.1 (Continued)

6. Questions for the physician:

_____

_____

_____

_____

_____

MEDICAL REPORT 18.1

EMERGENCY ROOM PROCEDURE REPORT

PATIENT NAME: Doe, John

ACCOUNT NUMBER:

ATTENDING MD: Smith, M.D.

ROOM NUMBER:

ADMITTED: 08/26

DATE OF OPERATION: 8/26

SURGEON: Smith, M.D.

ANESTHESIOLOGIST:

PRE-PROCEDURE DIAGNOSIS: Posterior superior dislocation of left hip.

POST-PROCEDURE DIAGNOSIS: Posterior superior dislocation of left hip.

ANESTHESIA: General with muscle relaxation.

PROCEDURE: Closed reduction of posterior superior dislocation of left hip. (Third dislocation.)

ESTIMATED BLOOD LOSS: None.

COMPLICATIONS: None.

DESCRIPTION OF PROCEDURE: Mr. Doe was taken to the operating room. A general anesthetic was initiated. Endotracheal tube was established and then secured. After administration of a muscle relaxant, traction/counter-traction technique was used to reduce the patient's hip. This is the patient's third dislocation in a two-week period. Given the apparent instability of the hip, the patient will be admitted and the patient will be scheduled for arthroscopic revision as soon as it can be arranged.

_____

Smith, MD

NOTES

REPORT OF OPERATION

PATIENT NAME:	Doe, John
ACCOUNT NUMBER:	
ATTENDING MD:	Smith, M.D.
ROOM NUMBER:	
ADMITTED:	08/26

DATE OF OPERATION: 8/26

SURGEON: Smith, M.D.

ANESTHESIOLOGIST:

PREOPERATIVE DIAGNOSIS: Recurrent posterior superior dislocation of left hip.

OPERATIVE PROCEDURE: Acetabular revision of left total hip.

POST-PROCEDURE DIAGNOSIS: Recurrent posterior superior dislocation of left hip.

ANESTHESIA: General.

ESTIMATED BLOOD LOSS: Approximately 1000 cc.

DRAINS: OrthoPak to the left hip.

COMPLICATIONS: None.

OPERATIVE NOTE IN DETAIL: Mr. Doe was taken to the operating room and placed in the supine position. A general anesthetic was initiated and endotracheal tube was established and then secured. The patient was placed in the right lateral decubitus position with the left hip up and left hip was then prepped and draped in the usual sterile fashion. The patient's left hip was incised. The subcutaneous tissue was incised and explored. The repaired iliotibial band was sharply incised in the plane of incision. Residual suture was removed as it was encountered. The hip was entered anteriorly with resection of what was the healing gluteus minimus and medius muscular structures. This was taken off at the level of the greater trochanteric region. The previously placed cable that had been placed for a stress fracture at the calcar at the time of the original surgery was removed as we explored the hip. The patient's hip joint was then identified. The hip was found to be easily dislocatable. The patient had prodigious amounts of scar tissue of the hip. The previously placed acetabular cup showed prodigious amounts of early bone formation, particularly in the margins of the cup. The screws and the cup were removed with a great deal of difficulty; first we had marginal bone and removing prodigious amounts of scar tissue. The scar tissue was very vascular. After removing the cup, the acetabular itself was inspected. It appears that there may have been some subsiding of the cup within the acetabular margin itself and this may have possibly led to instability that was noted. At this point, an attempt was made to stabilize the acetabular head with a spiked porous coated cup.

The spikes were found to be inadequate in obtaining this affixation because of the osteopenia in the patient's acetabular wall. At this point, we turned our attention to the multiple holed shell. We placed screws in multiple positions. The cup was brought into a more vertical attitude and a 20-degree lipped liner was placed to allow for distal stability. The cup was placed into position. The trial head and trial acetabular were placed and trial reductions were made. We obtained maximum stability by placing the head in increased vertical attitude and increased coverage enough to allow increased coverage in the forward flexed position. The patient's cup was noted to be stable. New cup and hip construct was noted to be stable in all planes of motion. The patient's gluteus minimus and medius were repaired to the level of the greater trochanteric ridge. A large-bore drain was placed in the deep surface of the wound. The iliotibial band was once again repaired using a 1-inch bias and the subcutaneous tissue was approximated with 0 Vicryl and 2-0 Vicryl and the skin was approximated with staples. The patient was placed in the abduction pillow and returned to the recovery room in stable and satisfactory condition.

Smith, MD

Case Study 18.2 (Coder/Abstract Summary Form)

Patient: **Kevin Johnson**

Patient documentation: **Review Medical Reports 18.3 and 18.4**

1. Principal diagnosis:

   _____

2. Secondary or other diagnoses:

   _____

3. Principal procedure:

   _____

4. Other procedures:

   _____

5. Additional documentation needed:

   _____

   _____

   _____

6. Questions for the physician:

   _____

   _____

   _____

   _____

   _____

HISTORY AND PHYSICAL

PATIENT NAME: Johnson, Kevin

ACCOUNT NUMBER:

ATTENDING MD: Smith, M.D.

ROOM NUMBER:

ADMITTED: 06/26

HISTORY OF PRESENT ILLNESS: Patient is a 72-year-old white male with a medical history of recently diagnosed coronary artery disease, status post CABG performed at ABC Hospital one week ago. Also history of polycystic kidney disease with history of gross hematuria in the past. History of liver cysts, small abdominal aortic aneurysm being followed up. The patient has history of depression being treated with Zoloft, recently widowed. His only daughter died. Patient is now admitted. Post-CABG, he apparently went to a nursing home for rehab. He was discharged home last week. He went home noticed onset of severe swelling, induration, warmth, as well as pain over the left thigh as well as the left groin incisional sites where the vein was harvested for bypass grafting. No history of any fever or chills, rigors. No history of any chest pain, shortness of breath, hemoptysis.

PAST MEDICAL HISTORY: As above.

PAST SURGICAL HISTORY: As above.

ALLERGIES: Penicillin.

HOME MEDICATIONS: Ecotrin 81 mg po q. day, Zoloft 200 mg po q. hs.

PHYSICAL EXAMINATION

GENERAL: Elderly white male lying in bed, appears in no acute distress.

VITAL SIGNS: T-afebrile. 98.2. p-72, pp 128/80, R-16.

HEENT: PERRLA, EOMI. Oral mucosa is moist.

NECK: Supple. No lymphadenopathy. No JVD.

CHEST: Healing surgical incisional site in the midline.

CARDIOVASCULAR: Normal S1 and S2, regular. No S3. No murmurs.

ABDOMEN: Soft, nontender, nondistended. Bowel sounds positive. No hepatosplenomegaly. No masses felt.

EXTREMITIES: Positive redness, warmth, with firm/brawny induration noted over the medial aspect of the mid thigh on the left side at the site of incision for vein harvesting. Also history of similar induration and swelling at the left groin site, although there are no palpable tender lymph nodes in the left groin region itself. There is also significant induration noted at the posterior medial aspect of the left thigh. No Homan's sign.

NEURO: Awake, alert and oriented × 3. Cranial nerves II–XII are grossly intact. Power 5/5 bilaterally in upper and lower limbs.

LABORATORY DATE: Preliminary report for bilateral venous Doppler done in the ER was negative for DVT. Initial CBC, CMP showed evidence of moderate anemia with hemoglobin and hematocrit of 8 and 27. Patient was also noted to have low albumin of 2.9, protein 5.7, calcium 8.2. AST is low at 12.

MEDICAL REPORT 18.3 (CONTINUED)

ASSESSMENT AND PLAN:

1. Left thigh induration and swelling, likely represents cellulitis at infected saphenous vein harvest site, post CABG. Other possibilities include underlying DVT that still remains a consideration in spite of negative venous Doppler. Place patient on subcu Lovenox 60mg q12h, continue home medications. IV Ancef 1 gram 18h. Will obtain repeat CBC, CMP in a.m. If hematocrit drops further, will consider blood transfusions. Will repeat venous Doppler on Monday morning. Will reassess patient in a.m.

Smith, MD

NOTES

MEDICAL REPORT 18.4

RADIOLOGICAL INTERPRETATION

PATIENT NAME: Johnson, Kevin

ACCOUNT NUMBER:

ATTENDING MD: Smith, M.D.

ROOM NUMBER:

ADMITTED: 06/26

HISTORY: CELLULITIS, LT LEG PAIN ER C1 VENOUS DOPPLER LT LOWER EXTREMITY LOWER LEG PAIN

LEFT LOWER EXTREMITY DOPPLER EVALUATION, 06/26

There is appropriate compressibility, flow in response to augmentation maneuvers throughout the deep venous system of the left lower extremity.

IMPRESSION:

1. No sonographic evidence of deep venous thrombosis is demonstrated within the left lower extremity.

_____

Exray, M.D.

NOTES

Case Study 18.3 (Coder/Abstract Summary Form)

Patient: **Jane Anderson**

Patient documentation: **Review Medical Reports 18.5 and 18.6**

1. Principal diagnosis:

   _____

2. Secondary or other diagnoses:

   _____

3. Principal procedure:

   _____

4. Other procedures:

   _____

5. Additional documentation needed:

   _____

   _____

   _____

   _____

6. Questions for the physician:

   _____

   _____

   _____

   _____

   _____

DISCHARGE SUMMARY

PATIENT NAME: Anderson, Jane

ACCOUNT NUMBER:

ATTENDING MD: Smith, M.D.

ROOM NUMBER:

ADMITTED: 06/26

DISCHARGED: 07/04

FINAL DIAGNOSIS:

1. Colostomy secondary to resection of obstructing colon carcinoma.

COMPLICATIONS:

1. Nasopharyngeal laceration secondary to NG tube.

2. Persistent postoperative atelectasis secondary to mucous plugging.

3. Pleural effusion.

OPERATIVE PROCEDURE: Closure of colostomy by resection and anastomosis by Dr. Smith. Nasopharyngoscopy by Dr. Nose. Bronchoscopy with bronchial lavage by Dr. Bronchos. Thoracentesis by Dr. Bronchos.

HISTORY: This is a 66-year-old white female who last year presented with obstructing carcinoma of her colon. She underwent resection of the cancer, but anastomosis was not feasible. End-colostomy and Hartman procedure was carried out. She has completed her course of chemotherapy in the interim and has had pre-operative colonoscopy both of the distal segment and proximal to the colostomy. These show no evident lesions. The remainder of her pre-operative workup is also within normal limits. Following appropriate bowel prep she was admitted for closure of her colostomy.

HOSPITAL COURSE: She was taken to surgery where an uneventful closure of her colostomy resection and anastomosis was carried out. In the course of placing a nasogastric tube, she developed a laceration of the right side of the nasopharynx. She developed some laryngospasm in the recovery room, which required positive pressure ventilation by mask, and from the nasopharyngeal laceration she developed subcutaneous emphysema of her face and neck. She was placed on appropriate antibiotics and consultation was obtained from Dr. Nose who carried out nasopharyngoscopy and revealed the small area of bruising and probable laceration in nasopharynx. She was continued on Unasyn and Levaquin and her subcutaneous emphysema resolved over the next 2 days. She also developed persisting right lower lobe atelectasis, which did not clear with bronchodilators and incentive spirometry. Dr. Bronchos was consulted and a bronchoscopy was carried out which showed considerable mucous plugging. Once these plugs were removed, no further atelectasis was encountered. Her abdomen continued to heal and progress quite nicely. She began passing flatus and her nasogastric tube was removed. A diet was begun. She was noted on follow up chest x-ray to have a moderate right sided pleural effusion and a very small left sided pleural effusion. Consultation was obtained with Dr. Bronchos and a right-sided thoracentesis was carried out. Results of these studies reveal no evidence of infection thus far. No abnormal cells. At the present time she is eating without difficulty. She is having bowel movements without problem. Her abdomen is soft and non-tender. She is breathing well. Chest is clear.

She is discharged home for follow-up in the office.

DISCHARGE DIET: Regular.

DISCHARGE MEDICATIONS: Lorcet Plus #24 1 every 4–6 hours prn pain.

MEDICAL REPORT 18.5 (CONTINUED)

DISCHARGE ACTIVITIES: Light. She may shower.

FOLLOW-UP APPOINTMENT: In 3 days for removal of her staples. 2–3 weeks for routine follow-up. She is to call for problems with increasing pain, nausea, vomiting, abdominal distension, wound redness or drainage, or fever.

CONDITION OF PATIENT ON DISCHARGE: Satisfactory.

_____

Smith, MD

NOTES

REPORT OF OPERATION

PATIENT NAME:	Anderson, Jane
ACCOUNT NUMBER:	
ATTENDING MD:	Smith, M.D.
ROOM NUMBER:	
SUR DATE:	06/26

SURGEON: Smith, M.D.

ANESTHESIOLOGIST:

PREOPERATIVE DIAGNOSIS: Status post resection of obstructing carcinoma of the transverse colon with end-colostomy and Hartmann procedure.

POSTOPERATIVE DIAGNOSIS: Status post resection of obstructing carcinoma of the transverse colon with end-colostomy and Hartmann procedure.

OPERATION: Closure of colostomy resection and anastomosis, lysis of adhesions, incidental appendectomy.

ANESTHESIA: General endotracheal.

INDICATIONS: 66-year-old female who last year had an obstructing carcinoma of her transverse colon. This was resected and the colostomy and Hartmann procedure done. She has finished her chemotherapy and returns now for closure of her colostomy.

DESCRIPTION: Under satisfactory general endotracheal anesthesia, the patient was placed into Allen stirrups and properly padded and positioned. The ostomy site was closed with a purse-string suture of 00 silk. The abdomen, perineum, groin, and thighs were thoroughly prepped with Betadine scrub and Betadine prep solution and draped sterilely. Midline incision was reopened and extended into the lower abdomen. The incision was carried down until the peritoneal cavity was entered. Numerous dense adhesions were carefully lysed. The small bowel was carefully inspected throughout its length and no evidence of entry or lead from the small bowel or colon was found. An elliptical incision was made in a transverse manner around it and the tissues were dissected free until the ostomy could be retracted into the peritoneal cavity, then the ostomy site was taken down. She had developed a parastomal hernia and the sac from the hernia was likewise resected. The ostomy was essentially in the proximal right colon at about the level of the hepatic flexure. This was freed up to allow for anastomosis and the ostomy site was resected with a 55.0-mm linear stapler cutter closing the enterotomy site with the TA-60 stapler. Bowel contents were passed across the anastomosis and were seen to flow freely into the distal segment without evidence of leak or obstruction. A 000 Vicryl suture was placed at the crotch of the anastomosis to reinforce it. The mesenteric defect was closed with interrupted sutures of 000 Vicryl. Since the cecum was in a somewhat higher position than normal, it was elected to carry out an appendectomy since appendicitis in this area would be very difficult to diagnose. The mesoappendix was divided between hemostats and ligated with 00 Chromic ties.

The base of the appendix was then stapled with the TA-60 stapler and the appendix was amputated. This gave a nice closure of the appendiceal stump at its junction with the cecum. Hemostasis was complete. There was no evidence of leak. There was no evidence of intraperitoneal metastasis. The gallbladder was without gallstones. There was no evidence of liver metastases. The stomach appeared normal. A nasogastric tube was positioned in the antrum of the stomach. The peritoneal cavity was then copiously irrigated with many liters of warm saline until it was clean. The peritoneum and posterior fascia at the ostomy site were closed with suture of PDS. Anterior fascial layers were closed with interrupted sutures of #1 PDS. A Penrose drain was placed in the depths of the ostomy site and brought through each end as a through and

MEDICAL REPORT 18.6 (CONTINUED)

through drain. The skin at the ostomy site was then closed with a surgical skin stapler. Omentum was placed over the anastomosis as an omental patch. The fascia was then closed in the midline with continuous sutures of #1 Novofil. The subcutaneous tissues were copiously irrigated with saline and the skin was closed with the surgical skin stapler. Sterile dressings were applied. Sponge, needle and instrument counts were reported to be correct. The patient tolerated the procedure well and was sent to the recovery room in satisfactory condition.

Smith, MD

NOTES

Coding for Mental Disorders

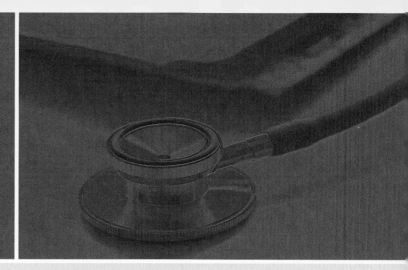

Chapter Outline

The *Diagnostic and Statistical Manual of Mental Disorders*

Types of Mental Disorders

Therapies for Mental Disorders, Including Treatments for Alcohol and/or Drug Abuse

Testing Your Comprehension

Coding Practice I: Chapter Review Exercises

Coding Practice II: Medical Record Case Studies

Chapter Objectives

▶ Identify common mental disorders.

▶ Identify common clinical therapies related to mental disorders.

▶ Recognize the typical manifestations of mental disorders and the clinical therapies used to treat them in terms of their implications for coding.

▶ Correctly code common mental disorders and related therapies by using the ICD-9-CM and medical records.

Mental disorders are included in code categories 290 to 319 of chapter 5 of the Tabular List of Diseases of ICD-9-CM. The human mind is complex, and its problems are not as readily understood as disorders of the structure or function of a tissue or organ. Unlike removing a diseased gallbladder, in which the pathology is readily seen and followed by definitive treatment, the cause of psychiatric disease is often uncertain. Treatment outcomes are generally measured over time, for example, when a patient demonstrates improved interrelationships and an increased ability to function in society.

Word Parts and Meanings of Terms Related to Mental Disorders

Word Part	Meaning	Example	Definition of Example
schiz/o-	split	schizoid; "oid" means *resembling*	A mild form of schizophrenia
phren/o	mind	Schizophrenia	Split mind; a psychosis involving a withdrawal from the external world (i.e., reality) that may include hallucinations, delusions, etc.
-phobia	fear	Claustrophobia	Fear of being in closed-in places (e.g., elevator, closet)
para-	abnormal	paranoia	An abnormal, irrational fear
psych/o-	mind	psychosis; psychotherapy	A condition wherein there is a significant impairment in reality testing; treatment of the mind
-ment/o	mind	dementia; "de-" means *a lack of, less*	Lack or loss of mental abilities
-thymia	mind	dysthymia; "dys-" means *bad, abnormal, painful*	Abnormal mind (i.e., usually depression with anxiety)
-phoria	feeling; mental state; bearing	euphoria; "eu-" means *good* or *normal*	An exaggerated feeling of well-being or good
cata-	down	catatonic	Decrease in reacting or responding to the environment; no physical movement or speech (mute)
anxi/o-	uneasy; apprehension; tension	anxiety	A feeling of tension or uneasiness
agora-	marketplace	agoraphobia	Fear of a marketplace (i.e., fear of crowded places)
iatr/o	treatment	psychiatrist	A physician who specializes in treating mental disorders
-mania	obsession; obsessive	kleptomania; "klept/o" means *to steal*	One who is obsessed with stealing

Measuring the results of psychotherapy can be difficult to quantify to insurance companies, and, as a result, payments to providers can be delayed or withheld. Provider documentation and medical coding are critical communication elements for patient care improvement and reimbursements to providers. To assist in your understanding of this material, the Word Parts Box on this page reviews common word parts, meanings, examples, and definitions of terms related to mental disorders.

The *Diagnostic and Statistical Manual of Mental Disorders*

Psychiatrists (doctors who specialize in the treatment of the mind and who can prescribe drugs), psychologists, licensed clinical social workers, and licensed mental health counselors (nonphysicians trained in psychotherapeutic methods) document the services they provide by using medical terminology from the *Diagnostic and Statistical Manual of Mental Disorders*, 4th Ed (DSM-IV), which is published by the American Psychiatric Association. Derived from ICD-9-CM, this manual provides codes for the classification of mental disorders and is also used as a diagnostic tool to help mental health professionals establish a patient's diagnosis.

To understand the terminology used by psychiatrists/psychologists, coders must understand the DSM. However, Medicare and other third-party payers mandate the use of ICD-9-CM for coding. Therefore, although mental health providers often use DSM terminology, patient cases are coded according to ICD-9-CM.

As a diagnostic tool, the DSM uses five axes to describe psychological functioning in the total context of a patient's medical condition(s) and psychosocial and environmental concerns. The five axes are often referred to in the mental health professional's documentation and include the following elements:

1. **axis I:** psychiatric disorder that receives the focus of treatment (e.g., clinical depression)
2. **axis II:** personality disorder(s) and mental retardation
3. **axis III:** other general medical conditions
4. **axis IV:** psychosocial and environmental issues
5. **axis V:** global assessment of functioning

Whether the mental disorder codes reported from ICD-9-CM are sequenced as the principal or secondary diagnosis depends on the circumstances of the admission and the health-care facility's main focus of care upon the patient's admission. For example, if a patient was admitted to a medical facility for medical evaluation and treatment for a condition such as alcoholic cirrhosis of the liver and also had a psychiatric disorder such as depression, then the alcoholic cirrhosis (as the main reason for admission and the main focus of care) would be sequenced as the principal diagnosis, and the psychiatric condition of depression would be sequenced as a secondary diagnosis. Depending on the circumstances of admission, the inverse could also be true. For example, if a patient was admitted to a medical facility for medical evaluation and treatment for confusion secondary to alcoholic psychosis and also had a medical disorder, such as chronic obstructive pulmonary disease, then the alcoholic psychosis (as the main reason for admission and the main focus of care) would be sequenced as the principal diagnosis, and the chronic obstructive pulmonary disease would be sequenced as a secondary diagnosis.

EXAMPLE

A patient was admitted with acute congestive heart failure. The patient also had a history of bipolar disorder that was under current medical therapy.

    Principal diagnosis: *428.0*
    Secondary diagnosis: *296.7*

A patient was admitted to a psychiatric facility for acute exacerbation of paranoid schizophrenia. The patient also had non-insulin-dependent diabetes mellitus and emphysema.

    Principal diagnosis: *295.34*
    Secondary diagnosis: *492.8 + 250.00*

Types of Mental Disorders

There are many types of mental disorders, but the most commonly encountered disorders are explained here. These include anxiety disorders; eating disorders; affective psychoses; delirium and dementia; schizophrenia; substance-related mental disorders; personality disorders; Alzheimer's disease; psychogenic disorders and psychic factors associated with diseases; and organic brain disease.

Anxiety Disorders

Anxiety is characterized by apprehension, distress, and fear or tension that can include physical symptoms such as heart palpitations, shortness of breath, sweating, dizziness, and shakiness. Examples of types of anxiety disorders include the following:

▶ anxiety with depression, also called **dysthymia** (code 300.4)
▶ phobic disorders, such as agoraphobia (code 300.22; fear of being in public places), claustrophobia (code 300.29; fear of being in closed-in places), and social anxiety disorder (code 300.23; e.g., fear of speaking in public)
▶ obsessive-compulsive disorder (code 300.3), in which the patient's anxiety produces recurrent thoughts (obsessions) and repetitive acts (compulsions)
▶ stress reactions, which can manifest as acute stress reactions that are transient or temporary (category 308) or adjustment stress reactions that are prolonged or chronic (category 309)

EXAMPLE	
	Anxiety in acute stress reaction: 308.0
	Acute posttraumatic stress disorder: 308.3
	Combat fatigue: 308.9
	Adjustment reaction with anxious mood: 309.24
	Prolonged posttraumatic stress disorder (e.g., post-Vietnam, Gulf or Iraq War syndrome): 309.81
	Prolonged grief reaction: 309.1

Eating Disorders

Anorexia nervosa and bulimia are common eating disorders. Most often seen in adolescent girls, anorexia nervosa (code 307.1) is classified as a mental disorder because it manifests in an individual's having a false self-perception of his or her weight. Affected individuals have an appetite, but they often excessively diet or exercise to stave off the fear of unwanted weight gain. These individuals may appear emaciated to others, but they continue to see themselves as overweight. Bulimia (code 307.51) is characterized by binge eating followed by self-induced vomiting or an overuse of laxatives to rid the body of food in order to lose weight (i.e., "binge and purge").

Affective Psychoses

Affective psychoses (code category 296) are characterized by severe disturbances of mood. The 296 category includes a fourth digit that indicates the type of affective disorder (e.g., manic, major depression, or bipolar). With the one exception of the four-digit code 296.7 (bipolar affective disorder, unspecified), all other affective disorder codes in the 296 category require a fifth digit that indicates the current phase of illness (e.g., mild, moderate, or severe with psychotic features) or classifies other specified or atypical affective psychoses.

Manic disorder is the manic episode of a manic-depressive psychosis disorder. In a manic episode, the individual exhibits extreme happiness or excitement that is exaggerated or out of context with his or her real circumstances.

Major depression is characterized by severe sadness that inhibits one's normal functioning and may include psychotic features (loss of contact with reality or failure of reality testing).

Bipolar disorder (circular type) is characterized by manic episodes or cycles (excessive elation) alternating with depressive episodes or cycles (excessive sadness).

Severe recurrent major depression with psychosis: 296.34

Bipolar disorder, currently moderately depressed: 296.52

Bipolar disorder: 296.80

Manic-depressive, currently manic: 296.40

Bipolar disorder, currently moderately manic: 296.42

Chronic major depression, severe: 296.33

Acute psychotic depression, first episode: 296.24

Mild manic depression, currently manic: 296.41

Manic depression, currently severely depressed: 296.53

Do not confuse the documentation of "depression" with that of "major depression." Depression not otherwise specified (NOS; code 311) is not an affective disorder, but involves a less severe depressed mood, and the individual exhibits no psychotic features. Depression NOS is a common secondary diagnosis for many inpatients enduring the acute stresses of illness and the associated psychosocial problems. It usually responds well to medication or other therapy.

Delirium and Dementia

Delirium is characterized by an acute transient (i.e., temporary) disturbance of one's mental state with acute (i.e., severe) confusion. It may occur as a result of head trauma, alcohol or drug intoxication, metabolic disturbances such as those caused by kidney failure (uremia), electrolyte imbalances, or infections (e.g., sepsis or pneumonia).

Be careful if following the cross reference for metabolic encephalopathy (348.31), which leads you to delirium in the Alphabetic Index to Diseases. Under the main term "Encephalopathy; metabolic," a cross-reference directs you to see also "Delirium, NOS," (code 780.09) which is coded from chapter 16 on Symptoms, Signs, and Ill-Defined Conditions. However, this may have been intended to be coded more specifically by the physician as "acute" or "subacute" delirium (acute confusion), which is coded to 293.0 or 293.1, respectively. **Acute** and **subacute** are given as subterms under the main term "Delirium." These codes indicate that the acute or subacute delirium is a transient mental disorder caused by an endocrinologic, metabolic, or infective disorder, as described in the inclusion notes under codes 293.0 and 293.1 in the *Tabular List of Diseases*. Clarify the coding of metabolic encephalopathy with the physician and, if necessary, have the physician add supporting documentation to the patient's medical record.

TABLE 19.1	Fifth Digits to Describe Phases of Schizophrenic Illness	
Digit	**Phase**	**Description**
0	Unspecified	—
1	Subchronic	<2-yr course of illness
2	Chronic	>2-yr course of illness
3	Subchronic with acute exacerbation	<2-yr course of illness with acute onset (exacerbation) of symptoms
4	Chronic with acute exacerbation	>2-yr course of illness with acute onset (exacerbation) of symptoms
5	In remission	No active symptoms of the disease

Dementia is characterized by the loss of mental ability (e.g., memory loss, personality changes, and impaired judgment) and intellectual ability because of a nonacute, chronic condition associated with permanent brain damage. Dementia often occurs from diseases such as Alzheimer's disease, Parkinson's disease, senile brain degeneration, brain injury, cerebrovascular disorders such as a stroke, and central nervous system neoplasms. Dementia often requires the assignment of two codes (i.e., mandatory dual coding) to describe first the underlying condition causing the dementia and then the associated dementia.

EXAMPLE	*Dementia attributable to Parkinson's disease: 331.82 + 294.10*
	Alzheimer's dementia with behavioral disturbances: 331.0 + 294.11

Schizophrenia

Schizophrenia (category code 295) is characterized by a person's withdrawal from reality. Symptoms include sensory hallucinations (e.g., hearing voices or seeing things that are not there), disorganized thinking (incoherence), impaired social functioning (e.g., detachment from others), delusions (false beliefs), and broadcasting (the belief that others can hear one's thoughts). The DSM-IV provides mental health practitioners with specific criteria that should be met before the diagnosis of schizophrenia is assigned; one criterion is that the patient must demonstrate continuous signs or symptoms of the illness for at least 6 months. The 295 category includes the use of a fourth digit to indicate the type of schizophrenia (e.g., paranoid or catatonic) and a fifth digit to indicate the current phase of illness. The phases or courses of schizophrenic illness are classified in Table 19.1.

EXAMPLE	*Chronic schizoaffective disorder: 295.72*
	Acute exacerbation of chronic schizophrenia: 295.34
	Chronic undifferentiated schizophrenia: 295.62

Substance-Related Disorders

ICD-9-CM classifies the conditions of alcohol abuse (problem drinking) or dependence (alcoholism) and drug abuse or dependence (e.g., of cannabis, cocaine, or opioids) in chapter 5 ("Mental Disorders") in the ICD-9-CM

Tabular List of Diseases. Abuse of drugs and/or alcohol is classified to category 305, dependence on alcohol is classified to category 303, and dependence on drugs is classified to category 304.

There is a distinction between substance abuse and dependence. Drug and/or alcohol **abuse** involves the nondependent psychological inclination to take a substance in excess despite its negative consequences to one's health and social functioning (e.g., problem drinker or drug abuser). However, drug and/or alcohol **dependence** is characterized by a physical reliance on the substance and withdrawal symptoms when no longer taking the substance.

Documentation of "alcohol use" is not the same as "alcohol abuse." Physician documentation of a patient's using alcohol or being a "social" drinker is not the same as the patient's being an abuser of alcohol. Do not automatically classify a patient who drinks alcohol as an alcohol abuser.

A common abbreviation for beverage alcohol is ETOH (ethyl alcohol), and many physicians simply document "ETOHism" for alcoholism or "ETOH abuse" to indicate alcohol abuse.

Fifth digits are provided for abuse and dependency codes to describe the current phase of the illness (Table 19.2).

Even though there are indented subterms for both "acute" and "chronic" under the main term "Alcoholism" in the *Alphabetic Index to Diseases*, code only the acute condition when the physician documents both "acute and chronic alcoholism" (correct: 303.0X; incorrect: 303.0X + 303.9X). Alcoholism, by its nature, is recognized within the medical community as a chronic disease, and this is therefore implied when acute alcoholism is coded.

Other conditions classified in the mental disorders chapter of ICD-9-CM can sometimes be associated with alcohol or drug dependence. These include alcoholic psychosis and drug psychosis disorders.

Alcohol-induced mental disorders (category 291) includes the following:

▶ alcoholic withdrawal delirium (i.e., delirium tremens): 291.0
▶ alcoholic dementia: 291.2
▶ alcohol withdrawal hallucinosis: 291.3

TABLE 19.2	Fifth Digits to Describe Phases of Substance Abuse and Dependency	
Digit	**Phase**	**Description**
0	Unspecified	—
1	Continuous	Prolonged consumption of excessive amounts of alcohol
2	Episodic	-Binge drinking; on-again, off-again, excessive weekend or social drinking, etc.
3	In remission	Not currently consuming alcohol

▶ alcoholic psychosis, NOS: 291.9
▶ alcohol induced sleep disorder: 291.82

Careful attention to the exclusion notes under each condition within category 291 will prevent redundant coding.

EXAMPLE	*Alcoholic withdrawal delirium with hallucinosis: 291.0*
	(Note—Do not code 291.0 [alcohol withdrawal delirium] + 291.3 [alcohol withdrawal hallucinosis], because code 291.3 excludes code 291.0; code 291.0 only.)

Drug-induced mental disorders (code category 292) includes the following:

▶ drug withdrawal syndrome: 292.0
▶ drug-induced hallucinosis: 292.12
▶ drug-induced delirium: 292.81
▶ drug-induced dementia: 292.82
▶ drug-induced sleep disorder: 292.85

SEQUENCING CODES FOR SUBSTANCE-RELATED DISORDERS

Recognizing the main focus of the treatment and considering the length of the patient's stay will help you determine whether to sequence the substance abuse and dependence code or the substance-related condition code as the principal diagnosis. For example, **detoxification** is a medical treatment that usually involves a short stay in a medical facility to manage alcohol and/or withdrawal symptoms. In this situation, sequence the alcohol- or drug-related psychosis (291 or 292) as the principal diagnosis because that is the principal focus of care. **Rehabilitation** for substance abuse and/or dependence usually involves a much longer inpatient stay (i.e., 28 days) or long-term outpatient management. In this case, sequence the alcohol and/or drug abuse or dependence (category 303, 304, or 305) as the principal diagnosis. **Combined detoxification and rehabilitation**, when provided during the same episode of care at the same facility, require you to sequence the alcohol and/or drug abuse or dependence codes (category 303, 304, or 305) as the principal diagnosis.

If the patient is admitted for evaluation and treatment of an acute medical condition associated with the alcohol abuse or dependence, sequence the acute medical condition as the principal diagnosis, followed by a code for the substance abuse or dependence disorder. Substance abuse and/or dependence codes should also be listed as additional codes when a patient is admitted for an unrelated condition.

EXAMPLE	*A patient was admitted to a hospital for detoxification therapy for acute alcoholic withdrawal syndrome with delirium tremens. The patient was a chronic alcoholic, continuous.*
	Principal diagnosis: 291.0 *Acute alcoholic withdrawal syndrome with delirium tremens*
	Secondary diagnosis: 303.91 *Chronic alcoholism, continuous*
	Procedure: 94.62 *Alcohol detoxification therapy*
	A patient was admitted to the hospital for treatment of acute on chronic alcoholic intoxication and received both alcoholic detoxification and rehabilitation therapy.
	Principal diagnosis: 303.00 *Acute on chronic alcoholic intoxication*
	Procedure: 94.63 *Alcohol detoxification and rehabilitation therapy*

A patient was admitted for treatment of alcoholic cirrhosis with ascites related to his alcoholism (continuous). A paracentesis to drain the ascites was performed, and detoxification therapy was given during the admission. The patient was given a referral to Alcoholics Anonymous at discharge.

Principal diagnosis:	*571.2 Alcoholic cirrhosis*
Secondary diagnoses:	*789.5 + 303.91 Ascites; and, alcoholism, continuous*
Procedures:	*54.91 + 94.62 Paracentesis; and, alcohol detoxification therapy*

(Note—For this case, sequence the medical condition of alcoholic cirrhosis as the principal diagnosis, with the type of substance abuse listed as an additional diagnosis. Even though the disease of alcoholic cirrhosis includes an assumption of alcoholism, you must code alcoholism separately because it is a separate disease that requires separate attention and treatment.)

A patient was admitted for femoral neck fracture from a fall, and the history revealed that the patient was a chronic alcoholic. The patient was taken to the operating room for an open reduction/internal fixation for the femoral fracture and also required detoxification therapy during his stay.

Principal diagnosis:	*820.8 Femoral neck fracture*
Secondary diagnosis:	*303.90 + E888.9 Chronic alcoholism; and , injury due to fall*
Procedures:	*79.35 + 94.62 ORIF femoral neck fracture; and, alcohol detoxification therapy*

Tobacco use disorder (code 305.1), which affects many people, and misuse of laxatives (code 305.9X), commonly seen in the elderly, are also coded to chapter 5 on mental disorders in the ICD-9-CM.

TIP Physicians will sometimes document the cumulative effects of a smoking habit in terms of "pack years" within the patient's medical record. To determine the number of pack years, the physician multiples the number of packs smoked per day times the number of years smoked. For example, a "50 pack year" smoker could mean either one pack per day for 50 years (1 pack × 50 years), or two packs per day for 25 years (2 packs × 25 years).

Personality Disorders

Personality disorders (category 301) are characterized by abnormal patterns of behavior and thinking about one's self and others that cause impairment in social functioning. Personality disorders include the following:

- ▶ borderline personality disorder (which causes unstable interpersonal relationships): 301.83
- ▶ antisocial personality disorder (showing a lack of concern for others): 301.7
- ▶ histrionic personality disorder (marked by emotional outbursts): 301.5
- ▶ paranoid personality disorder (persistent mistrust of others): 301.0
- ▶ passive-aggressive personality (aggression through passive means): 301.84

Alzheimer's Disease

Alzheimer's disease is a unique illness that often occurs in elderly people. Characterized by cerebral atrophy and central nervous system degeneration with neural plaques, this condition results in the progressive destruction of brain cells. Common symptoms accompanying the disease include memory and intellectual loss, emotional and behavioral disturbances, and wandering. ICD-9-CM provides a mandatory dual-coding mechanism for classifying Alzheimer's dementia with behavioral disturbance (code 331.0 + 294.11) and Alzheimer's dementia without behavioral disturbance (code 331.0 + 294.10).

Psychogenic Disorders and Psychic Factors Associated with Diseases

Psychogenic disorders (category codes 306 and 307) occur when a patient's mental conflicts are expressed as physical symptoms but do not involve tissue damage or organic illness. **Psychic factors associated with diseases** (category 316) occur when a patient's mental illness has played a major role in the cause of a physical condition that involves tissue damage and organic illness. Category code 316 requires the use of an additional code to identify the associated physical condition.

EXAMPLE	
Psychogenic vomiting: 306.4	
Psychogenic chest pain: 307.89	
Psychogenic paralysis: 306.0	
Psychogenic hyperventilation: 306.1	
Psychogenic asthma: 316 + 493.90	
Psychogenic dermatitis: 316 + 692.9	
Psychogenic gastric ulcer: 316 + 532.90	
Psychogenic ulcerative colitis: 316 + 556	

Organic Brain Syndrome

A **syndrome** is a group of symptoms that point to a particular disease. In organic brain syndrome (OBS), central nervous system symptoms after organic brain damage are apparent. The symptoms of OBS can include significant memory disturbances or lapses, intellectual impairment, personality changes (e.g., irritability and lethargy), and physical weakness. OBS can result from different causes, such as a traumatic brain injury (e.g., after concussion), alcoholism, and postencephalitic brain damage, or it can be associated with age (senility). Carefully review the physician's documentation in the medical record to determine whether the OBS is specified as psychotic or nonpsychotic, because this can affect the classification. Nonpsychotic mental disorders attributable to organic brain damage are classified to category 310, whereas OBS with psychosis is classified to the organic psychotic condition category (293 to 294).

EXAMPLE	
Organic brain syndrome, NOS (nonpsychotic): 310.9	
Organic personality syndrome (nonpsychotic): 310.1	
Organic postconcussion syndrome (nonpsychotic): 310.2	
Organic brain syndrome with psychosis: 294.9	
Organic brain syndrome, posttraumatic, with chronic psychosis: 294.8	
Organic brain syndrome, posttraumatic, with acute psychosis: 293.0	

Therapies for Mental Disorders, Including Treatments forAlcohol and/or Drug Abuse

Excluding alcohol and/or drug detoxification and rehabilitation therapy, common therapies for mental disorders include psychotherapy, electroconvulsive therapy, and psychotherapeutic drugs.

Types of **psychotherapy** include behavior therapy (code 94.33); group therapy (code 94.44); family therapy (code 94.42); and hypnosis (code 94.32). Psychotherapeutic play therapy (code 94.36) is often used with children, who cannot be as verbally expressive as adults.

Electroconvulsive therapy (code 94.27) is sometimes used in the treatment of major depression or the depressive cycle of bipolar disorder. In electroconvulsive therapy, electricity is applied to the brain to induce seizures and increase the level of dopamine in the brain. Dopamine is an intrinsic chemical neurotransmitter in the brain that may help to alleviate severe depression.

Psychotherapeutic drugs used to treat mental disorders include antidepressants (e.g., sertraline hydrochloride [Zoloft], amitriptyline [Elavil], and fluoxetine hydrochloride [Prozac]), antianxiety agents (e.g., alprazolam [Xanax], lorazepam [Ativan], and diazepam [Valium]), and antipsychotics (e.g., haloperidol [Haldol], chlorpromazine [Thorazine], thioridazine [Mellaril], and lithium).

Procedure subcategory 94.6X provides codes for alcohol and/or drug detoxification, rehabilitation, and combined detoxification and rehabilitation therapy. Correctly assigning these therapy codes is critically important for receiving reimbursement when reporting substance abuse and dependence diagnoses to third-party payers, who often question the medical necessity for substance-related patient admissions.

SUMMARY

This chapter has identified common emotional and mental disorders and the various clinical therapies used to treat these ailments. The manifestations that are symptomatic of these problems also have been referenced in this chapter, and an emphasis has been placed on proper coding practices to use through the use of ICD-9-CM and patient clinical records.

TESTING YOUR COMPREHENSION

1. Derived from ICD-9-CM, what manual provides codes for the classification of mental disorders and is also used as a tool to help mental health professionals establish a patient's diagnosis?

_____

2. To understand the terminology used by psychiatrists/psychologists, coders must understand the DSM. However, Medicare and other third-party payers mandate the use of which codes for the reporting of mental health diagnoses?

_____

3. What is a term used to describe a clinical condition in which anxiety is manifested with depression?

_____

4. What is another clinical term for an irrational fear?

_____

5. A false self-perception of one's weight is also clinically known as what?

_____

6. Binge eating followed by self-induced vomiting is referred to as what?

_____

7. Affective psychoses are included in which code category?

_____

8. An acute transient mental disturbance with acute confusion is referred to as what?

_____

9. The loss of thinking or intellectual capacity associated with brain damage or another clinical condition affecting the brain is referred to as what?

_____

10. Identify the proper code categories for conditions related to substance abuse and dependence: (a) abuse of drugs or alcohol; (b) dependence on alcohol; and (c) dependence on drugs.

_____

11. To which category is alcohol psychosis classified?

_____

12. A stay in an inpatient facility to manage one's withdrawal from a substance abuse condition is referred to as what?

_____

13. What clinical condition is characterized by abnormal patterns of behavior and thinking about one's self and others that cause impairment in social functioning?

_____

14. A group of symptoms pointing to a particular disease is referred to as what?

_____

15. Identify some common therapies used for various mental disorders.

_____

16. What is the clinical difference between substance abuse and substance dependence?

_____

CODING PRACTICE I   Chapter Review Exercises

Directions

By using your ICD-9-CM codebook, code the following diagnoses and procedures:

	DIAGNOSIS/PROCEDURES	CODE
1	Acute alcohol intoxication in chronic alcoholism. Depression. Alcohol detoxification and rehabilitation.	
2	Chronic paranoid schizophrenia.	
3	Acute delirium attributable to electrolyte imbalance. Alzheimer's disease with dementia. Emphysema with hypercapnia and mixed acid-base disorder.	
4	Anxiety with depression. Chronic fatigue syndrome. Hypochondriasis.	
5	Alcoholic cardiomyopathy. Alcohol dependence, continuous.	
6	Chest pain secondary to cocaine abuse.	
7	Bipolar disorder, currently depressed, severe.	
8	Recurrent major depression with psychotic episode. Electroconvulsive therapy.	
9	Phantom limb pain, status post above-the-knee amputation. Posttraumatic stress disorder. Gulf War veteran.	
10	Acute exacerbation of chronic schizoaffective disorder.	
11	Anorexia nervosa. Dehydration. Severe malnutrition. Total parenteral nutrition. Intravenous hydration.	

	DIAGNOSIS/PROCEDURES	CODE
12	Acute confusion secondary to multi-infarct dementia.	
13	Delirium tremens, alcohol-withdrawal seizures. Acute and chronic alcoholism, episodic. Detoxification therapy.	
14	Agoraphobia with panic attack. Psychogenic dermatitis.	
15	Attention-deficit disorder with hyperactivity.	
16	Tension headache. Adjustment reaction caused by academic stress. Emancipation disorder, college freshman; first time away from home and living in dormitory.	
17	Tourette's syndrome. Facial tics.	
18	Psychogenic diarrhea. Mild dehydration. Obsessive-compulsive personality disorder. Intravenous fluid hydration.	
19	Acute confusion secondary to propoxyphene (Darvon). Darvon prescribed after recent extraction of wisdom teeth.	
20	Organic brain syndrome secondary to chronic alcoholism. Scabies. Patient lives on the streets.	
21	Altered mental status, etiology unknown.	

CODING PRACTICE II   Medical Record Case Studies

Instructions

1. Carefully review the medical reports provided for each case study.
2. Research any abbreviations and terms that are unfamiliar or unclear.
3. Identify as many diagnoses and procedures as possible.
4. Because only part of the patient's total record is available, determine what additional documentation you might need.
5. If appropriate, identify any questions you might ask the physician to code this case correctly and completely.
6. Complete the appropriate blanks below for each case study.

CHAPTER 19 CASE STUDIES

Case Study 19.1 (Coder/Abstract Summary Form)

Patient: **Jane Doe**

Patient documentation: **Review Medical Report 19.1**

1. Principal diagnosis:

   _____

2. Secondary or other diagnoses:

   _____

3. Principal procedure:

   _____

4. Other procedures:

   _____

5. Additional documentation needed:

   _____

   _____

   _____

   _____

Case Study 19.1 (Continued)

6. Questions for the physician:

_____

_____

_____

_____

_____

MEDICAL REPORT 19.1

CONSULTATION

PATIENT: DOE, JANE

DOB:

MED REC:

PT ADMN:

ADMN DTE:

LOCATION:

PHYSICIAN:

DATE OF CONSULTATION:

REQUESTING PHYSICIAN:

CONSULTING PHYSICIAN:

HISTORY OF PRESENT ILLNESS: This is a 62-year-old white female, disabled, who was admitted because of generalized weakness and pain. The patient is well known to me. She has a long history of schizoaffective disorder, bipolar type. She has been hospitalized many times in psychiatric facilities. The patient has been taking Zyprexa as well as Zoloft. She apparently has been increasingly delusional. She has been having somatic delusions, believing that she has cancer. Her family apparently has been unable to care for her at home and wants her to be placed in a nursing home. She has been depressed, easily agitated and argumentative. The patient possibly was not compliant with her medications. She has been refusing treatment at the emergency room primarily because of her delusions.

PSYCHIATRIC HISTORY: The patient has been hospitalized several times. She has a history of chronic psychiatric illnesses, diagnosed with schizoaffective disorder bipolar type.

MEDICAL HISTORY: Hypothyroidism, hypercholesterolemia, hypertension, compensated congestive heart failure.

FAMILY HISTORY: No history of psychiatric illness.

PERSONAL AND SOCIAL HISTORY: The patient was living at home with youngest daughter. No history of alcohol or substance abuse.

MENTAL STATUS EXAMINATION: The patient is currently alert, overweight, white female. She is currently not in acute distress. She is coherent. Positive for somatic delusions. She is convinced that she has cancer. She also is making inappropriate remarks like asking me what happened to my baby. She also was making inappropriate remarks about her previous psychiatrist. She denies suicidal or homicidal ideations. Mood is depressed and irritable. Affect is restricted. Oriented to person, place, and partly to time. Concentration is impaired. Short term and long term memory intact. Insight and judgment impaired. She has poor understanding of her medical and psychiatric illness. Also does not have clear understanding of her inability to care for herself at home.

ASSESSMENT:
AXIS I   Schizoaffective disorder, depressed.

AXIS II   Deferred

AXIS III   As above.

Medical Report 19.1 (Continued)

RECOMMENDATIONS: This 62-year-old patient is currently acutely psychotic consistent with exacerbation of schizoaffective disorder.

I would recommend:

1. Given patient's weight problem, I would suggest discontinuing Zyprexa.
2. Use Risperdal 2 mg b.i.d.
3. Continue Zoloft 25 mg q.a.m.
4. Ativan 1 mg p.o. or IM q. 6h. p.r.n. for agitation.
5. Agree with placing patient in skilled nursing facility. I will also consider Baker Act.

I will follow patient with you. Thank you very much for allowing me to participate in the care of this patient.

SMITH, MD

NOTES

Case Study 19.2 (Coder/Abstract Summary Form)

Patient: **Trudy Jefferson**

Patient documentation: **Review Medical Report 19.2**

1. Principal diagnosis:

   _____

2. Secondary or other diagnoses:

   _____

3. Principal procedure:

   _____

4. Other procedures:

   _____

5. Additional documentation needed:

   _____

   _____

   _____

6. Questions for the physician:

   _____

   _____

   _____

   _____

   _____

MEDICAL REPORT 19.2

CONSULTATION

PATIENT: JEFFERSON, Trudy

DOB:

MED REC:

PT ADMN:

ADMN DTE:

LOCATION:

PHYSICIAN:

DATE OF CONSULTATION:

REFERRING PHYSICIAN:

CONSULTING PHYSICIAN:

REASON FOR CONSULTATION: The patient is a 72-year-old widowed white female who was referred for psychiatric consultation for evaluation and management as the patient was very confused and agitated and psychotic.

HISTORY OF PRESENT ILLNESS: I have reviewed the chart, discussed with staff and interviewed the patient. I also had a chance to speak to the patient's son who was visiting. The patient is known to me as I have seen her in the nursing home, mainly for depression, but here the patient was admitted for altered mental status and she was found to have a urinary tract infection and congestive heart failure. Yesterday, she was very confused, agitated and had symptoms of delirium, paranoia, very abusive to nursing staff, calling them whores and telling that they had syphilis and she was also very delusional stating that she was going to have a baby. She states that she is 29 years old. She did not know where she was and when I asked her who the president was, she said it was Kennedy. She had no idea where she was living before she came to the hospital. She is doing better today. She had been on Haldol p.r.n., which has made some positive effect on the patient, and the patient is not agitated and abusive but still confused and delusional. I explained to the patient and the son how medical problems can make patients with dementia delirious and it is not uncommon but they feel once she is medically better, she will improve and as noted, already improving. She denies depression but appears a little anxious.

PSYCHIATRIC HISTORY: History of depression and dementia. She has been on Prozac and Ambien in the nursing home.

SOCIAL HISTORY: The patient is widowed, resident of a nursing home. No history of alcohol abuse or drug abuse.

MEDICAL HISTORY: Please refer to History and Physical.

MENTAL STATUS EXAMINATION: The patient is well developed, fairly well nourished, alert, oriented to person only. She did not know the date or the month or the year. Her speech is coherent, spontaneous; normal tone and volume. Her mood is not depressed but anxious. The patient is not suicidal; the patient is not homicidal. The patient's thinking is not organized; evidence of confusion and delusional thinking is quite apparent. The patient's recent memory is impaired. Her concentration is impaired. Her retention and recall is impaired. Her insight and judgment are impaired. Impulse control was questionable.

DIAGNOSIS:
1. Dementia, but acute delirium improving.
2. Depressive disorder, stable.
3. Urinary tract infection.

Continued

MEDICAL REPORT 19.2 (CONTINUED)

RECOMMENDATIONS:

1. The patient will be started on Risperdal 0.25 mg twice a day, 1:00 PM and 5:00 PM and Haldol would be 1 mg by mouth or IM every four hours p.r.n.

2. For all of her medical needs, she will continue with her primary care physician.

3. I will follow the patient from a psychiatric point of view here in the hospital and then in the nursing home.

4. I will also recommence Prozac 20 mg every day and Ambien 5 mg h.s. p.r.n.

Thank you for consulting me.

_____

SMITH, MD

NOTES

Case Study 19.3 (Coder/Abstract Summary Form)

Patient: **Anne Connors**

Patient documentation: **Review Medical Report 19.3**

1. Principal diagnosis:

   _____

2. Secondary or other diagnoses:

   _____

3. Principal procedure:

   _____

4. Other procedures:

   _____

5. Additional documentation needed:

   _____

   _____

   _____

   _____

6. Questions for the physician:

   _____

   _____

   _____

   _____

   _____

MEDICAL REPORT 19.3

CONSULTATION

PATIENT: CONNORS, Anne

DOB:

MED REC:

PT ADMN:

ADMN DTE:

LOCATION:

PHYSICIAN:

CHIEF COMPLAINT: "I don't know!"

HISTORY OF PRESENT ILLNESS: This is an 74-year-old female patient, evaluated on the medicine unit. The patient was admitted from a local nursing home with an overall episode of decreasing level of consciousness, as well as increasing temperature and chest congestion. It is felt that the patient is aspirating which is very similar to the circumstances in which the patient was last seen by psychiatry. Since admission, the patient has been essentially lethargic and has not presented any type of behavior problems to the staff. This being said, the patient does have a long-term history of Alzheimer's type dementia, with chronic delusional thinking and has often been quite difficult to manage as she will become psychotic, as well as quite agitated and impulsive. During her last admission, her medications were decreased but did have to be increased once her medical problems cleared secondary to the above-mentioned behaviors.

The patient's history of cognitive decline is well detailed in previous reports but let it suffice to say that she has had a fairly typical decline that is seen with patients with Alzheimer's type dementia and has had associated psychotic and behavioral problems.

The patient's current psychotropic drug regimen consists of

1. Depakote ER 500 mg b.i.d.

2. Exelon 6 mg b.i.d.

3. Seroquel 200 mg h.s.

4. Seroquel 50 mg b.i.d.

5. The patient does have, as needed, doses of Desyrel 50 mg h.s. and also Haldol 2.5 mg q. 4 hours p.r.n. The patient has not received any doses of p.r.n. medications since admission.

MEDICAL AND PSYCHIATRIC HISTORY: The patient's first psychiatric contact was in the mid 1990s. The patient went on to develop Alzheimer's dementia and the patient has had several inpatient psychiatric admissions secondary to behavioral problems related to this. There is no history of alcohol or drug abuse.

Physical medical problems include atherosclerotic cardiovascular disease with coronary artery disease and hypertension, arthritis, diabetes, pacemaker, peripheral vascular disease.

FAMILY HISTORY: Reported as negative for neuropsychiatric illness.

PERSONAL AND SOCIAL HISTORY: She has a ninth-grade education. The patient was married once and did have 5 children. Her husband has been deceased for a little over 20 years. The patient has been residing in the nursing home setting for at least the last 7–8 years. The patient worked on her farm with her husband throughout her adult life.

MEDICAL REPORT 19.3 (CONTINUED)

STRENGTHS AND ASSETS: Good family support, stable premorbid adaptation, and no evidence of tardive dyskinesia.

MENTAL STATUS EXAMINATION: The patient is a well-developed, elderly female with white hair, who appears her stated age. The patient is asleep and, although she does arouse, she is still difficult to engage in the interview. Psychomotor slowing is noted. Speech is easily understandable. The patient is mildly hard of hearing. Mood is irritable. Affect is congruent. Thinking is quite disorganized at this point. Thought content without active hallucinations noted currently, although the patient is clearly delusional. Cognitively, the patient is oriented to herself, will orient to location with hints. No further aspect of the mental status examination was completed at this time.

DIAGNOSTIC IMPRESSION:

Axis I: Dementia, Alzheimer's type, with psychosis and depression.

Axis II: None.

Axis III: Likely Alzheimer's type dementia.

   Atherosclerotic cardiovascular disease with coronary artery disease and hypertension.

   Diabetes.

   Arthritis.

   Pacemaker.

   Peripheral vascular disease.

Axis IV: Stressors: primary cognitive and physical decline.

Axis V: 20.

DISCUSSION AND RECOMMENDATIONS: Currently it appears that the patient's medications were placed at their previous doses after return from her last hospitalization. It is known that the patient's behavior has been fairly stable in the nursing home setting, as well as her level of consciousness. This being said, clearly her mental status is suffering from her ongoing medical problems.

For now, will again decrease the patient's medication slightly and will monitor her behavior closely. Of course, the patient does still have her as-needed dose of Haldol if her behavior should suddenly change.

Thank you very much for the consultation. Please feel free to contact if you wish to discuss.

SMITH, MD

Case Study 19.4 (Coder/Abstract Summary Form)

Patient: **John Doe**

Patient documentation: **Review Medical Report 19.4**

1. Principal diagnosis:

_____

2. Secondary or other diagnoses:

_____

3. Principal procedure:

_____

4. Other procedures:

_____

5. Additional documentation needed:

_____

_____

_____

6. Questions for the physician:

_____

_____

_____

_____

_____

MEDICAL REPORT 19.4

CONSULTATION

PATIENT: DOE, JOHN

DOB:

MED REC:

PT ADMN:

ADMN DTE:

LOCATION:

PHYSICIAN:

CHIEF COMPLAINT: "I think had a stroke again!"

HISTORY OF PRESENT ILLNESS: The patient is a 78-year-old male, evaluated on telemetry. The patient does have a history of previous admissions related to neurologic symptoms, which include stroke-like episodes, transient ischemic attacks, and seizures. The attending Dr. has seen patient and he feels that this is a complex case, but is unable to say that there was definite neurologic pathology to his current presentation. Workup, including MRI of the brain, is negative. In fact, he only has mild small-vessel disease. The EEG does demonstrate some interictal epileptiform activity on the left side. However, the attending Dr. does not feel that this explains his presentation. This patient is known to me from a previous consultation. Unfortunately, these records are not available to me at this time.

The patient is a poor historian. However, he does state that he was initially admitted with an inability to speak and some shaking of his arm. These symptoms seem to have resolved rather rapidly.

The patient does readily relate anxiety and panic symptomatology. He notes that he often gets short of breath, has chest pain, chest tightness, feels shaky, and has heart palpitations. The patient attributes most of these to his chronic obstructive pulmonary disease.

Furthermore, the patient acknowledges some depression. He does have long-term difficulties with sleep. Appetite has not been a problem. The patient does complain that he cannot walk or do much of anything anymore and gets little enjoyment from his life. He denies suicidal ideation. He denies feeling helpless, hopeless, or worthless.

CURRENT PSYCHOTROPIC REGIMEN: Consists of:

1. Celexa 40 mg h.s.
2. Xanax 0.25 mg b.i.d.
3. Tegretol XR 400 mg b.i.d. The patient does have a therapeutic Tegretol level.

The patient is thought to be basically cognitively intact. He does acknowledge that he has difficulty with his memory.

MEDICAL AND PSYCHIATRIC HISTORY: The patient, in addition to psychiatric consultation here, did go to the XYZ Mental Health Center a number of years ago. Apparently, this was one visit. He states that he was told that there was nothing wrong. The patient denies any history of drug or alcohol abuse.

Physical medical problems are significant for history of seizure disorder, thought to be well controlled, chronic obstructive pulmonary disease, remote history of congestive heart failure, history of hypertension, prostatectomy, and osteoarthritis.

FAMILY HISTORY: Significant for two daughters and a son who he states is a "worthless bum and alcoholic!"

PERSONAL AND SOCIAL HISTORY: The patient reports a 6th-grade education and is illiterate. The patient was married for 40 or 50 years and worked in a factory. His wife died approximately 15 years ago from breast cancer. The patient is currently living with an old friend, who helps look after him. He also has the assistance of a home health nurse who loads his medication box.

The patient has three children that live in other states and he hasn't heard from them in awhile. The patient does not have much family support.

Continued

MEDICAL REPORT 19.4 (CONTINUED)

PATIENT STRENGTHS AND ASSETS: Cognitively intact, does have supportive living arrangements and no evidence of tardive dyskinesia.

MENTAL STATUS EXAMINATION: Alert, attentive, cooperative, easily engaged gentleman. He is a bit anxious about psychiatric evaluation and jokes, "you must think I'm nuts!" The patient is a well-developed, well-nourished, rotund-appearing gentleman. He is also hard of hearing. Speech is a bit rapid. Psychomotor activity displays his anxiety and mild agitation. The patient does make good eye contact. Mood is primarily anxious. Affect congruent. Thinking basically logical, goal-oriented, and relevant. Thought content without hallucinations of delusions. The patient did not appear to be guarded. Cognitively, he is fully oriented including year, month, and date. Memory was tested. He remembers three of four words instantly, one of four at 5 minutes. He does not get any others with hints. The patient's effort was rather poor at this point. The patient recalls the last two presidents without difficulties. The patient abstracts one of three simple proverbs.

DIAGNOSTIC IMPRESSION:

Axis I: Panic disorder without agoraphobia.

Probable generalized anxiety disorder.

Major depression. Recurrent, mild.

Axis II: None.

Axis III: Seizure disorder.

Chronic obstructive pulmonary disease.

Hypertension.

History of prostatectomy.

Osteoarthritis.

Axis IV: Stressors: the physical problems, perhaps, some degree of social and sensory isolation.

Axis V: 35.

DISCUSSION AND RECOMMENDATIONS: There is little doubt that the patient has a significant anxiety disorder. His history and symptom reporting is vague. Presentation is compatible with severe anxiety which is complicating his other medical issues. Patient also has an element of depression.

Do note that patient is on some steroids that could easily exacerbate his symptoms.

Recommendations will be to give him a trial of Effexor. Effexor can be quite helpful for the anxiety component. Plan to start low does of Effexor tomorrow morning. Monitor tolerance and titrate accordingly. Additionally, if he does well with the Effexor will taper out the Celexa.

All records are not available as far as I can recall. The patient did not follow up as an outpatient. I would be concerned that he will not follow up again. It may be useful for the patient to have a course of rehabilitation where medications can be fully adjusted and properly judged.

Thank you very much for the consultation. Please feel free to contact me if you wish to discuss. The patient will be followed.

SMITH, MD

PART III

THE IMPACT OF CODING ON HEALTH SERVICES ADMINISTRATION

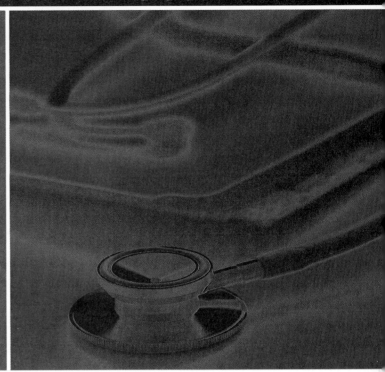

Chapter 20   Managed Health Care and Health Information Management

Managed Health Care and Health Information Management

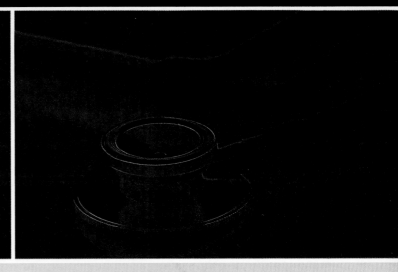

Chapter Objectives

▶ Describe the development of managed care from its beginnings.

▶ Explain how managed care has affected health information management (HIM) as a discipline.

▶ Identify the prominent types of managed care models.

▶ Explain the managed care reimbursement models being used.

▶ Explain the impact of managed care on the coding profession.

America's health-care delivery system is fundamentally sound and is arguably the best in the world. Our accomplishments in the fields of medical research and health care have established a standard to which other nations aspire, specifically the combination of professionally trained clinicians and vast clinical resources that are available to treat complex medical conditions.

The primary challenge confronting Americans today is how to make the health-care system responsive and more accessible to everyone. Before managed care, Americans enjoyed unimpeded access to health care through a more traditional fee-for-service system. The insurance industry provided indemnity health plans with nominal deductibles and unlimited visits to the physician(s) of choice. This pattern of insurance coverage mirrored Medicare's generous reimbursement structure. However, Medicare's skyrocketing costs contributed to significant deficit spending by the federal government and an inflationary spiral in health-care expenditures that necessitated significant changes. The changes did not come without debate, and many of the changes did not work as well as planned. Ultimately, the federal government instituted a series of legislative initiatives that became known as **managed care**.[1]

This chapter chronicles how these initiatives have led to the system of health care that we have today as exemplified by several legislative actions and how these laws have impacted the provision of health services in America. Also addressed will be the way in which the private insurance industry initiated many of the changes required by the Medicare program and how these changes have affected the health information management (HIM) and coding professions. This chapter also will address the managed care system and the effect of coding in the managed care environment.[2]

Origin, Emergence, and Early Development—Prepaid Health Care

Prepaid medical services first reached America's shores in a limited sense in 1798 when the Federal Marine Hospital Service was established to contain the spread of communicable diseases among members of the U.S. Merchant Marine Service. These transient seafaring laborers were highly susceptible to the numerous and highly contagious diseases that encircled the globe and claimed hundreds of unsuspecting victims. To fund this health program, 20 cents was taken from each seaman's monthly paycheck.[3]

The development of voluntary prepaid health plans began emerging during the California Gold Rush of 1849; one of those plans, sponsored by the Southern Pacific Railroad Company, survived well into the 20th century.[3] The number of such plans increased during the first half of the 20th century. In 1929, more than 1,500 Texas school teachers began paying 50 cents per person per month to become participating members of a prepaid hospital plan sponsored through Baylor Hospital.[4] During that same year, two Southern California physicians established a prepaid plan that served 2,000 members of the Los Angeles County Department of Water and Power. At the same time, proponents of fee-for-service medicine initiated an aggressive attack on prepaid health plans and what was characterized as their unethical advertising. An attack led by the Los Angeles County Medical Society and the California Medical Association vilified two of their own members—Drs. Donald Ross and Clifford Loos—for the unconventional practices of the Ross-Loos Clinic. This organized opposition to prepaid medical plans lasted for almost five decades.[4]

The infancy of prepaid medicine was further nurtured, although inadvertently, by a young surgeon, Sidney Garfield, who contracted to care for

5,000 medically neglected employees working along the Colorado River aqueduct, which ran 190 miles from the desert communities of Southern California to the suburbs of Los Angeles. His practice included a 12-bed hospital that he had developed. Initially, Dr. Garfield could not collect much more than the fees authorized through the workers' compensation program, and the insurance companies frequently objected to the claims submitted for payment.[5] Despite Garfield's obvious dedication, his experiment was losing money. His plight was noticed by two officers of the Industrial Indemnity Exchange, Harold Hatch and Alonzo Ordway, and they suggested paying Dr. Garfield $1.50 per employee per month as a prepayment for services to be rendered. In addition, Hatch, Ordway, and Garfield developed a prepayment plan for the workers, for illnesses and injuries unrelated to the workplace, at a rate of 5 cents per day. Nearly all of the workers joined, and Garfield employed 10 physicians and constructed 2 additional inpatient facilities.[4]

On the basis of his success in Southern California, Dr. Garfield accepted an offer in 1938 from Edgar Kaiser to develop a similar plan in Mason City, WA, where 5,000 Kaiser employees were constructing the Grand Coulee Dam. Kaiser prepaid a non-work-related voluntary health-care plan. In this case, however, most of the workers had families with no health coverage and without the means to pay a hospital bill if a family member became ill. In response, Garfield created a family plan in which spouses paid 50 cents per day and in which 25 cents per day was charged for each child. The plan became a financial success and formed the basis for a 30-year relationship between Kaiser and Garfield, until Kaiser's death in 1967.[4] The ultimate result of this relationship was the Kaiser Foundation Health Plan. By 1990, the Kaiser Foundation Health Plan had a membership in excess of 6 million subscribers. Today, that membership exceeds 7 million subscribers.

In addition to the Garfield/Kaiser effort, other lesser-known but equally important ventures into the prepaid arena were occurring. One in Elk City, OK, sought to make health-care services available to farm employees and their families. Dr. Michael Shadid, the plan's founder, established a rural farmers' health-care cooperative and strove to ensure that each participant received services to meet his or her basic health-care needs. To qualify, each participant purchased shares at $50 per share to build a hospital. In return, the subscribers received health-care services at a discount from Dr. Shadid.[6] In 1934, the Farmer's Union assumed responsibility for both the hospital and the health-care plan Dr. Shadid had established. In return for his efforts and unyielding commitment, Dr. Shadid was subsequently disqualified from the county medical society and was threatened with having his medical license revoked. Some 20 years later, as a result of a successful antitrust suit against the county and state medical societies, Dr. Shadid was absolved of any wrongdoing.[7]

Each of these ventures and others like them in the earliest days of prepaid health care had two distinct characteristics in common—establishing an accessible and affordable model of service delivery to large groups of individuals to bridge the gap in the availability of health-care services to everyone, regardless of ability to pay, and unselfishly approaching both medical practice and the financing of health care on the part of the respective founders.

Prepaid Health Care to Managed Health Care

How did America shift from a series of prepaid health plans to managed care? Events dating back to 1946 gradually and incrementally led to managed care, a reimbursement system emphasizing shortened hospital stays and limits on reimbursement for services provided. Getting to this point, however, was not a result of a single sweeping legislative action. Instead, the process took several years and included many new laws that gave the government greater control over reimbursement and that held providers more accountable for their actions.

The relevance of these legislative changes to the coding professions relates to the importance of structuring medical coding to conform to an increasing environment of federal oversight. The expectations and demands for consistency in clinical diagnoses and the proper documentation of care stress the importance of having coding professionals who can properly advise a clinician to avoid an inadvertent violation of proper billing practices.

Legislation Leading to Managed Care

Several legislative actions ultimately established what is known today as managed care.

The Hill-Burton Act

In 1946, Congress passed the Hill-Burton Act to alleviate an acute shortage of hospitals and beds. The result was an expansion of bed capacity that was intended to increase public access to needed health-care services.[8] The program was an unqualified success and resulted in a significant development of new hospitals and beds for an expectant public that included many returning World War II veterans and their growing families.

Subsequent to the Hill-Burton legislation, President Harry Truman expressed a desire for and a commitment to enacting a program of universal health-care coverage for all citizens of the United States. Although he was unsuccessful in his bid to see this legislation adopted, America's consciousness of the disparity of available health-care resources was aroused and continued through the subsequent Eisenhower, Kennedy, and Johnson administrations. The result in 1965 was the passage and enactment of Title 18 and Title 19 of the Social Security Act. These became known as the Medicare and Medicaid Amendments, and the programs fostered through this legislation opened for business January 1, 1966.

Medicare

Medicare represented the first substantive involvement of the federal government in actually paying for the health-care services of significant numbers of citizens—ultimately this population included the aged, the economically disadvantaged, and those with certain disabilities (e.g., renal failure). The implications of this legislation led to accountability among providers and payers alike that grew out of an exchange of fees paid for services rendered. Mountainous costs to the federal budget resulted from this important relationship between providers and our government.

After several amendments to the Medicare legislation were passed, there was a heightened awareness of the importance of involving coding specialists in the presentation of billing submissions. As evidenced by the incremental development of managed care, the importance of proper coding to the entire process was not immediately apparent in 1966. Rather, its importance and the dependence on coders developed out of necessity. As the complexity of Medicare legislation increased, it resulted in the growth of the numbers and types of facilities offering health care services beyond traditional hospital inpatient care (e.g., observation and step-down units, ambulatory surgery centers, ambulatory care medical clinics, home health agencies, physician group practices). This set the foundation for the spectrum of managed care.

As the cost of the Medicare program escalated, the concerns of legislators and payers similarly increased. Restraining the debt created from Medicare's burgeoning costs became essential. Shortly after the Medicare legislation was enacted, Congress passed separate acts that spurred comprehensive health planning (public law [PL] 89-749) and regional medical program development (PL 89-239) as priorities. The health-care planning legislation was intended to foster long-range planning and program development. The regional medical programs were focused on planning and establishing programs to treat heart disease, cancer, and stroke, the three primary causes of death in 1965. Unfortunately, these initiatives became rivals, and the subsequent turf wars resulted in disappointing progress.

UTILIZATION REVIEW AND PRECERTIFICATION

In 1972 and 1973, two new legislative efforts were undertaken—professional standards review organizations (PSROs) in 1972 (PL 92-603) and the Health Maintenance Organization (HMO) Act in 1973 (PL 93-222).[8] PSROs were independent peer review agencies (i.e., included physicians) contracted by the federal government to review the appropriateness and "medical necessity" of patient care under federally funded health programs such as Medicare and Medicaid. This was to ensure the government was protecting the solvency of the Medicare Trust Fund that was supported by working peoples' tax dollars. The Health Maintenance Organization Act was driven by a growing concern for the rising costs of employee health benefits and premiums. This Act established federal loans and grants for developing and implementing health care delivery organizations called health maintenance organizations (HMOs). An HMO is a prepaid voluntary health plan that provides an umbrella of various health care servcies to enrollees in retirn for a fixed monthly premium (i.e., capitation).

Both the PSRO and HMO legislative programs introduced **utilization review** (UR) and **precertification** to the language of medical practice and were the first attempt to establish accountability as a signal of the responsibilities of both providers and consumers. These laws also afforded an introduction to the challenges of gaining willing compliance and the active participation of medical providers. UR recognized that health-care resources are precious and expensive, and sought to ensure that the health-care resources used to treat a patient's condition were "medically necessary" and appropriate for the patient's needs. Precertification by the payer prior to a provider's services being rendered represented an external check to ensure that the medical necessity for expending health-care resources to treat the patient had been established. Additionally, this would help to avoid under-utilization or over-utilization of health-care resources.

The initial UR attempts were largely foiled by clinicians who saw government oversight as government control; this proved to be an unsuccessful venue in which to foster lasting professional behavioral change. HMOs also were experiencing many problems. The legislative product was a misunderstanding in Congress between liberals and conservatives: the liberal wing saw HMOs as fostering universal health-care coverage for all Americans, and conservatives saw HMOs as controlling and perhaps even reducing the cost of health care. Neither of the respective beliefs came to pass. Nonetheless, the seeds had been sown for two essential elements of managed care—UR and precertification—and this represented the beginning of health care UR and case management processes as we know it today.

THE EMPLOYEE RETIREMENT INCOME SECURITY ACT (ERISA)

Another legislative program adopted in 1974, the Employee Retirement Income Security Act (ERISA), was enacted to regulate the corporate use of pension funds to protect employees from misuse or fraud that could result in the loss of retirement funds. As part of this legislation, HMOs were granted a **preemption from oversight** by state departments of insurance.[8] ERISA allowed large employers (national corporations) to establish their own self-funded health plans that were not subject to state regulations that were disparate and cost prohibitive. In contrast to state oversight, the self-funded health plans were allowed federal oversight, and employers' organizations designed health plans using alternate delivery systems and cost-containment strategies such as UR and wellness care. Federally qualified HMOs were to come under the jurisdiction of the U.S. Department of Labor. As part of the preemption, HMOs were exempted from punitive damages arising from litigation involving their handling of care and other aspects of their relationships with subscribers. Although the legislation was certainly well intended, it contributed to a mentality among the expanding number of HMOs that they were above reproach when called to task for failing to act in a policyholder's interest under the contract of the health-care plan coverage. This attitude resulted in an inability of health-care plan operators to understand and accept that they had an obligation to respect the interests and rights of their subscribers, as well as the prerogatives of providers who cared for them. At the same time, this circumstance created enormous pressures on those responsible for billing services on behalf of health-care plan providers, and the level of contentiousness between payer and provider intensified.

Between 1975 and 1981, the legislative front became quiet, and activity subsided to a minimum. Jimmy Carter's presidency did not result in a significant number of legislative initiatives for either Congress or the American public to consider.

THE TAX EQUITY AND FISCAL RESPONSIBILITY ACT AND PROSPECTIVE PAYMENT (TEFRA)

With the election of Ronald Reagan in 1980, matters changed dramatically in terms of both the philosophy of our government and its engagement in the business of health care. The result was a more active approach to restraining both the cost and utilization of our nation's health-care resources. In 1983, the Tax Equity and Fiscal Responsibility Act (TEFRA) brought **prospective payment** to the forefront of the health-care debate. Under TEFRA, the reimbursement formula called Diagnosis Related Groups (DRGs) assigned fixed (prospective) payments to hospitals for inpatient services based on the average cost of treating the patient's condition which is reported through medical coding. This new reimbursement system changed the paradigm for health-care administrators and reinvented the financial systems that they had been operating under for years. Prior to TEFRA, providers were paid retrospectively (i.e., after services were provided) on the basis of the "usual and customary charges". With the introduction of TEFRA, this payment system was drastically realigned according to a prospective payment formula in which the patient's diagnoses and procedures, as reported through medical codes, determined the provider's reimbursement. While the retrospective payment formula was determined by financial systems and had little link to quality care, prospective payment formula was based on clinical systems that determined reimbursement, and required health-care administrators to provide quality care at a reduced cost in order to make a profit under the DRG fixed payment formula. Given these changes, it is little wonder that health-care administrators began to embrace the philosophy of continuous quality improvement in order to improve patient care outcomes and services at a reduced cost as it became profitable under the prospective payment system to do so.

Fully implemented in 1985, diagnosis-related groups (DRGs) provided separate and distinct reimbursement levels for 492 medical and surgical inpatient diagnoses. For the first time since the advent of Medicare, spending for inpatient health services began to decline. Also, under TEFRA, was a provision to change the PSRO construct to a Peer Review Organization (PRO). The PSRO reviewed medical necessity, utilization, and quality of care; the PRO now also reviewed the DRG validation function to ensure that the medical codes reported were based on the care documented in the patient's medical record to determine that proper payment was made. For FY2008, the DRG system was redefined and renamed Medicare Severity–DRGs (MS-DRG). MS-DRG (2008) represent one of 745 valid classifications in which patients (in the same classification group) demonstrate similar resource consumption and length of stay (LOS) patterns.

Outpatient Services and Payment

Outpatient services rapidly increased through the 1980s in reaction to inpatient cost-controls established through DRGs, advancing (less invasive) technology, consumers' demand for shorter hospital stays, and PRO denials of provider payment for inpatients whose care did not meet the criteria for medical necessity. Many patients who were not sick enough to qualify for inpatient status were still too sick to go home, and alternative health-care settings (i.e., non-acute care) flourished. The alternative settings included observation units, home health services, ambulatory surgery, hospice, and step-down units. This new spectrum of health care settings aided in the rise of managed care organizations to manage the new health-care paradigm. UR turned to case management because utilization of health-care resources was important in every setting; and health-care administrators realized that both a financial and clinical stake was tied to care throughout this new health-care continuum that subsequently advanced computer networking to share patient information as well.

Just as they had with inpatient prospective payment systems, legislators turned their attention to reducing the increases in outpatient medical services spending and developed an outpatient prospective payment system. As part of the Omnibus Budget Reconciliation Act, passed in 1989 and fully implemented in 1997, resource-based relative value scales (RBRVS) became a preferred method of controlling reimbursements to physicians in medical practices that were unattached to a hospital.[9]

With the implementation of RBRVS that reimbursed physicians for their professional services, one outpatient setting was still un-affected by managed care's development—Hospital-based outpatient care (surgical and medical) provided in an ambulatory setting. Therefore, in 2000, **Ambulatory payment classifications** (APC) established a prospective payment mechanism to hospitals for this type of service.

When combined with passage of the Emergency Medical Treatment and Active Labor Act (EMTALA) in 1985, the development of managed care as a system of reimbursement and increased federal oversight became a reality. EMTALA, known as the "anti-dumping" statute and criticized as an unfunded mandate, requires "participating hospitals" (those that accept payments under the federal Medicare program), must provide care to anyone needing emergency treatment regardless of their ability to pay. Whether a patient sought care in an inpatient or outpatient setting or in an emergency department, the reality of government involvement became omnipresent.[2]

Managed Care

The development of the patchwork known as managed care was now complete. Bounded by eight different milestones that directly impact medical coding protocols, and extending from legislative initiatives begun in 1972 and ever continuing, the managed care system now has a complete array of responsibilities extending through almost all settings of inpatient and outpatient care that frame the way in which clinicians are reimbursed for the services provided.

Milestones in the Development of Managed Care

- ▶ **1972: PSROs (professional standards review organizations) and UR (utilization review)**
- ▶ **1973: HMO Act and precertification**
- ▶ **1974: ERISA's (Employee Retirement Income Security Act) pre-emption of HMOs (health management organizations) from state insurance department oversight**
- ▶ **1983: TEFRA (Tax Equity and Fiscal Responsibility Act), DRGs (diagnosis related groups), and PRO (peer review organization); now called Quality Improvement Organizations (QIO)**
- ▶ **1985: Emergency Medical Treatment and Active Labor Act (EMTALA)**
- ▶ **1989: RBRVS (resource-based relative value scales)**
- ▶ **1997: Ambulatory payment classifications (APC)**
- ▶ **2008: Medicare Severity DRGs (MS-DRG)**

Each legislative initiative narrowed the differences between inpatient and outpatient reimbursement and ultimately resulted in the managed care system of today. Each of the legislative initiatives also increased the employment and technical opportunities for medical coding specialists and at the same time heightened the expectations of these professionals by management and oversight authorities.

Past and Present of Health Information Management

The emergence of HIM and coding as respected professions has occurred over several years. Begun as technical fields in which coders were expected to find appropriate numbers and insert them as a means of categorizing diseases and procedures for study and research, HIM and coding have now evolved to become essential to the financial survival of health-care facilities and the clinical health of patients; and both are tied to the compliance initiatives of hospitals and other types of health-care organizations (outpatient clinics, ambulatory surgery centers, and other specialty practices).

The change in expectations dates back to 1972 and the enactment of PSROs as part of PL 92-603. The resulting UR process changed forever the way in which health information managers would be used. UR spawned a process, **quality assurance**, which described new accountability expectations that are closely entwined with the expectations of clinicians participating as providers in the Medicare program. To accomplish these quality-assurance responsibilities, PSROs were formulated. The record-keeping function that was established resulted in a heightened awareness of the importance of and role in the process for HIM specialists (also known at that time as **medical record administrators and technicians**). The provisions of the PSRO legislation defined as its purpose the establishment of cost-control mechanisms for medical services paid through the Social Security Act (Medicare). The provisions specifically required the following responsibilities of providers and administrators: 1) to determine whether services are medically necessary; 2) to determine whether services meet professionally recognized standards of quality; and 3) to determine whether certain medical treatments can be provided more economically in an alternative setting.[10] This represented a new beginning for **peer review**—a process that continues today. This also afforded a significant opportunity for coding specialists to carve out a meaningful role for themselves as the stewards of the PSRO peer review process. Evolving from the PSRO to the PRO, it is only fitting that this independent agency is now known as the Quality Improvement Organization (QIO). It contracts with the federal Centers for Medicare and Medicaid Services to work collaboratively with providers to improve the condition of patient care throughout the United States by leading the development of best care practices for major illnesses (e.g., congestive heart failure, acute myocardial infarction, and pneumonia) that are most suited to the individual provider's patient case-mix (i.e., type of patient they treat) as identified by medical codes.

The evaluation of clinical records in terms of content and format fell to the medical records administrator; thus began the ascent of health information managers and coders as respected and indispensable parts of the health-care team. With the passage of additional legislation that affected reimbursements for medical services, the importance of HIM and coding to the entire process of billing and reimbursement accelerated.

In 1985, when DRGs were implemented, again in 1989, when RBRVS was implemented, and yet again in 2000 when APCs appeared on the horizon, HIM and coding professionals were considered invaluable resources in sorting out legitimate claims from those that would be considered inappropriate. Thus emerged a clear-cut role for health information managers and coding professionals and a recognition that the process of coding and billing would likely be flawed without the presence and active engagement of these experts.

The significant partnership between providers and coding specialists includes more of an expert power for the coder in preventing errant practices in billing. The stakes are simply too high for physicians and administrators to bill for services that have not been properly validated or that incorrectly represent the level of service(s) provided. In this regard, the coder has become irreplaceable as a partner in the processes of health-care delivery, code compliance, and management. The hospital or medical practice administrator who ignores the advice of a coding specialist is almost surely destined to experience failure and perhaps even charges of corrupt medical practice.

The bottom line for practitioners and managers, and most assuredly for HIM and coding professionals, is that the benefits of professional consultation provide a means of assurance that what is being done is in strict compliance with prevailing rules, regulations, and statutes. This in turn will significantly minimize the risk of creating a moral hazard that can damage or even destroy the integrity and financial fabric of a health-care organization.[11] Hence, the opportunities for success and for engagement of coders in the process of managing the health-care services responsibilities of an organization are unlimited and are bounded only by the personal limitations that the health information manager or coding professional sets for herself or himself.

For example, the importance of the HIM specialist to the processes of coding and reimbursement is seen in the work performed attendant to RBRVS. Originally, RBRVS was intended to equalize reimbursements and to narrow the disparity between physician specialists and family practitioners. It also accomplished a secondary goal of reducing expenses associated with outpatient services under the Medicare program.

The basis of RBRVS was the development of three fundamental criteria in establishing a value for each code: 1) the proportionate amount of work and skill required to complete a given procedure; 2) the proportionate overhead cost associated with a particular procedural code; and 3) the proportionate cost of professional liability insurance in relation to the completion of a given procedure. A unique feature of RBRVS is that each of the three components of a code is adjusted according to a geographic practice cost index, known as a GPCI (an acronym pronounced "gypsy"). This serves to differentiate each code according to the part of the country from which the billing is generated. This recognition of the unique cost and inflation factors affecting each part of the United States establishes a precedent for better understanding the cost pressures under which physicians from varying geographic locales are operating.[9]

The preciseness of the RBRVS formula established a clearer definition of what codes were appropriate for each service that was to be provided. This in turn created significant opportunities for coders because of their expertise and understanding of the parameters of the respective billing options. This also reaffirmed their importance to the health-care services team in managing proper compliance with established government regulations and in addressing the propriety of billing for services rendered.

With this recognition and additional duties have come heightened expectations of accountability for the coding professional. This raises the bar both in terms of value to the organization and in terms of the level of responsibility for ensuring that all billing is accurate, complete, and representative of the actual service(s) provided to each patient.

Types of Managed Care Organizations

The managed care system is made up of several different types of payer organizations. The most prominent managed care systems today include HMOs, preferred provider organizations (PPOs), physician hospital organizations (PHOs), point-of-service (POS) plans, and independent practice associations (IPAs).

Health Maintenance Organizations

HMOs are prepaid plans that provide a specific benefit package. Participants pay a defined monthly premium with certain deductibles and coinsurance requirements for those benefits. The HMO will have either a closed panel, with a requirement that the practitioners of that panel be used for benefits to be paid, or an open panel, with much less restrictive requirements for services to be covered. In either case, however, the affiliated providers must be used for full benefits to be recognized and paid. The open-panel plans tend to be more expensive, and the benefits tend to be less comprehensive. This is because the open-panel HMO can exert less control and oversight of the providers as compared with a closed-panel plan. The paperwork requirements of an HMO are typically reduced compared with other forms of coverage, such as a PPO or a POS plan.

One disadvantage of HMOs is a potential duality of relationships created through the organization, which serves as both a payer representing the subscriber and an employer of the provider. The role of the health information manager may become one of mediating the differences that exist and ensuring that the purchaser (HMO), the provider (clinician), and the subscriber (the insured) are treated fairly. This is accomplished through the correct assignment of billable codes that represent the health services provided, a fair interpretation of the benefits due each subscriber, and ensuring that the provider receives proper compensation for services rendered.

Preferred Provider Organizations

PPOs were first established in 1976 by the American Hospital Association. Hospital administrators were concerned that HMOs would significantly reduce the demand for hospital beds; hence, the early PPOs offered participating organizations discounted reimbursements (generally 20%) off their usual and customary rates. Over the next 25 years, PPOs grew to become the single largest type of payment system, and today they account for more than 40 million subscribers nationwide. The main advantage of a PPO is its relationship to the subscriber. The PPO permits a subscriber to seek treatment from a broad variety of providers in the PPO network. Recently, reimbursement rates have become more restrictive as the cost of care has increased. However, even with a higher premium than most HMOs, PPOs in many instances are a preferred alternative to the more restrictive utilization requirements of the typical HMO because of the ability to select from a broader range of providers.[12]

Physician Hospital Organizations

PHOs are a clinical care partnership between physician and hospital providers and, in some instances, an insurer. The PHO relationship can be characterized as either simple or complex. The simple PHO includes a group of physicians and a hospital. The complex PHO typically adds an insurance company or another form of payer organization to the physician/hospital partnership. The integration of the respective organizations creates both a payer obligation and a provider relationship that transcends the association that normally exists among provider, payer, and patient. Under a complex PHO, the patient purchases insurance coverage and receives the clinical services provided through that organization.

Point-of-Service Plans

POS plans have become popular because many people are reluctant to give up their primary care physician or specialist simply because that provider is not a member of the network. The POS model allows members flexibility: they can seek care within the network for a low deductible and low co-payment or can seek treatment outside the network and pay more. Because of the ability to go outside of the prescribed network for services, higher costs are associated with the POS model. Hence, the premiums are usually much higher as well. However, from a consumer perspective, the advantage of the POS plan is that it combines the benefits of managed care with those of more traditional insurance plans.[12]

Independent Practice Associations

IPAs are loose-knit networks in which a payer contracts with practitioners in several specialty groups, thus creating broad coverage for members. The IPA is disadvantaged as a consequence of a lack of control by the payer and a potential lack of incentives for the provider to make the most judicious decisions about services to be rendered. Typically, the costs associated with IPAs are much greater than those of other managed care plans.[12]

The Future of Managed Care and the Growing Role of Coding and Health Information Management

Managed care has significantly affected the HIM and coding professions. From a role that could have been characterized as clerical, in which clinicians dictated billing information and coders simply entered the required information on the appropriate form and submitted it for payment; health information managers and coding professionals now are an integral part of the health care team and the reimbursement process. They are routinely called upon to review the appropriateness of a series of billing codes. They are expected to correct errors that are observed in the preparation of a bill for submission. They are also involved in a host of other activities that are considered integral to the care/cure process of a hospital or a medical practice. For example, the coder may be asked to evaluate patient case-mix data to ensure that provider billings are consistent with the acuity level of the patients being served. An inconsistency between acuity level and bills that are submitted for payment can serve as a red flag to oversight agencies, and this could lead to investigation and prosecution if the claims are judged to be invalid.

A coder may also be expected to identify performance improvement activities being undertaken within an organization to enhance the skills of its clinicians. The work of a coding professional is seen as crucial in ensuring compliance with statutes, regulations, and standards of accreditation. In that regard, the coder is considered a partner of and an important contributor to the compliance officer of the hospital or medical practice. Without the competence and quality efforts of the coder, the compliance office would experience great difficulty in maintaining proper documentation to support its efforts to operate within the spirit and intent of the laws governing clinical service compliance.

The coder also plays a significant role in providing the data necessary to develop clinical practice standards (i.e., evidence-based medicine). Analyzing patient case-mix data is an essential function of the HIM professional. Exemplifying a best-practice model is a goal to which most—if not all—clinicians aspire. The health information manager and coding specialist can assist an organization in achieving that goal by seeking to provide insights into the clinical practice standards that will be viewed as exemplifying a firm commitment to excellence. In all instances, quality health care must represent the end goal in any recommendations that are submitted for consideration by clinicians. The coding professional is often in the best position to recognize the quality of the documentation that best evidences a binding commitment to quality services and care. In addition, coders play an indispensible role in collecting the data to comply with the new CMS requirement for recording present-on-admission (POA) indicators and Core Measures reporting (discussed in Chapter 18) that are part of a national initiative to promote "value-based purchasing" in healthcare (i.e., pay-for-performance [P4P] sytems). P4P incentivizes providers to apply evidence based protocols ("best care practices") that promote high quality clinical care and services at reduced cost and applies financial penalties for poor performance.

The health information manager and coding professional also play a substantial role in supporting the risk-management program of the organization. Exposure to liability is one of the more precarious risks faced by all clinical practitioners today. Proper and consistent coding can ensure that this risk is minimized, if not eliminated. In addition, participation in utilization and quality improvement studies can provide insights regarding where the organization may be strengthened in its ability to identify and correct potential problems. Also, in the process of reviewing patients' medical records, coders can screen records for the documentation of adverse patient occurrences to ensure that these cases have been brought to the proper attention of the risk manager for corrective action.

Strategic planning is an ongoing and important part of a health-care services organization's plans for future development to meet the health-care needs of the community and market it. The ability to align coded patient information with long-term strategic planning is an important goal. The efforts of the coding specialist to provide data to the planning team can ensure that the goals being formulated for future development are based on information that is consistent with the actual and ongoing clinical services of the organization. Without proper coding systems that are consistent and in line with the strategic initiatives of an organization, this could compromise the ultimate aim for a successful planning process. Pride in being associated with a development plan that seeks to showcase the strengths and contributions of an organization can be rewarding in the best sense of the word. The importance of the health information manager and coding professional in presenting that image to the employees of the organization should not be understated. The accuracy of the information that is presented is essential in ensuring that as many employees as possible will buy into the ongoing planning process and become its advocates.

The bottom line in health care today is outcomes management. Virtually all organizations providing health-care services are thoroughly focused on providing good outcomes relating to clinical care (i.e., patient evaluation and treatment), service, and cost. The accountability of health-care services organizations and the methods of measuring that accountability evoke considerable discussion and concern among health-care professionals at all levels of an organization. However, the expectation of excellence in treatment has become an indelible part of the care/cure process, and nothing less than a full and best effort in this arena is acceptable. The coder plays an integral role in measuring outcomes. The information generated through the daily work of the coder serves as data to either justify or refute claims of service excellence. Additionally, the information provided for quality reviews provides both a resource in support of the ongoing work of the committee and a road map to improve in those patient care areas deemed to be below par. This places the coder at the center of the process of evaluating the quality of care and the outcomes that are achieved for each patient served by a health-care organization.

Ultimately, satisfaction among health insurance consumers in all parts of America is influenced by several factors. Satisfaction can be maintained in part if cost, quality, and access remain essential elements for a health-care system. A turbulent environment in health care has been present and will continue to be present because of the numerous changes and adaptations needed for it to function efficiently. Costs must be contained before further damage is done to the infrastructure of our health-care delivery system. However, the combination of desiring flexibility and autonomy in the choice of providers while desiring quality health care within managed plans providing comprehensive services, continues to perplex purchasers, providers, and consumers of health-care services alike.

When choice is taken away, one must look at the pros and cons of each health-care plan. Reimbursement rates are also affected in each type of health-care plan, depending on the use of the benefits provided. A cost-effective and accessible environment for consumers is the goal.

Employers in increasing numbers are evaluating the total cost of providing health care to their employees. This expenditure is increasing each year and is not expected to decrease soon. Case studies and results of surveys have verified health insurance cost increases when compared with earlier years. This information is needed to put into perspective the possibility of increases in the years to come. Premiums, deductibles, co-payments, and exclusions from coverage itself are all affected in one way or another by the pricing of insurance products in relation to the benefits that are purchased by a client. Although a company must be assured that the insurance plan(s) offered to their employees will not adversely affect their capital base and ultimate financial goals, simply passing health-care costs on to employees is not a viable strategy. The disadvantages of an inadequate health-care benefit program far outweigh the benefits of coverage.

The ultimate goal of almost any organization is to maintain profitability, retain good employees, and remain competitive in its particular marketplace. If a managed care plan's options are not suitable, alternatives must be found that meet the objectives of cost-effectiveness and quality.

Several states are attempting to develop health benefit programs that are realistically priced and available to everyone interested in purchasing the product. However, the efforts to align quality with cost-effectiveness have proven to be elusive at best.

In time, America's system of health insurance coverage will have to undergo substantive changes in order to survive. Public officials will have to work with consumers and employers to identify a medium that is acceptable to providers, payers, consumers, and elected public officials in each state and geographic region. This likely will include a series of programs that will both stabilize costs and provide a mechanism of health insurance availability for those who presently are disenfranchised and excluded from coverage. The latest numbers suggest that more than 47 million Americans are uninsured at any given time.

The health information manager and coding professional will play key roles in providing patient data that fosters these necessary changes. They will contribute significantly to the development and implementation of a system complemented by responsible coding practices and attention to the rules and regulations that now comprise our nation's systems of health insurance for the aged, the disabled, and the poor. Coders and other HIM professionals will demonstrate required leadership skills through proper handling of patient records, through accuracy in coding each patient's record, and through their contributions to improved patient outcomes.

The hallmark of continuous quality improvement, as mirrored in the work of W. Edwards Deming, is to root out faulty systems and replace them with efficient and effective care/cure mechanisms that enhance the quality of care provided. Quality data ultimately provide the fuel that drives competence; the coder serves as the engineer responsible for ensuring that the needed data meet the tests of reliability and appropriateness. Coded medical data produces information to help health-care administrators measure patient outcomes in order to realize opportunities and make decisions that promote internal performance improvement activities that serve to improve the health-care services to patients. This is in line with the mission of all providers.

All competent leaders recognize that good-quality patient information is necessary for making competent decisions. Each coded patient chart tells an important story; your success as a coder or HIM specialist contributes immeasurably to the collective ability of the health-care organization and its professional staff to understand the conditions and needs of patients who are being served. Complementing the health-care provider's ultimate objective of ensuring the delivery of quality care is quality-coded data, which provide the infrastructure of support for the accomplishment of that objective. According to systems theory, if feedback from the system demonstrates poor patient outcomes (e.g., nosocomial infections), it is the administrator's ultimate responsibility to manage resources to improve the internal structures, processes, and outcomes through continuous quality improvement methods to improve patient care.

A Recent Addition to the Managed Care Jargon

The dynamic transition of our nations health delivery system continues unabated, just as it has since the advent of the Medicare program; and with this continuing transition we have added a new acronym to the managed care glossary of important terms. This time the terminology addition is referred to as RHIO (Regional Health Information Organization).

RHIO is used to signify a group of healthcare providers, purchasers of care, manufacturers, and vendors that have come together under the umbrella of a common and significant interest—that of a network serving a particular population of healthcare consumers. According to Laura Gater, the purpose of RHIOs is to connect various healthcare communities by improving quality, safety, and efficiencies in delivering healthcare services.[13]

Because RHIO as a concept has no defining or government mandated characteristics at this time, it is not possible to definitively say how such an organization should appear to an interested observer. Therefore, simply stated, a RHIO represents a group of stakeholders that is connected by a common interest or a series of integrated commitments to a particular community or region.[13]

It is not possible at this time to determine whether RHIOs will have a sustained presence or exert a significant influence on America's healthcare delivery system. Indeed, during the past 45 years the American healthcare scene has welcomed a number of organizations and concepts that were implemented with great fanfare, only to be discontinued without much impact having been experienced from their presence. Comprehensive Health Planning Agencies (CHPs), Regional Medical Programs (RMPs), and Professional Standards Review Organizations (PSROs) are but a few of the programs of yesteryear that have failed in terms of their intent and longevity.

Therefore, as students and as Health Information Managers we would be well advised to view this latest acronym with both hope and guarded optimism that it will possess the necessary requisite characteristics to significantly improve our ability as leaders in our professions to continue providing top quality services to our constituent communities.

SUMMARY

This chapter has focused on the origin, emergence, and early development of prepaid health care in America. This was followed by a discussion of how health care came to be known as managed care. The most prominent types of managed care organizations were then identified and explained. This was followed by a discussion of the role of the health information manager and coding professional in ensuring the success of a health-care organization. The uses of coded information were highlighted: 1) evaluating patient case-mix data; 2) identifying performance-improvement activities; 3) complying with regulations and accreditation standards; 4) developing superior clinical practice standards (i.e., best care practices); 5) identifying potential risks to the organization; and 6) aligning coded information systems with strategic organizational planning.

REFERENCES

1. Code of Federal Regulations, October 1, 2001, Title 42, vol 3 (42 CFR 489.24), 945–951.
2. Rotarius T, Fottler M, Morrison S, et al. Uncompensated care and emergency department utilization: an analysis of two central Florida hospitals. Health Care Manager, 2002.
3. Hendricks RA. A Model for National Health Care: The History of Kaiser Permanente. New Brunswick, NJ: Rutgers University Press, 1993.

4. Fein R. Medical Care, Medical Costs: The Search for a Health Insurance Policy. Cambridge, MA: Harvard University Press, 1989.

5. Calkins D, Fernandopulle R, Marino B. Health Care Policy. Cambridge, MA: Blackwell Science, 1995.

6. Fox PD. An overview of managed care. In: Kongstvedt P, ed. Essentials of Managed Health Care. Gaithersburg, MD: Aspen Publishers, 2001:4.

7. Mayer TR, Mayer GG. HMOs: origins and development. N Engl J Med 1985;312:590–594.

8. Liberman A, Rotarius T. Managed care evolution—where did it come from and where is it going? Health Care Manager 1999;18:50–57.

9. McMenamin P, Heald R, eds. Medicare RBRVS: The Physicians' Guide. Chicago: American Medical Association, 1998.

10. Liberman A, Bustamante M, Melvin C, et al. A community services approach to quality assurance. Med Rec News 1978;49:64–72.

11. Vaughan E, Vaughan T. Fundamentals of Risk and Insurance. New York: Wiley, 1999.

12. Kongstvedt P. Essentials of Managed Health Care. Gaithersburg, MD: Aspen Publishers, 2001.

13. Gater, L. The RHIO World. For the Record 2005, July 18: 17.

TESTING YOUR COMPREHENSION

1. Provide a specific example of how our government responded to the growing 1985 perception that patients were being dumped and bypassed by crowded hospital emergency departments.

2. Prepaid medical services first reached American shores in what year and under what auspices?

3. Who was the physician who teamed with Edgar Kaiser to establish the Kaiser Health Plan?

4. If managed care is not a system of care, what is it considered to be first and foremost?

5. Federal legislation in 1972 and 1973 established utilization review and precertification, respectively. Please identify these laws.

6. In 1983, the Tax Equity and Fiscal Responsibility Act brought prospective payment to the forefront of the health-care debate. Please name the product of that legislation.

7. In 1989 and 1997, two additional pieces of prominent reimbursement legislation were passed. Please name the products of these legislative initiatives.

8. The basis of RBRVS was the development of three fundamental criteria for establishing a value for each code. List the three criteria.

9. Please identify the prominent types of managed care organizations.

10. What uses of coded information are considered vital to the success of a health-care organization?

11. What is the primary challenge confronting Americans today in the health-care system?

12. What do all competent leaders recognize?

Medicare Severity-Adjusted Diagnosis-Related Groups (DRGs)

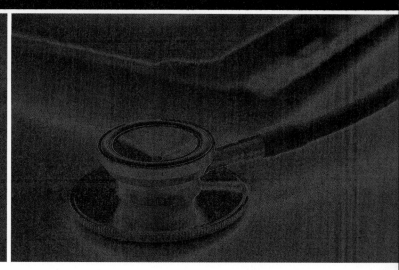

DEFINITIONS OF MS-DRG TERMS

Arithmetic Mean LOS (AMLOS)   The average number of days patients within a given DRG stay in the hospital, also referred to as the average length of stay. The AMLOS is used to determine payment for outlier cases.

Base Rate (i.e., blended rate)   A number assigned to a hospital used to calculate MS-DRG reimbursement. Base rates vary from hospital to hospital. The base rate adjusts reimbursement to allow for such individual characteristics of the hospital as geographic location, status (urban, rural, teaching), and local labor costs. The base rate is multiplied against the DRG/MS-DRG weight to convert it to dollars to establish a payment to the provider. FY2008 will begin with a 50/50 (DRG/MS-DRG) payment blend. MS-DRG weights will be fully implemented in 2009.

Case-Mix   The type of patents treated by the facility.

Case-Mix Index (CMI)   The sum of all MS-DRG relative weights, divided by the number of Medicare cases. A low CMI may denote MS-DRG assignments that do not adequately reflect the resources used to treat Medicare patients. *Healthcare administrators should follow the case-mix index trends (i.e., "peaks and valleys") for their facilities over time and be able to investigate and determine the cause for any significant changes. The case-mix index represents a statistical number that describes the resources used by the facility to treat their patients. The higher the case-mix index, the more resources were utilized in order to treat patients that are sicker (i.e., higher acuity level) than average (e.g., a case-mix index of 1.0 equals the resources needed to treat the average Medicare patient [a baseline value]; therefore, a case-mix index of >1.0 represents patients that consume more resources than average and a case-mix index of less than 1.0 represent patients that consume fewer resources than average).*

EXAMPLE OF CASE-MIX INDEX (CMI) FORMULA

MS-DRG	Description	Number of Patients	CMS Relative Weight	Total CMS Relative Weight
292	Heart failure and shock w/ CC	49	1.0053	49.256
194	Simple pneumonia & pleurisy age >17 w/ CC	45	1.0041	45.185
065	Intracranial hemorrhage or cerebral infarction	21	1.1748	24.671
178	Respiratory infections & inflammations age >17 w/ CC	19	1.4979	28.460
191	COPD w/ CC	17	0.9734	16.548
470	Major joint replacement or reattachment of lower extremity	16	2.0144	32.230
378	GI hemorrhage w/ CC	11	1.0048	11.053
392	Esophagitis, GE & misc. digestive disorders age >17 w/ CC	10	0.6685	6.685
641	Nutritional & misc. metabolic disorders age >17 w/ CC	8	0.6798	5.438
309	Cardiac arrhythmia & conduction disorders w/ CC	4	0.8320	3.328
	Total	**200**	**10.855**	**222.854**

$$\text{CMI} = 222.854 \div 200 = 1.1143$$

EXAMPLE OF CASE-MIX TRENDS

EXAMPLE

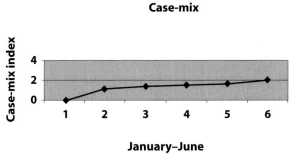

"MS-DRG creep." Possible explanation: Trend showing possible "upcoding."

EXAMPLE

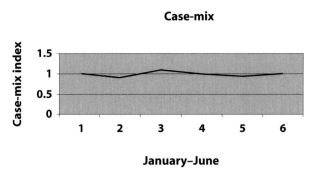

Steady case-mix trend. Possible explanation: Normal findings as health-care facilities commonly tend to treat similar types of patients that use similar resources over time.

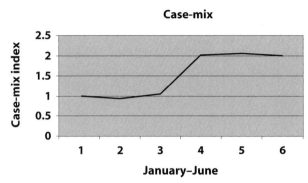

Case-mix

Drastic rise in case-mix. Possible explanation: Hospital is outsourcing coding, and "upcoding" may possibly be occurring or perhaps a better job in the coding section is being done. Hospital is providing new service or new physician line opened (recruited cardiovascular surgeon).

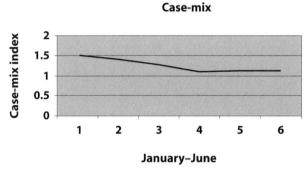

Case-mix

Slow drop in case-mix. Possible explanation: Hospital has stopped providing a clinical service, retirement of key physician admitter, loss of market share to competitor, or loss of expert coders.

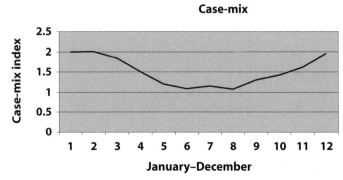

Case-mix

Fluctuation in case-mix. Possible explanation: Seasonal trend (physicians on vacation, Florida transient population).

Charges   The dollar amount of hospital bills (reflects provider markup to the consumer).

Comorbidity   A preexisting condition that because of its presence with a specific diagnosis can increase the LOS or cause the facility to expend more resources to treat the patient. It may effect the MS-DRG payment to the hospital. MS-DRGs established a three-tiered system that includes distinguishing between a MAJOR complication or comorbidity (MCC); a REGULAR complication of comorbidity (C/C); or, NO complication or comorbidity.

Complication   A condition that arises during the hospital stay that because of its presence with a specific diagnosis can increase the LOS or cause the facility to expend more resources to treat the patient. It may effect the MS-DRG payment to the hospital. MS-DRGs established a three-tiered system that includes distinguishing between a MAJOR complication or comorbidity (MCC); a REGULAR complication of comorbidity (C/C); or, NO complication or comorbidity

Core measures As part of the Reporting Hospital Quality Data for Annual Payment Update (RHQDAPU) update for 2008, CMS required hospitals to report on 27 different quality of care measures, which it makes available to the public in order for consumers to compare the performance of hospitals. Results data can soon be accessed on a dedicated web site (www.hospitalcompare.hhs.gov). Examples of measures include results of patient satisfaction surveys, 30–Day Risk Adjusted Heart Attack Mortality, 30–Day Risk Adjusted Heart Failure Mortality, and appropriate initial antibiotic selection for pneumonia. Hospitals can receive up to a two percent (2%) reduction in payment for FY2008 for nonparticipation and poor scores. At the time of this textbook's publishing, CMS is proposing to add 43 more measures to the mandatory quality reporting for FY2009.

Costs   The expenses associated with providing treatment to a given patient.

Diagnosis-Related Groups (DRG)   Now called MS-DRG (Medicare Severity-DRG). One of 745 valid classifications (for FY 2008) in which patients demonstrate similar resource consumption and LOS patterns.

Discharge Status   Disposition of the patient at discharge (for example: left against medical advice, discharged home, transferred to an acute care hospital, expired).

Fiscal Year (FY)   The Federal fiscal year (i.e., budget year) runs from October 1 to September 30 of every calendar year.

Geometric Mean Length of Stay (GMLOS)   Used to compute reimbursement, the GMLOS is a statistically adjusted value for all cases for a given DRG, allowing for outliers, transfer cases, and negative outlier cases that would normally skew the data. The GMLOS is used to determine payment only for transfer cases, i.e., the per diem rate.

Grouper   The software program that assigns DRGs.

Major Diagnostic Category (MDC)   Broad classification of diagnoses typically grouped by body system.

Other Diagnosis All conditions (secondary) that exist at the time of admission or that develop subsequently that affect the treatment received and/or the LOS. Diagnoses that relate to an earlier episode and that have no bearing on the current hospital stay are not to be reported.

Outliers There are two types of outliers: day outliers and cost outliers. Payment for day outliers has been eliminated with discharges occurring on or after October 1, 1997. A cost outlier is a case in which the costs for treating the patient are extraordinarily high in relation to the costs for other patients in the MS-DRG. An increase in cost outlier payments will compensate for the elimination of day outlier payments.

Per Diem Rate (per day payment) Payments to the hospital are calculated for each day of the patient's stay. Per diem rate is determined by dividing the MS- DRG payment by the GMLOS for the MS-DRG. The payment rate for the first day of stay is twice the per diem rate, and subsequent days are paid at the per diem rate up to the full MS-DRG amount. This per diem calculation is used when the patient is transferred from the hospial to a PPS exempt or skilled nursing facility, or the hospital stay is followed by a home health agency visit.

Present-on admission (POA) indicator Starting October 1, 2007, CMS requires hospitals to report whether or not diagnoses were POA. For FY2008, together with the Centers for Disease Control and Prevention, CMS identified 8 high- volume, hospital-acquired conditions that could have reasonably been prevented. October 1, 2008, CMS will begin imposing financial penalties for their occurrence (e.g., pressure ulcers code 707.0X; catheter-associated urinary tract infections code 996.64; object left in surgery code 998.4; air embolism code 999.1; surgical-site infections code 998.59 and mediastinitis after CABG surgery code 519.2; vascular catheter-associated infection code 999.31; blood incompatibility code 999.6; and, falls with injuries).

Principal Diagnosis The condition established after study to be chiefly responsible for occasioning the admission of the patient to the hospital for care.

Principal Procedure A procedure performed for definitive treatment rather than diagnostic or exploratory purposes, or that was necessary to treat a complication. The principal procedure usually is related to the principal diagnosis.

Relative Weight (RW) An assigned weight that is intended to reflect the relative resource consumption associated with each MS-DRG. The higher the relative weight, the greater the payment to the hospital. The relative weights are calculated by CMS (United States Centers for Medicare and Medicaid Services) and published in the final prospective payment system rule.

Remittance The amount that is paid by the insurer or individual to the provider for services rendered to the patient.

MEDICARE SEVERITY-ADJUSTED DIAGNOSIS-RELATED GROUPS (MS-DRGS) FOR 2009

Excerpted from The Centers for Medicare & Medicaid Services, August 19, 2008 Federal Register, final MS-DRGs effective October 1, 2008. The following is a list of MS-DRG assignments and their descriptions for Fiscal Year 2009.

MS-DRG Description	MS-DRG Description
001. Heart transplant or implant of heart assist system w MCC.	037. Extracranial procedures w MCC
002. Heart transplant or implant of heart assist system w/o MCC.	038. Extracranial procedures w CC
003. ECMO or trach w MV 961 hrs or PDX exc face, mouth & neck w maj O.R.	039. Extracranial procedures w/o CC/MCC
004. Trach w MV 96 hrs or PDX exc face, mouth & neck w/o maj O.R.	040. Periph/cranial nerve & other nerv syst proc w MCC.
005. Liver transplant w MCC or intestinal transplant.	041. Periph/cranial nerve & other nerv syst proc w CC or periph neurostim.
006. Liver transplant w/o MCC.	042. Periph/cranial nerve & other nerv syst proc w/o CC/MCC.
007. Lung transplant.	052. Spinal disorders & injuries w CC/MCC
008. Simultaneous pancreas/kidney transplant.	053. Spinal disorders & injuries w/o CC/MCC.
009. Bone marrow transplant.	054. Nervous system neoplasms w MCC
010. Pancreas transplant.	055. Nervous system neoplasms w/o MCC
011. Tracheostomy for face, mouth & neck diagnoses w MCC.	056. Degenerativenervous system disorders w MCC.
012. Tracheostomy for face, mouth & neck diagnoses w CC.	057. Degenerative nervous system disorders w/o MCC.
013. Tracheostomy for face, mouth & neck diagnoses w/o CC/MCC.	058. Multiple sclerosis & cerebellar ataxia w MCC.
020. Intracranial vascular procedures w PDX hemorrhage w MCC.	059. Multiple sclerosis & cerebellar ataxia w CC.
021. Intracranial vascular procedures w PDX hemorrhage w CC.	060. Multiple sclerosis & cerebellar ataxia w/o CC/MCC.
022. Intracranial vascular procedures w PDX hemorrhage w/o CC/MCC.	061. Acute ischemic stroke w use of thrombolytic agent w MCC.
023. Cranio w major dev impl/acute complex CNS PDX w MCC or chemo implant.	062. Acute ischemic stroke w use of thrombolytic agent w CC.
024. Cranio w major dev impl/acute complex CNS PDX w/o MCC.	063. Acute ischemic stroke w use of thrombolytic agent w/o CC/MCC.
025. Craniotomy & endovascular intracranial procedures w MCC.	064. Intracranial hemorrhage or cerebral infarction w MCC.
026. Craniotomy & endovascular intracranial procedures w CC.	065. Intracranial hemorrhage or cerebral infarction w CC.
027. Craniotomy & endovascular intracranial procedures w/o CC/MCC.	066. Intracranial hemorrhage or cerebral infarction w/o CC/MCC.
028. Spinal procedures w MCC.	067. Nonspecific cva & precerebral occlusion w/o infarct w MCC.
029. Spinal procedures w CC or spinal neurostimulators.	068. Nonspecific cva & precerebral occlusion w/o infarct w/o MCC.
030. Spinal procedures w/o CC/MCC	069. Transient ischemia
031. Ventricular shunt procedures w MCC	070. Nonspecific cerebrovascular disorders w MCC.
032. Ventricular shunt procedures w CC	071. Nonspecific cerebrovascular disorders w CC.
033. Ventricular shunt procedures w/o CC/MCC.	072. Nonspecific cerebrovascular disorders w/o CC/MCC.
034. Carotid artery stent procedure w MCC	073. Cranial & peripheral nerve disorders w MCC.
035. Carotid artery stent procedure w CC .	074. Cranial & peripheral nerve disorders w/o MCC.
036. Carotid artery stent procedure w/o CC/MCC.	075. Viral meningitis w CC/MCC
	076. Viral meningitis w/o CC/MCC
	077. Hypertensive encephalopathy w MCC
	078. Hypertensive encephalopathy w CC

MS-DRG Description	MS-DRG Description
079. Hypertensive encephalopathy w/o CC/MCC.	133. Other ear, nose, mouth & throat O.R. procedures w CC/MCC.
080. Nontraumatic stupor & coma w MCC	134. Other ear, nose, mouth & throat O.R. procedures w/o CC/MCC.
081. Nontraumatic stupor & coma w/o MCC.	135. Sinus & mastoid procedures w CC/MCC.
082. Traumatic stupor & coma, coma $1 hr w MCC.	136. Sinus & mastoid procedures w/o CC/MCC.
083. Traumatic stupor & coma, coma $1 hr w CC.	137. Mouth procedures w CC/MCC
084. Traumatic stupor & coma, coma $1 hr w/o CC/MCC.	138. Mouth procedures w/o CC/MCC
085. Traumatic stupor & coma, coma ,1 hr w MCC.	139. Salivary gland procedures
086. Traumatic stupor & coma, coma ,1 hr w CC.	146. Ear, nose, mouth & throat malignancy w MCC.
087. Traumatic stupor & coma, coma ,1 hr w/o CC/MCC.	147. Ear, nose, mouth & throat malignancy w CC.
088. Concussion w MCC	148. Ear, nose, mouth & throat malignancy w/o CC/MCC.
089. Concussion w CC	149. Dysequilibrium
090. Concussion w/o CC/MCC	150. Epistaxis w MCC
091. Other disorders of nervous system w MCC.	151. Epistaxis w/o MCC
092. Other disorders of nervous system w CC.	152. Otitis media & URI w MCC
093. Other disorders of nervous system w/o CC/MCC.	153. Otitis media & URI w/o MCC
094. Bacterial & tuberculous infections of nervous system w MCC.	154. Nasal trauma & deformity w MCC
095. Bacterial & tuberculous infections of nervous system w CC.	155. Nasal trauma & deformity w CC
096. Bacterial & tuberculous infections of nervous system w/o CC/MCC.	156. Nasal trauma & deformity w/o CC/MCC
097. Non-bacterial infect of nervous sys exc viral meningitis w MCC.	157. Dental & Oral Diseases w MCC
098. Non-bacterial infect of nervous sys exc viral meningitis w CC.	158. Dental & Oral Diseases w CC
099. Non-bacterial infect of nervous sys exc viral meningitis w/o CC/MCC.	159. Dental & Oral Diseases w/o CC/MCC
100. Seizures w MCC	163. Major chest procedures w MCC
101. Seizures w/o MCC	164. Major chest procedures w CC
102. Headaches w MCC	165. Major chest procedures w/o CC/MCC
103. Headaches w/o MCC	166. Other resp system O.R. procedures w MCC
113. Orbital procedures w CC/MCC	167. Other resp system O.R. procedures w CC
114. Orbital procedures w/o CC/MCC	168. Other resp system O.R. procedures w/o CC/MCC
115. Extraocular procedures except orbit	175. Pulmonary embolism w MCC
116. Intraocular procedures w CC/MCC	176. Pulmonary embolism w/o MCC
117. Intraocular procedures w/o CC/MCC	177. Respiratory infections & inflammations w MCC.
121. Acute major eye infections w CC/MCC	178. Respiratory infections & inflammations w CC.
122. Acute major eye infections w/o CC/MCC.	179. Respiratory infections & inflammations w/o CC/MCC.
123. Neurological eye disorders	180. Respiratory neoplasms w MCC
124. Other disorders of the eye w MCC	181. Respiratory neoplasms w CC
125. Other disorders of the eye w/o MCC	182. Respiratory neoplasms w/o CC/MCC
129. Major head & neck procedures w CC/MCC or major device.	183. Major chest trauma w MCC
130. Major head & neck procedures w/o CC/MCC.	184. Major chest trauma w CC
131. Cranial/facial procedures w CC/MCC	185. Major chest trauma w/o CC/MCC
132. Cranial/facial procedures w/o CC/MCC.	186. Pleural effusion w MCC
	187. Pleural effusion w CC
	188. Pleural effusion w/o CC/MCC
	189. Pulmonary edema & respiratory failure
	190. Chronic obstructive pulmonarydisease w MCC

MS-DRG Description	MS-DRG Description
191. Chronic obstructive pulmonarydisease w CC	231. Coronary bypass w PTCA w MCC
192. Chronic obstructive pulmonarydisease w/o CC/MCC	232. Coronary bypass w PTCA w/o MCC
193. Simple pneumonia & pleurisy w MCC	233. Coronary bypass w cardiaccath w MCC.
194. Simple pneumonia & pleurisy w CC . . .	234. Coronary bypass w cardiac cath w/o MCC.
195. Simple pneumonia & pleurisy w/o CC/	235. Coronary bypass w/o cardiac cath w MCC.
196. Interstitial lung disease w MCC	236. Coronary bypass w/o cardiac cath w/o MCC.
197. Interstitial lung disease w CC	237. Major cardiovasc procedures w MCC or thoracic aortic anuerysm repair.
198. Interstitial lung disease w/o CC/MCC	238. Major cardiovasc procedures w/o MCC.
199. Pneumothorax w MCC	239. Amputation for circ sys disorders exc upper limb & toe w MCC.
200. Pneumothorax w CC	240. Amputation for circ sys disorders exc upper limb & toe w CC.
201. Pneumothorax w/o CC/MCC	241. Amputation for circ sys disorders exc upper limb & toe w/o CC/MCC.
202. Bronchitis & asthma w CC/MCC	
203. Bronchitis & asthma w/o CC/MCC	242. Permanent cardiac pacemaker implant w MCC.
204. Respiratory signs & symptoms	243. Permanent cardiac pacemaker implant w CC.
205. Other respiratory system diagnoses w MCC.	244. Permanent cardiac pacemaker implant w/o CC/MCC.
206. Other respiratory system diagnoses w/o MCC	245. AICD generator procedures
207. Respiratory system diagnosis w ventilator support 961 hours.	246. Perc cardiovasc proc w drug-eluting stent w MCC or 41 vessels/stents.
208. Respiratory system diagnosis w ventilator support 96 hours.	247. Perc cardiovasc proc w drug-eluting stent w/o MCC.
215. Other heart assist system implant	248. Perccardiovascproc w non-drug-eluting stent w MCC or stents.
216. Cardiac valve & oth maj cardiothoracic proc w card cath w MCC	249. Perc cardiovasc proc w non-drug-eluting stent w/o MCC.
217. Cardiac valve & oth maj cardiothoracic proc w card cath w CC	250. Perc cardiovasc proc w/o coronary artery stent or AMI w MCC.
218. Cardiac valve & oth maj cardiothoracic proc w card cath w/o CC/MCC	251. Perc cardiovasc proc w/o coronary artery stent or AMI w/o MCC.
219. Cardiac valve & oth maj cardiothoracic proc w/o card cath w MCC	252. Other vascular procedures w MCC
220. Cardiac valve & oth maj cardiothoracic proc w/o card cath w CC	253. Other vascular procedures w CC
221. Cardiac valve & oth maj cardiothoracic proc w/o card cath w/o CC/MCC	254. Other vascular procedures w/o CC/MCC.
222. Cardiac defib implant w cardiac cath w AMI/HF/shock w MCC	255. Upper limb & toe amputation for circ system disorders w MCC.
223. Cardiac defib implant w cardiac cath w AMI/HF/shock w/o MCC	256. Upper limb & toe amputation for circ system disorders w CC.
224. Cardiac defib implant w cardiac cath w/o AMI/HF/shock w MCC	257. Upper limb & toe amputation for circ system disorders w/o CC/MCC.
225. Cardiac defib implant w cardiac cath w/o AMI/HF/shock w/o MCC	258. Cardiac pacemaker device replacement w MCC.
226. Cardiac defibrillator implant w/o cardiac cath w MCC	259. Cardiac pacemaker device replacement w/o MCC.
227. Cardiac defibrillator implant w/o cardiac cath w/o MCC	260. Cardiac pacemaker revision except device replacement w MCC.
228. Other cardiothoracic procedures w MCC.	261. Cardiac pacemaker revision except device replacement w CC.
229. Other cardiothoracic procedures w CC	
230. Other cardiothoracic procedures w/o CC/MCC.	

MS-DRG Description	MS-DRG Description
262. Cardiac pacemaker revision except device replacement w/o CC/MCC.	313. Chest pain
263. Vein ligation & stripping	314. Other circulatory system diagnoses w MCC.
264. Other circulatory system O.R. procedures.	315. Other circulatory system diagnoses w CC.
265. AICD lead procedures	316. Other circulatory system diagnoses w/o CC/MCC.
280. Acute myocardial infarction, discharged alive w MCC.	326. Stomach, esophageal & duodenal proc w MCC.
281. Acute myocardial infarction, discharged alive w CC.	327. Stomach, esophageal & duodenal proc w CC.
282. Acute myocardia infarction, discharged alive w/o CC/MCC.	328. Stomach, esophageal & duodenal proc w/o CC/MCC.
283. Acute myocardial infarction, expired w MCC.	329. Major small & large bowel procedures w MCC.
284. Acute myocardial infarction, expired w CC.	330. Major small & large bowel procedures w CC.
285. Acute myocardial infarction, expired w/o CC/MCC.	331. Major small & large bowel procedures w/o CC/MCC.
286. Circulatory disorders except AMI, w card cath w MCC.	332. Rectal resection w MCC
287. Circulatory disorders except AMI, w card cath w/o MCC.	333. Rectal resection w CC
	334. Rectal resection w/o CC/MCC
288. Acute & subacute endocarditis w MCC.	335. Peritoneal adhesiolysis w MCC
289. Acute & subacute endocarditis w CC	336. Peritoneal adhesiolysis w CC
290. Acute & subacute endocarditis w/o CC/MCC.	337. Peritoneal adhesiolysis w/o CC/MCC
291. Heart failure & shock w MCC	338. Appendectomy w complicated principal diag w MCC.
292. Heart failure & shock w CC	339. Appendectomy w complicated principal diag w CC.
293. Heart failure & shock w/o CC/MCC	340. Appendectomy w complicated principal diag w/o CC/MCC.
294. Deep vein thrombophlebitis w CC/MCC.	341. Appendectomy w/o complicated principal diag w MCC.
295. Deep vein thrombophlebitis w/o CC/MCC.	342. Appendectomy w/o complicated principal diag w CC.
296. Cardiac arrest, unexplained w MCC	343. Appendectomy w/o complicated principal diag w/o CC/MCC.
297. Cardiac arrest, unexplained w CC	
298. Cardiac arrest, unexplained w/o CC/MCC.	344. Minor small & large bowel procedures w MCC.
299. Peripheral vascular disorders w MCC	345. Minor small & large bowel procedures w CC.
300. Peripheral vascular disorders w CC	346. Minor small & large bowel procedures w/o CC/MCC.
301. Peripheral vascular disorders w/o CC/MCC.	347. Anal & stomal procedures w MCC ...
302. Atherosclerosis w MCC	348. Anal & stomal procedures w CC ...
303. Atherosclerosis w/o MCC	349. Anal & stomal procedures w/o CC/MCC.
304. Hypertension w MCC	350. Inguinal & femoral hernia procedures w MCC.
305. HYPERTENSION W/O MCC ...	351. Inguinal & femoral hernia procedures w CC.
306. Cardiac congenital & valvular disorders w MCC.	352. Inguinal & femoral hernia procedures w/o CC/MCC.
307. Cardiac congenital & valvular disorders w/o MCC.	353. Hernia procedures except inguinal & femoral w MCC.
308. Cardiac arrhythmia & conduction disorders w MCC.	354. Hernia procedures except inguinal & femoral w CC.
309. Cardiac arrhythmia & conduction disorders w CC.	355. Hernia procedures except inguinal &femoral w/o CC/MCC.
310. Cardiac arrhythmia & conduction disorders w/o CC/MCC.	
311. Angina pectoris	
312. Syncope & collapse	

MS-DRG Description	MS-DRG Description
356. Other digestive system O.R. procedures w MCC.	413. Cholecystectomy w c.d.e. w/o CC/MCC.
357. Other digestive system O.R. procedures w CC.	414. Cholecystectomy except by laparoscope w/o c.d.e. w MCC
358. Other digestive system O.R. procedures w/o CC/MCC.	415. Cholecystectomy except by laparoscope w/o c.d.e. w CC
368. Major esophageal disorders w MCC	416. Cholecystectomy except by laparoscope w/o c.d.e. w/o CC/MCC
369. Major esophageal disorders w CC	417. Laparoscopic cholecystectomy w/o c.d.e. w MCC.
370. Major esophageal disorders w/o CC/MCC.	418. Laparoscopic cholecystectomy w/o c.d.e. w CC.
371. Major gastrointestinal disorders & peritoneal infections w MCC.	419. Laparoscopic cholecystectomy w/o c.d.e. w/o CC/MCC.
372. Major gastrointestinal disorders & peritoneal infections w CC.	420. Hepatobiliary diagnostic procedures w MCC.
373. Major gastrointestinal disorders & peritoneal infections w/oCC/MCC	421. Hepatobiliary diagnostic procedures w CC.
374. Digestive malignancy w MCC	422. Hepatobiliary diagnostic procedures
375. Digestive malignancy w CC	423. Other hepatobiliary or pancreas O.R. procedures w MCC
376. Digestive malignancy w/o CC/MCC	424. Other hepatobiliary or pancreas O.R. procedures w CC
377. G.I. hemorrhage w MCC	425. Other hepatobiliary or pancreas O.R. procedures w/o CC/MCC
378. G.I. hemorrhage w CC	432. Cirrhosis & alcoholic hepatitis w MCC
379. G.I. hemorrhage w/o CC/MCC	433. Cirrhosis & alcoholic hepatitis w CC
380. Complicated peptic ulcer w MCC	434. Cirrhosis & alcoholic hepatitis w/o CC/MCC.
381. Complicated peptic ulcer w CC	435. Malignancy of hepatobiliary system or pancreas w MCC
382. Complicated peptic ulcer w/o cc/MCC	436. Malignancy of hepatobiliary system orpancreas w CC.
383. Uncomplicated peptic ulcer w MCC	437. Malignancy of hepatobiliary system opancreas w/o CC/MCC.
384. Uncomplicated peptic ulcer w/o MCC	438. Disorders of pancreas except malignancyw MCC.
385. Inflammatory bowel disease w MCC	439. Disorders of pancreas except malignancy w CC.
386. Inflammatory bowel disease w CC	440. Disorders of pancreas except malignancy w/o CC/MCC.
387. Inflammatory bowel disease w/o CC/MCC	441. Disorders of liver except malig, cirr, alc hepa w MCC.
388. G.I. obstruction w MCC	442. Disorders of liver except malig, cirr, alc hepa w CC.
389. G.I. obstruction w CC	443. Disorders of liver except malig, cirr, alchepa w/o CC/MCC.
390. G.I. obstruction w/o CC/MCC	444. Disorders of the biliary tract w MCC
391. Esophagitis, gastroent & misc digest disorders w MCC	445. Disorders of the biliary tract w CC
392. Esophagitis, gastroent & misc digest disorders w/o MCC	446. Disorders of the biliary tract w/o CC/MCC.
393. Other digestive system diagnoses w MCC	453. Combined anterior/posterior spinal fusion W MCC
394. Other digestive system diagnoses w CC	454. Combined anterior/posterior spinal fusion w CC.
395. Other digestive system diagnoses w/o CC/MCC	455. Combined anterior/posterior spinal fusionw/o CC/MCC.
405. Pancreas, liver & shunt procedures w MCC	456. Spinal fus exc cerv w spinal curv/malig/infec or 91 fus w MCC.
406. Pancreas, liver & shunt procedures w CC	457. Spinal fus exc cerv w spinal curv/malig/infec or 91 fus w MCC.
407. Pancreas, liver & shunt procedures w/o CC/MCC.	
408. Biliary tract proc except only cholecyst w or w/o c.d.e. w MCC.	
409. Biliary tract proc except only cholecyst w or w/o c.d.e. w CC.	
410. Biliary tract proc except only cholecyst w or w/o c.d.e. w/o CC/MCC.	
411. Cholecystectomy w c.d.e. w MCC	
412. Cholecystectomy w c.d.e. w CC	

MS-DRG Description	MS-DRG Description
458. Spinal fus exc cerv w spinal curv/malig/infec or 9 fus w CC.	487. Knee procedures w pdx of infection w/ o CC/MCC.
458. Spinal fus exc cerv w spinal curv/malig/infec or 9 fus w/o CC/MCC	488. Knee procedures w/o pdx of infection w CC/MCC.
459. Spinal fusion except cervical w MCC	489. Knee procedures w/o pdx of infection w/o CC/MCC.
460. Spinal fusion except cervical w/o MCC	490. Back & neck proc exc spinal fusion w CC/MCC or disc device/neurostim.
461. Bilateral or multiple major joint procs of lower extremity w MCC.	491. Back & neck proc exc spinal fusion w/o CC/MCC.
462. Bilateral or multiple major joint procs of lower extremity w/o MCC.	492. Lower extrem & humer proc except hip, foot, femur w MCC.
463. Wnd debrid & skn grft exc hand, for musculo-conn tiss dis w MCC.	493. Lower extrem & humer proc except hip , foot, femur w CC.
464. Wnd debrid & skn grft exc hand, for musculo-conn tiss dis w CC.	494. Lower extrem & humer proc except hip, foot, femur w/o CC/MCC.
465. Wnd debrid & skn grft exc hand, for musculo-conn tiss dis w/o CC/MCC.	495. Local excision & removal int fix devices exc hip & femur w MCC.
466. Revision of hip or knee replacement w MCC.	496. Local excision & removal int fix devices exc hip & femur w CC.
467. Revision of hip or knee replacement w CC	497. Local excision & removal int fix devices exc hip & femur w/o CC/MCC.
468. Revision of hip or knee replacement w/o CC/MCC	498. Local excision & removal int fix devices of hip & femur w CC/MCC.
469. Revision of hip or knee replacement w/o CC/MCC	499. Local excision & removal int fix devices of hip & femur w/o CC/MCC.
470. Major joint replacement or reattachment of lower extremity w/o MCC.	500. Soft tissue procedures w MCC
471. Cervical spinal fusion w MCC	501. Soft tissue procedures w CC
472. Cervical spinal fusion w CC	502. Soft tissue procedures w/o CC/MCC
473. Cervical spinal fusion w/o CC/MCC	503. Foot procedures w MCC
474. Amputation for musculoskeletal sys & conn tissue dis w MCC	504. Foot procedures w CC
475. Amputation for musculoskeletal sys & conn tissue dis w CC.	505. Foot procedures w/o CC/MCC
476. Amputation for musculoskeletal sys & conn tissue dis w/o CC/MCC.	506. Major thumb or joint procedures
477. Biopsies of musculoskeletal system & connective tissue w MCC.	507. Major shoulder or elbow joint procedures w CC/MCC.
478. Biopsies of musculoskeletal system & connective tissue w CC.	508. Major shoulder or elbow joint procedures w/o CC/MCC.
479. Biopsies of musculoskeletal system & connective tissue w/o CC/MCC.	509. Arthroscopy
480. Hip & femur procedures except major joint w MCC	510. Shoulder,elbowor forearm proc,exc major joint proc w MCC.
481. Hip & femur procedures except major joint w CC.	511. Shoulder,elbowor forearm proc,exc major joint proc w CC.
482. Hip & femur procedures except major joint w/o CC/MCC.	512. Shoulder,elbow or forearm proc,exc major joint proc w/o CC/MCC.
483. Major joint & limb reattachment proc of upper extremity w CC/MCC.	513. Hand or wrist proc, except major thumb or joint proc w CC/MCC.
484. Major joint & limb reattachment proc of upper extremity w/o CC/MCC.	514. Hand or wrist proc, except major thumb or joint proc w/o CC/MCC.
485. Knee procedures w pdx of infection w MCC.	515. Other musculoskelet sys & conn tiss O.R. proc w MCC.
486. Knee procedures w pdx of infection w CC.	516. Other musculoskelet sys & conn tiss O.R. proc w CC.

MS-DRG Description	MS-DRG Description
517. Other musculoskelet sys & conn tiss O.R. proc w/o CC/MCC.	566. Other musculoskeletal sys & connective tissue diagnoses w/o CC/MCC.
533. Fractures of femur w MCC	573. Skin graft &/or debrid for skn ulcer or cellulitis w MCC.
534. Fractures of femur w/o MCC	574. Skin graft &/or debrid for skn ulcer or cellulitis w CC.
535. Fractures of hip & pelvis w MCC	
536. Fractures of hip & pelvis w/o MCC	575. Skin graft &/or debrid for skn ulcer or cellulitis w/o CC/MCC.
537. Sprains, strains, & dislocations of hip, pelvis & thigh w CC/MCC.	576. Skin graft &/or debrid exc for skin ulcer or cellulitis w MCC.
538. Sprains, strains, & dislocations of hip, pelvis & thigh w/o CC/MCC.	577. Skin graft &/or debrid exc for skin ulcer or cellulitis w CC.
539. Osteomyelitis w MCC	578. Skin graft &/or debrid exc for skin ulcer or cellulitis w/o CC/MCC.
540. Osteomyelitis w CC	
541. Osteomyelitis w/o CC/MCC	579. Other skin, subcut tiss & breast proc w MCC.
542. Pathological fractures & musculoskelet & conn tiss malig w MCC.	580. Other skin, subcut tiss & breast proc w CC.
543. Pathological fractures & musculoskelet & conn tiss malig w CC.	581. Other skin, subcut tiss & breast proc w/o CC/MCC.
544. Pathological fractures & musculoskelet & conn tiss malig w/o CC/MCC	582. Mastectomy for malignancy w CC/ MCC.
545. Connective tissue disorders w MCC	583. Mastectomy for malignancy w/o CC/MCC.
546. Connective tissue disorders w CC	584. Breast biopsy, local excision & other breast procedures w CC/MCC.
547. Connective tissue disorders w/o CC/MCC.	585. Breast biopsy, local excision & other breast procedures w/o CC/MCC.
548. Septic arthritis w MCC	
549. Septic arthritis w CC	592. Skin ulcers w MCC
550. Septic arthritis w/o CC/MCC	593. Skin ulcers w CC
551. Medical back problems w MCC	594. Skin ulcers w/o CC/MCC
552. Medical back problems w/o MCC	595. Major skin disorders w MCC
553. Bone diseases & arthropathies w MCC	596. Major skin disorders w/o MCC
554. Bone diseases & arthropathies w/o MCC.	597. Malignant breast disorders w MCC
555. Signs & symptoms of musculoskeletal system & conn tissue w MCC.	598. Malignant breast disorders w CC
	599. Malignant breast disorders w/o CC/MCC.
556. Signs & symptoms of musculoskeletal system & conn tissue w/o MCC.	600. Non-malignant breast disorders w CC/MCC.
557. Tendonitis, myositis & bursitis w MCC	601. Non-malignant breast disorders w/o CC/MCC.
558. Tendonitis, myositis & bursitis w/o	602. Cellulitis w MCC
559. Aftercare, musculoskeletal system & connective tissue w MCC.	603. Cellulitis w/o MCC
	604. Trauma to the skin, subcut tiss & breast w MCC.
560. Aftercare, musculoskeletal system & connective tissue w CC.	605. Trauma to the skin, subcut tiss & breast w/o MCC.
561. Aftercare, musculoskeletal system & connective tissue w/o CC/MCC.	606. Minor skin disorders w MCC
	607. Minor skin disorders w/o MCC
562. Fx, sprn, strn & disl except femur, hip, pelvis & thigh w MCC.	614. Adrenal & pituitary procedures w CC/MCC.
563. Fx, sprn, strn & disl except femur, hip, pelvis & thigh w/o MCC.	615. Adrenal & pituitary procedures w/o CC/MCC.
	616. Amputatof lower limb for endocrine, nutrit, & metabol dis w MCC.
564. Other musculoskeletal sys & connective tissue diagnoses w MCC.	617. Amputat of lower limb for endocrine, nutrit, & metabol dis w CC.
565. Other musculoskeletal sys & connective tissue diagnoses w CC.	618. Amputat of lower limb for endocrine, nutrit, & metabol dis w/o CC/MCC.

MS-DRG Description	MS-DRG Description
619. O.R. procedures for obesity w MCC	665. Prostatectomy w MCC
620. O.R. procedures for obesity w CC	666. Prostatectomy w CC
621. O.R. procedures for obesity w/o CC/MCC.	667. Prostatectomy w/o CC/MCC
622. Skin grafts & wound debrid for endoc, nutrit & metab dis w MCC.	668. Transurethral procedures w MCC
623. Skin grafts & wound debrid for endoc, nutrit & metab dis w CC.	669. Transurethral procedures w CC
624. Skin grafts & wound debrid for endoc, nutrit & metab dis w/o CC/MCC.	670. Transurethral procedures w/o CC/MCC.
625. Thyroid, parathyroid & thyroglossal procedures w MCC.	671. Urethral procedures w CC/MCC
626. Thyroid, parathyroid &thyroglossal procedures w CC.	672. Urethral procedures w/o CC/MCC
627. Thyroid, parathyroid& thyroglossal procedures w/o CC/MCC.	673. Other kidney & urinary tract procedures w MCC.
628. Other endocrine, nutrit & metab O.R. proc w MCC.	674. Other kidney & urinary tract procedures w CC.
629. Other endocrine, nutrit & metab O.R. proc w CC.	675. Other kidney & urinary tract procedures w/o CC/MCC.
630. Other endocrine, nutrit & metab O.R. proc w/o CC/MCC.	682. Renal failure w MCC
637. Diabetes w MCC	683. Renal failure w CC
638. Diabetes w CC	684. Renal failure w/o CC/MCC
639. Diabetes w/o CC/MCC	685. Admit for renal dialysis
640. Nutritional & misc metabolic disorders w MCC.	686. Kidney & urinary tract neoplasms w MCC.
641. Nutritional & misc metabolic disorders w/o MCC.	687. Kidney & urinary tract neoplasms w CC.
642. Inborn errors of metabolism	688. Kidney & urinary tract neoplasms w/o CC/MCC.
643. Endocrine disorders w MCC	689. Kidney & urinary tract infections w MCC.
644. Endocrine disorders w CC	690. Kidney & urinary tract infections w/o MCC.
645. Endocrine disorders w/o CC/MCC	691. Urinary stones w esw lithotripsy w CC/MCC.
652. Kidney transplant	692. Urinary stones w esw lithotripsy w/o CC/MCC.
653. Major bladder procedures w MCC	693. Urinary stones w/o esw lithotripsy w MCC.
654. Major bladder procedures w CC	694. Urinary stones w/o esw lithotripsy w/o MCC.
655. Major bladder procedures w/o CC/MCC.	695. Kidney & urinary tract signs & symptoms w MCC.
656. Kidney & ureter procedures for neoplasm w MCC.	696. Kidney & urinary tract signs & symptoms w/o MCC.
657. Kidney & ureter procedures for neo-	697. Urethral stricture
658. Kidney & ureter procedures for neoplasm w/o CC/MCC.	698. Other kidney & urinary tract diagnoses w MCC.
659. Kidney & ureter procedures for non-Neoplasm w MCC.	699. Other kidney & urinary tract diagnoses w CC.
660. Kidney & ureter procedures for non-neoplasm w CC.	700. Other kidney & urinary tract diagnoses w/o CC/MCC.
661. Kidney & ureter procedures for non-neoplasm w/o CC/MCC.	707. Major male pelvic procedures w CC/MCC.
662. Minor bladder procedures w MCC	708. Major male pelvic procedures w/o CC/MCC.
663. Minor bladder procedures w CC	709. Penis procedures w CC/MCC
664. Minor bladder procedures w/o CC/MCC.	710. Penis procedures w/o CC/MCC
	711. Testes procedures w CC/MCC
	712. Testes procedures w/o CC/MCC
	713. Transurethral prostatectomy w CC/MCC.
	714. Transurethral prostatectomy w/o CC/MCC.
	715. Other male reproductive system O.R. proc for malignancy w CC/MCC.
	716. Other male reproductive system O.R. proc for malignancy w/o CC/MCC.
	717. Other male reproductive system O.R. proc exc malignancy w CC/MCC.

MS-DRG Description	MS-DRG Description

718. Other male reproductive system O.R. proc exc malignancy w/o CC/MCC.

722. Malignancy, male reproductive system w MCC.

722. Malignancy, male reproductive system w CC.

723. Malignancy, male reproductive system w/o CC/MCC.

724. Benign prostatic hypertrophy w MCC

725. Benign prostatic hypertrophy w/o MCC.

726. Inflammation of the male reproductive system w MCC

727. Inflammation of the male reproductive system w/o MCC.

728. Other male reproductive system diagnoses w CC/MCC.

729. Other male reproductive system diagnoses w/o CC/MCC.

730. Other male reproductive system diagnoses w/o CC/MCC

734. Pelvic evisceration, rad hysterectomy & rad vulvectomy w CC/MCC.

735. Pelvic evisceration, rad hysterectomy & rad vulvectomy w/o CC/MCC

736. Uterine & adnexa proc for ovarian or adnexal malignancy w MCC.

737. Uterine & adnexa proc for ovarian or adnexal malignancy w CC.

738. Uterine & adnexa proc for ovarian or adnexal malignancy w/o CC/MCC.

739. Uterine, adnexa proc for non-ovarian/adnexal malig w MCC

740. Uterine,adnexa proc for non-ovarian/adnexal malig w CC.

741. Uterine, adnexa proc for non-ovarian/adnexal malig w/o CC/MCC.

742. Uterine & adnexa proc for non-malignancyw CC/MCC.

743. Uterine & adnexa proc for non-malignancyw/o CC/MCC.

744. D&C, conization, laparascopy & tubalinterruption w CC/MCC.

745. D&C, conization, laparascopy & tubalinterruption w/o CC/MCC.

746. Vagina, cervix & vulva procedures w CC/MCC.

747. Vagina, cervix & vulva procedures w/o CC/MCC.

748. Female reproductive system reconstructive procedures.

749. Other female reproductive system O.R. procedures w CC/MCC.

750. Other female reproductive system O.R. procedures w/o CC/MCC.

754. Malignancy, female reproductive system w MCC.

755. Malignancy, female reproductive system w CC.

756. Malignancy, female reproductive system w/o CC/MCC.

757. Infections, female reproductive system w MCC.

758. Infections, female reproductive system w CC.

759. Infections, female reproductive system w/o CC/MCC.

760. Menstrual & other female reproductive system disorders w CC/MCC.

761. Menstrual & other female reproductive system disorders w/o CC/MCC.

765. Cesarean section w CC/MCC

766. Cesarean section w/o CC/MCC

767. Vaginal delivery w sterilization &/or D&C.

768. Vaginal delivery w O.R. proc except steril &/or D&C.

769. Postpartum & post abortion diagnoses w O.R. procedure.

770. Abortion w D&C, aspiration curettage or hysterotomy.

774. Vaginal delivery w complicating diagnoses.

775. Vaginal delivery w/o complicating diagnoses.

776. Postpartum & post abortion diagnoses w/o O.R. procedure.

777. w/o O.R. procedure.

778. Threatened abortion

779. Abortion w/o D&C

780. False labor

781. Other antepartum diagnoses w medical complications.

782. Other antepartum diagnoses w/o medical complications.

789. Neonates, died or transferred to another acute care facility.

790. Extreme immaturity or respiratory distress syndrome, neonate.

791. Prematurity w major problems

792. Prematurity w/o major problems

793. Full term neonate w major problems

794. Neonate w other significant problems

795. Normal newborn

799. Splenectomy w MCC

800. Splenectomy w CC

801. Splenectomy w/o CC/MCC

802. Other O.R. proc of the blood & blood forming organs w MCC.

803. Other O.R. proc of the blood & blood forming organs w CC.

804. Other O.R. proc of the blood & blood forming organs w/o CC/MCC.

MS-DRG Description	MS-DRG Description
808. Major hematol/immun diag exc sickle cell crisis & coagul w MCC.	843. Other myeloprolif dis or poorly diff neopl diag w MCC.
809. Major hematol/immun diag exc sickle cell crisis & coagul w CC.	844. Other myeloprolif dis or poorly diff neopl diag w CC.
810. Major hematol/immun diag exc sickle cell crisis & coagul w/o CC/MCC.	845. Other myeloprolif dis or poorly diff neopl diag w/o CC/MCC.
811. Red blood cell disorders w MCC	846. Chemotherapy w/o acute leukemia as secondary diagnosis w MCC.
812. Red blood cell disorders w/o MCC	847. Chemotherapy w/o acute leukemia as secondary diagnosis w CC.
813. Coagulation disorders	848. Chemotherapy w/o acute leukemia as secondary diagnosis w/o CC/MCC.
814. Reticuloendothelial & immunity disorders w MCC.	849. Radiotherapy
815. Reticuloendothelial & immunity disorder w/o CC/MCC.	853. Infectious & parasitic diseases w O.R. procedure w MCC.
816. Reticuloendothelial & immunity disorders w/o CC/MCC.	854. Infectious & parasitic diseases w O.R. procedure w CC.
820. Lymphoma & leukemia w major O.R procedure w MCC	855. Infectious & parasitic diseases w O.R. procedure w/o CC/MCC.
821. Lymphoma & leukemia w major O.R. procedure w CC.	856. Postoperative or post-traumatic infections w O.R. proc w MCC.
822. Lymphoma & leukemia w major O.R. procedure w/o CC/MCC.	857. Postoperative or post-traumatic infections w O.R. proc w CC.
823. Lymphoma & non-acute leukemia w other O.R. proc w MCC.	858. Postoperative or post-traumatic infections w O.R. proc w/o CC/MCC.
824. Lymphoma & non-acute leukemia w other O.R. proc w CC.	862. Postoperative & post-traumatic infections w MCC.
825. Lymphoma & non-acute leukemia w other O.R. proc w/o CC/MCC.	863. Postoperative & post-traumatic infections w/o MCC.
826. Myeloprolif disord or poorly diff neopl w maj O.R. proc w MCC.	864. Fever of unknown origin
827. Myeloprolif disord or poorly diff neopl w maj O.R. proc w CC.	865. Viral illness w MCC
828. Myeloprolif disord or poorly diff neopl w maj O.R. proc w/o CC/MCC.	866. Viral illness w/o MCC
829. Myeloprolif disord or poorly diff neopl w other O.R. proc w CC/MCC.	867. Other infectious & parasitic diseases diagnoses w MCC.
830. Myeloprolif disord or poorly diff neopl w other O.R. proc w/o CC/MCC.	868. Other infectious & parasitic diseases diagnoses w CC.
834. Acute leukemia w/o major O.R. procedure w MCC.	869. Other infectious & parasitic diseases diagnoses w/o CC/MCC.
835. Acute leukemia w/o major O.R. procedure w CC.	870. Septicemia or severe sepsis w MV 961 hours
836. Acute leukemia w/o major O.R. procedure w/o CC/MCC.	871. Septicemia or severe sepsis w/o MV 961 hours w MCC
837. Chemo w acute leukemia as sdx or w high dose chemo agent w MCC.	872. Septicemia or severe sepsis w/o MV 961 hours w/o MCC
838. Chemo w acute leukemia as sdx w CC or high dose chemo agent.	880. O.R. procedure w principal diagnoses of mental illness.
839. Chemo w acute leukemia as sdx w/o CC/MCC.	881. Acute adjustment reaction & psychosocial dysfunction.
840. Lymphoma & non-acute leukemia w MCC.	882. Depressive neuroses
841. Lymphoma & non-acute leukemia w CC.	883. Neuroses except depressive
842. Lymphoma & non-acute leukemia w/o CC/MCC	884. Disorders of personality & impulse control.
	885. Organic disturbances & mental retardation.

MS-DRG Description	MS-DRG Description
886. Psychoses	945. Rehabilitation w CC/MCC
887. Behavioral & developmental disorders	946. Rehabilitation w/o CC/MCC
894. Other mental disorder diagnoses	947. Signs & symptoms w MCC
895. Alcohol/drug abuse or dependence, left ama.	948. Signs & symptoms w/o MCC
896. Alcohol/drug abuse or dependence w rehabilitation therapy.	949. Aftercare w CC/MCC
897. Alcohol/drug abuse or dependence w/o rehabilitation therapy w MCC.	950. Aftercare w/o CC/MCC
901. Wound debridements for injuries w MCC.	951. Other factors influencing health status
902. Wound debridements for injuries w CC.	955. Craniotomy for multiple significant trauma.
903. Wound debridements for injuries w/o CC/MCC.	956. Limb reattachment, hip & femur proc for multiple significant trauma.
904. Skin grafts for injuries w CC/MCC	957. Other O.R. procedures for multiple significant trauma w MCC.
905. Skin grafts for injuries w/o CC/MCC	958. Other O.R. procedures for multiple significant trauma w CC.
906. Hand procedures for injuries	959. Other O.R. procedures for multiple significant trauma w/o CC/MCC.
907. Other O.R. procedures for injuries w MCC.	
908. Other O.R. procedures for injuries w CC.	963. Other multiple significant trauma w MCC.
909. Other O.R. procedures for injuries w/o CC/MCC.	964. Other multiple significant trauma w CC.
913. Traumatic injury w MCC	965. Other multiple significant trauma w/o CC/MCC.
914. Traumatic injury w/o MCC	969. HIV w extensive O.R. procedure w MCC.
915. Allergic reactions w MCC	970. HIV w extensive O.R. procedure w/o MCC.
916. Allergic reactions w/o MCC	974. HIV w major related condition w MCC
917. Poisoning & toxic effects of drugs w MCC.	975. HIV w major related condition w CC
918. Poisoning & toxic effects of drugs w/o MCC.	976. HIV w major related condition w/o CC/MCC.
919. Complications of treatment w MCC	977. HIV w or w/o other related condition
920. Complications of treatment w CC	981. Extensive O.R. procedure unrelated to principal diagnosis w MCC.
921. Complications of treatment w/o CC/MCC.	982. Extensive O.R. procedure unrelated to principal diagnosis w CC.
922. Other injury, poisoning & toxic effect diag w MCC.	983. Extensive O.R. procedure unrelated to principal diagnosis w/o CC/MCC.
923. Other injury, poisoning & toxic effect diag w/o MCC.	984. Prostatic O.R. procedure unrelated to principal diagnosis w MCC.
927. Extensive burns or full thickness burns w MV 961 hrs w skin graft.	985. Prostatic O.R. procedure unrelated to principal diagnosis w CC.
928. Full thickness burn w skin graft or inhal inj w CC/MCC.	986. Prostatic O.R. procedure unrelated to principal diagnosis w/o CC/MCC.
929. Full thickness burn w skin graft or inhal inj w/o CC/MCC.	987. Non-extensive O.R. proc unrelated to principal diagnosis w MCC.
933. Extensive burns or full thickness burns w MV 961 hrs w/o skin graft.	988. Non-extensive O.R. proc unrelated to principal diagnosis w CC.
934. Full thickness burn w/o skin grft or inhal inj.	989. Non-extensive O.R. proc unrelated to principal diagnosis w/o CC/MCC.
935. Non-extensive burns	998. Principal diagnosis invalid as discharge diagnosis.
939. O.R. proc w diagnoses of other contact w health services w MCC.	999. Ungroupable
940. O.R. proc w diagnoses of other contact w health services w CC.	
941. O.R. proc w diagnoses of other contact w health services w/o CC/MCC.	

Laboratory Reference Range Values

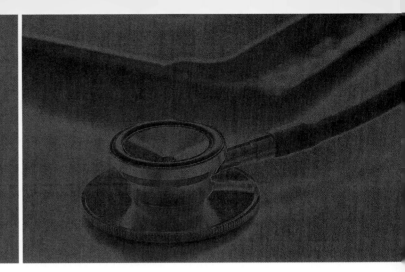

Show-Hong Duh, PhD, DABCC, Department of Pathology
University of Maryland School of Medicine
Janine Denis Cook, PhD, Department of Medical and Research Technology
University of Maryland School of Medicine

Reference range values are for apparently healthy people and often overlap significantly with values for those who are sick. Actual values may vary significantly due to differences in assay methodologies and standardization. Institutions may also set up their own reference ranges based on the particular populations they serve; thus, regional differences may exist. Consequently, values reported by individual laboratories may differ from those listed in this appendix.

All values are given in conventional and SI units. However, where the SI units have not been widely accepted, conventional units are used. In case of the heterogenous nature of the materials measured or uncertainty about the exact molecular weight of the compounds, the SI system cannot be followed, and mass per volume is used as the unit of concentration.

Abbreviations

ACD, acid-citrate-dextrose; **CHF,** congestive heart failure; **Cit,** citrate; **Cl,** chloride; **CNS,** central nervous system; **CSF,** cerebrospinal fluid; **cyclic AMP,** adenosine 3′,5′-cyclic phosphate; **EDTA,** ethylenediaminetetraacetic acid; **HDL,** high-density lipoprotein; **Hep,** heparin; **LDL-C,** low-density lipoprotein-cholesterol; **Ox,** oxalate; **RBC,** red blood cell(s); **RIA,** radioimmunoassay; **SD,** standard deviation; **WBC,** white blood cell(s).

REFERENCES

Burtis CA, Ashwood ER, eds. Tietz textbook of clinical chemistry, 3rd ed. Philadelphia: WB Saunders, 1998.

Children's Hospital, St. Louis, The Department of Clinical Laboratories. High Density Lipoprotein Lipid Panel: Cholesterol, HDL, Cholesterol, LDL (calculated), Cholesterol, Total, Triglycerides. Parathyroid Hormone (PTH). Available at: http://webserver01.bjc.org/slch/pro/Professional.htm? http://webserver01.bjc.org/labtestguide/Lab%20Test%20Guidebook/guide .htm. Accessed April 20, 2004.

Clinical chemistry laboratory: Reference range values in clinical chemistry. Professional services manual. Baltimore, Department of Pathology, University of Maryland Medical System, 1999.

Harmening DM, ed. Hematologic values in clinical hematology and fundamentals of hemostasis, 2nd ed. Philadelphia: FA Davis, 1992.

Laboratory Corporation of America. Erythrocyte Sedimentation Rate, Westergren. Available at: http://www.labcorp.com/datasets/labcorp/html/ chapter/mono/he005000.htm. Accessed April 20, 2004.

Laboratory Corporation of America. Fecal Fat, Quantitative. Available at: http://www. labcorp.com/datasets/labcorp/html/chapter/mono/sc008000 .htm. Accessed April 20, 2004.

National cholesterol education program: Report of the expert panel on detection, evaluation, and treatment of high blood cholesterol in adults. *Arch Intern Med* 1988;148:36–99.

Triglyceride, high density lipoprotein, and coronary heart disease. National Institute of Health Consensus Statement, NIH Consensus Development Conference, 1992;10(2).

University of Texas Health Center at San Antonio. Neonatal Bilirubin. Available at: http://labs-sec.uhs-sa.com/clinical_ext/dols/soprefrange.asp. Accessed April 20, 2004.

University of Texas Medical Branch. Erythrocyte Sedimentation Rate, Wintrobe. Available at: http://www.utmb.edu/lsg/LabSurvivalGuide/hem/ Sedimentation_Rate.htm. Accessed April 20, 2004.

University of Virginia Children's Medical Center. Therapy Review: Warfarin (Coumadin®). *Pediatric Pharmacotherapy*. January 1995;1(5). Available at: http://www.people.virginia. edu/~smb4v/cmchome.html. Accessed April 20, 2004.

Warfarin Therapy in Children Who Require Long-Term Total Parenteral Nutrition *Pediatrics* [electronic article]. November 2003;112(5):386. Available at: http://pediatrics. aappublications.org/cgi/content/full/112/ 5/e386. Accessed April 20, 2004.

Test	Conventional Units	SI Units
Acetaminophen, serum or plasma (Hep or EDTA)		
Therapeutic	10–30 μg/mL	66–199 μmol/L
Toxic	>200 μg/mL	>1324 μmol/L
Acetone		
Serum		
Qualitative	Negative	Negative
Quantitative	0.3–2.0 mg/dL	0.05–0.34 mmol/L
Urine		
Qualitative	Negative	Negative
Acid hemolysis test (Ham)	<5% lysis	<0.05 lysed fraction
Adrenocorticotropin (ACTH), plasma		
8 AM	<120 pg/mL	<26 pmol/L
Midnight (supine)	<10 pg/mL	<2.2 pmol/L
*alanine aminotransferase (ALT, SGPT), serum		
Male	13–40 U/L (37°C)	0.22–0.68 μkat/L (37° C)
Female	10–28 U/L (37°C)	0.17–0.48 μkat/L (37° C)
Albumin		
Serum		
Adult	3.5–5.2 g/dL	35–52 g/L
>60 y	3.2–4.6 g/dL	32–46 g/L
	Avg. of 0.3 g/dL higher in upright individuals	Avg. of 3 g/dL higher in upright individuals
Urine		
Qualitative	Negative	Negative
Quantitative	50–80 mg/24 h	50–80 mg/24 h
CSF	10–30 mg/dL	100–300 mg/dL
*Aldolase, serum	1.0–7.5 U/L (30° C)	0.02–0.13 μkat/L (30° C)
Aldosterone		
Serum		
Supine	3–16 ng/dL	0.08–0.44 nmol/L
Standing	7–30 ng/dL	0.19–0.83 nmol/L
Urine	3–19 μg/24 h	8–51 nmol/24 h
Amikacin, serum or plasma (EDTA)		
Therapeutic		
Peak	25–35 μg/mL	43–60 μmol/L
Trough		
Less severe infection	1–4 μg/mL	1.7–6.8 μmol/L
Life-threatening infection	4–8 μg/mL	6.8–13.7 μmol/L
Toxic		
Peak	>35–40 μg/mL	>60–68 μmol/L
Trough	>10–15 μg/mL	>17–26 μmol/L
∂-Aminolevulinic acid, urine	1.3–7.0 mg/24 h	10–53 μmol/24 h
Amitriptyline, serum or plasma (Hep or EDTA); trough (≥12 h after dose)		
Therapeutic	80–250 ng/mL	289–903 nmol/L
Toxic	>500 ng/mL	>1805 nmol/L
Ammonia		
Plasma (Hep)	9–33 μmol/L	9–33 μmol/L

*Test values depend on laboratory methods.

Test	Conventional Units	SI Units
*Amylase		
Serum	27–131 U/L	0.46–2.23 μkat/L
Urine	1–17 U/h	0.017–0.29 μkat/h
Amylase:creatine clearance ratio	1–4%	0.01–0.04
Androstenedione, serum		
Male	75–205 ng/dL	2.6–7.2 nmol/L
Female	85–275 ng/dL	3.0–9.6 nmol/L
Anion gap		
$(Na - (Cl + HCO_3))$	7–16 mEq/L	7–16 mmol/L
$((Na + K) - (Cl + HCO_3))$	10–20 mEq/L	10–20 mmol/L
α_1-Antitrypsin, serum	78–200 mg/dL	0.78–2.00 g/L
Apolipoprotein A-1		
Male	94–178 mg/dL	0.94–1.78 g/L
Female	101–199 mg/dL	1.01–1.99 g/L
Apolipoprotein B		
Male	63–133 mg/dL	0.63–1.33 g/L
Female	60–126 mg/dL	0.60–1.26 g/L
Arsenic		
Whole blood (Hep)	0.2–2.3 μg/dL	0.03–0.31 μmol/L
Chronic poisoning	10–50 μg/dL	1.33–6.65 μmol/L
Acute poisoning	60–930 μg/dL	7.98–124 μmol/L
Urine, 24 h	5–50 μg/d	0.07–0.67 μmol/d
Ascorbic acid, plasma (Ox, Hep, EDTA)	0.4–1.5 mg/dL	23–85 μmol/L
*Aspartate aminotransferase (AST, (37°C) SGOT), serum	10–59 U/L (37°C)	0.17–1.00 −2 to +3 kat/L
Base excess, blood (Hep)	−2 to +3 mmol/L	−2 to +3 mmol/L
Bicarbonate, serum (venous)	22–29 mmol/L	22–29 mmol/L
*†Bilirubin		
Bilirubin, direct		
Birth–death	0.0–0.4 mg/dL	
Bilirubin, total		
Birth–1 day	1.0–6.0 mg/dL	
1–2 days	6.0–7.5 mg/dL	
2–5 days	4.0–13.5 mg/dL	
5 days–death	0.2–1.2 mg/dL	
Total bilirubin, neonatal		
Birth–1 day	1.0–6.0 g/dL	
1–2 days	6.0–7.5 g/dL	
2–5 days	4.0– 13.5 g/dL	
5 days–1 month	0.0–1.8 g/dL	
1 month–death	0.0–1.8 g/dL	
Bone marrow, differential cell count		
Adult		
Undifferentiated cells	0–1%	0–0.01
Myeloblast	0–2%	0–0.02
Promyelocyte	0–4%	0–0.04
Myelocytes		
Neutrophilic	5–20%	0.05–0.20
Eosinophilic	0–3%	0–0.03
Basophilic	0–1%	0–0.01

*Test values depend on laboratory methods.

†Bilirubin data—Source: http://labs-sec.uhs-sa.com/clinical_ext/dols/soprefrange.asp

Test	Conventional Units	SI Units
Metamyelocytes and bands		
Neutrophilic	5–35%	0.05–0.35
Eosinophilic	0–5%	0–0.05
Basophilic	0–1%	0–0.01
Segmented neutrophils	5–15%	0.05–0.15
Pronormoblast	0–1.5%	0–0.015
Basophilic normoblast	0–5%	0–0.05
Polychromatophilic normoblast	5–30%	0.05–0.30
Orthochromatic normoblast	5–10%	0.05–0.10
Lymphocytes	10–20%	0.10–0.20
Plasma cells	0–2%	0–0.02
Monocytes	0–5%	0–0.05
CA 125, serum	<35 U/mL	<35 kU/L
CA 15–3, serum	<30 U/mL	<30 kU/L
CA 19–9, serum	<37 U/mL	<37 kU/L
Cadmium, whole blood (Hep)	0.1–0.5 µg/dL	8.9–44.5 nmol/L
Toxic	10–300 µg/dL	0.89–26.70 µmol/L
Cadmium, urine, 24 h	<15 µg/d	<0.13 µmol/d
Calcitonin, serum or plasma		
Male	≤100 pg/mL	≤100 ng/L
Female	≤30 pg/mL.	≤30 ng/L
Calcium, serum	8.6–10.0 mg/dL (Slightly higher in children)	2.15–2.50 mmol/L (Slightly higher in children)
Calcium, ionized, serum	4.64–5.28 mg/dl	1.16–1.32 mmol/L
Calcium, urine		
Low calcium diet	50–150 mg/24 h	1.25–3.75 mmol/24 h
Usual diet; trough	100–300 mg/24 h	2.50–7.50 mmol/24 h
Carbamazepine, serum or plasma (Hep or EDTA); trough		
Therapeutic	4–12 µg/mL	17–51 µmol/L
Toxic	>15 µg/mL	>63 µmol/L
Carbon dioxide, total serum/plasma	22–28 mmol/L	22–28 mmol/L (Hep)
Carbon dioxide (PCO_2), blood arterial	Male 35–48 mmHg Female 32–45 mmHg	4.66–6.38 kPa 4.26–5.99 kPa
Carbon monoxide as carboxyhemoglobin (HbCO), whole blood (EDTA)		
Nonsmokers	0.5–1.5% total Hb	0.005–0.015 HbCO fraction
Smokers		
1–2 packs/d	4–5% total Hb	0.04–0.05 HbCO fraction
>2 packs/d	8–9% total Hb	0.08–0.09 HbCO fraction
Toxic	>20% total Hb	>0.20 HbCO fraction
Lethal	>50% total Hb	>0.50 HbCO fraction
Carotene, serum	10–85 µg/dL	0.19–1.58 µmol/L
Catecholamines, plasma (EDTA)		
Dopamine	<30 pg/mL	<196 pmol/L
Epinephrine	<140 pg/mL	<764 pmol/L
Norepinephrine	<1700 pg/mL	<10,047 pmol/L
Catecholamines, urine		
Dopamine	65–400 µg/24 h	425–2610 nmol/24 h
Epinephrine	0–20 µg/24 h	0–109 nmol/24
Norepinephrine	15–80 µg/24 h	89–473 nmol/24

Test	Conventional Units		SI Units
CEA, serum			
Nonsmokers	<5.0 ng/mL		<5.0 µg/L
*Cell counts, adult			
RBC Male	$4.7–6.1 \times 10^6/\mu L$		$4.7–6.1 \times 10^{12}/L$
Female	$4.2–5.4 \times 10^6/\mu L$		$4.2–5.4 \times 10^{12}/L$
WBC			
Total	$4.8–10.8 \times 10^3/\mu L$		$4.8–10.8 \times 10^6/L$
Differential	Percentage	Absolute	Absolute (SI)
Myelocytes	0	$0/\mu L$	0/L
Neutrophils			
Bands	3–5	$150–400/\mu L$	$150–400 \times 10^6/L$
Segmented	54–62	$3000–5800/\mu L$	$3000–5800 \times 10^6/L$
Lymphocytes	20.5–51.1	$1.2–3.4 \times 10^3/\mu L$	$1.2–3.4 \times 10^9/L$
Monocytes	1.7–9.3	$0.11–0.59 \times 10^3/\mu L$	$0.11–0.59 \times 10^9/L$
Granulocytes	42.2–75.2	$1.4–6.5 \times 10^3/\mu L$	$1.4–6.5 \times 10^9/L$
Eosinophils		$0.07 \times 10^3/\mu L$	$0.07 \times 10^9/L$
Basophils		$0–0.2 \times 10^3/\mu L$	$0–0.2 \times 10^9/L$
Platelets		$130–400 \times 10^3/\mu L$	$130–400 \times 10^9/L$
Cell counts, adult (continued)			
Reticulocytes	0.5–1.5% red cells		0.005–0.015 of RBC
	$24,000–84,000/\mu L$		$24–84 \times 10^9/L$
Cells, CSF	0–10 lymphocytes /mm³		0–10 lymphocytes /mm³
	0 RBC/ mm³		0 RBC/ mm³
Ceruloplasmin, serum	20–60 mg/dL		0.2–6.0 g/L
Chloramphenicol, serum or plasma (Hep or EDTA); trough			
Therapeutic	10–25 µg/mL		31–77 µmol/L
Toxic	>25 µg/mL		>77 µmol/L
Chloride			
Serum or plasma	98–107 mmol/L		98–107 mmol/L
Sweat			
Normal	5–35 mmol/L		5–35 mmol/L
Cystic fibrosis	60–200 mmol/L		60–200 mmol/L
Urine, 24 h (vary greatly with Cl intake)			
Infant	2–10 mmol/24 h		2–10 mmol/24 h
Child	15–40 nmol/24 h		15–40 mmol/24 h
Adult	110–250 mmol/24 h		110–250 mmol/24 h
CSF	118–332 mmol/L (20 mmol/L higher than serum)		118–332 mmol/L (20 mmol/L higher than serum)
Cholesterol, serum			
Adult desirable	<200 mg/dL		<5.2 mmol/L
borderline	200–239 mg/dL		5.2–6.2 mmol/L
high risk	≥240 mg/dL		≥6.2 mmol/L
*Cholinesterase, serum	4.9–11.9 U/mL		4.9–11.9 kU/L
Dibucaine inhibition	79–84%		0.79–0.84
Fluoride inhibition	58–64%		0.58–0.64
*Chorionic gonadotropin, intact			
Serum or plasma (EDTA)			
Male and nonpregnant female	<5.0 mIU/mL		<5.0 IU/L
Pregnant female	Varies with gestational age		
Urine, qualitative			
Male and nonpregnant female	Negative		Negative
Pregnant female	Positive		Positive

*Test values depend on laboratory methods.

Test	Conventional Units	SI Units
Clonazepam, serum or plasma (Hep or EDTA); trough		
Therapeutic	15–60 ng/mL	48–190 nmol/L
Toxic	>80 ng/mL	>254 nmol/L
Coagulation tests		
Antithrombin III (synthetic substrate)	80–120% of normal	0.8–1.2 of normal
Bleeding time (Duke)	0–6 min	0–6 min
Bleeding time (Ivy)	1–6 min	1–6 min
Bleeding time (template)	2.3–9.5 min	2.3–9.5 min
Clot retraction, qualitative	50–100% in 2 h	0.5–1.0/2 h
Coagulation time (Lee-White)	5–15 min (glass tubes)	5–15 min (glass tubes)
	19–60 min (siliconized tubes)	19–60 min (siliconized tubes)
Cold hemolysin test (Donath-Landsteiner)	No hemolysis	No hemolysis
Complement components		
Total hemolytic complement activity, plasma (EDTA)	75–160 U/mL	75–160 kU/L
Total complement decay rate (functional), plasma (EDTA)	10–20%	Fraction decay rate: 0.10–0.20
	Deficiency: >50%	>0.50
C1q, serum	14.9–22.1 mg/dL	149–221 mg/L
C1r, serum	2.5–10.0 mg/dL	25–100 mg/L
C1s(C1 esterase), serum	5.0–10.0 mg/dL	50–100 mg/L
C2, serum	1.6–3.6 mg/dL	16–36 mg/L
C3, serum	90–180 mg/dL	0.9–1.8 g/L
C4, serum	10–40 mg/dL	0.1–0.4 g/L
C5, serum	5.5–11.3 mg/dL	55–113 mg/L
C6, serum	17.9–23.9 mg/dL	179–239 mg/L
C7, serum	2.7–7.4 mg/dL	27–74 mg/L
C8, serum	4.9–10.6 mg/dL	49–106 mg/L
C9, serum	3.3–9.5 mg/dL	33–95 mg/L
Coombs test		
Direct	Negative	Negative
Indirect	Negative	Negative
Copper		
Serum		
Male	70–140 μg/dL	11–22 μmol/L
Female	80–155 μg/dL	13–24 μmol/L
Urine	3–35 μg/24 h	0.05–0.55 μmol/24 h
Corpuscular values of RBC (values are for adults; in children values vary with age)		
Mean corpuscular hemoglobin (MCH)	27–31 pg	0.42–0.48 fmol
Mean corpuscular hemoglobin concentration (MCHC)	33–37 g/dL	330–370 g/L
Mean corpuscular volume (MCV)	Male 80–94 μ^3	80–94 fL
	Female 81–99 μ^3	81–99 fL
Cortisol, serum		
Plasma (Hep, EDTA, Ox)		
8 AM	5–23 μg/dL	138–635 nmol/L
4 PM	3–16 μg/dL	83–441 nmol/L
10 PM	<50% of 8 AM value	<0.5 of 8 AM value
Free, urine	<50 μg/24 h	<138 mmol/24 h
†*Creatine kinase (CK), serum		
Male	15–105 U/L (30°C)	0.26–1.79 μkat/L (30°C)
Female	10–80 U/L (30°C)	0.17–1.36 μkat/L (30°C)

Note: Strenuous exercise or intramuscular injections may cause transient elevation of CK.

| *Creatine kinase MB isoenzyme, serum | 0–7 ng/mL | 0–7 μg/l |

Test	Conventional Units	SI Units
*Creatinine		
Serum or plasma, adult		
Male	0.7–1.3 mg/dL	62–115 μmol/L
Female	0.6–1.1 mg/dL	53–97 μmol/L
Urine		
Male	14–26 mg/kg body weight/24 h	124–230 μmol/kg body weight/24 h
Female	11–20 mg/kg body weight/24 h	97–177 μmol/kg body weight/24 h
*Creatinine clearance, serum or plasma and urine		
Male	94–140 mL/min/1.73 m^2	0.91–1.35 mL/s/m^2
Female	72–110 mL/min/1.73 m^2	0.69–1.06 mL/s/m^2
Cryoglobulins, serum	0	0
Cyanide		
Serum		
Nonsmokers	0.004 mg/L	0.15 μmol/L
Smokers	0.006 mg/L	0.23 μmol/L
Nitroprusside therapy	0.01–0.06 mg/L	0.38–2.30 μmol/L
Toxic	>0.1 mg/L	>3.84 μmol/L
Whole blood (Ox)		
Nonsmokers	0.016 mg/L	0.61 μmol/L
Smokers	0.041 mg/L	1.57 μmol/L
Nitroprusside therapy	0.05–0.5 mg/L	1.92–19.20 μmol/L
Toxic	>1 mg/L	>38.40 μmol/L
Cyclic AMP		
Plasma (EDTA)		
Male	4.6–8.6 ng/mL	14–26 nmol/L
Female	4.3–7.6 ng/mL	13–23 nmol/L
Urine, 24 h	0.3–3.6 mg/d or 0.29–2.1 mg/g creatinine	100–723 μmol/d or 100–723 μmol/mol creatinine
Cystine or cysteine, urine, qualitative	Negative	Negative
*C-Peptide, serum	0.78–1.89 ng/mL	0.26–0.62 nmol/L
C-Reactive protein, serum	<0.5 mg/dL	<5 mg/L
‡*Cyclosporine, whole blood		
Therapeutic, trough	100–200 ng/mL	83–166 nmol/L
Dehydroepiandrosterone (DHEA), serum		
Male	180–1250 ng/dL	6.2–43.3 nmol/L
Female	130–980 ng/dL	4.5–34.0 nmol/L
Dehydroepiandrosterone sulfate (DHEAS) serum or plasma (Hep, EDTA)		
Male	59–452 μg/dL	1.6–12.2 μmol/L
Female		
Premenopausal	12–379 μg/dL	0.8–10.2 μmol/L
Postmenopausal	30–260 μg/dL	0.8–7.1 μmol/L
Desipramine, serum or plasma (Hep or EDTA); trough (12 h after dose)		

*Test values depend on laboratory methods.

†Test values depend on patient's race.

‡Actual therapeutic range should be adjusted for individual patient.

Test	Conventional Units	SI Units
Therapeutic	75–300 ng/mL	281–1125 nmol/L
Toxic	>400 ng/mL	>1500 nmol/L
Diazepam, serum or plasma (Hep or EDTA); trough		
Therapeutic	100–1000 ng/mL	0.35–3.51 μmol/L
Toxic	>5000 ng/mL	>17.55 μmol/L
Digitoxin, serum or plasma (Hep or EDTA); 7.8 h after dose)		
Therapeutic	20–35 ng/mL	26–46 nmol/L
Toxic	>45 ng/mL	>59 nmol/L
Digoxin, serum or plasma (Hep or EDTA): ≥12 h after dose		
Therapeutic		
CHF	0.8–1.5 ng/mL	1.0–1.9 nmol/L
Arrhythmias	1.5–2.0 ng/mL	1.9–2.6 nmol/L
Toxic		
Adult	>2.5 ng/mL	>3.2 nmol/L
Child	>3.0 ng/mL	>3.8 nmol/L
Disopyramide, serum or plasma (Hep or EDTA); trough		
Therapeutic arrhythmias		
Atrial	2.8–3.2 μg/mL	8.3–9.4 μmol/L
Ventricular	3.3–7.5 μg/mL	9.7–22 μmol/L
Toxic	> 7 μg/mL	20.7 μmol/L
Doxepin, serum or plasma (Hep or EDTA); trough (≥12 h after dose)		
Therapeutic	150–250 ng/mL	537–895 nmol/L
Toxic	>500 ng/mL	>1790 nmol/L
*Estradiol, serum		
Adult		
Male	10–50 pg/mL	37–184 pmol/L
Female	Varies with menstrual cycle	
Ethanol (alcohol), whole blood (Ox) or serum		
Depression of CNS	>100 mg/dL	>21.7 mmol/L
Fatalities reported	>400 mg/dL	>86.8 mmol/L
Ethosuximide, serum or plasma (Hep or EDTA): trough		
Therapeutic	40–100 μg/mL	283–708 μmol/L
Toxic	>150 μg/mL	1062 μmol/L
Euglobin lysis	No lysis in 2 h	No lysis in 2 h
α-Fetoprotein (AFP), serum	<15 ng/mL	<15 μg/L
§Fat, fecal, F, 72 h		
Infant, breast-fed	<1 g/d	
Pediatrics (0–6 y)	<2 g/d	
Adults	<7 g/d	
Adult (fat-free diet)	<4 g/d	
‖Fatty acids, total, serum	190–240 mg/dL	7–15 mmol/L
Nonesterified, serum	8–25 mg/dL	0.28–0.89 mmol/L

‖"Fatty acids" include a mixture of different aliphatic acids of varying molecular weight; a mean molecular weight of 284 D has been assumed.

*Test values depend on laboratory methods.

§NOTE on fecal fat: Reference values vary from laboratory to laboratory, but are generally found within the range of 5–7 g/d. It should be noted that children, especially infants, cannot ingest the 100 g/d of fat that is suggested for the test. Therefore, a fat retention coefficient is determined by measuring the difference between ingested fat and fecal fat, and expressing that difference as a percentage. The figure, called the fat retention coefficient, is 95% or greater in healthy children and adults. A low value indicates steatorrhea. *http://www.labcorp.com/datasets/labcorp/html/chapter/mono/sc008000.htm*

Test	Conventional Units	SI Units
Ferritin, serum		
Male	20–150 ng/mL	20–250 μg/L
Female	10–120 ng/mL	10–120 μg/L
Ferritin values of <20 ng/mL (20 μg/L) have been reported to be generally associated with depleted iron stores.		
Fibrin degradation products	<10 μg/mL	<10 mg/L
‡Fibrinogen, plasma (NaCit)	200–400 mg/dL	2–4 g/L
Fluoride		
Plasma (Hep)	0.01–0.2 μg/mL	0.5–10.5 μmol/L
Urine	0.2–3.2 μg/mL	10.5–168 μmol/L
Urine, occupational exposure	<8 μg/mL	<421 μmol/L
*Folate, Serum	3–20 ng/mL	7–45 nmol/L
Erythrocytes	140–628 ng/mL RBC	317–1422 nmol/L RBC
Follicle-stimulating hormone (FSH), serum and plasma (Hep)		
Male	1.4–15.4 mIU/mL	1.4–15.4 IU/L
Female		
Follicular phase	1–10 mIU/mL	1–10 IU/L
Midcycle	6–17 mIU/mL	6–17 IU/L
Luteal phase	1–9 mIU/mL	1–9 IU/L
Postmenopausal	19–100 mIU/mL	19–100 IU/L
‡Free Thyroxine Index (FTI), serum	4.2–13	4.2–13
Gastrin, serum	<100 pg/mL	<100 ng/L
Gentamicin, serum or plasma (EDTA)		
Therapeutic		
Peak		
Less severe infection	5–8 μg/mL	10.4–16.7 μmol/L
Severe infection	8–10 μg/mL	16.7–20.9 μmol/L
Trough		
Less severe infection	<1μg/mL	<2.1 μmol/L
Moderate infection	<2 μg/mL	<4.2 μmol/L
Severe infection	<2–4 μg/mL	<4.2–8.4 μmol/L
Toxic		
Peak	>10–12 μg/mL	>21–25 μmol/L
Trough	>2–4 μg/mL	>4.2–8.4 μmol/L
Glucose (fasting)		
Blood	65–95 mg/dL	3.5–5.3 mmol/L
Plasma or serum	74–106 mg/dL	4.1–5.9 mmol/L
Glucose, 2 h postprandial, serum	<120 mg/dL	<6.7 mmol/L
Glucose, urine		
Quantitative	<500 mg/24 h	<2.8 mmol/24 h
Qualitative	Negative	Negative
Glucose, CSF	40–70 mg/dL	2.2–3.9 mmol/L
*Glucose-6-phosphate dehydrogenase (G-6-PD) in RBC, whole blood (ACD, EDTA, or Hep)	12.1 ± 2.1 U/g Hb (SD)	0.78 ± 0.13 mU/mol Hb
	351 ± 60.6 U/10^{12} RBC	0.35 ± 0.06 nU/RBC
	4.11 ± 0.71 U/mL RBC	4.11 ± 0.71 kU/L RBC
γ-Glutamyltransferase (GGT), serum		
Males	2–30 U/L (37°C)	0.03–0.51 μkat/L (37°C)
Females	1–24 U/L (37°C)	0.02–0.41 μkat/L (37°C)

‡Actual therapeutic range should be adjusted for individual patient.
*Test values depend on laboratory methods.

Test	Conventional Units	SI Units
Glutethimide, serum		
Therapeutic	2–6 µg/mL	9–28 µmol/L
Toxic	>5 µg/mL	>23 µmol/L
Glycated hemoglobin (Hemoglobin A1c), whole blood (EDTA)	4.2%–5.9%	0.042–0.059
Growth hormone, serum		
Male	<5 ng/mL	<5 µg/L
Female	<10 ng/mL	<10 µg/L
Haptoglobin, serum	30–200 mg/dL	0.3–2.0 g/L
†HDL-lipid panel		
Cholesterol, HDL	>40 mg/dL	
Cholesterol, LDL (calculated)		
optimal	<100 mg/dL	
near optimal	100–129 mg/dL	
borderline high	130–159 mg/dL	
high	>160 mg/dL	
Cholesterol, total		
0–1 y	50–120 mg/dL	
1–2 y	70–190 mg/dL	
2–16 y	120–220 mg/dL	
>16 y	0–199 mg/dL	
desirable	<200 mg/dL	
borderline	200–239 mg/dL	
high	>240 mg/dL	
¶Triglycerides		
desirable	<150 mg/dL	
borderline high	150–199 mg/dL	
high	>200 mg/dL	
Hematocrit		
Males	42–52%	0.42–0.52
Females	37–47%	0.37–0.47
Newborns	53–65%	0.53–0.65
Children (varies with age)	30–43%	0.30–0.43
Hemoglobin (Hb)		
Males	14.0–18.0 g/dL	2.17–2.79 mmol/L
Females	12.0–16.0 g/dL	1.86–2.48 mmol/L
Newborn	17.0–23.0 g/dL	2.64–3.57 mmol/L
Children (varies with age)	11.2–16.5 g/dL	1.74–2.56 mmol/L
Hemoglobin, fetal	≥1 y old: <2% of total Hb	≥1 y old: <0.02% of total Hb
Hemoglobin, plasma	<3 mg/dL	<0.47 µmol/L
Hemoglobin and myoglobin, urine, qualitative	Negative	Negative
Hemoglobin electrophoresis, whole blood (EDTA, Cit, or Hep)		
HbA	>95%	>0.95 Hb fraction
HbA$_2$	1.5–3.7%	0.015–0.37 Hb fraction
HbF	<2%	<0.02 Hb fraction
Homogentisic acid, urine, qualitative	Negative	Negative
β-Hydroxybutyric acids, serum, plasma	0.21–2.81 mg/dL	20–270 µmol/L

†Test values depend on patient's race.

¶NOTE: If the triglyceride value is >400 mg/dL, the LDL calculation is invalid.

http://webserver01.bjc.org/slch/pro/Professional.htm?http://webserver01.bjc.org/labtestguide/Lab%20Test%20Guidebook/slchlabsiteonline.htm

Test	Conventional Units	SI Units
17-Hydroxycorticosteroids		
Urine		
Males	3–10 mg/24 h	8.3–27.6 μmol/24 h (as cortisol)
Females	2–8 mg/24 h	5.5–22 μmol/24 h (as cortisol)
5-Hydroxylindoleacetic acid, urine		
Qualitative	Negative	Negative
Quantitative	2–7 mg/24 h	10.4–36.6 μmol/24 h
Imipramine, serum or plasma (Hep or EDTA); trough (≥12 h after dose)		
Therapeutic	150–250 ng/mL	536–893 nmol/L
Toxic	>500 ng/mL	>1785 nmol/L
Immunoglobulins, serum		
IgG	700–1600 mg/dL	7–16 g/L
IgA	70–400 mg/dL	0.7–4.0 g/L
IgM	40–230 mg/dL	0.4–2.3 g/L
IgD	0–8 mg/dL	0–80 mg/L
IgE	3–423 mg/dL	3–423 kIU/L
Immunoglobulin G (IgG), CSF	0.5–6.1 mg/dL	0.5–6.1 g/L
Insulin, plasma (fasting)	2–25 μU/mL	13–174 pmol/L
*Iron, serum		
Males	65–175 μg/dL	11.6–31.3 μmol/L
Females	50–170 μg/dL	9.0–30.4 μmol/L
Iron binding capacity, serum total (TBIC)	250–425 μg/dL	44.8–71.6 μmol/L
Iron saturation, serum		
Male	20–50%	0.2–0.5
Female	15–50%	0.15–0.5
17-Ketosteroids, urine		
Males	10–25 mg/24 h	38–87 μmol/24 h
Females	6–14 mg/24 h (decreases with age)	21–52 μmol/24 h (decreases with age)
L-Lactate		
Plasma (NaF)		
Venous	4.5–19.8 mg/dL	0.5–2.2 mmol/L
Arterial	4.5–14.4 mg/dL	0.5–1.6 mmol/L
Whole blood (Hep), at bed rest		
Venous	8.1–15.3 mg/dL	0.9–1.7 mmol/L
Arterial	<11.3 mg/dL	<1.3 mmol/L
Urine, 24 h	496–1982 mg/d	5.5–22 mmol/d
CSF	10–22 mg/dL	1.1–2.4 mmol/L
*Lactate dehydrogenase (LDH)		
Total (L0P), 37°C, serum		
Newborn	290–775 U/L	4.9–13.2 μkat/L
Neonate	545–2000 U/L	9.3–34 μkat/L
Infant	180–430 U/L	3.1–7.3 μkat/L
Child	110–295 U/L	1.9–5 μkat/L
Adult	100–190 U/L	1.7–3.2 μkat/L
>60 y	110–210 U/L	1.9–3.6 μkat/L
*Isoenzymes, serum by agarose gel electrophoresis		
Fraction 1	14–26% of total	0.14–0.26 fraction of total
Fraction 2	29–39% of total	0.29–0.39 fraction of total
Fraction 3	20–26% of total	0.20–0.26 fraction of total

*Test values depend on laboratory methods.

Test	Conventional Units	SI Units
Fraction 4	8–16% of total	0.08–0.16 fraction of total
Fraction 5	6–16% of total	0.06–0.16 fraction of total
*Lactate dehydrogenase, CSF	10% of serum value	0.10 fraction of serum value
LDL-cholesterol (LDL-C), serum or plasma (EDTA)		
Adult desirable	<130 mg/dL	<3.37 mmol/L
borderline	130–159 mg/dL	3.37–4.12 mmol/L
high risk	≥160 mg/dL	≥ 4.13 mmol/L
Lead		
Whole blood (Hep)	<25 μg/dL	<1.2 μmol/L
Urine, 24 h	<80 μg/d	<0.39μmol/d
Lecithin:sphingomyelin (L:S) ratio, amniotic fluid	2.0–5.0 indicates probable fetal lung maturity; >3.5 in diabetic patients	2.0–5.0 indicates probable fetal lung maturity; >3.5 in diabetic patients
Lidocaine, serum or plasma (Hep or EDTA); 45 min after bolus dose		
Therapeutic	1.5–6.0 μg/mL	6.4–26 μmol/L
Toxic		
CNS, cardiovascular depression	6–8 μg/mL	26–34.2 μmol/L
Seizures, obtundation, decreased cardiac output	>8 μg/mL	>34.2μmol/L
*Lipase, serum	23–300 U/L (37°C)	0.39–5.1 μkat/L (37°C)
Lithium, serum or plasma (Hep or EDTA); 12 h after last dose		
Therapeutic	0.6–1.2 mmol/L	0.6–1.2 mmol/L
Toxic	>2 mmol/L	>2 mmol/L
Lorazepam, serum or plasma (Hep or EDTA) therapeutic	50–240 ng/mL	156–746 nmol/L
*Luteinizing hormone (LH), serum or plasma (Hep)		
Male	1.24–7.8 mIU/mL	1.24–7.8 IU/L
Female		
Follicular phase	1.68–15.0 mIU/mL	1.68–15.0 IU/L
Midcycle peak	21.9–56.6 mIU/mL	21.9–56.6 IU/L
Luteal phase	0.61–16.3 mIU/mL	0.61–16.3 IU/L
Postmenopausal	14.2–52.5 mIU/mL	14.2–52.3 IU/L
Magnesium		
Serum	1.3–2.1 mEq/L	0.65–1.07 mmol/L
	1.6–2.6 mg/dL	16–26 mg/L
Urine	6.0–10.0 mEq/24 h	3.0–5.0 mmol/24 h
Mercury		
Whole blood (EDTA)	0.6–59 μg/L	<0.29 μmol/L
Urine, 24 h	<20 μg/d	<0.01 μmol/d
Toxic	>150 μg/d	>0.75 μmol/d
Metanephrines, total, urine	0.1–1.6 mg/24 h	0.5–8.1 μmol/24 h
Methemoglobin, (MetHb, hemoglobin), whole blood (EDTA, Hep or ACD)	0.06–0.24 g/dL or 0.78 ± 0.37% of total Hb (SD)	9.3–37.2 μmol/L or mass fraction of total Hb: 0.008 ± 0.0037 (SD)
Methotrexate, serum or plasma (Hep or EDTA)		
Therapeutic	Variable	Variable

*Test values depend on laboratory methods.

Test	Conventional Units	SI Units
Toxic		
1–2 wk after low-dose therapy	≥0.02 μmol/L	≥0.02 μmol/L
post-IV infusion 24 h	≥5 μmol/L	≥5 μmol/L
48 h	≥0.5 μmol/L	≥0.5 μmol/L
72 h	≥0.05 μmol/L	≥0.05 μmol/L
Myelin basic protein, CSF	<2.5 ng/mL	<2.5 μg/L
Myoglobin, serum	<85 ng/mL	<85 μg/L
Nortriptyline, serum or		
plasma (Hep or EDTA); trough		
(≥12 h after dose)		
Therapeutic	50–150 ng/mL	190–570 nmol/L
Toxic	>500 ng/mL	>1900 nmol/L
*5′-Nucleotidase, serum	2–17 U/L	0.034–0.29 μkat/L
N-Acetylprocainamide, serum or plasma		
(Hep or EDTA); trough		
Therapeutic	5–30 μg/mL	18–108 μmol/L
Toxic	>40 μg/mL	>144 μmol/L
Occult blood, feces, random	Negative (<2 mL blood/150 g)	Negative (<13.3 mL blood/kg
Qualitative, urine, random	stool/d	stool/d)
	Negative	Negative
Osmolality		
Serum	275–295 mOsm/kg serum water	275–295 mmol/kg serum water
Urine	50–1200 mOsm/kg water	50–1200 mmol/kg water
Ratio, urine:serum	1.0–3.0,	1.0–3.0,
	3.0–4.7 after 12 h fluid restriction	3.0–4.7 after 12 h fluid restriction
Osmotic fragility of RBC	Begins in 0.45–0.39% NaCl	Begins in 77–67 mmol/L NaCl
	Complete in 0.33–0.30% NaCl	Complete in 56–51 mmol/L NaCl
Oxazepam, serum or plasma	0.2–1.4 μg/mL	0.70–4.9 μmol/L
(Hep or EDTA), therapeutic		
Oxygen, blood		
Capacity	16–24 vol% (varies with	7.14–10.7 mmol/L (varies with
	hemoglobin)	hemoglobin)
Content		
Arterial	15–23 vol%	6.69–10.3 mmol/L
Venous	10–16 vol%	4.46–7.14 mmol/L
Saturation		
Arterial and capillary	95–98% of capacity	0.95–0.98 of capacity
Venous	60–85% of capacity	0.60–0.85 of capacity
Tension		
pO_2 arterial and capillary	83–108 mmHg	11.1–14.4 kPa
Venous	35–45 mmHg	4.6–6.0 kPa
P50, blood	25–29 mmHg (adjusted to	3.33–3.86 kPa
	pH 7.4)	
Partial thromboplastin time activated	<35 sec	<35 sec (APTT)
Pentobarbital, serum or plasma (Hep or		
EDTA); trough		
Therapeutic		
Hypnotic	1.5 μg/mL	4–22 μmol/L
Therapeutic coma	20–50 μg/mL	88–221 μmol/L
Toxic	>10 μg/mL	>44 μmol/L

*Test values depend on laboratory methods.

Test	Conventional Units	SI Units
pH		
Blood, arterial	7.35–7.45	7.35–7.45
Urine	4.6–8.0 (depends on diet)	Same
Phenacetin, plasma (EDTA)		
Therapeutic	1.30 µg/mL	6–167 µmol/L
Toxic	50–250 µg/mL	279–1395 µmol/L
Phenobarbital, serum or plasma (Hep or EDTA); trough		
Therapeutic	15–40 µg/mL	65–172 µmol/L
Toxic		
Slowness, ataxia, nystagmus	35–80 µg/mL	151–345 µmol/L
Coma with reflexes	65–117 µg/mL	280–504 µmol/L
Coma without reflexes	>100 µg/mL	>430 µmol/L
Phenosulfonphthalein excretion (PSP), urine	28–51% in 15 min 13–24% in 30 min 9–17% in 60 min 3–10% in 2 h (After injection of 1 mL PSP intravenously)	0.28–0.51 in 15 min 0.13–0.24 in 30 min 0.09–0.17 in 60 min 0.03–0.10 in 2 h (After injection of 1 mL PSP intravenously)
Phenylalanine, serum	0.8–1.8 mg/dL	48–109 µmol/L
Phenytoin, serum or plasma (Hep or EDTA); trough		
Therapeutic	10–20 µg/mL	40–79 µmol/L
Toxic	>20 µg/mL	>79 µmol/L
*Phosphatase, acid, prostatic, serum RIA	<3.0 ng/mL	<3.0 µg/L
*Phosphatase, alkaline, total, serum	38–126 U/L (37°C)	0.65–2.14 µkat/L
Phosphate, inorganic, serum		
Adults	2.7–4.5 mg/dL	0.87–1.45 mmol/L
Children	4.5–5.5 mg/dL	1.45–1.78 mmol/L
Phosphatidylglycerol (PG), amniotic fluid		
Fetal lung immaturity	Absent	Same
Fetal lung maturity	Present	Same
Phospholipids, serum	125–275 mg/dL	1.25–2.75 g/L
Phosphorus, urine	0.4–1.3 g/24 h	12.9–42 mmol/24 h
Porphobilinogen, urine		
Qualitative	Negative	Negative
Quantitative	<2.0 mg/24 h	<9 µmol/24 h
Porphyrins, urine		
Coproporphyrin	34–230 µg/24 h	52–351 nmol/ 24 h
Uroporphyrin	27–52 µg/24 h	32–63 nmol/ 24 h
Potassium, plasma (Hep)		
Males	3.5–4.5 mmol/L	3.5–4.5 mmol/L
Females	3.4–4.4 mmol/L	3.4–4.4 mmol/L
Potassium		
Serum		
Premature		
Cord	5.0–10.2 mmol/L	5.0–10.2 mmol/L
48 h	3.0–6.0 mmol/L	3.0–6.0 mmol/L
Newborn cord	5.6–12.0 mmol/L	5.6–12.0 mmol/L

*Test values depend on laboratory methods.

Test	Conventional Units	SI Units
Newborn	3.7–5.9 mmol/L	3.7–5.9 mmol/L
Infant	4.1–5.3 mmol/L	4.1–5.3 mmol/L
Child	3.4–4.7 mmol/L	3.4–4.7 mmol/L
Adult	3.5–5.1 mmol/L	3.5–5.1 mmol/L
Urine, 24 h	25–125 mmol/d; varies with diet 70% of plasma level or	25–125 mmol/d; varies with diet 0.70 of plasma level;
CSF	2.5–3.2 mmol/L; rises with plasma hyperosmolality	rises with plasma hyperosmolality
Prealbumin (transthyretin), serum	10–40 mg/dL	100–400 mg/L
Primidone, serum or plasma (Hep or EDTA); trough		
Therapeutic	5–12 µg/mL	23–55 µmol/L
Toxic	>15 µg/mL	>69 µmol/L
Procainamide, serum or plasma (Hep or EDTA); trough		
Therapeutic	4–10 µg/mL	17–42 µmol/L
Toxic (also consider effect of metabolite (NAPA)	>10–12 µg/mL	>42–51 µmol/L
*Progesterone, serum		
Adult		
Male	13–97 ng/dL	0.4–3.1 nmol/L
Female		
Follicular phase	15–70 ng/dL	0.5–2.2 nmol/L
Luteal phase	200–2500 ng/dL	6.4–79.5 nmol/L
Pregnancy	Varies with gestational week	
*Prolactin, serum		
Males	2.5–15.0 ng/mL	2.5–15.0 µg/L
Females	2.5–19.0 ng/mL	2.5–19.0 µg/L
Propoxyphene, plasma (EDTA)		
Therapeutic	0.1–0.4 µg/mL	0.3–1.2 µmol/L
Toxic	>0.5 µg/mL	>1.5 µmol/L
Propranolol, serum or plasma (Hep or EDTA); trough		
Therapeutic	50–100 ng/mL	193–386 nmol/L
*Prostate-specific antigen (PSA), serum		
Male	<4.0 ng/mL	<4.0 µg/L
*Protein, serum		
Total	6.4–8.3 g/dL	64–83 g/L
Albumin	3.9–5.1 g/dL	39–51 g/L
Globulin		
α_1	0.2–0.4 g/dL	2–4 g/L
α_2	0.4–0.8 g/dL	4–8 g/L
β	0.5–1.0 g/dL	5–10 g/L
γ	0.6–1.3 g/dL	6–13 g/L

*Test values depend on laboratory methods.

NOTE: INR=[(Patient PT)/(Normal PT)] *ISI where ISI is the international sensitivity index, a value provided by the reagent manufacturer. NOTE: …target therapeutic range (international normalized ratio) of 2.0–3.0. http://pediatrics.aappublications.org/cgi/content/full/112/5/e386

NOTE: The American College of Chest Physicians has recommended a therapeutic INR range for adults of 2.0–3.0, except in patients with mechanical cardiac valves who should have an INR of 2.5–3.5. 1 …target INR range of 2.6–3.8 for children with heart disease and a slightly lower range of 2.1–3.3 for treating children with established venous thrombosis. Clinicians at Toronto's Hospital for Sick Children used an INR range of 2.0–3.0 initially but later found that a lower target of 1.3–1.8 was as effective and resulted in no bleeding complications. http://www.healthsystem.virginia.edu/internet/pediatrics/pharma-news/jan95.pdf

NOTE: The recommended therapeutic target for the treatment and prevention of venous thromboembolisms and pulmonary embolisms is an INR of 2.5 with a range between 2.0–3.0, and children with mechanical prosthetic heart valves have a recommended therapeutic INR range of 3.0 INR range between 2.5–3.5. Evaluate at that time. http://www.warfarinfo.com/pediatrics.htm

#http://www.labcorp.com/datasets/labcorp/html/chapter/mono/he005000.htm; http://www.utmb.edu/lsg/LabSurvivalGuide/hem/Sedimentation_Rate.htm

Test	Conventional Units	SI Units
Urine		
Qualitative	Negative	Negative
Quantitative	50–80 mg/24 h (at rest)	50–80 mg/24 h (at rest)
CSF, total	8–32 mg/dL	80–320 mg/dL
Prothrombin, consumption	>20 sec	>20 sec
Prothrombin time-international normalized ratio (see NOTES below)		
INR: birth–6 mo	1.0–1.6 INR: 6 mo–adult	0.9–1.2
Protoporphyrin, total, WB	<60 μg/dL	<600 μg/L
Pyruvate, blood	0.3–0.9 mg/dL	34–103 μmol/L
Quinidine, serum or plasma (Hep or EDTA); trough		
Therapeutic	2–5 μg/mL	6–15 μmol/L
Toxic	>6 μg/mL	>18 μmol/L
Salicylates, serum or plasma (Hep or EDTA); trough		
Therapeutic	150–300 μg/mL	1.09–2.17 mmol/L
Toxic	>500 μg/mL	>3.62 mmol/L
#Sedimentation rate, erythrocyte (ESR, sed rate)		
Westergren		
Male: 0–50 y	0–15 mm/h	
Male: 50 y	0–20 mm/h	
Female: 0–50 y	0–20 mm/h	
Female: 50 y	0–30 mm/h	
Wintrobe		
Males	<10 mm/h	
Females	<20 mm/h	
Critical value	>75 mm/h	
Sodium		
Serum or plasma (Hep)		
Premature		
Cord	116–140 mmol/L	116–140 mmol/L
48 h	128–148 mmol/L	128–148 mmol/L
Newborn, cord	126–166 mmol/L	126–166 mmol/L
Newborn	133–146 mmol/L	133–146 mmol/L
Infant	139–146 mmol/L	139–146 mmol/L
Child	138–145 mmol/L	138–145 mmol/L
Adult	136–145 mmol/L	136–145 mmol/L
Urine, 24 h	40–220 mEq/d (diet dependent)	40–220 mmol/d (diet dependent)
Sweat		
Normal	10–40 mmol/L	10–40 mmol/L
Cystic fibrosis	70–190 mmol/L	70–190 mmol/L
Specific gravity, urine	1.002–1.030	1.002–1.030
*Testosterone, serum		
Male	280–1100 ng/dL	0.52–38.17 nmol/L
Female	15–70 ng/dL	0.52–2.43 nmol/L
Pregnancy	3–4 × normal	3–4 × normal
Postmenopausal	8–35 ng/dL	0.28–1.22 nmol/L

*Test values depend on laboratory methods.

Test	Conventional Units	SI Units
Theophylline, serum or plasma (Hep or EDTA)		
Therapeutic		
Bronchodilator	8–20 µg/mL	44–111 µmol/L
Prem. apnea	6–13 µg/mL	33–72 µmol/L
Toxic	>20 µg/mL	>110 µmol/L
Thiocyanate, serum or plasma (EDTA)		
Nonsmoker	1–4 µg/mL	17–69 µmol/L
Smoker	3–12 µg/mL	52–206 µmol/L
Therapeutic after nitroprusside infusion	6–29 µg/mL	103–499 µmol/L
Urine		
Nonsmoker	1–4 mg/d	17–69 µmol/d
Smoker	7–17mg/d	120–292 µmol/d
Thiopental, serum or plasma (Hep or EDTA); trough		
Hypnotic	1.0–5-0 µg/mL	4.1–20.7 µmol/L
Coma	30–100 µg/mL	124–413 µmol/L
Anesthesia	7–130 µg/mL	29–536 µmol/L
Toxic concentration	>10 µg/mL	>41 µmol/L
*Thyroid-stimulating hormone (TSH), serum	0.4–4.2 µU/mL	0.4–4.2 mU/L
Thyroxine (T_4) serum	5–12 µg/dL (varies with age, higher inchildren and pregnant women)	65–155 nmol/L (varies with age, higher in children and pregnant women)
*Thyroxine, free, serum	0.8–2.7 ng/dL	10.3–35 pmol/L
Thyroxine binding globulin (TBG), serum	1.2–3.0 mg/dL	12–30 mg/L
Tobramycin, serum or plasma (Hep or EDTA)		
Therapeutic		
Peak		
Less severe infection	5–8 µg/mL	11–17 µmol/L
Severe infection	8–10 µg/mL	17–21 µmol/L
Trough		
Less severe infection	<1 µg/mL	<2 µmol/L
Moderate infection	<2 µg/mL	<4 µmol/L
Severe infection	<2–4 µg/mL	<4–9 µmol/L
Toxic		
Peak	>10–12 µg/mL	>21–26 µmol/L
Trough	>2–4 µg/mL	>4–9 µmol/L
Transferrin, serum		
Newborn	130–275 mg/dL	1.30–2.75 g/L
Adult	212–360 mg/dL	2.12–3.60 g/L
>60 yr	190–375 mg/dL	1.9–3.75 g/L
Triglycerides, serum, fasting		
Desirable	<250 mg/dL	<2.83 mmol/L
Borderline high	250–500 mg/dL	2.83–5.67 mmol/L
Hypertriglyceridemia	>500 mg/dL	>5.65 mmol/L
*Triiodothyronine, total (T_3) serum	100–200 ng/dL	1.54–3.8 nmol/L
*Troponin-I, cardiac, serum	undetectable	undetectable
Troponin-T, cardiac, serum	undetectable	undetectable
Urea nitrogen, serum	6–20 mg/dL	2.1–7.1 mmol urea/L

*Test values depend on laboratory methods.

Test	Conventional Units	SI Units
Urea nitrogen/creatinine ratio, serum	12:1 to 20:1	48–80 urea/creatinine mole ratio
*Uric acid		
Serum, enzymatic		
Male	4.5–8.0 mg/dL	0.27–0.47 mmol/L
Female	2.5–6.2 mg/dL	0.15–0.37 mmol/L
Child	2.0–5.5 mg/dL	0.12–0.32 mmol/L
Urine	250–750 mg/24 h (with normal diet)	1.48–4.43 mmol/24 h (with normal diet)
Urobilinogen, urine	0.1–0.8 Ehrlich unit/2 h 0.5–4.0 EU/d	0.1–0.8 EU/2 h 0.5–4.0 EU/d
Valproic acid, serum or plasma (Hep or EDTA); trough		
Therapeutic	50–100 µg/mL	347–693 µmol/L
Toxic	>100 µg/mL	>693 µmol/L
Vancomycin, serum or plasma (Hep or EDTA)		
Therapeutic		
Peak	20–40 µg/mL	14–28 µmol/L
Trough	5–10 µg/mL	3–7 µmol/L
Toxic	>80–100 µg/mL	>55–69 µmol/L
Vanillylmandelic acid (VMA), urine (4-hydroxy-3-methoxymandelic acid)	1.4–6.5 mg/24h	7–33 µmol/d
Viscosity, serum	1.00–1.24 cP	1.00–1.24 cP
Vitamin A, serum	30–80 µg/dL	1.05–2.8 µmol/L
Vitamin B12, serum	110–800 pg/mL	81–590 pmol/L
Vitamin E, serum		
Normal	5–18 µg/mL	12–42 µmol/L
Therapeutic	30–50 µg/mL	69.6–116 µmol/L
Zinc, serum	70–120 µg/dL	10.7–18.4 µmol/L

*Test values depend on laboratory methods.

Medical Prefixes, Suffixes, and Combining Forms: The Building Blocks of Medical Language

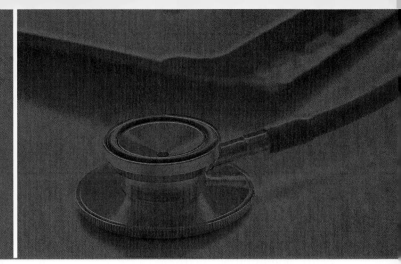

a- not, without, -less

ab-, abs- from, away from, off

acanth(o)- thorn

acou- hearing

acr(o)- extremity

acu- hearing; needle

ad- increase, adherence, motion toward

-ad toward, in the direction of; -ward

aden(o)- gland

adip(o)- fat

-agog, -agogue promoter, stimulator

aidoio- genitals

-al pertaining to

alb(o)- white

alge(si)-, algio-, algo- pain

allo- other, different

ambi- around, on (both) sides, on all sides, both

ambly(o)- dull

amyl(o)- starch, polysaccharide

an- not, without, -less

ana- up, toward, apart

andr(o)- male

angi(o)- vessel

ankylo- crooked

ante- before

anthraco- coal, carbon

anthropo- human (either gender)

anti- against, opposing; curative; antibody

apo- separated from, derived from

aque(o)- water

-ar pertaining to

-arche beginning

arteri(o)- artery

arthr(o)- joint, articulation

-ary pertaining to

-ase an enzyme

-ate a salt or ester of an "-ic" acid

athero- pasty, fatty

atto- one-quintillionth (10^{-18})

audi(o)- hearing

aur(i)-, auro- ear

aut(o)- self, same

bacteri(o)- bacteria

balan(o)- glans penis

bi- twice, double

bio- life

blasto- budding by cells or tissue

blephar(o)- eyelid

brachi(o)- arm

brachy- short

bronch- bronchus

brady- slow

bronch(i)-, bronch(i)o- bronchus

carcin(o)- cancer

cardi(o)- heart; esophageal opening of stomach

carpo- wrist

cata- down

caud(o)- tail, lower part of body

-cele hernia, swelling

celio- abdomen

-centesis surgical puncture

centi- one-hundredth (10^{-2})

cephal(o)- the head

cervic(o)- neck; uterine cervix

cheil(o)- lip

cheir(o)- hand

chem(o)- chemistry; drug

chir(o)- hand

chlor(o)- green; chlorine

chol(e)- bile

chondrio-, chondr(o)- cartilage; granular; gritty

chrom-, chromat-, chromo- color

chron(o)- time

-cidal, -cide killing, destroying

cis- on this side, on the near side

-clast breaker

-clysis washing

co- with, together, in association, complete

col- with, together, in association, complete

colp(o)- vagina

com-, con- with, together, in association, complete

conio- dust

cor- with, together, in association, complete

coreo- pupil

cost(o)- rib

crani(o)- cranium

-crine secretion

cry(o)- cold

crypt(o)- hidden

culdo- cul-de-sac

cyan(o)- blue; cyanide

cycl- circle, cycle; ciliary body

cyst(i)-, cysto- bladder; cyst; cystic duct

cyt-, -cyte, cyto- cell

dacry(o)- tears

dactyl(o)- finger, toe

de- away from; cessation

deca- ten

deci- one-tenth (10^{-1})

deka- ten

dent(i)- tooth

derm-, derma-, dermat(o)-, dermo- skin

-desis binding

dextr(o)- right, toward or on the right side

di- separation, taking apart, reversal, not, un-

dif- separation, taking apart, reversal, not, un-

dipso- thirst

dir-, dis- separation, taking apart, reversal, not, un-

duo- two

duodeno- duodenum

-dynia pain

dynamo- force, energy

dys- bad, difficult, wrong

ect- outer, on the outside

-ectasia, -ectasis dilation, stretching

ecto- outer, on the outside

-ectomy excision

-emphraxis obstruction

encephal(o)- brain

end(o)- within, inner

enter(o)- intestine

ent(o)- inner, within

ep-, epi- upon, following, subsequent to

ergo- work

erythr(o)- red, redness

eso- inward

esthesio- sensation, perception

eu- good, well

ex- out of, from, away from

exo- exterior, external, outward

extra- without, outside of

ferri- ferric ion (Fe^{3+})

ferro- metallic iron; ferrous ion (Fe^{2+})

fibr(o)- fiber

-form in the form or shape of

galact(o)- milk

gastr(o)- stomach; belly

gen-, -gen producing, coming to be; precursor

giga- one billion (10^9)

gingiv(o)- gums

gloss(o)- tongue

gluco- glucose

glyco- sugars

gnath(o)- jaw

gon- seed, semen

gonio- angle

gono- seed, semen

-gram writing, recording

granul(o)- granular, granule

-graph recording instrument

gyn(e)-, gyneco-, gyno- woman

hecto- one hundred (10^2)

hem(a)-, hemat(o)- blood

hemi- one-half

hemo- blood

hepat-, hepatico-, hepato- liver

hept(a)- seven

hidr(o)- sweat

hist-, histio-, histo- tissue

homeo- same, constant

hydr(o)- water; hydrogen

hyper- above normal, excessive

hypo- below normal, deficient

hyster(o)- uterus; hysteria; late, following

-ia condition

-iasis condition, infestation, infection

-ic pertaining to

-ics organized knowledge, practice, treatment

ileo- ileum

ilio- ilium

in- in; not

-in chemical suffix

-ine chemical suffix

infra- below

inguino- groin

inter- between, among

intra-, intro- within

irid(o)- iris

ischi(o)- ischium

-ism condition, disease; practice, doctrine

-ismus spasm; contraction

iso- equal, like; isomer; sameness

-ite of the nature of, resembling

-ites -y, -like

-itides plural of -itis

-itis inflammation

kal(i)- potassium

kary(o)- nucleus

kerat(o)- cornea, cornified epithelium

kilo- one thousand (10^3)

kin(e)-, kinesi(o)-, kineso-, kino- movement

labio- lip

lacrim(o)- tears

lact(i)-, lacto- milk

laparo- abdomen, abdominal wall

laryng(o)- larynx

lateri-, latero- lateral, to one side, side

-lepsis, -lepsy seizure

lepto- light, slender, thin, frail

leuk(o)- white

lien(o)- spleen

linguo- tongue

lip(o)- fat, lipid

lith(o)- stone, calculus, calcification

-log speech, words

log(o)- speech, words

-logy study of; collecting

lymph(o)- lymph; lymphocyte

lys(o)-, -lysis, -lytic dissolution, disintegration; release

macr(o)- large; long

mal- bad, deficient

-malacia softening

mamm-, mamm(a)-, mammo- breast

mast(o)- breast

meg- large, oversize

mega- large, oversize; one million (10^6)

megal(o)- large

-megaly enlargement

melan(o)- black

men- menstruation

mening(o)- meninges

meno- menstruation

ment(o)- chin

-mer member of a series

mes(o)- middle, mean, intermediate; attaching membrane

meta- after, behind; joint action, sharing

-meter measurement, measuring device

metr(o)- uterus

micr- small, microscopic

micro- small, microscopic; one-millionth (10^{-6})

milli- one-thousandth (10^{-3})

mon(o)- single

morph(o)- form, shape, structure

my(o)- muscle

myel(o)- bone marrow; spinal cord

myring(o)- tympanic membrane

myx(o)- mucus

nano- dwarf; one-billionth (10^{-9})

nas(o)- nose

natr(i)- sodium

necr(o)- death, necrosis

neo- new

nephr(o)- kidney

neur(i)-, neuro- nerve, nervous system

norm(o)- normal

octo- eight

oculo- eye

odont(o)- tooth

odyn(o)-, -odynia pain

-oid resemblance to

olig(o)- few, little

-oma tumor, neoplasm

-omata plural of -oma

oncho-, onco- tumor, bulk, volume

-one ketone (-CO- group)

onych(o)-, -onychia fingernail, toenail

oo- ovum, oocyte, ovary

oophor(o)- ovary

ophthalm(o)- eye

-opia, -opsia, -opsis vision

or- mouth

orchi-, orchid(o)-, orchio- testis

ori-, oro- mouth

-ose sugar

-oses plural of -osis

-osis process, condition, state

osseo- bony

ossi- bone

ost(e)-, osteo- bone

ovari(o)- ovary

ov(i)-, ovo- ovum, oocyte

ox(a)-, oxo- oxygen

oxy- sharp, acid; acute, shrill, quick; oxygen

pachy- thick

pan-, pant(o)- all, entire

para- beside, near; similar; subordinate; abnormal

pari- equal

path(o)- disease, abnormality

-pathy disease, abnormality

ped(i)-, pedo- child; foot

-penia deficiency

penta- five

per- through, thoroughly, intensely

peri- around, about

-pexy fixation, usually surgical

phaco- lens

-phage, -phagia, phago-, -phagy eating, devouring

phako- lens

phanero- visible, evident

pharmaco- drug, medicine

pharyng(o)- pharynx

phil- attraction; chemical affinity

-philia attraction; chemical affinity

philo- attraction; chemical affinity

phleb(o)- vein

-phobe, -phobia fear; chemical repulsion

phon(o)- sound, speech

phor(o)- carrying, bearing

phos-, phot(o)- light

phren(i)- diaphragm; mind; phrenic

-phrenia mind

phrenico-, phreno- diaphragm; mind; phrenic

-phylaxis protection

phyll(o)- leaf

physi(o)- physical; natural

physo- swelling, inflation; air, gas

phyt(o)- plants

pico- one-trillionth (10^{-12})

plan(i)-, plano- flat

-plasia formation

plasm(a)-, plasmat(o)-, plasmo- plasma

platy- wide, flat

-plegia paralysis

pleo- more

plesio- near, similar

pleur(a)-, pleuro- rib, side, pleura

pluri- several, more

-pnea breath, respiration

pneo- breath, respiration

pneum(a)-, pneumat(o)- air, gas; lung; breathing

pod(o)- foot, foot-shaped

-poiesis, -poietic production

poikilo- irregular, variable

polio- gray

poly- many, multiple; polymer

post- after, behind, posterior

pre- anterior, before

presby- old

pro- before, forward; precursor

proct(o)- anus, rectum

prot(o)- first

pseud(o)- false

psych(e)-, psycho- mind

-ptosis sagging, falling

pyel(o)- (renal) pelvis

pykn(o)- dense, compact

pyo- suppuration, pus

pyreto- fever

pyro- fire, heat, fever

quadr(i)- four

rachi(o)- spinal column

radio- radiation, x-ray; radius

re- again, back, backward

rect(i)- straight

rect(o)- rectum

ren(o)- kidney

retro- backward, behind

rhin(o)- nose

-rrhagia discharge, bleeding

-rrhaphy surgical suturing

-rrhea flow

-rrhexis rupture

salping(o)- tube

sarco- flesh, muscle

schisto-, schiz(o)- split, cleft, division

scler(o)- hardness, sclerosis; ocular sclera

scolio- crooked

-scope instrument for viewing

-scopy viewing

scot(o)- shadow, darkness

semi- one-half; partly

sept- seven; septum; sepsis, infection

septi- seven

septo- seven; septum; sepsis, infection

sial(o)- saliva, salivary gland

sider(o)- iron

sigmoid(o)- S-shaped; sigmoid colon

sin-, sin(o)-, sinu- sinus

sito- food, grain

somat-, somato-, somatico- body, bodily

somno- sleep

son(o)- sound; ultrasound

spasmo- spasm

sperm(a), spermat(o), spermo- semen, sperm

sphygmo- pulse

spir(o)- breathing

splanchn(i)-, splanchno- viscera

splen(o)- spleen

staphyl(o)- grape, bunch of grapes; staphylococci

-stasis stopping

-stat arresting change or movement

steno- narrowness, constriction

stereo- solid

stheno- strength, force, power

stom(a)-, stomat(o)- mouth

sub- beneath, less than normal, inferior

super- above, in excess, superior

supra- above

sy-, syl-, sym-, syn-, sys- together

tachy- rapid

tel(e)- distant

ten-, tendin-, teno-, tenont(o)- tendon

tera- one quadrillion (10^{15})

tetra- four

thel(o)- nipple

therm(o)- heat

thora-, thorac(i)-, thoracico, thoraco- chest, thorax

thromb(o)- blood clot

thyre(o)-, thyr(o)- thyroid gland

toco-, toko- childbirth

-tome cutting instrument; segment, section

-tomy cutting operation

tono- tone, tension, pressure

top(o)- place, topical

tox(i)-, toxico-, toxo- toxin, poison

trache(o)- trachea

trans- across, through, beyond

tri- three

trich(i)- hair

-trichia, tricho- hair

tris- three

-trophic, tropho-, -trophy food, nutrition

-tropia, -tropic, -tropy turning, tendency, affinity

ultra- beyond

uni- one, single

uri- uric acid

-uria urine, urination

uric(o)- uric acid

uro- urine; urinary tract

vas- duct; blood vessel

vasculo- blood vessel

vaso- duct, blood vessel

vesic(o)- urinary bladder, vesicle

xanth(o)- yellow

xero- dry

zo(o)- animal; life

zym(o)- fermentation, enzyme

Common Medical Abbreviations and Acronyms

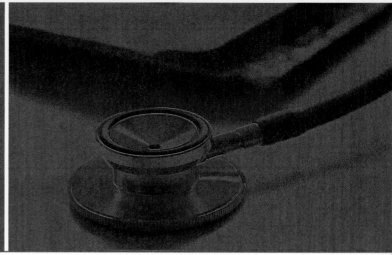

ā	before
A2 or A.	aortic valve closure (heart sound)
AAA	abdominal aortic aneurysm
AAL	anterior axillary line
AB	abortion
ab	antibody
abd	abdomen; abduction
ABG	arterial blood gas
ax.	before meals (*ante* cibum)
ACE	angiotensin-converting enzyme
ACh	acetylcholine (neurotransmitter)
ACTH	adrenocorticotropic hormone
AD	right ear (*auris* dextra); Alzheimer disease
ADD	attention deficit disorder
add	adduction
ADH	antidiuretic hormone; vasopressin
ADHD	attention-deficit hyperactivity disorder
ADL	activities of daily living
ADT	admission, discharge, transfer
ad fib	as desired
AF	atrial fibrillation
AFB	acid-fast bacillus (bacilli)
AFO	ankle foot orthosis (device for stabilization)
AFP	alpha-fetoprotein

AHF	antihemophilic factor (coagulation factor XIII)
AI	aortic insufficiency; artificial insemination
AIDS	acquired immunodeficiency syndrome
AIHA	autoimmune hemolytic anemia
AKA	above-knee amputation
alb	albumin (protein)
alk phos	alkaline phosphatase (elevated in liver disease)
ALL	acute lymphocytic leukemia
ALS	arnyotrophic lateral sclerosis (Lou Gehrig disease)
ALT	alanine aminotransferase (elevated in liver and heart disease)
Amb	ambulate, ambulatory (walking)
AML	acute myelocytic (myelogenous) leukemia
ANC	absolute neutrophil count
AODL	activities of daily living
AP, A.P., A/P	anteroposterior
A&P	auscultation and percussion
aq.	water *(aqua)*; aqueous
ARDS	adult respiratory distress syndrome
ARF	acute renal failure
ARMD	age related macular degeneration
AROM	active range of motion

AS	left ear *(auris sinistra)*; aortic stenosis
ASA	acetylsalicylic acid (aspirin)
ASD	atrial septal defect
ASH	asymmetrical septal hypertrophy
ASHD	arteriosclerotic heart disease
AST	aspartate aminotransferase (elevated in liver and heart disease)
AU	both ears *(auris uterque)*
Au	gold
AV	arteriovenous; atrioventricular
AVM	arteriovenous malformation
AVR	aortic valve replacement
A&W	alive and well
Ba	barium
bands	banded neutrophils
baso	basophils
BBB	bundle branch block
BC	bone conduction
B cells	lymphocytes produced in the bone marrow
BE	barium enema
bid, b.i.d.	twice a day (bis *in die*)
BKA	below knee amputation
BM	bowel movement
BMR	basal metabolic rate
BMT	bone marrow transplant
BP	blood pressure
BPH	benign prostatic hyperplasia (hypertrophy
BRBPR	bright red blood per rectum; hernatochezia
BSE	breast self examination
BSO	bilateral salpingo-oophorectomy
BSP	bromsulphalein (dye used in liver function test)
BT	bleeding time
BUN	blood urea nitrogen
Bx, bx	biopsy
C	Celsius or centigrade; calorie
ĉ	with (cum)
C1, C2	first, second cervical vertebra
CA	chronological age; cardiac arrest
Ca	calcium; cancer
CABG	coronary artery bypass graft

CAD	coronary artery disease
CAO	chronic airway obstruction
CAPD	continuous ambulatory peritoneal dialysis
cap	capsule
Cath	catheter; catheterization
CAT scan	computed (axial) tomography
CBC, c.b.c.	complete blood count
cc	chief complaint
cc	cubic centimeter (unit of volume; 1/1000 liter)
CCU	coronary care unit
CDH	congenital dislocated hip
CEA	carcinoembryonic antigen
cf.	compare
CF	cystic fibrosis
cGy	centigray (one hundredth of a gray; a rad)
CHD	coronary heart disease
chemo	chemotherapy
CHF	congestive heart failure
chol	cholesterol
chr	chronic
μci	microcurie
CIN	cervical intraepithelial neoplasia
cis	carcinoma *in situ*
CK	creatine kinase
Cl	chlorine
CLD	chronic liver disease
CLL	chronic lymphocytic leukemia
cm	centimeter (1/100 meter)
CMG	cystometrograrn
CML	chronic myelogenous leukemia
CMV	cytornegalovirus
CNS	central nervous system
CO	cobalt
C/O	complains of
CO2	carbon dioxide
COPD	chronic obstructive pulmonary disease
CP	cerebral palsy; chest pain
CPA	costophrenic angle
CPD	cephalopelvic disproportion
CPK	creatine phosphokinase
CPR	cardiopulmonary resuscitation

CR	complete response	**DSA**	digital subtraction angiography
CRF	chronic renal failure	**DSM**	Diagnostic and Statistical Manual of Mental Disorders
CS	cesarean section	**DT**	delirium tremens (caused by alcohol withdrawal)
C&S	culture and sensitivity		
C-section	cesarean section	**DTR**	deep tendon reflexes
CSF	cerebrospinal fluid	**DUB**	dysfunctional uterine bleeding
C-spine	cervical spine films	**DVT**	deep venous thrombosis
ct.	count	**Dx**	diagnosis
CTA	clear to auscultation		
CTS	carpal tunnel syndrome	**EBV**	Epstein-Barr virus
CT scan	computed tomography	**ECC**	endocervical curettage; extracorporeal circulation
CVA	cerebrovascular accident; costovertebral angle	**ECF**	extended-care facility
CVP	central venous pressure	**ECG**	electrocardiogram
CVS	cardiovascular system; chorionic villus sampling	**ECHO**	echocardiography
		ECMO	extracorporeal membrane oxygenation
c/w	compare with; consistent with	**ECT**	electroconvulsive therapy
CX (CXR)	chest x-ray	**ED**	emergency department
Cx	cervix	**EDC**	estimated date of confinement
cysto	cystoscopy	**EEG**	electroencephalogram
		EENT	eyes, ears, nose & throat
D/C	discontinue; discharge	**EGD**	esophagogastroduodenoscopy
D&C	dilatation (dilation) and curettage	**EKG**	electrocardiogram
DCIS	ductal carcinoma in situ	**ELISA**	enzyme-linked immunosorbent assay (AIDS Test)
DD	discharge diagnosis		
Decub.	decubitus (lying down)	**EM**	electron microscope
Derm	dermatology	**EMB**	endometrial biopsy
DES	diethylstilbestrol; diffuse esophageal spasm	**EMG**	electromyograrn
		ENT	ear, nose, and throat
DI	diabetes insipidus; diagnostic imaging	**EOM**	extraocular movement; extraocular muscles
DIC	disseminated intravascular coagulation	**eos.**	eosinophil (type of white blood cell)
		Epo	erythropoietin
diff.	differential count (white blood cells)	**ER**	emergency room; estrogen receptor
DIG	digoxin; digitalis	**ERCP**	endoscopic retrograde cholangiopancreatography
dL, d1	deciliter (1/10 liter)		
DLE	discoid lupus erythernatosus	**ERT**	estrogen replacement therapy
DM	diabetes mellitus	**ESR**	erythrocyte sedimentation
DNA	deoxyribonucleic acid	**ESRD**	end-stage renal disease
DNR	do not resuscitate	**ESWL**	extracorporeal shock wave lithotripsy
D.O.	Doctor of Osteopathy		
DOA	dead on arrival	**ETOH**	alcohol
DOB	date of birth	**ETT**	exercise tolerance test
DOE	dyspnea on exertion	**F**	Fahrenheit
DPT	diphtheria, pertussis, tetanus (vaccine)		
DRE	digital rectal exam		
DRG	diagnosis-related group		

FACP	Fellow, American College of Physicians
FACS	Fellow, American College of Surgeons
FB	fingerbreadth; foreign body
FBS	fasting blood sugar
FDA	Food and Drug
Fe	iron
FEF	forced expiratory flow
FEV	forced expiratory volume
FH	family history
FHR	fetal heart rate
FROM	full range of movement/motion
FSH	follicle-stimulating hormone
F/u	follow-up
5-FU	5-fluorouracil (used in cancer chemotherapy)
FUO	fever of undetermined origin
Fx	fracture
μg	microgram (one-millionth of a gram)
G	gravida (pregnant)
g, gm	gram
Ga	gallium
GABA	gamma-aminobutyric acid
GB	gallbladder
GBS	gallbladder series (x-rays)
GC	gonorrhea
G-CSF	granulocyte colony stimulating factor
GERD	gastroesophageal reflux
GFR	glomerular filtration rate
GH	growth hormone
GI	gastrointestinal
Grav. 1, 2, 3	first, second, third pregnancy
GTT	glucose tolerance test
gt, gft	drop (gutta), drops (guttae)
GU	genitourinary
Gy	gray (unit of radiation and equal to 100 rads)
GYN	gynecology
H	hydrogen
h, hr	hour
H2 blocker	H2 (histamine) receptor antagonist
HBV	hepatitis B virus

HCG (hCG)	human chorionic gonadotropin
HCI	hydrochloric acid
HCO3	bicarbonate
Hct (HCT)	hernatocrit
HCV	hepatitis C virus
HCVD	hypertensive cardiovascular disease
HD	hemodialysis (artificial kidney machine)
HDL	high-density lipoprotein
He	helium
HEENT	head, eyes, ears, nose, and throat
Hg	mercury
Hgb	hemoglobin
hGH	human growth hormone
H&H	hernatocrit and hemoglobin
HIV	human immunodeficiency virus
HLA	histocompatibility locus antigen
HNP	herniated nucleus pulposus
h/o	history of
H20	water
hpf	high-power field (microscope)
HPI	history of present illness
HPV	human papillomavirus
HRT	hormone replacement therapy
h.s.	at bedtime (hora somni)
HSG	hysterosalpingography
HSV	herpes simplex virus
ht	height
HTN	hypertension (high blood pressure)
Hx	history
I	iodine
131I	radioactive isotope of iodine
IBD	inflammatory bowel disease
ICP	intracranial pressure
ICSH	interstitial cell-stimulating hormone
ICU	intensive care unit
I&D	incision and drainage
ID	infectious disease
IDDM	insulin-dependent diabetes mellitus
IgA, IgD, IgE, IgG, IgM	immunoglobulins
IHD	ischernic heart disease

IHSS	idiopathic hypertrophic subaortic stenosis		**LLL**	left lower lobe (lung)
IM	intramuscular; infectious mononucleosis		**LLQ**	left lower quadrant (abdomen)
			LMP	last menstrual period
IMV	intermittent mandatory ventilation		**LOC**	loss of consciousness
inf.	infusion; inferior		**LOS**	length of stay
INH	isoniazid (drug used to treat tuberculosis)		**LP**	lumbar puncture
			lpf	low-power field (microscope)
inj.	injection		**LPN**	licensed practical nurse
I & O	intake and output		**LS**	lumbosacral spine
IOL	intraocular lens (implant)		**LSD**	lysergic acid diethylamide
IOP	intraocular pressure		**LSK**	liver, spleen, and kidneys
I.Q.	intelligence quotient		**LTB**	laryngotracheal bronchitis
IUD	intrauterine device		**LTC**	long-term care
IUP	intrauterine pregnancy		**LTH**	luteotropic hormone (prolactin)
IV	intravenous (injection)		**LUL**	left upper lobe (lung)
IVP	intravenous pyelogram		**LUQ**	left upper quadrant (abdomen)
			LV	left ventricle
K	potassium		**L&W**	living and well
kg	kilogram (1000 grams)		**lymphs**	lymphocytes
KJ	knee jerk		**lytes**	electrolytes
KS	Kaposi sarcoma			
KUB	kidney, ureter, and bladder (x-ray exam)		**MA**	mental age
			MAI	Mycobacterium avium intracellulare
L, l	liter; left; lower		**MAOI**	monoamine oxidase inhibitor
L1, L2	first, second lumbar vertebra		**MBD**	minimal brain dysfunction
LA	left atrium		**mcg**	microgram
LAD	left anterior descending (coronary artery)		**MCH**	mean corpuscular hemoglobin
			MCHC	mean corpuscular hemoglobin concentration
lat	lateral		**mci**	millicurie
LAVH	laparoscopic assisted vaginal hysterectomy		**uCi**	microcurie
			MCP	metacarpophalangeal joint
LB	large bowel		**MCV**	mean corpuscular volume (average size of a RBC)
LBBB	left bundle branch block (heart block)			
LD	lethal dose		**M.D.**	Doctor of Medicine
LDH	lactate dehydrogenase		**MED**	minimum effective dose
LDL	low-density lipoprotein		**mEq**	milliequivalent
L-dopa	levodopa (used to treat Parkinson disease)		**mEq/L**	milliequivalent per liter
			mets	metastases
L.E.	lupus erythernatosus		**Mg**	magnesium
LEEP	loop electrocautery excision procedure		**mg**	milligram (1/1000 gram)
			mg/CC	milligram per cubic centimeter
LES	lower esophageal sphincter		**mg/dl**	milligram per deciliter
LFTs	liver function tests		**μg**	microgram (one-millionth of a gram)
LH	luteinizing hormone		**MH**	marital history; mental health

MI	myocardial infarction; mitral insufficiency
mL, ml	milliliter (1/1000 liter)
mm	millimeter (1/1000 meter; 0.039 inch)
mmHg	millimeters of mercury
MMPI	Minnesota Multiphasic Personality Inventory
MMR	measles-mumps-rubella (vaccine)
MMT	manual muscle testing
Mμ	millimicron (1y1000 micron; a micron is 10-3mm
μM	micrometer (one-millionth of a meter)
mono	monocyte (white blood cell)
MR	mitral regurgitation
MRI	magnetic resonance imaging
mRNA	messenger RNA
MS	multiple sclerosis; mitral stenosis
MSL	midsternal line
MTX	methotrexate
MUGA	multiple-gated acquisition scan (of heart)
multip	multipara; multiparous
MVP	mitral valve prolapse
N	nitrogen
Na	sodium
NB	newborn
NBS	normal bowel or breath sounds
ND	normal delivery; normal development
NED	no evidence of disease
neg.	negative
NG tube	nasogastric tube
NHL	non-Hodgkin lymphoma
NIDDM	non- insulin-dependent diabetes mellitus (type 2)
NK cells	natural killer cells
NKDA	no known drug allergies
NPO	nothing by mouth (non per os)
NSAID	nonsteroidal anti-inflammatory drug
NSR	normal sinus rhythm (of heart)
NTP	normal temperature and pressure
O	oxygen
OA	osteoarthritis
OB/GYN	obstetrics and gynecology
OCPS	oral contraceptive pills

O.D.	Doctor of Optometry; overdose; right eye (oculus dexter)
OR	operating room
ORIF	open reduction internal fixation
ORTH; ortho	orthopedics
O.S.	left eye (oculus sinister)
os	opening; mouth; bone
O.T.	occupational therapy
O.U.	each eye (oculus uterque)
OZ.	ounce
P	phosphorus; posterior; pressure; pulse; pupil
p	after
P2	pulmonary valve closure (heart sound)
PA	pulmonary artery; posteroanterior
P-A	posteroanterior
P&A	percussion and auscultation
PAC	premature atrial contraction
PaCO2	partial pressure of carbon dioxide
palp.	palpable; palpation
PALS	pediatric advanced life support
Pa02, P02	partial pressure of oxygen
Pap smear	Papanicolaou smear (cells from cervix and vagina)
Para 1, 2, 3	unipara, bipara, tripara (number of viable births)
P.C.	after meals (post cibum)
PCP	Pneumocystis carinii pneumonia; phencyclidine
PCR	polymerase chain reaction (process allows making copies of genes)
PD	peritoneal dialysis
PDA	patent ductus arteriosus
PDR	Physicians' Desk Reference
PE	physical examination; pulmonary embolism
PEEP	positive end-expiratory pressure
PEG	percutaneous endoscopic gastrostomy (a feeding tube)
PEJ	percutaneous endoscopic jejunostomy (a feeding tube)
per os	by mouth
PERRLA	pupils equal, round, react to light and accomodation

PET	positron emission tomography		**PVC**	premature ventricular contraction
PE tube	ventilating tube for eardrum		**PVD**	peripheral vascular disease
PFT	pulmonary function test		**PWB**	partial weight bearing
PG	prostaglandin		**q**	every (quaque)
PH	past history		**q.d.**	every day (quaque die)
PH	hydrogen ion concentration (alkalinity and acidity measurement)		**q.h.**	every hour (quaque hora)
PI	present illness		**q.i.d.**	four times daily (quater in die)
PID	pelvic inflammatory disease		**q.n.**	each night (quaque nox)
PIP	proximal interphalangeal joint		**q.s.**	as much as suffices (quantum sufficit)
PKU	phenylketonuria		**qt**	quart
p.m.	afternoon (post meridian)			
PMH	past medical history		**R**	respiration; right
PAIN	polymorphonuclear leukocyte		**RA**	rheumatoid arthritis; right atrium
PMS	premenstrual syndrome		**Ra**	radium
PND	paroxysmal nocturnal dyspnea		**rad**	radiation absorbed dose
P/O	postoperative		**RBBB**	right bundle branch block
P.O.	by mouth (per os)		**RBC, rbc**	red blood cell (corpuscle); red blood count
poly	polymorphonuclear leukocyte		**R.D.D.A.**	recommended daily dietary allowance
postop	postoperative (after surgery)		**RDS**	respiratory distress syndrome
PPBS	postprandial blood sugar		**REM**	rapid eye movement
PPD	purified protein derivative (test for tuberculosis)		**RF**	rheumatoid factor
preop	preoperative		**Rh**	rhesus (monkey) factor in blood
prep	prepare for		**RIA**	radioirnmunoassay (minute quantities are measured)
PR	partial response		**RIND**	reversible ischernic neurologic deficit/defect
primip	primipara		**RLL**	right lower lobe (lung)
PRL	prolactin		**RLQ**	right lower quadrant (abdomen)
p.r.n.	as required (pro re nata)		**RML**	right middle lobe (lung)
procto	proctoscopy		**RNA**	ribonucleic acid
prot.	protocol		**WO**	rule out
Pro. time	prothrombin time (test of blood clotting)		**ROM**	range of motion
PSA	prostate-specific antigen		**ROS**	review of systems
PT	prothrombin time; physical therapy		**RRR**	regular rate and rhythm (of the heart)
PTA	prior to admission (to hospital)		**RT**	right; radiation therapy
PTC	percutaneous transhepatic cholangiography		**RUL**	right upper lobe (lung)
PTCA	percutaneous transluminal coronary angioplasty		**RUQ**	right upper quadrant (abdomen)
PTH	parathyroid hormone		**RV**	right ventricle
PTT	partial thromboplastin time (test of blood clotting)		**Rx**	treatment; therapy; prescription
PU	pregnancy urine		**ŝ**	without (sine)
PUVA	psoralen ultraviolet A (treatment for psoriasis)		**SI, S2**	first, second sacral vertebra
			S-A node	sinoatrial node (pacemaker of heart)
			SAD	seasonal affective disorder

SBE	subacute bacterial endocarditis
SBFT	small bowel follow-through (x-rays of small intestine)
sed. rate	sedimentation rate (rate of erythrocyte sedimentation)
segs	segmented neutrophils; polys
SERM	selective estrogen receptor modifier
SGOT (AST)	serum glutarnic-oxaloacetic transaminase
SGPT (ALT)	serum glutamic-pyruvic transaminase
SIADH	syndrome of inappropriate antidiuretic hormone
SIDS	sudden infant death syndrome
Sig.	let it be labeled
SLE	systemic lupus erythernatosus
SMA 12	twelve blood chemistries
SOAP	subjective, objective, assessment, and plan
SOB	shortness of breath
s.o.s.	if necessary (si opus sit)
S/P	status post (previous disease condition)
SPECT	single-photon emission computed tomography
sp. gr.	specific gravity
SSRI	selective serotonin reuptake inhibitor (antidepressant)
staph.	staphylococci (berry-shaped bacteria in clusters)
stat.	immediately (statim)
STD	sexually transmitted disease
STH	somatotropin (growth hormone)
Strep.	streptococci (berry-shaped bacteria in twisted chains)
Subcu	subcutaneous
SVC	superior vena cava
SVD	spontaneous vaginal delivery
Sx	symptoms
T	temperature; time
TI, T2	first, second thoracic vertebra
T3	triiodothyronine test
T,	thyroxine test
TA	therapeutic abortion
T&A	tonsillectomy and adenoidectomy

TAH	total abdominal hysterectomy
TAT	Thematic Apperception Test
TB	tuberculosis
Tc	technetium
T cells	lymphocytes produced in the thymus gland
TEE	transesophageal echocardiogram
TENS	transcutaneous electrical nerve stimulation
TFT	thyroid function test
TIA	transient ischernic attack
t.i.d.	three times daily (ter in die)
TLC	total lung capacity
TM	tympanic membrane
TMJ	temporomandibular joint
TNM	tumor, nodes, and metastases
tPA	tissue plasminogen activator
TPN	total parenteral nutrition
TPR	temperature, pulse, and respiration
TRUS	transrectal ultrasound
TSH	thyroid-stimulating hormone
TSS	toxic shock syndrome
TUR, TURP	transurethral resection of the prostate
TVH	total vaginal hysterectomy
Tx	treatment
U	unit
UA	urinalysis
UAO	upper airway obstruction
UC	uterine contractions
UE	upper extremity
UGI	upper gastrointestinal
umb.	navel (umbilicus)
U/O	urinary output
URI	upper respiratory infection
U/S	ultrasound
UTI	urinary tract infection
UV	ultraviolet
VA	visual acuity
VC	vital capacity (of lungs)
VCUG	voiding cystourethrogram
VF	visual field
Vis a Vis	as compared with; in relation to

V/Q scan   ventilation-perfusion scan

V/S   vital signs; versus

VSD   ventricular septa defect

VT   ventricular tachycardia (abnormal heart rhythm)

WAIS   Wechsler Adult Intelligence Scale

WBC, wbc   white blood cell; white blood count

WDWN   well developed, well nourished

WISC   Wechsler Intelligence Scale for Children

WNL   within normal limits

Wt   weight

XRT   radiation therapy

Y/0, yrs   year(s) old

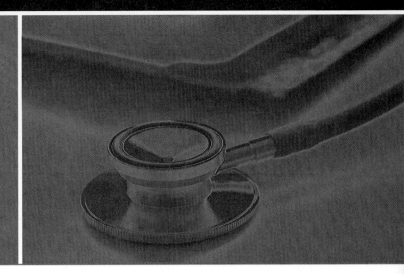

ICD-9-CM Codes for 2009

Excerpted from The Centers for Medicare & Medicaid Services, August 19, 2008 Federal Register, final code changes effective October 1, 2008 for ICD-9-CM. The following is a list of new ICD-9-CM codes for Fiscal Year 2009 only. Be sure to review deleted codes, revised code descriptions, and subterms that can make significant differences.

New Diagnosis Codes, Effective October 1, 2008

The final addendum providing complete information on changes to the diagnosis part of ICD-9-CM is posted on CDC's webpage at: www.cdc.gov/nchs/icd9.htm

038.12 Methicillin resistant Staphylococcus aureus septicemia

041.12 Methicillin resistant Staphylococcus aureus in conditions classified elsewhere and of unspecified site

046.11 Variant Creutzfeldt-Jakob disease

046.19 Other and unspecified Creutzfeldt-Jakob disease

046.71 Gerstmann-Sträussler-Scheinker syndrome

046.72 Fatal familial insomnia

046.79 Other and unspecified prion disease of central nervous system

051.01 Cowpox

051.02 Vaccinia not from vaccination

059.00 Orthopoxvirus infection, unspecified

059.01 Monkeypox

059.09 Other orthopoxvirus infections

059.10 Parapoxvirus infection, unspecified

059.11 Bovine stomatitis

059.12 Sealpox

059.19 Other parapoxvirus infections

059.20 Yatapoxvirus infection, unspecified

059.21 Tanapox

059.22 Yaba monkey tumor virus

059.8 Other poxvirus infections

059.9 Poxvirus infections, unspecified

078.12 Plantar wart

136.21 Specific infection due to acanthamoeba

136.29 Other specific infections by free-living amebae

199.2 Malignant neoplasm associated with transplant organ

203.02 Multiple myeloma, in relapse

203.12 Plasma cell leukemia, in relapse

203.82 Other immunoproliferative neoplasms, in relapse

204.02 Acute lymphoid leukemia, in relapse

204.12 Chronic lymphoid leukemia, in relapse

204.22 Subacute lymphoid leukemia, in relapse

204.82 Other lymphoid leukemia, in relapse

204.92 Unspecified lymphoid leukemia, in relapse

205.02 Acute myeloid leukemia, in relapse

205.12 Chronic myeloid leukemia, in relapse

205.22 Subacute myeloid leukemia, in relapse

205.32 Myeloid sarcoma, in relapse

205.82 Other myeloid leukemia, in relapse

205.92 Unspecified myeloid leukemia, in relapse

206.02 Acute monocytic leukemia, in relapse

206.12 Chronic monocytic leukemia, in relapse

206.22 Subacute monocytic leukemia, in relapse

206.82 Other monocytic leukemia, in relapse

206.92 Unspecified monocytic leukemia, in relapse

207.02 Acute erythremia and erythroleukemia, in relapse

207.12 Chronic erythremia, in relapse

207.22 Megakaryocytic leukemia, in relapse

207.82 Other specified leukemia, in relapse

208.02 Acute leukemia of unspecified cell type, in relapse

208.12 Chronic leukemia of unspecified cell type, in relapse

208.22 Subacute leukemia of unspecified cell type, in relapse

208.82 Other leukemia of unspecified cell type, in relapse

208.92 Unspecified leukemia, in relapse

209.00 Malignant carcinoid tumor of the small intestine, unspecified portion

209.01 Malignant carcinoid tumor of the duodenum

209.02 Malignant carcinoid tumor of the jejunum

209.03 Malignant carcinoid tumor of the ileum

209.10 Malignant carcinoid tumor of the large intestine, unspecified portion

209.11 Malignant carcinoid tumor of the appendix

209.12 Malignant carcinoid tumor of the cecum

209.13 Malignant carcinoid tumor of the ascending colon

209.14 Malignant carcinoid tumor of the transverse colon

209.15 Malignant carcinoid tumor of the descending colon

209.16 Malignant carcinoid tumor of the sigmoid colon

209.17 Malignant carcinoid tumor of the rectum

209.20 Malignant carcinoid tumor of unknown primary site

209.21 Malignant carcinoid tumor of the bronchus and lung

209.22 Malignant carcinoid tumor of the thymus

209.23 Malignant carcinoid tumor of the stomach

209.24 Malignant carcinoid tumor of the kidney

209.25 Malignant carcinoid tumor of foregut, not otherwise specified

209.26 Malignant carcinoid tumor of midgut, not otherwise specified

209.27 Malignant carcinoid tumor of hindgut, not otherwise specified

209.29 Malignant carcinoid tumor of other sites

209.30 Malignant poorly differentiated neuroendocrine carcinoma, any site

209.40 Benign carcinoid tumor of the small intestine, unspecified portion

209.41 Benign carcinoid tumor of the duodenum

209.42 Benign carcinoid tumor of the jejunum

209.43 Benign carcinoid tumor of the ileum

209.50 Benign carcinoid tumor of the large intestine, unspecified portion

209.51 Benign carcinoid tumor of the appendix

209.52 Benign carcinoid tumor of the cecum

209.53 Benign carcinoid tumor of the ascending colon

209.54 Benign carcinoid tumor of the transverse colon

209.55 Benign carcinoid tumor of the descending colon

209.56 Benign carcinoid tumor of the sigmoid colon

209.57 Benign carcinoid tumor of the rectum

209.60 Benign carcinoid tumor of unknown primary site

209.61 Benign carcinoid tumor of the bronchus and lung

209.62 Benign carcinoid tumor of the thymus

209.63 Benign carcinoid tumor of the stomach

209.64 Benign carcinoid tumor of the kidney

209.65 Benign carcinoid tumor of foregut, not otherwise specified

209.66 Benign carcinoid tumor of midgut, not otherwise specified

209.67 Benign carcinoid tumor of hindgut, not otherwise specified

209.69 Benign carcinoid tumor of other sites

238.77 Post-transplant lymphoproliferative disorder (PTLD)

249.00 Secondary diabetes mellitus without mention of complication, not stated as uncontrolled, or unspecified

249.01 Secondary diabetes mellitus without mention of complication, uncontrolled

249.10 Secondary diabetes mellitus with ketoacidosis, not stated as uncontrolled, or unspecified

249.11 Secondary diabetes mellitus with ketoacidosis, uncontrolled

249.20 Secondary diabetes mellitus with hyperosmolarity, not stated as uncontrolled, or unspecified

249.21 Secondary diabetes mellitus with hyperosmolarity, uncontrolled

249.30 Secondary diabetes mellitus with other coma, not stated as uncontrolled, or unspecified

249.31 Secondary diabetes mellitus with other coma, uncontrolled

249.40 Secondary diabetes mellitus with renal manifestations, not stated as uncontrolled, or unspecified

249.41 Secondary diabetes mellitus with renal manifestations, uncontrolled

249.50 Secondary diabetes mellitus with ophthalmic manifestations, not stated as uncontrolled, or unspecified

249.51 Secondary diabetes mellitus with ophthalmic manifestations, uncontrolled

249.60 Secondary diabetes mellitus with neurological manifestations, not stated as uncontrolled, or unspecified

249.61 Secondary diabetes mellitus with neurological manifestations, uncontrolled

249.70 Secondary diabetes mellitus with peripheral circulatory disorders, not stated as uncontrolled, or unspecified

249.71 Secondary diabetes mellitus with peripheral circulatory disorders, uncontrolled

249.80 Secondary diabetes mellitus with other specified manifestations, not stated as uncontrolled, or unspecified

249.81 Secondary diabetes mellitus with other specified manifestations, uncontrolled

249.90 Secondary diabetes mellitus with unspecified complication, not stated as uncontrolled, or unspecified

249.91 Secondary diabetes mellitus with unspecified complication, uncontrolled

259.50 Androgen insensitivity, unspecified

259.51 Androgen insensitivity syndrome

259.52 Partial androgen insensitivity

275.5 Hungry bone syndrome

279.50 Graft-versus-host disease, unspecified

279.51 Acute graft-versus-host disease

279.52 Chronic graft-versus-host disease

279.53 Acute on chronic graft-versus-host disease

289.84 Heparin-induced thrombocytopenia (HIT)

337.00 Idiopathic peripheral autonomic neuropathy, unspecified

337.01 Carotid sinus syndrome

337.09 Other idiopathic peripheral autonomic neuropathy

339.00 Cluster headache syndrome, unspecified

339.01 Episodic cluster headache

339.02 Chronic cluster headache

339.03 Episodic paroxysmal hemicrania

339.04 Chronic paroxysmal hemicrania

339.05 Short lasting unilateral neuralgiform headache with conjunctival injection and tearing

339.09 Other trigeminal autonomic cephalgias

339.10 Tension type headache, unspecified

339.11 Episodic tension type headache

339.12 Chronic tension type headache

339.20 Post-traumatic headache, unspecified

339.21 Acute post-traumatic headache

339.22 Chronic post-traumatic headache

339.3 Drug induced headache, not elsewhere classified

339.41 Hemicrania continua

339.42 New daily persistent headache

339.43 Primary thunderclap headache

339.44 Other complicated headache syndrome

339.81 Hypnic headache

339.82 Headache associated with sexual activity

339.83 Primary cough headache

339.84 Primary exertional headache

339.85 Primary stabbing headache

339.89 Other headache syndromes

346.02 Migraine with aura, without mention of intractable migraine with status migrainosus

346.03 Migraine with aura, with intractable migraine, so stated, with status migrainosus

346.12 Migraine without aura, without mention of intractable migraine with status migrainosus

346.13 Migraine without aura, with intractable migraine, so stated, with status migrainosus

346.22 Variants of migraine, not elsewhere classified, without mention of intractable migraine with status migrainosus

346.23 Variants of migraine, not elsewhere classified, with intractable migraine, so stated, with status migrainosus

346.30 Hemiplegic migraine, without mention of intractable migraine without mention of status migrainosus

346.31 Hemiplegic migraine, with intractable migraine, so stated, without mention of status migrainosus

346.32 Hemiplegic migraine, without mention of intractable migraine with status migrainosus

346.33 Hemiplegic migraine, with intractable migraine, so stated, with status migrainosus

346.40 Menstrual migraine, without mention of intractable migraine without mention of status migrainosus

346.41 Menstrual migraine, with intractable migraine, so stated, without mention of status migrainosus

346.42 Menstrual migraine, without mention of intractable migraine with status migrainosus

346.43 Menstrual migraine, with intractable migraine, so stated, with status migrainosus

346.50 Persistent migraine aura without cerebral infarction, without mention of intractable migraine without mention of status migrainosus

346.51 Persistent migraine aura without cerebral infarction, with intractable migraine, so stated, without mention of status migrainosus

346.52 Persistent migraine aura without cerebral infarction, without mention of intractable migraine with status migrainosus

346.53 Persistent migraine aura without cerebral infarction, with intractable migraine, so stated, with status migrainosus

346.60 Persistent migraine aura with cerebral infarction, without mention of intractable migraine without mention of status migrainosus

346.61 Persistent migraine aura with cerebral infarction, with intractable migraine, so stated, without mention of status migrainosus

346.62 Persistent migraine aura with cerebral infarction, without mention of intractable migraine with status migrainosus

346.63 Persistent migraine aura with cerebral infarction, with intractable migraine, so stated, with status migrainosus

346.70 Chronic migraine without aura, without mention of intractable migraine without mention of status migrainosus

346.71 Chronic migraine without aura, with intractable migraine, so stated, without mention of status migrainosus

346.72 Chronic migraine without aura, without mention of intractable migraine with status migrainosus

346.73 Chronic migraine without aura, with intractable migraine, so stated, with status migrainosus

346.82 Other forms of migraine, without mention of intractable migraine with status migrainosus

346.83 Other forms of migraine, with intractable migraine, so stated, with status migrainosus

346.92 Migraine, unspecified, without mention of intractable migraine with status migrainosus

346.93 Migraine, unspecified, with intractable migraine, so stated, with status migrainosus

349.31 Accidental puncture or laceration of dura during a procedure

349.39 Other dural tear

362.20 Retinopathy of prematurity, unspecified

362.22 Retinopathy of prematurity, stage 0

362.23 Retinopathy of prematurity, stage 1

362.24 Retinopathy of prematurity, stage 2

362.25 Retinopathy of prematurity, stage 3

362.26 Retinopathy of prematurity, stage 4

362.27 Retinopathy of prematurity, stage 5

364.82 Plateau iris syndrome

372.34 Pingueculitis

414.3 Coronary atherosclerosis due to lipid rich plaque

482.42 Methicillin resistant pneumonia due to Staphylococcus aureus

511.81 Malignant pleural effusion

511.89 Other specified forms of effusion, except tuberculous

530.13 Eosinophilic esophagitis

535.70 Eosinophilic gastritis, without mention of hemorrhage

535.71 Eosinophilic gastritis, with hemorrhage

558.41 Eosinophilic gastroenteritis

558.42 Eosinophilic colitis

569.44 Dysplasia of anus

571.42 Autoimmune hepatitis

599.70 Hematuria, unspecified

599.71 Gross hematuria

599.72 Microscopic hematuria

611.81 Ptosis of breast

611.82 Hypoplasia of breast

611.83 Capsular contracture of breast implant

611.89 Other specified disorders of breast

612.0 Deformity of reconstructed breast

612.1 Disproportion of reconstructed breast

625.70 Vulvodynia, unspecified

625.71 Vulvar vestibulitis

625.79 Other vulvodynia

649.70 Cervical shortening, unspecified as to episode of care or not applicable

649.71 Cervical shortening, delivered, with or without mention of antepartum condition

649.73 Cervical shortening, antepartum condition or complication

678.00 Fetal hematologic conditions, unspecified as to episode of care or not applicable

678.01 Fetal hematologic conditions, delivered, with or without mention of antepartum condition

678.03 Fetal hematologic conditions, antepartum condition or complication

678.10 Fetal conjoined twins, unspecified as to episode of care or not applicable

678.11 Fetal conjoined twins, delivered, with or without mention of antepartum condition

678.13 Fetal conjoined twins, antepartum condition or complication

679.01 Maternal complications from in utero procedure, delivered, with or without mention of antepartum condition

679.02 Maternal complications from in utero procedure, delivered, with mention of postpartum complication

679.03 Maternal complications from in utero procedure, antepartum condition or complication

679.04 Maternal complications from in utero procedure, postpartum condition or complication

679.10 Fetal complications from in utero procedures, unspecified as to episode of care or not applicable

679.11 Fetal complications from in utero procedures, delivered, with or without mention of antepartum condition

679.12 Fetal complications from in utero procedures, delivered, with mention of postpartum complication

679.13 Fetal complications from in utero procedures, antepartum condition or complication

679.14 Fetal complications from in utero procedures, postpartum condition or complication

695.10 Erythema multiforme, unspecified

695.11 Erythema multiforme minor

695.12 Erythema multiforme major

695.13 Stevens-Johnson syndrome

695.14 Stevens-Johnson syndrome-toxic epidermal necrolysis overlap syndrome

695.15 Toxic epidermal necrolysis

695.19 Other erythema multiforme

695.50 Exfoliation due to erythematous condition involving less than 10 percent of body surface

695.51 Exfoliation due to erythematous condition involving 10-19 percent of body surface

695.52 Exfoliation due to erythematous condition involving 20-29 percent of body surface

695.53 Exfoliation due to erythematous condition involving 30-39 percent of body surface

695.54 Exfoliation due to erythematous condition involving 40-49 percent of body surface

695.55 Exfoliation due to erythematous condition involving 50-59 percent of body surface

695.56 Exfoliation due to erythematous condition involving 60-69 percent of body surface

695.57 Exfoliation due to erythematous condition involving 70-79 percent of body surface

695.58 Exfoliation due to erythematous condition involving 80-89 percent of body surface

695.59 Exfoliation due to erythematous condition involving 90 percent or more of body surface

707.20 Pressure ulcer, unspecified stage

707.21 Pressure ulcer, stage I

707.22 Pressure ulcer, stage II

707.23 Pressure ulcer, stage III

707.24 Pressure ulcer, stage IV

707.25 Pressure ulcer, unstageable

729.90 Disorders of soft tissue, unspecified

729.91 Post-traumatic seroma

729.92 Nontraumatic hematoma of soft tissue

729.99 Other disorders of soft tissue

733.96 Stress fracture of femoral neck

733.97 Stress fracture of shaft of femur

733.98 Stress fracture of pelvis

760.61 Newborn affected by amniocentesis

760.62 Newborn affected by other in utero procedure

760.63 Newborn affected by other surgical operations on mother during pregnancy

760.64 Newborn affected by previous surgical procedure on mother not associated with pregnancy

777.50 Necrotizing enterocolitis in newborn, unspecified

777.51 Stage I necrotizing enterocolitis in newborn

777.52 Stage II necrotizing enterocolitis in newborn

777.53 Stage III necrotizing enterocolitis in newborn

780.60 Fever, unspecified

780.61 Fever presenting with conditions classified elsewhere

780.62 Postprocedural fever

780.63 Postvaccination fever

780.64 Chills (without fever)

780.65 Hypothermia not associated with low environmental temperature

780.72 Functional quadriplegia

788.91 Functional urinary incontinence

788.99 Other symptoms involving urinary system

795.07 Satisfactory cervical smear but lacking transformation zone

795.10 Abnormal glandular Papanicolaou smear of vagina

795.11 Papanicolaou smear of vagina with atypical squamous cells of undetermined significance (ASC-US)

795.12 Papanicolaou smear of vagina with atypical squamous cells cannot exclude high grade squamous intraepithelial lesion (ASC-H)

795.13 Papanicolaou smear of vagina with low grade squamous intraepithelial lesion (LGSIL)

795.14 Papanicolaou smear of vagina with high grade squamous intraepithelial lesion (HGSIL)

795.15 Vaginal high risk human papillomavirus (HPV) DNA test positive

795.16 Papanicolaou smear of vagina with cytologic evidence of malignancy

795.18 Unsatisfactory vaginal cytology smear

795.19 Other abnormal Papanicolaou smear of vagina and vaginal HPV

796.70 Abnormal glandular Papanicolaou smear of anus

796.71 Papanicolaou smear of anus with atypical squamous cells of undetermined significance (ASC-US)

796.72 Papanicolaou smear of anus with atypical squamous cells cannot exclude high grade squamous intraepithelial lesion (ASC-H)

796.73 Papanicolaou smear of anus with low grade squamous intraepithelial lesion (LGSIL)

796.74 Papanicolaou smear of anus with high grade squamous intraepithelial lesion (HGSIL)

796.75 Anal high risk human papillomavirus (HPV) DNA test positive

796.76 Papanicolaou smear of anus with cytologic evidence of malignancy

796.77 Satisfactory anal smear but lacking transformation zone

796.78 Unsatisfactory anal cytology smear

796.79 Other abnormal Papanicolaou smear of anus and anal HPV

997.31 Ventilator associated pneumonia

997.39 Other respiratory complications

998.30 Disruption of wound, unspecified

998.33 Disruption of traumatic injury wound repair

999.81 Extravasation of vesicant chemotherapy

999.82 Extravasation of other vesicant agent

999.88 Other infusion reaction

999.89 Other transfusion reaction

V02.53 Carrier or suspected carrier of Methicillin susceptible Staphylococcus aureus

V02.54 Carrier or suspected carrier of Methicillin resistant Staphylococcus aureus

V07.51 Prophylactic use of selective estrogen receptor modulators (SERMs)

V07.52 Prophylactic use of aromatase inhibitors

V07.59 Prophylactic use of other agents affecting estrogen receptors and estrogen levels

V12.04 Personal history of Methicillin resistant Staphylococcus aureus

V13.51 Personal history of pathologic fracture

V13.52 Personal history of stress fracture

V13.59 Personal history of other musculoskeletal disorders

V15.21 Personal history of undergoing in utero procedure during pregnancy

V15.22 Personal history of undergoing in utero procedure while a fetus

V15.29 Personal history of surgery to other organs

V15.51 Personal history of traumatic fracture

V15.59 Personal history of other injury

V23.85 Pregnancy resulting from assisted reproductive technology

V23.86 Pregnancy with history of in utero procedure during previous pregnancy

V28.81 Encounter for fetal anatomic survey

V28.82 Encounter for screening for risk of pre-term labor

V28.89 Other specified antenatal screening

V45.11 Renal dialysis status

V45.12 Noncompliance with renal dialysis

V45.87 Transplanted organ removal status

V45.88 Status post administration of tPA (rtPA) in a different facility within the last 24 hours prior to admission to current facility

V46.3 Wheelchair dependence

V51.0 Encounter for breast reconstruction following mastectomy

V51.8 Other aftercare involving the use of plastic surgery

V61.01 Family disruption due to family member on military deployment

V61.02 Family disruption due to return of family member from military deployment

V61.03 Family disruption due to divorce or legal separation

V61.04 Family disruption due to parent-child estrangement

V61.05 Family disruption due to child in welfare custody

V61.06 Family disruption due to child in foster care or in care of non-parental family member

V61.09 Other family disruption

V62.21 Personal current military deployment status

V62.22 Personal history of return from military deployment

V62.29 Other occupational circumstances or maladjustment

V87.01 Contact with and (suspected) exposure to arsenic

V87.09 Contact with and (suspected) exposure to other hazardous metals

V87.11 Contact with and (suspected) exposure to aromatic amines

V87.12 Contact with and (suspected) exposure to benzene

V87.19 Contact with and (suspected) exposure to other hazardous aromatic compounds

V87.2 Contact with and (suspected) exposure to other potentially hazardous chemicals

V87.31 Contact with and (suspected) exposure to mold

V87.39 Contact with and (suspected) exposure to other potentially hazardous substances

V87.41 Personal history of antineoplastic chemotherapy

V87.42 Personal history of monoclonal drug therapy

V87.49 Personal history of other drug therapy

V88.01 Acquired absence of both cervix and uterus

V88.02 Acquired absence of uterus with remaining cervical stump

V88.03 Acquired absence of cervix with remaining uterus

V89.01 Suspected problem with amniotic cavity and membrane not found

V89.02 Suspected placental problem not found

V89.03 Suspected fetal anomaly not found

V89.04 Suspected problem with fetal growth not found

V89.05 Suspected cervical shortening not found

V89.09 Other suspected maternal and fetal condition not found

New Procedure Codes, Effective October 1, 2008

The final addendum which describes all changes to the procedure part of ICD-9-CM is posted on CMS' webpage at: www.cms.hhs.gov/ICD9ProviderDiagnosticCodes

00.49 SuperSaturated oxygen therapy

00.58 Insertion of intra-aneurysm sac pressure monitoring device (intraoperative)

00.59 Intravascular pressure measurement of coronary arteries

00.67 Intravascular pressure measurement of intrathoracic arteries

00.68 Intravascular pressure measurement of peripheral arteries

00.69 Intravascular pressure measurement, other specified and unspecified vessels

17.11 Laparoscopic repair of direct inguinal hernia with graft or prosthesis

17.12 Laparoscopic repair of indirect inguinal hernia with graft or prosthesis

17.13 Laparoscopic repair of inguinal hernia with graft or prosthesis, not otherwise specified

17.21 Laparoscopic bilateral repair of direct inguinal hernia with graft or prosthesis

17.22 Laparoscopic bilateral repair of indirect inguinal hernia with graft or prosthesis

17.23 Laparoscopic bilateral repair of inguinal hernia, one direct and one indirect, with graft or prosthesis

17.24 Laparoscopic bilateral repair of inguinal hernia with graft or prosthesis, not otherwise specified

17.31 Laparoscopic multiple segmental resection of large intestine

17.32 Laparoscopic cecectomy

17.33 Laparoscopic right hemicolectomy

17.34 Laparoscopic resection of transverse colon

17.35 Laparoscopic left hemicolectomy

17.36 Laparoscopic sigmoidectomy

17.39 Other laparoscopic partial excision of large intestine

17.41 Open robotic assisted procedure

17.42 Laparoscopic robotic assisted procedure

17.43 Percutaneous robotic assisted procedure

17.44 Endoscopic robotic assisted procedure

17.45 Thoracoscopic robotic assisted procedure

17.49   Other and unspecified robotic assisted procedure

33.72   Endoscopic pulmonary airway flow measurement

37.36   Excision or destruction of left atrial appendage (LAA)

37.55   Removal of internal biventricular heart replacement system

37.60   Implantation or insertion of biventricular external heart assist system

38.23   Intravascular spectroscopy

45.81   Laparoscopic total intra-abdominal colectomy

45.82   Open total intra-abdominal colectomy

45.83   Other and unspecified total intra-abdominal colectomy

48.40   Pull-through resection of rectum, not otherwise specified

48.42   Laparoscopic pull-through resection of rectum

48.43   Open pull-through resection of rectum

48.50   Abdominoperineal resection of the rectum, not otherwise specified

48.51   Laparoscopic abdominoperineal resection of the rectum

48.52   Open abdominoperineal resection of the rectum

48.59   Other abdominoperineal resection of the rectum

53.42   Laparoscopic repair of umbilical hernia with graft or prosthesis

53.43   Other laparoscopic umbilical herniorrhaphy

53.62   Laparoscopic incisional hernia repair with graft or prosthesis

53.63   Other laparoscopic repair of other hernia of anterior abdominal wall with graft or prosthesis

53.71   Laparoscopic repair of diaphragmatic hernia, abdominal approach

53.72   Other and open repair of diaphragmatic hernia, abdominal approach

53.75   Repair of diaphragmatic hernia, abdominal approach, not otherwise specified

53.83   Laparoscopic repair of diaphragmatic hernia, with thoracic approach

53.84   Other and open repair of diaphragmatic hernia, with thoracic approach

80.53   Repair of the anulus fibrosus with graft or prosthesis

80.54   Other and unspecified repair of the anulus fibrosus

85.70   Total reconstruction of breast, not otherwise specified

85.71   Latissimus dorsi myocutaneous flap

85.72   Transverse rectus abdominis myocutaneous (TRAM) flap, pedicled

85.73   Transverse rectus abdominis myocutaneous (TRAM) flap, free

85.74   Deep inferior epigastric artery perforator (DIEP) flap, free

85.75   Superficial inferior epigastric artery (SIEA) flap, free

85.76   Gluteal artery perforator (GAP) flap, free

85.79   Other total reconstruction of breast

Answers to Testing Your Comprehension

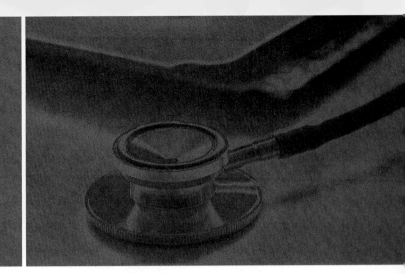

CHAPTER 1

1. ICD-9-CM (volumes 1, 2, 3) and CPT/HCPCS.
2. International Classification of Diseases, 9th Revision, Clinical Modification.
3. It emphasizes chronic diseases rather than acute infectious diseases that are more prevalent in developing countries.
4. Diagnosis-related groups for inpatient hospital services.
5. Principal diagnosis; complications; comorbidities; necessity of operating room procedures; age and sex of patient; and discharge status.
6. MS-DRG relative weight × hospital's base rate = amount reimbursed. Example: For MS-DRG 195 [pneumonia], $0.7301 \times \$4,922.73 = \$3,594.09$.
7. (a) Single classification principle; (b) categories are exhaustive; (c) categories are mutually exclusive.
8. A coder should never code from the index.
9. Subterm, also known as an essential modifier.
10. Clarifies code selection but does not change code assignment.
11. The *Tabular List of Diseases*.
12. To describe other factors influencing health care (e.g., V45.01 indicates that the patient has a cardiac pacemaker) and to describe the reasons for contact with health services (e.g., V58.11 indicates the patient was admitted for the purpose of receiving chemotherapy).
13. Cause of injury; cause of poisoning; adverse effects of medications.
14. Hypertension Table; Neoplasm Table; Table of Drugs and Chemicals.
15. ICD-10.
16. UB-04 or CMS 1450.
17. CMS 1500.
18. ICD-9-CM.
19. ICD-9-CM and CPT/HCPCS.
20. ICD-9-CM and CPT/HCPCS.
21. Yes, ICD-10 is used for the coding of causes of death as a required content for death certificates.

CHAPTER 2

1. Learn how to locate the codes by using the ICD-9-CM codebook.
2. Not elsewhere classified. This indicates that the documentation used was specific and that a more precise classification code is not available.
3. Notes that appear in all three ICD-9-CM volumes to assist in issuing correct code assignments.
4. Cross references direct the coder to refer to an alternative main term.
5. Slanted brackets are used to display a manifestation code when dual coding is required.
6. "Code first underlying condition" signifies that the code for the underlying condition must be sequenced before the italicized manifestation of the disease code.
7. Brackets enclose synonyms, abbreviations, alternative wording, or explanatory phrases.

8. Braces connect a series of terms to a common stem.

9. A colon signifies an incomplete term or root term or stem requiring at least one modifier.

10. The Uniform Hospital Discharge Data Set (UHDDS) presents a common core of data on individual hospital discharges in the Medicare and Medicaid programs.

11. The procedure performed for a definitive treatment and most closely related to the principal diagnosis.

12. (a) Mandatory dual coding or classification; (b) use additional codes as may be required; (c) use combination codes when necessary.

13. (a) Look up main term in the alphabetic index; (b) review all subterms under the main term; (c) review all nonessential modifiers; (d) follow all cross-references; (e) locate the code numerically in the procedure tabular information; (f) select the operative or procedure code.

14. V codes (a) explain the reasons for the healthcare encounter and (b) explain other factors influencing health care.

15. E codes (a) report the external cause of a poisoning; (b) report the adverse effect of a medication taken as prescribed; (c) report the external cause of an injury.

CHAPTER 3

1. (a) Database; (b) problem list; (c) initial plans; (d) progress notes.

2. Forms are organized by department (e.g., laboratory, x-ray, and nurse and physician progress notes are separated).

3. Various forms and caregiver notes are arranged in strict chronological order to allow for a quick assessment of the patient at any moment in time.

4. (a) Patient identification; (b) insurance information; (c) sometimes admitting/final diagnosis.

5. Consultant Report.

6. When there is no supporting documentation from the attending physician.

7. Physician/Coder Query/Clarification Form.

8. Size of the patient record, length of stay, sex, age, and admitting diagnosis.

CHAPTER 4

1. (a) **Sign** is an abnormality indicative of a disease discovered by the physician during an examination; (b) **symptom** is a subjective sign of disease

as expressed by the patient; and (c) **ill-defined condition** is a condition that does not clearly indicate a specific diagnosis.

2. (a) Definitive diagnosis is not identified; (b) patient is transferred to another facility or signs out against medical advice before a workup has been completed.

3. It is considered vague and a questionable cause for an inpatient hospitalization.

4. Codes 790 to 796 of chapter 16.

5. It means that the diagnosis is no longer a possibility because after study it was determined that the condition did not occur.

6. (a) DO code symptoms if they are not routinely associated with a disease; (b) DO NOT code symptoms that are routinely associated with a disease.

CHAPTER 5

1. No, because type 2 diabetics may also take insulin.

2. Excess antidiuretic hormone is secreted from the pituitary gland, and this results in too much water retention in the body.

3. Cystic fibrosis.

4. Hypokalemia.

5. High-fat diet.

6. Dehydration.

7. Code the diabetes code first, followed by the code for the complication or manifestation.

8. Graves disease.

9. Improper digestion of fats and excess respiratory mucous discharge.

10. Diets high in sugar and carbohydrates but deficient in protein.

11. Osteomalacia (softening of the bones).

12. Rickets (a metabolic bone disease).

13. Metabolism.

14. Nerves and muscles.

15. It influences the number of resources required to care for a patient.

CHAPTER 6

1. Both the organism and the condition.

2. Hemodynamic collapse and multiorgan system failure.

3. Code the septicemia first and the urinary tract infection second.

4. Code the septicemia first and the septic shock second.

5. The terms **sepsis** or **SIRS** must be present.
6. When the physician documents bacterial infection of an unspecified site.
7. Through inhaling airborne droplets or coming into contact with infected individuals.
8. Cell death.
9. (a) Contaminated food or water; (b) no significant long-term liver damage.
10. (a) Needlesticks; (b) chronic liver disease.
11. (a) Transmitted through the blood or as a result of sexual contact; (b) chronic hepatitis, cirrhosis, and liver failure.
12. Stiff neck, fever, headache, and sensitivity to light.
13. Tubercle bacilli.
14. Hemoptysis, persistent coughing, and weight loss.

Chapter 7

1. The colon.
2. Colonoscopy and barium enema.
3. An open sore on the skin or epithelial tissue lining the internal organs.
4. Peptic ulcer.
5. Review the complete medical record for the exact site of the ulcer.
6. Upper GI bleed.
7. Esophagitis
8. GERD.
9. Bile.
10. Inflammation.
11. Cholecystitis.
12. Pancreatitis.
13. Gallstones and alcoholism.
14. Hernia.
15. The bowel is protruding and thereby causing an intestinal obstruction.
16. The stomach protrudes through the esophageal opening in the diaphragm.

Chapter 8

1. Pneumonia, also called pneumonitis.
2. Gram-negative.
3. Aspiration pneumonia.
4. An asthma attack that is not responding to conventional treatment and is hard to control.
5. A cardiac cause, usually congestive heart failure.
6. Atelectasis.
7. Congestive heart failure.
8. Adult or acute respiratory distress syndrome.

9. (a) Insertion of a needle through the skin into the pleural space to drain fluid from the pleural cavity (b) to obtain fluid for analysis.
10. Tracheostomy is a therapeutic procedure that creates an open airway so the patient can breathe.

Chapter 9

1. (a) Kidneys, (b) bladder, (c) ovaries, (d) prostate gland.
2. (a) Endometriosis, (b) cervical dysplasia, (c) genital prolapse, (d) dysfunctional uterine bleeding, (e) breast diseases such as fibrocystic disease.
3. Disorders of the prostate gland.
4. (a) Hematuria, (b) urinary incontinence, (c) painful urination, (d) obstructive uropathy, (e) renal colic.
5. (a) Filtration, (b) absorption, (c) elimination.
6. Erythropoietin.
7. Renal failure.
8. The kidneys fail to eliminate excess water and sodium.
9. Heart failure.
10. (a) Hemodialysis and (b) peritoneal dialysis.
11. (a) Vascular access device or (b) arteriovenous fistula.
12. A solution is infused into a patient's peritoneal cavity from a plastic bag through a catheter.
13. Kidney transplantation.
14. Sharp flank pain, referred to as *renal colic*.
15. Extracorporeal shockwave lithotripsy; transurethral endoscopic procedures.
16. Bowman's capsule.
17. (a) Blood urea nitrogen and (b) creatinine.
18. TURP (transurethral resection of the prostate).

Chapter 10

1. Protective covering for the body.
2. Production of sebum to keep skin lubricated.
3. Production of sweat to cool the body.
4. (a) Cellulitis, (b) ulcers, (c) gangrene, (d) dermatitis, (e) some erythematous conditions.
5. Infection can spread to the lymph nodes and the bloodstream and result in sepsis.
6. Signifies a breakdown of the skin and an impending ulcer. This is particularly problematic for bedridden and wheelchair-bound patients.
7. Diabetes mellitus and atherosclerotic peripheral vascular disease.

8. (a) Poison ivy, (b) topical drugs, (c) contact with an allergen such as dust, (d) sunburn, (e) diaper rash.
9. (a) Foods eaten and (b) medications ingested or injected.
10. Toxic epidermal necrolysis (scalded skin syndrome).
11. Stevens-Johnson syndrome.
12. Debridement.
13. Excision of a skin lesion.
14. No: specific codes can identify the site and type of graft.

CHAPTER 11

1. Degenerative joint disease.
2. The fifth digit assignment will specify the joint involved.
3. Joint-replacement surgery.
4. It will be coded twice, because there is no single combination code.
5. No. Instead it should be coded as acute posthemorrhagic anemia (285.1).
6. (a) Inflammatory drugs, (b) gold compounds, (c) analgesics, (d) physical therapy, (e) joint-replacement surgery.
7. Podagra (painful big toe).
8. Determine whether the injury is chronic (recurrent or old) or acute (current or new).
9. External injury.
10. Weakening of the bone by disease.
11. Vertebrae and hip.
12. (a) Intravenous antibiotics, (b) incision and drainage, (c) excisional debridement, (d) amputation of the affected limb.
13. Necrotizing fasciitis.
14. Injury or strain to the chest muscles.
15. Hospital admission for surgical intervention.
16. (a) Systemic lupus erythematosus; (b) systemic scleroderma.
17. (a) Joint pain, (b) fever, (c) skin rash.
18. (a) Steroids to reduce inflammation and tissue damage, (b) immunosuppressive drugs, (c) physical therapy.
19. Systemic sclerosis or scleroderma.

CHAPTER 12

1. (a) Bacteria, (b) viruses, (c) fungi.
2. A lumbar puncture (spinal tap).
3. Encephalitis.
4. Spinal tap or blood culture.

5. Levodopa.
6. Senses of person, place, and time.
7. (a) Muscle weakness, (b) numbness, (c) paralysis.
8. The coder can report the residual conditions specifically attributable to each CVA.
9. Grand mal epilepsy.
10. Whether the epilepsy is intractable.
11. (a) Cornea, (b) sclera, (c) conjunctiva.
12. (a) Choroid, (b) ciliary body, (c) iris.
13. (a) Retina, (b) optic disc.
14. (a) Inability to determine the effect on patient care, (b) inability to determine the effect on health services resource use, (c) inability to determine appropriateness of provider reimbursement.
15. (a) Increased intraocular pressure, (b) excavation, (c) atrophy of the optic nerve.
16. Buildup of aqueous humor in the anterior chamber of the eye that cannot drain properly.
17. Inability of the eyes to remain balanced or parallel when looking in the same direction.
18. Loss of central vision.
19. (a) Auricle, (b) external auditory canal.
20. (A) Malleus, (b) incus, (c) stapes.
21. (a) Cochlea, (b) organ of Corti, (c) vestibule and semicircular canals, (d) auditory fluids, (e) cilia.
22. Hardening of bone tissue around the oval window.
23. Inflammation of the inner ear.

CHAPTER 13

1. (a) Arteries, (b) arterioles, (c) veins, (d) venules, and (e) capillaries.
2. (a) Anemia and (b) coagulopathy.
3. Heart tissue that dies is not replaced.
4. Coronary artery disease.
5. Unstable angina.
6. Acute myocardial infarction.
7. Coronary artery disease with preinfarction angina as an additional code.
8. Heart catheterization.
9. It provides a distinct picture of the coronary vessels.
10. It maintains perfusion of the heart and systemic circulation in an unstable patient with an occluded vessel.
11. (a) Cardiopulmonary bypass, (b) temporary pacemaker implant, (c) cardioplegia, and (d) hypothermia.
12. No, because some minor procedures are considered integral to the coronary artery bypass graft.

13. No.
14. It causes the heart to contract more forcefully.
15. Heart failure.
16. It causes a mechanical contraction.
17. Drugs or electrical cardioversion.
18. V53.32.
19. Electrical impulses are completely blocked through the atrioventricular node.
20. (a) Incompatible codes for the pulse generator and lead insertion and (b) pulse generator is inserted without the lead insertion.
21. (a) Systolic more than 140; (b) diastolic more than 90.
22. (a) Papilledema and (b) history of spontaneous nosebleeds.
23. Because of the damage it causes to the heart and kidneys.
24. (a) Tricuspid, (b) pulmonary, (c) mitral, and (d) aortic.
25. Percutaneous balloon valvuloplasty.
26. A progressive degenerative disease of the heart muscle.
27. Alcoholism.
28. A decreased supply of blood to the brain caused by cerebral thrombus, embolism, or hemorrhage.
29. An abnormal localized widening of an artery.
30. This affects its ability to carry oxygen effectively.
31. Erythropoietin.
32. Pancytopenia.

CHAPTER 14

1. An abnormal growth of tissue that arises from normal tissue.
2. True.
3. They are slow growing and noninvasive.
4. They crowd surrounding organs and can sometimes transform to a cancerous condition.
5. It seeks to identify where the cancer began, because the originating source can continue seeding secondary cancer sites.
6. They are solid tumors, and only solid tumors can metastasize.
7. It is referred to as **contiguous** or **overlapping** sites.
8. It represents a secondary spread to the lungs with an unknown primary cancer site.
9. It serves as a localized radiologic kill of tumor cells while minimizing radiation damage to healthy tissue.

10. The cancer code is sequenced as the principal diagnosis, and the symptoms are listed as additional codes.
11. Hair loss, nausea, and anemia.
12. The part of the body that is irradiated.
13. Maturity of the neoplasm when viewed under a microscope.
14. The amount of spread (has the cancer metastasized?).
15. (a) Grade 1 = tumor is well structured; (b) grade 2 = tumor is moderately differentiated; (c) grade 3 = tumor is poorly differentiated; (d) grade 4 = tumor is very poorly differentiated.

CHAPTER 15

1. From the point of conception to 6 weeks after delivery of the neonate.
2. Because pregnancy complicates almost all other conditions.
3. Three main sections: (a) prenatal section, (b) labor and delivery section, and (c) postpartum section.
4. Between 22 completed weeks and 36 completed weeks.
5. (a) Stage 1, from the beginning of uterine contractions to full dilation of the cervical os; (b) stage 2, from full dilation to delivery; (c) stage 3, from delivery of the placenta to the end of uterine contractions.
6. The main complication of the delivery.
7. False.
8. Code 75.69.
9. Episiotomy.
10. Cesarean section.
11. This fact should be reported to the medical record or patient care review committee.
12. V25.2—Request for sterilization.
13. Abortive outcome.
14. (a) Spontaneous abortion, (b) legal abortion, (c) illegal abortion, (d) unspecified abortion, and (e) failed (legal) abortion.
15. Stillbirth.
16. Outside of its normal location.
17. Tubal pregnancy.

CHAPTER 16

1. From before birth through day 28 of life.
2. (a) Genetic factors, (b) complications of the pregnancy or delivery, and (c) maternal conditions affecting the neonate.

3. Physical status at 1 and 5 minutes after birth.
4. (a) Down's syndrome, (b) cleft lip and palate, (c) Marfan's syndrome, (d) congenital hip dislocation, and (e) fractured clavicle.
5. Birth weight of less than 1,000 g.
6. Jaundice.
7. Coombs' test.
8. Meconium.
9. Neonatal cyanosis.
10. Shunting of blood from one side of the heart to the other.
11. Projectile vomiting during feeding.
12. Congenital hydrocephalus.
13. Hemangioma.
14. Spina bifida.
15. Hepatitis B.

CHAPTER 17

1. The most severe injury.
2. For reporting to the state trauma registry, because this helps legislators to set policy relating to serious-injury reduction.
3. Unexpected circumstances that cause serious injury or death while a patient is under the care of a health-care facility.
4. Motor vehicle collision, because of the order of precedence.
5. A traumatic fracture results from an injury; a pathologic fracture results from a bone weakened because of disease.
6. To bring the bone back into anatomic alignment.
7. Manipulative procedure preceded by an incision into the site of the fracture.
8. Shoulder and hip joints.
9. Closed or open reduction of the dislocation.
10. Tendons.
11. The circumstances of each admission.
12. Injury chapter.
13. System chapter.
14. Codes 900 to 904.
15. Codes 950 to 957.
16. The "rule of nines."
17. It assesses the threat to life and the probability of survival.
18. (a) Allergic reaction, (b) drug hypersensitivity, (c) idiosyncratic reaction, (d) drug toxicity.
19. To a poisoning.

CHAPTER 18

1. Category 996 to 999.
2. There is no time limit.

3. Hip replacement surgery.
4. No.
5. It is a complication resulting from patient care.
6. Infection and inflammation; mechanical; and other complications.
7. To add to the supply of healthy blood cells.
8. No additional code is required to add detail.
9. The medical records and billing must be combined under the inpatient stay.

CHAPTER 19

1. DSM-IV.
2. ICD-9-CM.
3. Dysthymia.
4. A phobic disorder.
5. Anorexia nervosa.
6. Bulimia.
7. 296.
8. Delirium.
9. Dementia.
10. (a) 305; (b) 303; (c) 304.
11. 291.
12. Detoxification.
13. Personality disorder.
14. A syndrome.
15. (a) Psychotherapy; (b) electroconvulsive therapy; (c) psychotropic medications.
16. **Abuse** involves the nondependent psychological inclination to take the substance regardless of the negative consequences; **dependence** involves a physical reliance on the substance and withdrawal symptoms when the substance is discontinued.

CHAPTER 20

1. Emergency Medical Treatment and Active Labor Act of 1985.
2. 1798; Federal Marine Hospital Service.
3. Sidney Garfield, MD.
4. A reimbursement mechanism.
5. The PSRO Act and the HMO Act.
6. DRGs.
7. RBRVS and ambulatory payment classifications.
8. The three criteria include the following: (a) the proportional amount of work and skill required to complete a given procedure; (b) the proportionate overhead cost associated with a particular procedural code; and (c) the proportinate cost of professional liability insurance in relation to the completion of a given procedure.

9. HMOs, PPOs, PHOs, POS plans, and IPAs.

10. (a) Evaluating patient-mix data; (b) identifying performance-improvement activities; (c) complying with regulations and accrediting body standards; (d) developing superior clinical practice standards; (e) identifying potential sources of risk; and (f) aligning coded information systems with strategic organizational objectives and planning.

11. How to make health-care systems responsive and more accessible to everyone.

12. Good-quality patient information is necessary for making competent decisions.

Answers to Coding Practice I: Chapter Review Exercises

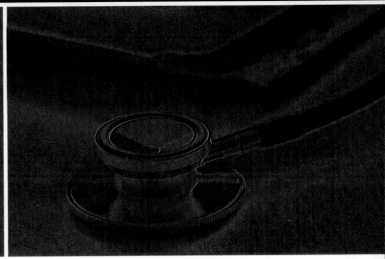

CHAPTER 2

1. 595.0
   041.4
2. 482.41
3. 250.71
   443.81
4. 426.2
5. 440.23
   707.10
6. 913.1
7. 733.42
   733.14
8. 286.7
9. 558.9
10. 204.02
11. 281.0
12. 410.71
    427.31
    V58.61
13. 441.4
    V45.01
    38.44
14. 292.81
15. 414.00
    411.1
    37.23
    88.57
    88.53
16. 532.00
    280.0
17. 428.0
18. 357.0
19. 574.00
    51.23
    87.53
20. 813.42, E960.0
    79.02
21. 715.95
    81.51
22. 780.2
    427.89
    458.0
23. 997.4
    560.1
24. 453.40
25. 487.1
    786.3
26. V58.11
    174.9
    196.3
    99.25
27. 820.8
    E881.0
    E849.0
28. 845.00
    E927
29. V58.0
    162.3
    92.23
30. 881.00
    E920.3
    86.59

CHAPTER 3

1. 682.6
2. 493.90
3. 821.30
   79.35
4. 047.9
5. 396.3
6. 714.0
7. 617.0
8. 287.30
9. 727.61
   83.63
10. 717.6
    80.16
11. 250.30
12. 276.1
13. 882.0
    86.59
14. 331.0
    294.11
15. 428.0

CHAPTER 4

1. 571.2
   789.59
   303.91
   54.91
2. 780.2
3. 789.00
   575.10
   558.9

4. 780.4
   386.30
   346.10
5. 428.0
   466.0
6. 599.0
7. 486
8. 595.9
9. 785.1
   427.89
   306.2
10. 787.01
    E942.1
    427.31
11. 782.0
    905.2
12. 781.3
    909.4
13. 780.31
14. 780.60
    794.8
15. 992.0
16. 715.96
17. 434.11
    784.3
18. 782.0
19. 786.59
20. 787.91
21. 401.9
    784.7
22. 780.79
    781.0
23. 250.90
24. 783.41
25. 458.0

Chapter 5

1. 250.60
   536.3
   43.11
2. 250.61
   357.2
3. 250.80
4. 242.00
   06.39
5. 244.1
6. 253.6
7. 486
   277.02
8. 263.9
   438.82, 787.20
   43.19

9. 276.51
   536.2
10. 278.01, V85.4
    44.69
11. 414.00
    272.0
12. 402.91
    428.21
    276.8
13. 250.31
14. 250.72
    440.24
15. 242.91
16. 250.41
    583.81
17. 252.1
18. 250.70
    443.81
    707.10
19. 307.1
    262
20. 183.0
    197.7
    197.6
    197.5
    199.0
    261
    68.49
    65.61
    50.12
    54.23
    45.26

Chapter 6

1. 038.49
   785.52
2. 595.0
   041.4
3. 079.99
4. 009.0
   276.52
5. 466.11
6. 042
   078.5
   363.13
   112.0
7. 820.8
   E881.0
   042
   176.0
   79.35

8. V30.00
   795.71
9. 070.21
10. 088.81
    320.7
11. 112.83
12. 091.81
    03.31
13. 011.24
    V09.0
14. 042
    115.05
15. 574.00
    998.59
    038.9
    995.91
    V08
    51.23
    87.53
16. 022.3
17. 094.0
18. 098.40
19. 078.5
    573.1
20. 513.0
    041.11
    786.3
21. 038.49
    995.92
    785.52
    584.9
    518.81

Chapter 7

1. 577.0
   574.10
   272.0
   278.01
   V64.41
   51.22
   51.51
   87.53
2. 532.40
   280.0
   45.13
3. 535.41
   280.0
4. 535.30
   303.90
5. 550.11
   53.05

6. 562.13
   280.0
7. 530.11
   276.51
8. 531.00
   285.1
9. 556.9
   48.63
10. 540.0
    997.4
    560.1
    47.01
11. 531.10
    44.41
12. 560.39
    96.38
13. 537.83
14. 562.13
    285.1
    45.75
    46.11
    47.19
    99.04
15. V55.3
    V12.79
    998.89
    780.62
    46.52
16. 530.81
    553.3
    44.66
17. 531.20
    43.7
18. 578.9
19. 553.21
    53.61
20. 555.1

CHAPTER 8

1. 428.0
2. 518.81
   491.21
   96.71
   96.04
3. 482.1
   511.1
   34.91
4. 493.22
5. 491.21
   33.24

6. 507.0
   438.82, 787.20
   438.20
7. 162.3
   997.39
   518.0
   32.49
8. 410.71
   518.81
9. 518.5
10. 428.0
    511.9 (significant)
    34.04
11. 002.0
    484.8
12. 434.11
    518.81
13. 518.81
    482.84
14. 806.00 ("includes" notes
    contain quadriplegia)
    518.81
    E828.2
    E849.4
    31.29
    96.72
15. 470
    473.0
    21.5
16. 518.84
    492.8
    96.71
    96.04
17. 493.01
18. 508.1
    V10.11
    V15.3
    E879.2
19. 512.0
    34.04
20. 042
    136.3
    33.24
21. 506.1
    E864.3
    E849.6

CHAPTER 9

1. 600.11
   596.0
   788.20
   60.29

2. 592.1
   591
   56.0
3. 584.9
   585.9
   276.7
   38.95
   39.95
4. 599.0
   041.04
5. V56.0
   403.91, 585.6
   39.27
   39.95
6. 618.5
   59.5
7. 626.8
   V16.49
   69.09
8. 617.9
   622.10
   68.23
   69.09
   67.2
9. 788.20
10. 598.9
    601.9
    58.6
    57.32
11. 618.01
    625.6
    70.50
12. 590.10
    599.70
13. 600.01
    788.20
    585.9
    57.32
14. 220
    614.6
    65.29
    54.59
15. 218.1
    625.9
    614.6
    625.6
    68.49
    65.61
    59.5
16. 622.7
    68.59
17. 604.90
    99.21

18. 607.84
401.9
64.97
19. 584.9
276.51
20. 584.9
599.60

CHAPTER 10

1. 707.05, 707.24
496
331.0
294.10
428.0
593.9
86.70
2. 707.8
682.3
86.22
99.21
3. 693.0
599.0
E931.0
4. 692.74
V15.82
5. 701.4
86.3
6. 459.81
707.10
7. 440.24
707.10
84.15
8. 682.3
913.5
E906.4
99.21
9. 692.4
10. 695.10
99.23
11. 702.0
86.3
12. 708.0
13. 973.0
980.0
708.0
780.4
E858.4
E860.0
305.00
14. 242.00
250.00
709.01

15. 681.11
86.27
16. 694.4
17. 706.2
86.04
18. 696.1
99.83
19. 684
041.00
99.21
20. 683
041.10
99.21
21. 707.15
250.02
401.9
86.28
99.21

CHAPTER 11

1. 715.95
285.1
81.52
2. 733.82
905.4
79.36
3. 722.10
03.09
4. 733.13
721.3
5. 710.0
323.81
6. 728.86
83.44
7. 726.10
83.63
8. 717.83
81.45
9. 711.01
99.21
10. 733.6
11. 733.42
81.51, 00.74
12. 250.81
731.8
730.07
84.11
13. 724.02
80.51
81.08

14. 710.1
530.5
43.11
15. 719.06
81.91
16. 714.0
736.20
81.71
17. 726.73
77.68
18. 722.73
80.51
19. 722.51
20. 733.13
733.01

CHAPTER 12

1. 378.01
15.11
2. 389.20
20.98
3. 331.0
294.11
4. 780.39
5. 370.00
6. 361.03
14.52
14.49
7. 353.6
V49.75
8. 345.10
9. 331.3
294.11
10. 333.94
11. 336.1
12. 386.00
13. 324.0
14. 366.10
13.59
13.71
15. 365.22
16. 349.0
780.60
17. 354.0
04.43
18. 382.9
20.01
19. 340
20. 346.01
21. 350.1
22. 320.3
03.31

CHAPTER 13

1. 427.81
   37.83
   37.72
2. 414.01
   411.1
   36.12
   36.16
   39.61
   37.23
   88.53
   88.57
3. 434.11
   342.90
   438.11
4. 433.10
   38.12
5. 428.0
   427.1
   414.8
6. 414.01
   411.1
   00.66
   36.06, 00.40, 00.45
7. 440.23
   707.10
   39.50, 00.40
8. 401.9
   784.7
   21.02
9. 410.01
   404.93, 585.6
   428.0
   414.00
   443.9
   V45.11
   V45.81
10. 427.41
    427.5
    492.8
    250.00
    414.00
    244.9
    37.94
    37.26
11. 578.9
    E934.2
    V43.3
    V58.61
12. 441.03
    38.45
    38.44

13. 404.92, 585.6
    285.21
14. 428.0
    401.9
    396.1
15. 430
    780.39
16. 451.19
    38.7
17. 194.0
    405.99
18. 414.00
    411.1
    410.42
    V45.81
19. 434.01
    781.2
20. 444.22
    39.29

CHAPTER 14

1. 185
   788.20
   60.29
2. 174.8
   196.3
   85.43
3. 285.22
   153.9
   99.04
4. 162.3
   786.3
   33.27
5. 276.51
   536.2
   157.9, E933.1
   99.29
6. V58.11
   162.9
   197.7
   99.25
7. 188.9
   599.70
   57.49
   57.32
8. 198.3
   V10.3
9. 155.0
   576.2
10. 233.0
    85.21

11. 198.3
    162.9
    780.39
12. 153.6
    560.89
    45.73
13. 198.5
    733.13
    199.1
    338.3
14. 189.0
    55.51
    55.23
15. 204.02
    41.31
16. 202.80
17. 183.0
    196.6
    197.7
    218.1
    68.49
    65.61
    40.3
    50.12
18. 150.5
    787.20
    263.9
    45.16
    43.11
19. 211.3
    V10.05
    45.42
20. 239.0
    88.01

CHAPTER 15

1. 654.21
   V27.0
   73.6
2. 664.11
   658.11
   V27.0
   75.69
   73.4
3. 659.71
   645.11
   V27.0
   74.1
   73.4
   75.32
   75.34

4. 650
   V27.0
   73.59
5. 652.21
   V27.0
   74.1
6. 664.31
   648.81
   653.51
   V27.0
   75.62
7. 633.10
   66.62
8. 643.13
9. 634.91
   69.02
10. 675.24
11. 642.33
12. 642.51
    644.21
    V27.0
    74.1
13. 632
    96.49
14. 646.63
    590.80
15. 660.41
    656.11
    666.22
    648.22
    280.0
    V27.0
    72.1
    99.11
    99.04
16. 653.41
    660.11
    648.11
    244.9
    648.22
    285.1
    V27.0
    74.1
17. 661.21
    659.61
    V25.2
    V27.0
    74.1
    66.32

18. 665.51
    645.11
    V27.0
    75.61
    73.09
19. 644.21
    656.41
    V27.1
    73.59
    73.4
20. 656.31
    644.21
    651.01
    V27.2
    74.0
    73.59

Chapter 16

1. V30.01
   754.31
2. V30.01
   765.27
   765.17
   769
   774.2
   96.72
   96.04
   38.92
   99.83
3. V30.00
   V05.3
   64.0
   99.55
4. V30.00
   766.1
   775.0
5. 749.22
   27.54
   27.62
6. V31.00 (Twin A)
   765.18
   765.28
   V29.0
   V31.01 (Twin B)
   765.18
   765.28
   768.3
   770.6
   V29.0

7. V30.00
   767.2
   766.1
8. V30.00
   747.0
9. V30.01
   763.82
   762.5
10. V30.00
    766.21
    758.0
    745.4
11. V30.00
    778.6
    752.61
12. V30.01
    770.89
    771.81
    773.1
    38.92
    99.21
    99.01
13. V30.00
    765.18
    765.28
    779.5
    770.6
14. V30.1
15. V30.00
    764.07
    760.71
    779.3
16. 765.18
    783.41
17. 741.00
    02.34
18. V30.00
    228.01
    86.3
19. 746.5
    759.82
    35.24
20. 343.9

Chapter 17

1. 820.09
   E880.9
   E849.6
   81.52

2. 831.01
   E884.0
   E849.4
   79.71
3. 845.00
   E927
   E849.0
4. 847.2
   E927
   E849.1
5. 852.22
   E888.1
   E849.0
   87.03
6. 860.0
   807.05
   922.1
   E819.0
   34.04
7. 903.2
   881.00
   E920.1
   39.31
8. 955.6
   883.0
   E920.2
   04.3
9. 806.06
   E883.0
   96.04, 96.72
   762.5
10. 924.01
    E888.9
11. 928.20
    826.0
    E916
    E849.4
12. 824.9
    922.1
    924.01
    921.2
    E828.2
    79.36
    79.66
13. 882.1
    E906.3
14. 887.2
    958.4
    E919.8
    E849.1
    84.06

15. 942.32
    941.20
    E894
16. 969.0
    E950.3
    786.09
    780.8
    781.0
    311
17. 578.9
    E934.2
    427.31
    428.0
    496
    403.90
    585.9
    305.1
    V58.61
18. 701.4
    906.5
    E929.4
    86.84
19. 824.4
    E826.1
    79.36
20. 692.76
    E926.2
    E849.8
21. 947.1
    E869.8
    E849.4
22. 820.8
    E885.9
    E849.0
    78.55
23. 882.1
    E920.1
    E849.3
    82.09
24. 866.01
    599.71
    E960.0
25. 836.0
    E917.0
    80.6
    80.26
26. 941.35
    941.29
    942.22
    948.30
    E924.0
    E849.0

CHAPTER 18

1. 997.39
   518.0
2. 997.4
   560.1
3. 996.64
   599.0
   041.4
   438.20
   596.54
4. 996.42
   V43.65
   79.76
5. 999.2
6. 996.73
   403.91
   585.6
   39.42
7. 996.77
   V43.65
   00.80
8. 997.62
   250.70
   443.81
   84.3
9. 414.01
   411.1
   998.12
   37.22
   88.53
   88.57
10. 560.81
    496
    401.9
    998.2
    54.59
    46.73
11. 998.32
12. 440.23
    414.00
    401.9
    250.01
    997.1
    410.91
    518.5
    V45.81
    84.17
    96.71
    96.04

13. 433.30
401.9
997.02
38.12
00.40
14. 626.8
218.9
280.0
625.2
997.5
788.20
68.49
65.62
15. 996.62
038.9
995.91
250.40
585.9
16. 574.10
530.81
244.9
998.89
780.62
51.23
87.53
17. 996.81
584.9
403.91, 585.6
250.40
581.81
38.95
39.95
18. 999.5
280.0
626.2
218.9
99.04

19. 996.61
V45.01
37.79
20. 998.83
V54.9
99.21

CHAPTER 19

1. 303.00
311
94.63
2. 295.32
3. 276.4
293.0
492.8
331.0
294.10
4. 300.4
780.71
300.7
5. 425.5
303.91
6. 305.60
786.50
7. 296.53
8. 296.34
94.27
9. 353.6
V49.76
309.81
10. 295.74
11. 307.1
276.51
261
99.15
99.29

12. 290.41
13. 291.0
780.39
303.02
94.62
14. 300.21
316
692.9
15. 314.01
16. 339.10
309.23
309.22
17. 307.23
18. 306.4
276.51
300.3
99.29
19. 292.81
E935.8
20. 291.2
303.90
133.0
V60.0
21. 780.97

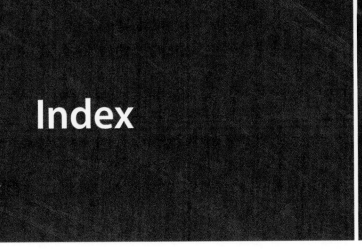
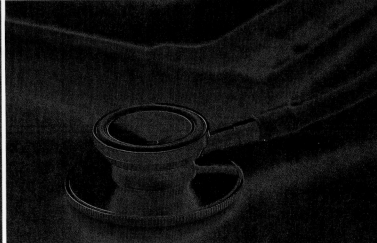

Index

Page numbers in italics denote figures. Those followed by "t" denote tables; those followed by "mr" denote medical reports.

A

a-, 372t
Abbreviations, 729–736
Abdominal aortic aneurysm, 398
Abnormal findings, 74
Abortion, 487–488
Abuse, 578–579
Accelerated hypertension, 391
Acquired immunodeficiency syndrome, 126–127
Acronyms, 729–736
Acute coronary occlusion, 378
Acute exacerbation of chronic obstructive pulmonary disease, 193–194
Acute infective polyneuritis, 339–340
Acute lymphocytic leukemia, 438
Acute myeloid leukemia, 438
Acute myocardial infarction, 379–380
Acute renal failure, 231–232
aden/o-, 723t
Adenoviral meningitis, 332
Adjustment reaction, 642
Admission history and physical report, 463–464mr
Admission symptom, 72–73
Admission-for-birth codes, 526–527
Admission/registration record, 556mr
Adult abuse, 578–579
Adult respiratory distress syndrome, 200
Adverse effect
  definition of, 575
  iatrogenic, 612–613
  nosocomial, 612–613
Affective psychoses, 642–643
Age-related macular degeneration, 344
agora-, 640t

Agoraphobia, 642
AHA (*see* American Hospital Association)
AHIMA (*see* American Health Information Management Association)
-al, 524t
Alcohol abuse, 644–645
Alcohol dependence, 644–645
Alcoholic cardiomyopathy, 394
Alcoholic psychosis, 645
Alcoholism, 644–646
Allergic asthma, 194
Alphabetic Index to Diseases
  abnormal findings coding, 74
  coding conventions used in, 26–28
  description of, 8–10
  late effects, 577–578
Alphabetic Index to External Cause of Injury, 10
Alphabetic Index to Procedures, 12–14
Aluminum overloading, dialysis dementia caused by, 237
Alzheimer's dementia, 334, 644
Alzheimer's disease, 333–334, 647–648
Ambulatory payment classifications, 676
American Health Information Management Association, 15
American Hospital Association, 15
Amputations, 568–569
Amyotrophic lateral sclerosis, 334
an-, 372t
ana-, 430t
"And," 30
Anemia
  aplastic, 400–401
  blood-loss, 152
  definition of, 400